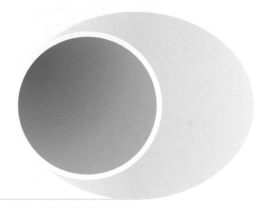

Atlas of Orthopedic Pathology

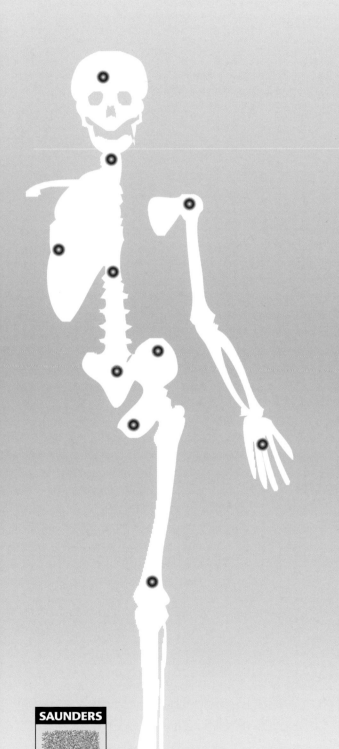

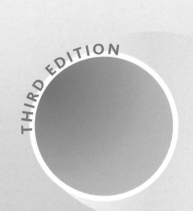

THIRD EDITION

Atlas of Orthopedic Pathology

Lester E. Wold, MD

Professor and Emeritus Chairman
Department of Laboratory Medicine and Pathology
Mayo Clinic, Rochester, Minnesota

K. Krishnan Unni, MD

Professor and Emeritus Staff
Department of Laboratory Medicine and Pathology
Mayo Clinic, Rochester, Minnesota

Franklin H. Sim, MD

Consultant, Department of Orthopedic Surgery
Chair, Division of Orthopedic Oncology
Mayo Clinic, Rochester, Minnesota

Murali Sundaram, MD

Department of Radiology
Cleveland Clinic, Cleveland, Ohio

Claus-Peter Adler, MD

Institute of Pathology
University of Freiburg,
Freiburg, Germany

SAUNDERS

ELSEVIER

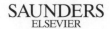

1600 John F. Kennedy Blvd.
Ste 1800
Philadelphia, PA 19103-2899

ATLAS OF ORTHOPEDIC PATHOLOGY, THIRD EDITION   ISBN: 978-1-4160-5328-6

Notice

Neither the Publisher nor the authors assume any responsibility for any loss or injury and/or damage to persons or property arising out of or related to any use of the material contained in this book. It is the responsibility of the treating practitioner, relying on independent expertise and knowledge of the patient, to determine the best treatment and method of application for the patient.

The Publisher

Library of Congress Cataloging-in-Publication Data

Atlas of orthopedic pathology / Lester E. Wold ... [et al.]. — 3rd ed.
   p. ; cm.
Includes bibliographical references and index.
ISBN 978-1-4160-5328-6
1. Bones—Diseases—Atlases. 2. Orthopedics—Atlases. I. Wold, Lester E. (Lester Eugene), 1949-
[DNLM: 1. Bone Diseases—pathology—Atlases. WE 17 A88062 2008]

RC930.A85 2008
616.7'1070222—dc22

2007031065

Acquisitions Editor: William Schmitt
Developmental Editor: Katie DeFrancesco
Project Manager: Bryan Hayward
Design Direction: Lou Forgione

Printed in China

Last digit is the print number: 9 8 7 6 5 4 3 2 1

Working together to grow
libraries in developing countries

www.elsevier.com | www.bookaid.org | www.sabre.org

ELSEVIER   BOOK AID International   Sabre Foundation

This text is dedicated to the memory of our mentors, who helped us learn how to be better physicians and human beings. We value their advice and strive to ensure that their wisdom is passed on to subsequent generations of orthopedic surgeons, radiologists, and pathologists. In particular, we dedicate this text to Dr. David C. Dahlin, who was a guiding force in our lives and in the development of the body of knowledge related to orthopedic pathology.

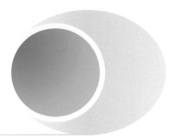

Preface

This atlas of orthopedic tumors and non-tumorous conditions is intended as an introduction to the complex subject of orthopedic pathology. It offers a starting point for pathology residents, orthopedic residents, and radiology residents to learn about the clinical, radiographic, and pathologic features of common and uncommon orthopedic conditions. This atlas is organized into sections of related conditions. Each chapter within a section is organized in a manner to succinctly display data and information.

The third edition of this atlas includes additional chapters on tumor-like conditions as well as updated references for most chapters. Clinical signs, symptoms, major radiographic features, radiographic differential diagnosis, gross and microscopic pathologic differential diagnosis, and treatment sections are organized in outline format. Only the major features are presented. For more information the reader is referred to an abbreviated list of references that follows the outlined information. These references are by no means complete, but offer a starting point for a more in-depth review of each condition. This atlas complements many texts that contain abundant information concerning both tumors and tumor-like conditions of bone.

Lester E. Wold, MD
K. Krishnan Unni, MD
Franklin H. Sim, MD
Murali Sundaram, MD
Claus-Peter Adler, MD

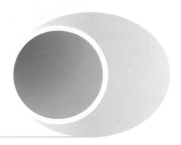

Contents

SECTION 1:
Metabolic, Developmental, and Inflammatory Conditions of Bone

1. Hyperparathyroidism — 3
2. Osteoporosis — 11
3. Renal Osteodystrophy — 17
4. Rickets — 23
5. Osteomalacia — 31
6. Oncogenic Osteomalacia (Phosphaturic Mesenchymal Tumor) — 37
7. Paget's Disease — 45
8. Camurati-Engelmann Disease (Progressive Diaphyseal Dysplasia) — 53
9. Hypertrophic Osteoarthropathy — 59
10. Melorheostosis — 67
11. Osteopetrosis — 73
12. Osteogenesis Imperfecta — 81
13. Fluorosis — 89
14. Gaucher's Disease — 93
15. Osteoarthritis — 99
16. Neuropathic Joint (Charcot's Joint) — 105
17. Rheumatoid Arthritis — 111
18. Ochronosis—Disorder of Tyrosine and Phenylalanine Catabolism Secondary to Homogentisic Acid and Related Compounds — 121
19. Gout — 125
20. Chondrocalcinosis (Pseudogout, Calcium Pyrophosphate Dihydrate Crystal Deposition Disease) — 135
21. Amyloidosis — 139
22. Xanthomatosis — 145
23. Fibrous Dysplasia — 151
24. Osteofibrous Dysplasia — 159
25. Ankylosing Spondylitis — 167
26. Synovial Chondromatosis — 173
27. Pigmented Villonodular Synovitis — 179
28. Arthroplasty Effect — 189

SECTION 2:
Bone Tumors and Tumorlike Conditions

Section 2A: Bone-Forming Tumors

29. Osteoid Osteoma — 195
30. Osteoblastoma — 203
31. Osteosarcoma (Conventional) — 211
32. Parosteal Osteosarcoma — 219
33. Periosteal Osteosarcoma — 227
34. High-Grade Surface Osteosarcoma — 235
35. Telangiectatic Osteosarcoma — 241
36. Low-Grade Central Osteosarcoma — 247
37. Small Cell Osteosarcoma — 251

Section 2B: Cartilage-Forming Tumors

38. Osteochondroma — 258
39. Chondroma — 265
40. Chondroblastoma — 273
41. Chondromyxoid Fibroma — 279
42. Multiple Chondromas — 285
43. Periosteal Chondroma — 291
44. Chondrosarcoma — 297
45. Chondrosarcoma Arising in Osteochondroma — 305
46. Dedifferentiated Chondrosarcoma — 313
47. Mesenchymal Chondrosarcoma — 319
48. Clear Cell Chondrosarcoma — 325

Section 2C: Fibrous and Fibrohistiocytic Tumors

49. Benign Fibrous Histiocytoma — 332
50. Fibrosarcoma — 337
51. Malignant Fibrous Histiocytoma — 343

Section 2D: Hematopoietic Tumors

52. Malignant Lymphoma — 350
53. Myeloma — 361
54. Mastocytosis (Mast Cell Disease) — 367
55. Langerhans' Cell Histiocytosis (Histiocytosis X) — 373

Section 2E: Vascular Tumors

56. Hemangioma — 380
57. Hemangioendothelioma, Epithelioid Hemangioendothelioma, and Angiosarcoma — 387

Section 2F: Tumors of Unknown Origin

58. Hemangiopericytoma — 396
59. Giant Cell Tumor — 403
60. Malignancy in Giant Cell Tumor (Malignant Giant Cell Tumor) — 411
61. Adamantinoma — 415
62. Chordoma — 421
63. Ewing's Sarcoma — 427

Section 2G: Secondary Sarcomas

64. Paget's Sarcoma — 438
65. Postradiation Sarcoma — 443

Section 2H: Tumorlike Conditions

66. Neurilemmoma — 448
67. Aneurysmal Bone Cyst — 453
68. Unicameral Bone Cyst (Simple Cyst) — 459

69. Giant Cell Reaction (Giant Cell Reparative Granuloma) — 465
70. Fibroma (Metaphyseal Fibrous Defect) — 471
71. Avulsive Cortical Irregularity (Fibrous Cortical Defect, Periosteal Desmoid) — 477
72. Mesenchymal Hamartoma of the Chest Wall. — 481
73. Osteomyelitis — 485
74. Avascular Necrosis — 495
75. Massive Osteolysis (Gorham's Disease) — 503
76. Hemophilia — 509
77. Metastatic Carcinoma — 513
78. Sarcoidosis — 519
79. Bizarre Parosteal Osteochondromatous Proliferation (BPOP) — 525
80. Erdheim-Chester Disease — 533

Index — 539

Metabolic, Developmental, and Inflammatory Conditions of Bone

Hyperparathyroidism

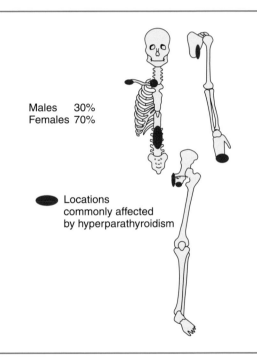

Males 30%
Females 70%

Locations
commonly affected
by hyperparathyroidism

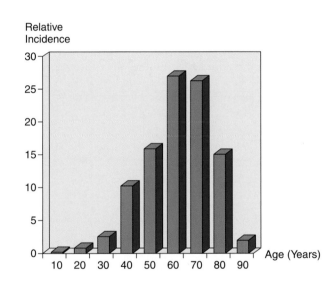

Clinical Signs

1. Most cases are asymptomatic and detected biochemically on screening studies. (Of all cases of hypercalcemia, 90% result from malignancy and hyperparathyroidism, in that order.)
2. Biochemical studies reveal increased serum calcium and decreased serum phosphorus concentrations in cases of primary hyperparathyroidism. (Secondary hyperparathyroidism is initially characterized by increased serum phosphorus concentrations.)
3. Renal stones may be present. (Incidence has decreased from approximately 65% in the mid 1970s to approximately 5% in the mid 1990s.)

4. Hypertension is present in approximately 20% of patients.
5. Depression, psychosis, or severe neurosis is seen in approximately 20% of patients.
6. Osteoporosis is seen in approximately 10% of patients.

Clinical Symptoms

1. Bone and joint pain and tenderness are present in about 15% of patients.
2. Flank pain associated with renal stones may occur (present in approximately one third of patients but depends on the prevalence of screening calcium determinations done in the population).

3. Constipation, indigestion, or ulcer symptoms are present in approximately 30% of patients.
4. Muscle pain is present in approximately 15% of patients.
5. Fatigue is the most common complaint and is mentioned by about half the patients.
6. Polyuria and polydipsia may occur.
7. Nausea and vomiting may be seen in patients with severe hypercalcemia.
8. Approximately 50% of patients are asymptomatic.

Major Radiographic Features

1. Diffuse osteopenia can be seen.
2. Radiographs of the hand show erosion of the tufts of the phalanges and subperiosteal cortical resorption particularly prominent on the radial aspect of the phalangeal shafts.
3. Subperiosteal resorption may be evident in the region of the symphysis pubis, proximal and distal clavicles, ischial tuberosity, scapula, and the plates of the vertebral bodies.
4. Periarticular erosions, particularly of the bones of the hands, wrists, and feet (most commonly involving the distal interphalangeal joint), may be noted.
5. Loss of the lamina dura surrounding the tooth roots may occur.
6. Occasionally, patients present with a lytic bony lesion ("brown tumor").
7. Renal calculi may be seen.
8. Bone changes may not be identified in the early stages of the disease.
9. Soft tissue calcification may be present.
10. Decreased cortical bone density may be evident.

Radiographic Differential Diagnosis

1. Ankylosing spondylitis (when the disease involves the sacroiliac joints).
2. Primary bone tumor when a brown tumor of hyperparathyroidism is present.
3. Osteomalacia.

Major Pathologic Features

1. Osteoclasts are increased on the bone surface.
2. In longstanding cases, there is "tunneling" resorption of the trabeculae.

3. With secondary hyperparathyroidism resulting from renal failure, marrow fibrosis and increased woven bone may be prominent.
4. The brown tumor of hyperparathyroidism is histologically a giant cell reparative granuloma consisting of numerous multinucleated giant cells lying in a spindle cell, mononuclear cell stroma.

Pathologic Differential Diagnosis

1. Giant cell tumor of bone (in cases of brown tumor).
2. Myelofibrosis.
3. Fibrous dysplasia.
4. Paget's disease.

Treatment

1. Parathyroid tissue (adenoma or hyperplastic glands) can be surgically removed.
2. Intravenous bisphosphonates (zoledronate and pamidronate) are of major value in treating hypercalcemia.
3. Cinacalcet can be used to control the hypercalcemia in patients with parathyroid cancer who cannot be cured surgically.
4. Bone disease (osteitis fibrosa cystica) will heal with treatment of the primary parathyroid disease. Occasional large lesions (brown tumors) may require curettage and grafting. Pathologic fractures may require internal fixation.

References

Cohen-Solal M, Sebert JL: Renal osteodystrophy and hypercalcemia [review]. *Curr Opin Rheumatol* 5(3):357–362, 1993.
Heath H, Hodgson SF, Kennedy MA: Primary hyperparathyroidism: incidence, morbidity, and potential economic impact in a community. *N Engl J Med* 302:189–193, 1980.
Kearns AE, Thompson GB: Medical and surgical management of hyperparathyroidism. *Mayo Clinic Proc* 77:87–91, 2002.
Palmer M, Jakobsson S, Akerstrom G, et al: Prevalence of hypercalcaemia in a health survey: a 14-year follow-up study of serum calcium values. *Eur J Clin Invest* 18:39–46, 1988.
Resnick DL: Erosive arthritis of the hand and wrist in hyperparathyroidism. *Radiology* 110:263–269, 1974.

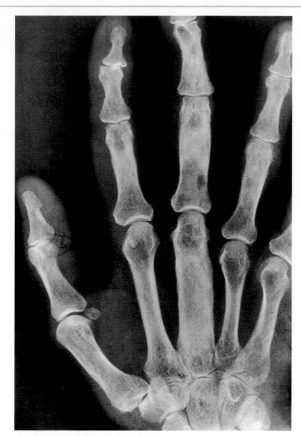

Figure 1–1 Radiograph of the hand illustrating the features of hyperparathyroidism. Note the erosive changes involving the phalangeal tufts and diffuse osteopenia. Subperiosteal resorption of bone is often most prominent on the radial side of the middle and proximal phalanges.

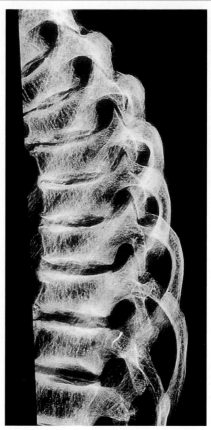

Figure 1–3 Radiograph of the vertebrae and ribs illustrating diffuse osteopenia associated with primary hyperparathyroidism.

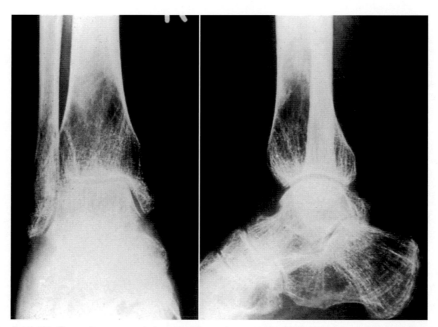

Figure 1–2 Radiograph of the distal tibia illustrating an osteolytic defect. The patient was identified as having primary hyperparathyroidism, and the defect shown is the result of a "brown tumor" of hyperparathyroidism. Such lesions may be seen in any skeletal location and may be confused pathologically with a giant cell tumor. If a lesion pathologically resembles a giant cell tumor but is not in an epiphyseal location, then hyperparathyroidism should be excluded.

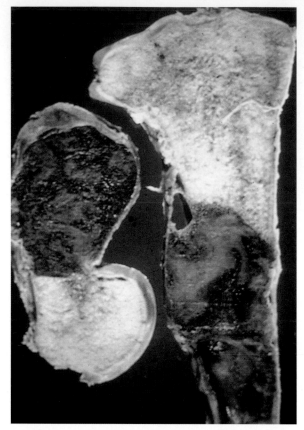

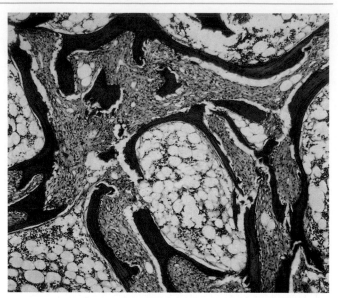

Figure 1–6 The marked dissecting osteitis or "tunneling" associated with longstanding hyperparathyroidism is illustrated in this photomicrograph. The bony trabeculae have been replaced at their center by fibrovascular connective tissue. The marrow in this example remains active but may even be replaced by fibrovascular connective tissue as the disease progresses, particularly in cases of secondary hyperparathyroidism related to renal failure.

Figure 1–4 This gross photograph of the proximal tibia illustrates the appearance of a brown tumor. Although grossly this lesion may resemble a giant cell tumor, its diaphyseal location is helpful in excluding giant cell tumor from the pathologic differential diagnosis. Brown tumors are at present uncommonly seen because most patients with hyperparathyroidism are identified early in the course of their disease.

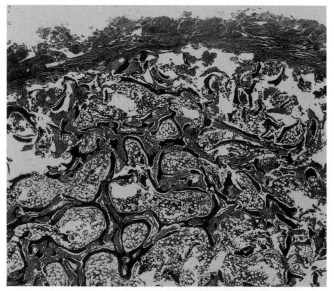

Figure 1–5 The histologic appearance of well-developed primary hyperparathyroidism is illustrated in this photomicrograph. The low-power histologic pattern shows irregular bony trabeculae that have been significantly remodeled. Figure 1–6 shows the pattern at higher magnification.

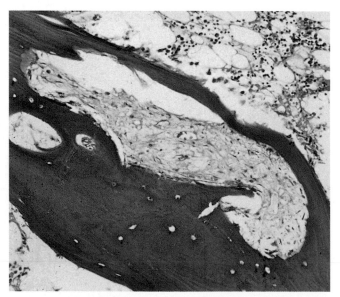

Figure 1–7 Earlier tunneling is shown in this photomicrograph from a patient with primary hyperparathyroidism. Active osteoclastic resorption may be identified in the region of the central trabecular bony destruction.

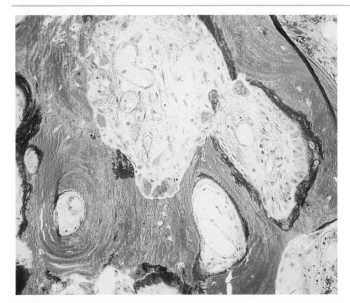

Figure 1–8 Hyperparathyroidism results in greater bony destruction than production. No tunneling is seen in this bone, which shows the earliest effects of changes from primary hyperparathyroidism.

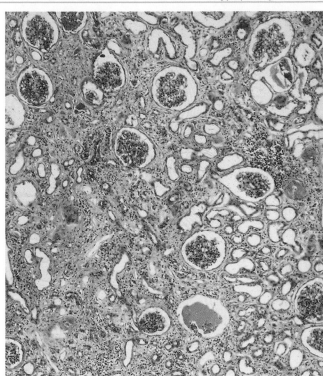

Figure 1–10 This photomicrograph illustrates the histologic appearance of the kidney in a patient with primary hyperparathyroidism.

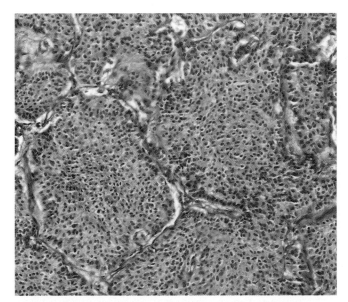

Figure 1–9 Parathyroid adenoma is the most common cause of primary hyperparathyroidism. This photomicrograph illustrates the histologic features of a parathyroid adenoma. Parathyroid hyperplasia is a less common cause of primary hyperparathyroidism, and the pathologist may have trouble distinguishing an adenoma from a hyperplastic gland because the histologic features of these conditions overlap significantly. Communication with the surgeon to identify how many glands are grossly enlarged is necessary to minimize errors in classification of the parathyroid pathology.

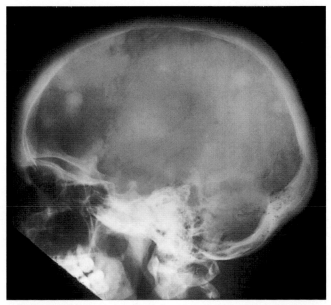

Figure 1–11 This radiograph of the skull is from a patient with renal osteodystrophy. Regions of radiolucency and some regions of increased mineralization are apparent, resulting in a "salt and pepper" appearance. The radiographic features of such examples of secondary hyperparathyroidism may overlap entirely with those seen in patients with primary hyperparathyroidism.

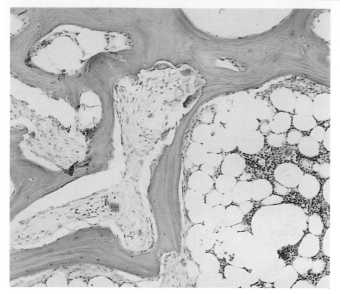

Figure 1–12 This photomicrograph reveals the histologic pattern seen in secondary hyperparathyroidism. Note that the trabecular tunneling previously illustrated in primary hyperparathyroidism (Fig. 1–6) is also evident in this condition. Osteoclastic resorption is also shown.

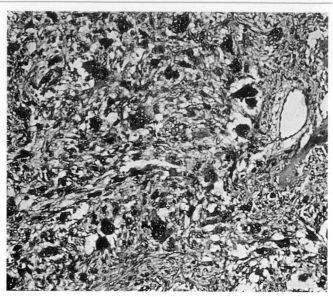

Figure 1–14 At higher magnification, brown tumors show a greater tendency to spindling of the mononuclear stromal cells than is seen in giant cell tumors. Reactive new bone may be present in these cases.

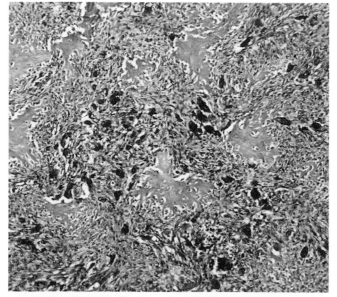

Figure 1–13 This low-power photomicrograph illustrates the features of a brown tumor. Although numerous osteoclast-type giant cells are present, this amount of fibrosis would be uncommon in giant cell tumors of bone. Another feature that helps distinguish such reactive lesions from giant cell tumors is the relative clustering of the giant cells in a brown tumor compared with their more uniform distribution in a giant cell tumor.

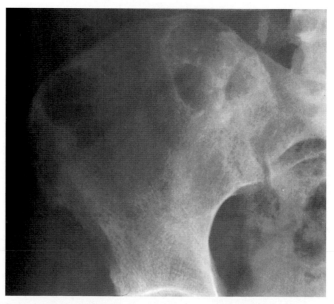

Figure 1–15 This radiograph illustrates a brown tumor of hyperparathyroidism involving the ilium.

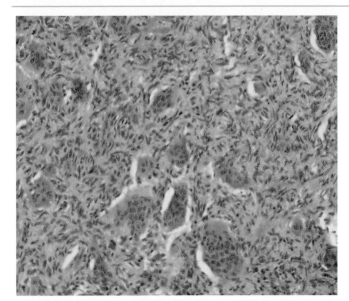

Figure 1–16 This photomicrograph illustrates the histologic pattern of the lesion shown in Figure 1–15. The fibrogenic stroma and greater degree of spindling of the mononuclear cells help differentiate this lesion from a giant cell tumor of the bone.

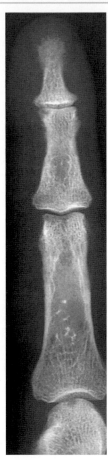

Figure 1–18 AP roentgenogram of the finger in a patient with hyperparathyroidism. Note the subperiosteal resorption of the phalanges. Note also the acro-osteolysis of the tuft and demineralization. Cortical tunneling with coarse trabeculae is present.

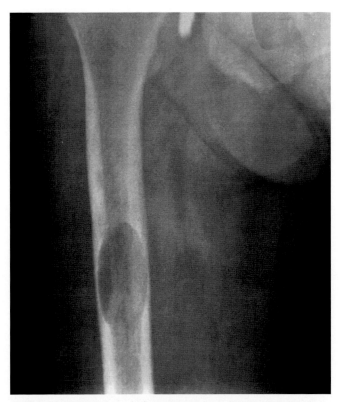

Figure 1–17 Anteroposterior (AP) roentgenogram of the right femur in a 59-year-old male patient with hyperparathyroidism. There is a large, well-defined lytic lesion in the diaphysis, with endosteal erosion and bony expansion.

2

Osteoporosis

Clinical Signs

1. Osteoporosis occurs most commonly in postmenopausal, slender women older than 65 years of age. Other associated clinical features include the following:
   a. Fair complexion.
   b. Freckles.
   c. Blond hair.
   d. Scoliosis.
2. Hip and forearm fracture with minor trauma.
3. Spasm of the paraspinal musculature is related to pathologic fracture of the vertebrae.
4. Loss of height (related to vertebral collapse) may occur.
5. Dietary intake of calcium is poor.

Clinical Symptoms

1. Back pain may be present.
2. Hip pain resulting from hip fracture after minor trauma (e.g., fall) may occur.
3. Osteoporosis may be related to estrogen deficiency, Cushing's syndrome, hyperthyroidism, diabetes mellitus, or immobilization. Clinical symptoms related to these conditions thus may be associated with osteoporosis.

Imaging Features

1. Dual-energy x-ray absorptiometry (DEXA) scanning is the examination of choice to determine bone mass, establish the diagnosis of osteoporosis, and monitor treatment of osteopenia and osteoporosis.
2. Cortical bone shows thinning.
3. Generalized osteopenia may be seen.
4. In vertebrae, there may be thinning and eventual disappearance of the vertical trabeculae.

5. Thoracic vertebrae may exhibit wedge fractures.
6. Lumbar vertebrae may exhibit crush fractures.
7. Intervertebral disc spaces may show widening.

Radiographic Differential Diagnosis

1. Multiple myeloma.

Major Pathologic Features

1. Trabecular bone volume is decreased. (Although morphometric studies show a significant difference in the population distribution of trabecular bone volume in individuals with and without osteoporosis, the overlap between the two groups is so great that this measure cannot be used alone to identify patients with osteoporosis.)
2. Osteoid volume is decreased.

Pathologic Differential Diagnosis

1. Cushing's syndrome.
2. Osteogenesis imperfecta.
3. Homocystinuria.
4. Turner's syndrome.
5. Malabsorption.
6. Immobilization.

Treatment

Medical

1. Treatment varies with cause. Nonpharmacologic measures include dietary, supplemental calcium salts, vitamin D, and exercise.

2. Bisphosphonates are the treatment of choice for most patients.
3. Selective estrogen receptor modulators (i.e., raloxifene) can be considered for younger patients to prevent vertebral fractures and breast cancer.
4. Calcitonin is a weak antiresorptive agent and is rarely used.
5. Teriparatide is the only approved agent that is capable of stimulating bone formation and should be considered for patients with severe osteoporosis or with osteoporosis that has failed to respond to bisphosphomalin.
6. Supportive care for vertebral fractures should be provided—analgesics, spinal support, and physical therapy.
7. Vertebroplasty should be considered for patients with vertebral compression fractures who do not respond to conservative management.

Surgical

1. For hip fractures, treatment is internal fixation versus prosthetic replacement.
2. For Colles' fractures, long bone fractures, treatment is closed reduction versus open reduction and internal fixation.

References

Andrew SM, Freemont AJ: Skeletal mastocytosis. *J Clin Pathol* 46(11):1033–1035, 1993.

Arnala I: Use of histological methods in studies of osteoporosis. *Calcif Tissue Int* 49 (Suppl):S31–S32, 1991.

Ashton-Key M, Gallagher PJ: The value of simple morphometric techniques in the diagnosis of osteoporosis. *Pathol Res Pract* 188(4–5):616–619, 1992.

Bronner F: Calcium and osteoporosis [review]. *Am J Clin Nutr* 60(6):831–836, 1994.

Chappard D, Plantard B, Petitjean M: Alcoholic cirrhosis and osteoporosis in men: a light and scanning electron microscopy study. *J Stud Alcohol* 52(3):269–274, 1991.

Chines A, Pacifici R, Avioli LV: Systemic mastocytosis presenting as osteoporosis: a clinical and histomorphometric study. *J Clin Endocrinol Metab* 72(1):140–144, 1991.

Chines A, Pacifici R, Avioli LA: Systemic mastocytosis and osteoporosis. *Osteoporos Int* 3(Suppl 1):147–149, 1993.

Compston JE, Croucher PI: Histomorphometric assessment of trabecular bone remodelling in osteoporosis [review]. *Bone Miner* 14(2):91–102, 1991.

Cosman F, Schnitzer MB, McCann PD: Relationships between quantitative histological measurements and noninvasive assessments of bone mass. *Bone* 13(3):237–242, 1992.

Croucher PI, Vedi S, Motley RJ: Reduced bone formation in patients with osteoporosis associated with inflammatory bowel disease. *Osteoporos Int* 3(5):236–241, 1993.

Dennison E, Cole Z, Cooper C: Diagnosis and epidemiology of osteoporosis. *Curr Opin Rheumatol* 17:456–461, 2005.

Diebold J, Batge B, Stein H: Osteoporosis in longstanding acromegaly: characteristic changes of vertebral trabecular architecture and bone matrix composition. *Virchows Arch A Pathol Anat Histopathol* 419(3):209–215, 1991.

Hain SF: DXA scanning for osteoporosis. *Clin Med* 6(3):254–258, 2006.

Jayasinghe JA, Jones SJ, Boyde A: Scanning electron microscopy of human lumbar vertebral trabecular bone surfaces. *Virchows Arch A Pathol Anat Histopathol* 422(1):25–34, 1993.

Lane JM, Vigorita VJ: Osteoporosis. *J Bone Joint Surg (Am)* 65:274, 1983.

Lin JT, Lane JM: Osteoporosis: a review. *Clin Orthop Relat Res* 425: 126–134, 2004.

Magaro M, Tricerri A, Piane D: Generalized osteoporosis in non–steroid treated rheumatoid arthritis. *Rheumatol Int* 11(2):73–76, 1991.

Mauck KF, Clarke BL: Diagnosis, screening, prevention, and treatment of osteoporosis. *Mayo Clin Proc* 81(5):662–672, 2006.

Motley RJ, Clements D, Evans WD: A four-year longitudinal study of bone loss in patients with inflammatory bowel disease. *Bone Miner* 23(2):95–104, 1993.

Ott SM: Clinical effects of bisphosphonates in involutional osteoporosis [review]. *J Bone Miner Res* 8 (Suppl 2):S597–S606, 1993.

Recker RR: Bone biopsy and histomorphometry in clinical practice. *Rheum Dis Clin North Am* 20(3):609–627, 1994.

Rillo OL, Di Stefano CA, Bermudez J, et al: Idiopathic osteoporosis during pregnancy. *Clin Rheumatol* 13(2):299–304, 1994.

Wilkinson JM, Cotton DW, Harris SC, et al: Assessment of osteoporosis at autopsy: mechanical methods compared to radiological and histological techniques. *Med Sci Law* 31(1):19–24, 1991.

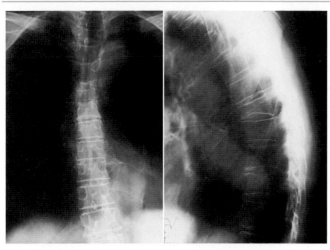

Figure 2–1 Anteroposterior (AP) (left) and lateral (right) radiographs of the thorax in a patient with osteoporosis. Note the diffuse osteopenia and the compression fracture of the thoracic vertebra. Exaggeration of the vertical striations in osteoporotic vertebrae also may be present.

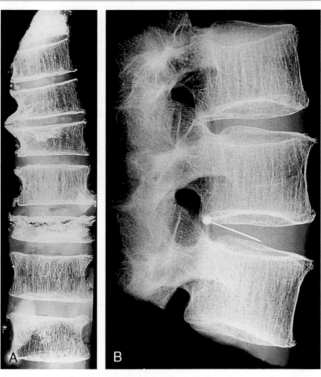

Figure 2–3 *A* and *B*: These radiographs illustrate the exaggerated vertical striations as well as compression fractures commonly seen in osteoporotic vertebrae.

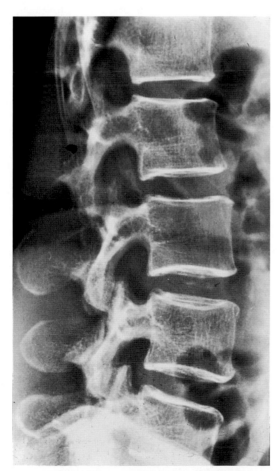

Figure 2–2 This radiograph of the lumbar vertebrae illustrates the exaggerated pattern of vertical striations that can be seen in patients with osteoporosis.

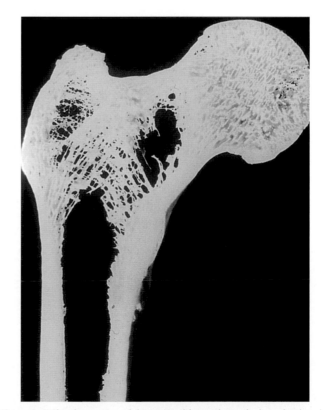

Figure 2–4 This thin section of the proximal femur shows the loss of trabecular bone seen in patients with osteoporosis. Figures 2–5 and 2–6 also illustrate the gross pathologic features seen in osteoporotic bone.

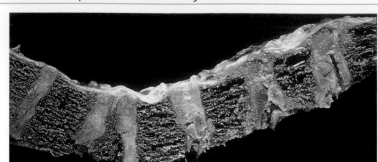

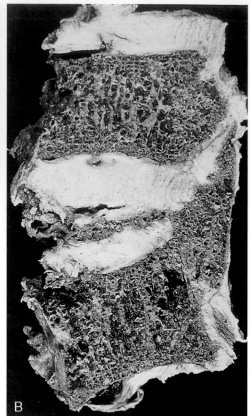

Figure 2–5 *A* and *B:* These illustrate the gross pathology that results in the radiographic features of osteoporotic vertebrae. Compression fractures are present in both of these specimens.

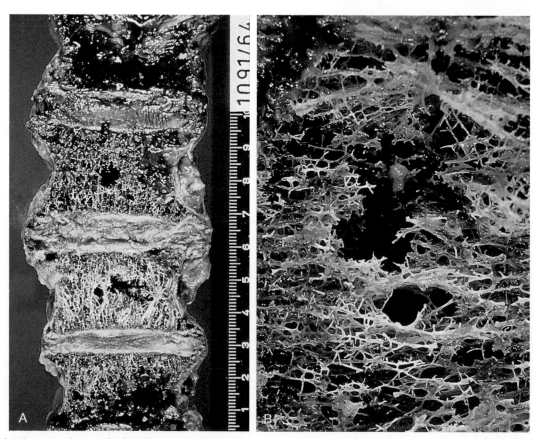

Figure 2–6 *A* and *B:* These two photographs show the loss of trabecular bone in osteoporotic vertebrae. Microfractures of the thinned trabecular bone are common. Histologically, a healing reaction may be present in these regions.

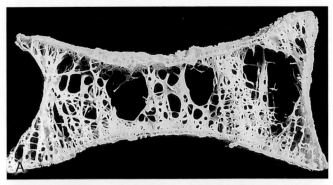

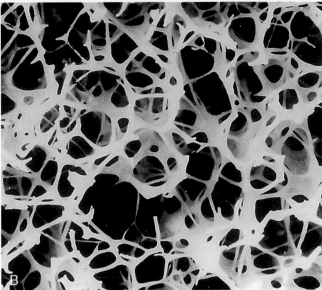

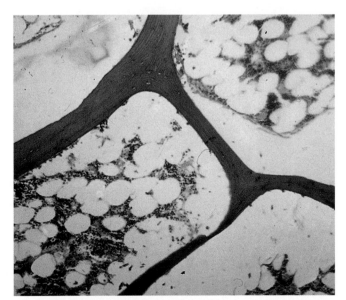

Figure 2–7 *A* and *B*: These two specimens have been carefully prepared to illustrate the marked thinning or loss of trabecular bone in osteoporosis. Compression of the vertebra is also present in this case.

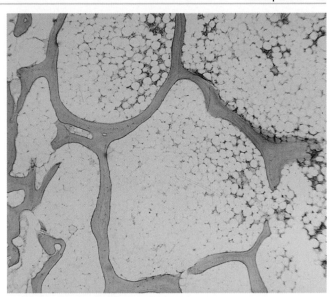

Figure 2–9 Cortical bone loss is a feature of osteoporotic bone, as shown in this photomicrograph. Thinning of the trabecular bone is also present.

Figure 2–8 This photomicrograph of osteoporotic bone reveals the thinning of trabecular bone without changes in the medullary content. In this case, little osteoblastic or osteoclastic activity is present. Such cases may be described as "inactive."

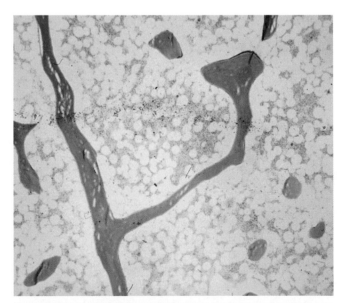

Figure 2–10 This photomicrograph illustrates the features of low turnover or inactive osteoporosis. Little osteoblastic or osteoclastic activity is evident in this biopsy specimen stained with trichrome stain. High turnover or active osteoporosis is characterized by excessive osteoclastic activity in the presence of normal or increased osteoblastic activity.

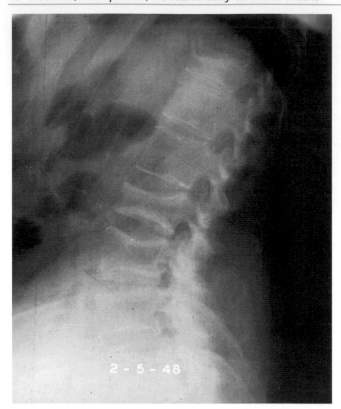

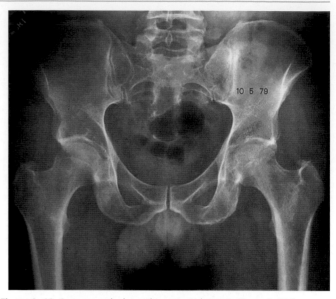

Figure 2–13 Seven months later, the patient shown in Figure 2–12 has experienced resolution of the pain and improvement in the radiograph.

Figure 2–11 Osteoporotic changes in the vertebrae are well illustrated in this x-ray film from a patient with Cushing's disease. Note the widened intervertebral spaces.

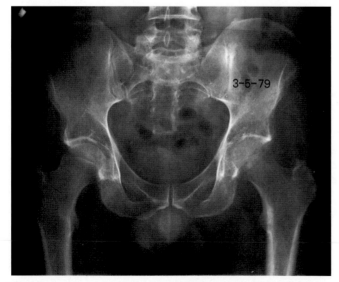

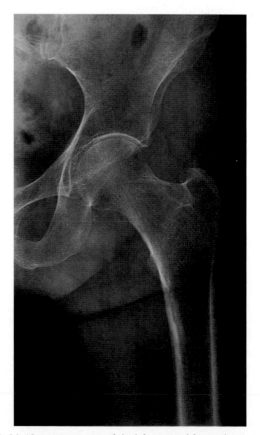

Figure 2–12 AP roentgenogram of the pelvis and proximal femora in a patient with transient osteoporosis. Demineralization of the bone in the proximal femur and acetabulum can be seen.

Figure 2–14 AP roentgenogram of the left proximal femur showing osteoporosis of the hip with diffuse demineralization of the bones and loss of trabeculae. Note the thinning of the cortex.

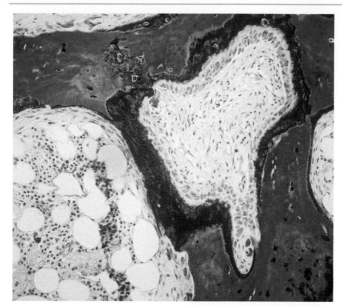

Figure 3–7 Osteoclastic resorption and osteoblastic deposition of new bone are seen in this example of renal osteodystrophy. Bony tunneling is also present (van Giesen stain).

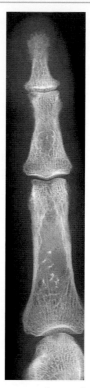

Figure 3–9 Subperiosteal bone resorption, particularly prominent in the phalangeal tufts, is characteristic of renal osteodystrophy.

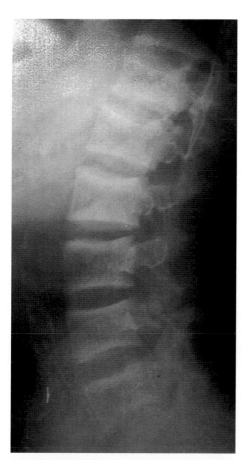

Figure 3–8 This radiograph of the spine illustrates the vertebral end plate sclerosis associated with renal osteodystrophy in a 41-year-old man with renal failure.

Rickets

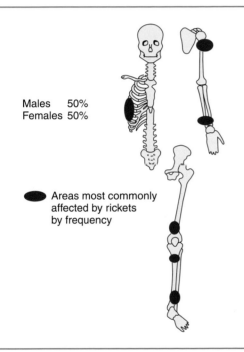

Males   50%
Females 50%

Areas most commonly
affected by rickets
by frequency

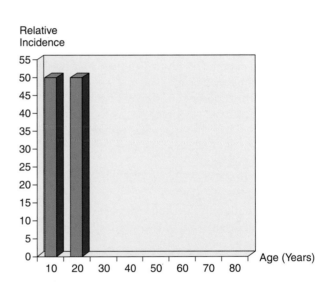

Clinical Signs

1. Widespread skeletal deformities in a child are present. (Rachitic abnormalities result from disturbances in the orderly mineralization and development of the growth plate; these disturbances are seen only prior to closure of the growth plates.)
2. The fontanelles bulge in patients during the first year of life. (During the first months of life, the skull is most severely affected.)
3. "Beading" of the costochondral junction (rachitic rosary) is seen.
4. Depression along the line of the diaphragmatic attachment to the ribs (Harrison's groove) is evident.

5. Wrists and ankles are enlarged secondary to flaring of the metaphysis.
6. The long bones exhibit anterior curvature. (During infancy and early childhood, the long bones show the greatest abnormality.)
7. Spinal abnormalities include dorsal kyphosis, scoliosis, and lumbar lordosis. (These are the result of upright weightbearing and thus are more common in older children.)
8. Muscle weakness is present.
9. Waddling gait is seen.
10. The serum phosphate concentration is decreased.

11. Some common signs by age of the affected child include the following:
    a. Infant: frontal bossing and flattening of the occipital portion of the skull.
    b. Young child: thickening of the forearm at the wrist, rachitic rosary, and Harrison's groove.
    c. Older child: bowing of the tibia and fibula.

Clinical Symptoms

1. Bone pain may occur.
2. Growth failure may be exhibited.
3. Lethargy may be experienced.
4. Muscle weakness may be present.

Major Radiographic Features

1. A wide and irregular growth plate (slight widening of the growth plate is an early sign of rickets) is best identified in those most active growth regions.
2. The metaphyseal end of the bone may flare.
3. Bone density is diminished (particularly in the metaphyseal region adjacent to affected growth plates).
4. Widening and cupping of the growth plate may be seen.
5. Cortical thinning may be evident.
6. Pseudofractures (Looser zones) may be seen.
7. Coarse trabeculae may be present.
8. The calvarium in neonates may show posterior flattening.
9. The frontal and parietal bones in neonates may have a squared configuration.
10. The intervertebral discs may expand, with resultant concavity of the vertebrae.
11. Basilar invagination of the skull may be evident.
12. The horizontal orientation of the sacrum is greater than normal.
13. Scoliosis and long bone bowing deformity occur in later childhood.

Radiographic Differential Diagnosis

1. Fanconi's syndrome.
2. Secondary hyperparathyroidism.
3. In patients younger than 1 year of age: biliary atresia and hypophosphatasia.
4. In patients resistant to the usual vitamin D therapy: renal disease, hypophosphatasia, and tumor-associated rickets (oncogenic osteomalacia).
5. X-linked hypophosphatemic rickets.

Major Pathologic Features

1. Disorganization of the growth plate (disorderly columns of proliferating cartilage) and adjacent metaphysis is evident.

2. The growth plate exhibits widening.
3. Defective mineralization of the bone may be seen immediately subjacent to the growth plate.
4. Pseudofractures may occur.
5. Large amounts of nonmineralized bone are present.

Pathologic Differential Diagnosis

1. Osteomalacia.

Pathogenesis

1. Abnormalities of vitamin D metabolism:
    a. Vitamin D deficiency: nutritional, malabsorption, lack of sun exposure for conversion of vitamin D to active metabolites. (In the United States, vitamin D deficiency is most commonly related to malabsorption.)
    b. Deficient dermal vitamin D conversion: renal failure, aging.
    c. Deficient hepatic synthesis: primary biliary cirrhosis, biliary atresia.
    d. Defective renal synthesis: hypoparathyroidism, renal failure, oncogenic osteomalacia.
2. Phosphate deficiency:
    a. Deficient intake.
    b. Impaired renal resorption of phosphate.
3. Defects in mineralization:
    a. Enzyme deficiencies: hypophosphatasia.
    b. Circulating inhibitors of bone mineralization: drugs, bisphosphonates, fluoride, aluminum.
4. States of rapid bone formation: osteopetrosis, renal bone disease (osteitis fibrosa cystica).
5. Other conditions: parenteral hyperalimentation.

Treatment

Medical

1. Treatment depends on the underlying cause but may include both medical and surgical approaches.
2. Medical approaches include the following:
    a. Nutritional rickets: cholecalciferol or ergocalciferol
    b. Vitamin D dependent rickets: Vitamin D and Vitamin D analogs, supplemental calcium. Hypophosphatemia vitamin-D-resistant rickets: phosphate and vitamin D supplementation.

Surgical

1. Surgical approaches are individualized depending on the type of fracture or deformity present but may include the following:
    a. Protected weightbearing for painful stress fracture.
    b. Closed versus open treatment of fracture.
    c. Corrective osteotomies for skeletal deformity.
    d. Epiphysiodesis in selected cases.

References

Gazit D, Tieder M, Liberman UA: Osteomalacia in hereditary hypophosphatemic rickets with hypercalciuria: a correlative clinical histomorphometric study. *J Clin Endocrinol Metab* 72(1):229–235, 1991.

Kaplan FS, August CS, Fallon MD: Osteopetrorickets. The paradox of plenty. Pathophysiology and treatment. *Clin Orthop Rel Res* 294:64–78, 1993.

Klein GL, Simmons DJ: Nutritional rickets: thoughts about pathogenesis. *Ann Med* 25(4):379–384, 1993.

Pitt MJ: Rickets and osteomalacia are still around [review]. *Radiol Clin North Am* 29(1):97–118, 1991.

Sullivan W, Carpenter T, Glorieux F: A prospective trial of phosphate and 1,25-dihydroxyvitamin D3 therapy in symptomatic adults with X-linked hypophosphatemic rickets. *J Clin Endocrinol Metab* 75(3):879–885, 1992.

Weidner N: Review and update: oncogenic osteomalacia-rickets [review]. *Ultrastruct Pathol* 15(4–5):317–333, 1991.

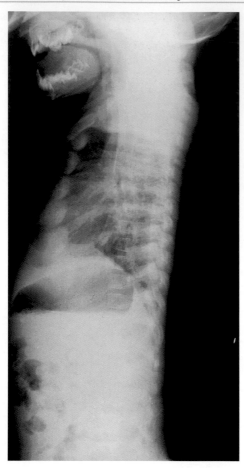

Figure 4–1 This lateral radiograph from a young child with rickets illustrates poor mineralization of the ribs, particularly in the region of the costochondral junction.

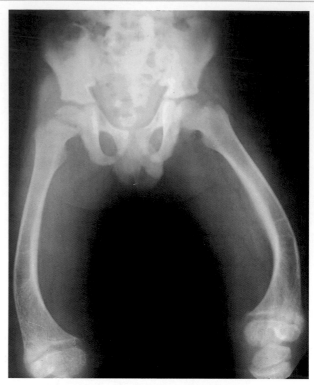

Figure 4–3 This radiograph shows bowing deformity of the femora in a 6-year-old patient with rickets. Some metaphyseal flaring is evident in the distal femora, and a thickened bony cortex is present on the concave side of the bony deformity.

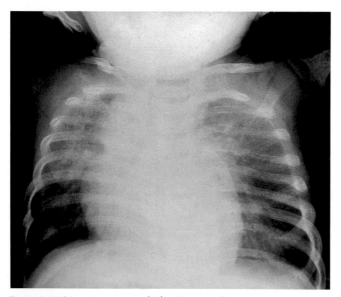

Figure 4–2 This anteroposterior (AP) radiograph of the chest from a young patient with rickets illustrates the irregular and poor mineralization of the ribs seen in this condition. In longstanding cases, the ribs may be deformed in the region of the diaphragmatic attachment, resulting in a groove (Harrison's groove).

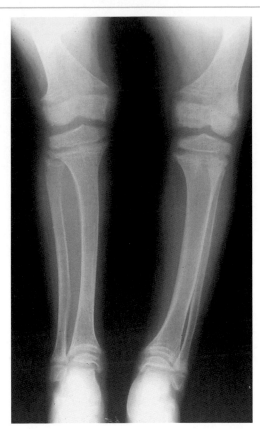

Figure 4–4 This radiograph illustrates widened growth plates and metaphyseal flaring in the distal femora and proximal tibiae bilaterally. Slight bowing of the tibia is evident in this 8-year-old girl with vitamin D–resistant rickets.

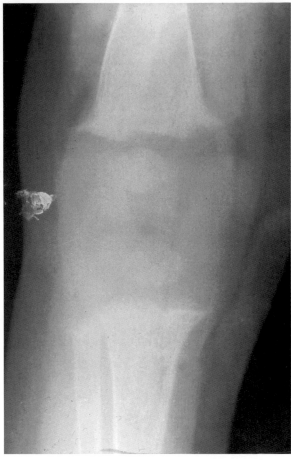

Figure 4–5 Marked rachitic changes are evident in this radiograph of the knee of a 3-year-old patient. Metaphyseal flaring and some cupping deformity are present. The irregular appearance of the metaphyseal bone may be the result of irregularly shaped penetrations of the epiphyseal cartilage into the metaphyseal bone.

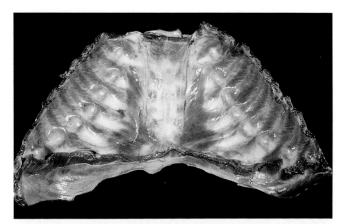

Figure 4–6 This photograph of the rib cage of a young patient who died with rickets illustrates the bilaterally symmetric enlargement of the costochondral cartilage that produces the so-called rachitic rosary.

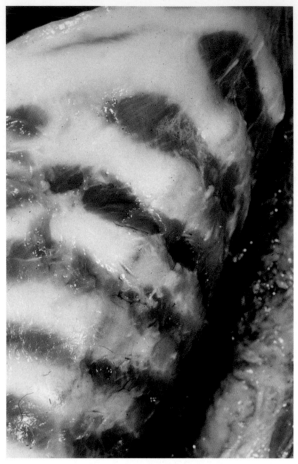

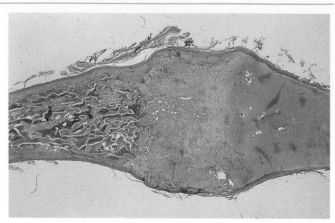

Figure 4–9 This histologic cross-section of a rib from the costochondral region shows an irregular proliferation of cartilage forming an enlarged mass of uncalcified cartilage.

Figure 4–7 This photograph shows at higher magnification the enlargement of the costochondral cartilage that produces the characteristic rachitic rosary.

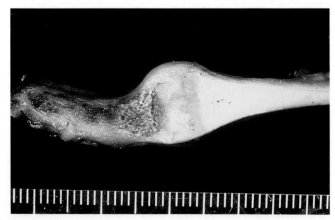

Figure 4–8 A cross-section of rib illustrates an abundance of cartilage forming an ellipsoid mass at the costochondral junction.

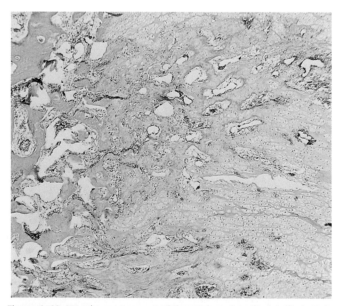

Figure 4–10 Irregular arrangement of the epiphyseal cartilage is illustrated in this photomicrograph. Note the absence of normal calcification of the cartilage.

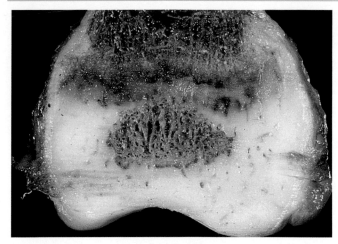

Figure 4–11 This cross-section of the distal femur in a young child who suffered from rickets shows widening of the epiphyseal growth plate and irregular masses of cartilage extending into the metaphyseal portion of the bone. These changes are typical of rickets.

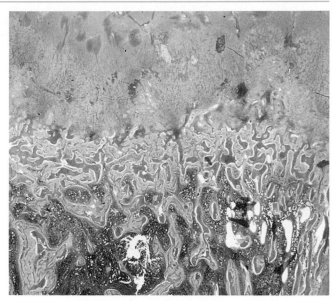

Figure 4–13 Irregular masses of cartilage with extension to involve the metaphyseal portion of the bone are illustrated in this low-magnification photomicrograph from the region of the epiphysis. In addition to the widened growth plate, poor mineralization of the cartilage, typical of rickets, is present.

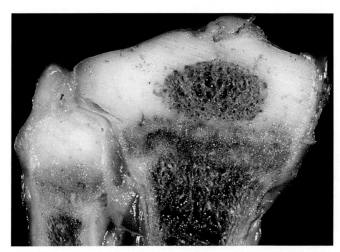

Figure 4–12 This cross-section of the proximal tibia and fibula illustrates features similar to those shown in Figure 4–11.

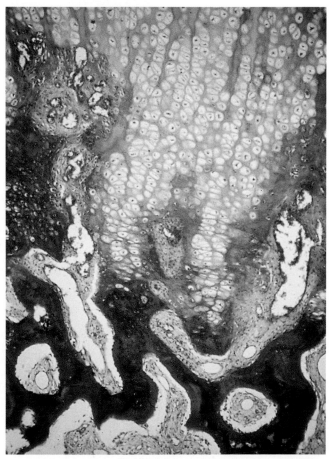

Figure 4–14 This photomicrograph illustrates the irregular interface between the epiphyseal cartilage and the adjacent bone at higher magnification than shown in Figure 4–13.

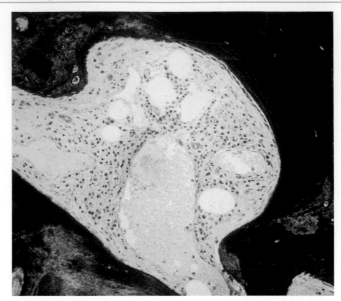

Figure 4–15 Poor mineralization is illustrated in this photomicrograph of rachitic bone stained with a von Kossa stain. Mineralized matrix stains black, and unmineralized osteoid, predominating in this specimen, stains red.

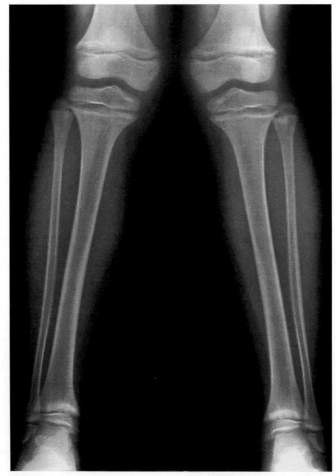

Figure 4–16 AP roentgenogram of both knees and tibiae in a patient with hypophosphatemic rickets. Note the widened growth plates and sclerosis on the metaphyseal side of the growth plate on the distal femur.

Osteomalacia

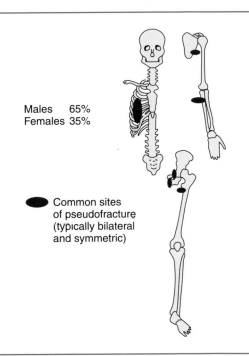

Males 65%
Females 35%

⬤ Common sites
of pseudofracture
(typically bilateral
and symmetric)

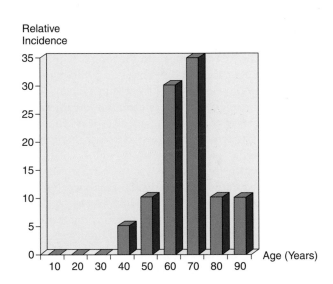

Clinical Signs

1. Patients may be symptomatic but typically have diffuse bone pain.
2. Dull, aching bone pain is worse with weightbearing (typically involves the ribs, lower back, knees, or legs).
3. Bone tenderness is present in approximately one third of patients.
4. Bowing of the limbs is seen in approximately 10% of patients.
5. Pigeon chest may be present.
6. Gibbus may be seen.
7. Lumbar scoliosis, thoracic kyphosis, or both may be seen.

8. Urinary excretion of hydroxyproline is increased.
9. Antalgic gait occurs in approximately 50% of patients.
10. Muscle weakness is found in approximately one third of patients.
11. Osteomalacia may be related to other conditions; therefore, the signs and symptoms related to Fanconi's syndrome, malabsorption, hypophosphatemia, tumor (oncogenic osteomalacia), hypochloremic acidosis, or skeletal resistance to vitamin D may be present in a given patient.
12. Biochemical abnormalities include the following:
    a. Elevated serum alkaline phosphatase concentration (in more than 90% of patients).

b. Low serum calcium or phosphate concentration (in approximately 50% of patients, with about one in eight patients having both).

c. Decreased urinary calcium excretion (in approximately one third of patients).

d. Elevated serum concentrations of parathyroid hormone (PTH) (in approximately 40% of patients).

e. Decreased serum concentrations of 1,25-dihydroxyvitamin D3 (in approximately 50% of patients).

Clinical Symptoms

1. Dull, aching bone pain may be vague initially but may become severe with longstanding disease.
2. Muscle weakness, more common in the proximal musculature, may be experienced.

Major Radiographic Features

1. Generalized osteopenia is present in approximately two thirds of cases, but this is a nonspecific finding.
2. Multiple bilaterally symmetric cortical lucent areas that are typically perpendicular to the long axis of the affected bone (so-called Looser zones and Milkman's syndrome) can be seen. These lucent zones incompletely span the affected bone. Most common sites are the axillary margin of the scapulae, lower ribs, pubic rami, neck of the femora, and posterior margin of the proximal ulnae.
3. The axial skeleton (vertebrae, pelvis, ribs, and sternum) is more affected than the appendicular skeleton. Concave deformity of the vertebrae ("codfish" vertebrae) occurs most commonly late in the course of the disease.
4. Vertebral bodies lose the distinctness of their trabecular pattern.
5. Vertebral discs appear to be enlarged as a result of vertebral end plates being depressed.
6. Pseudofractures or cortical lucent areas may show increased uptake on isotope bone scan (in approximately 20% of cases), particularly of the long bones and wrists.
7. Bone scan may be more sensitive in identifying multiple abnormal areas of increased isotope uptake.
8. Bone mass is decreased, as measured by single- and dual-photon absorptiometry.
9. Physiologic response to osteomalacia results in secondary hyperparathyroidism; therefore, radiographically the changes of hyperparathyroidism may be superimposed on those of osteomalacia (e.g., subperiosteal resorption of the phalanges).

Radiographic Differential Diagnosis

1. Stress fracture.
2. Hyperparathyroidism.

3. Radiolucent areas similar to pseudofractures (such areas can be seen in Paget's disease and fibrous dysplasia).

Major Pathologic Features

1. Increased nonmineralized osteoid lining the bony trabeculae can be seen.
2. Increased osteoid lining the haversian canals in the cortical bone is also identified.
3. Excessive nonmineralized osteoid may be seen in subperiosteal regions of the bone.
4. Morphometric analysis typically shows that more than 10% of the bone mass is nonmineralized.
5. Reduced osteoblastic and osteoclastic activity is seen in low-turnover osteomalacia.
6. Reduced tetracycline uptake is also seen in low-turnover osteomalacia.

Pathologic Differential Diagnosis

1. Rickets.

Pathogenesis

1. Abnormalities of vitamin D metabolism:
   a. Vitamin D deficiency: nutritional, malabsorption, lack of sun exposure for conversion of vitamin D to active metabolites.
   b. Deficient dermal vitamin D conversion: renal failure, aging.
   c. Deficient hepatic synthesis: primary biliary cirrhosis, biliary atresia.
   d. Defective renal synthesis: hypoparathyroidism, renal failure, oncogenic osteomalacia.
2. Phosphate deficiency:
   a. Deficient intake: excess aluminum hydroxide ingestion.
   b. Impaired renal resorption of phosphate.
3. Defects in mineralization:
   a. Enzyme deficiencies: hypophosphatasia.
   b. Circulating inhibitors of bone mineralization: drugs, bisphosphonates, fluoride, aluminum.
4. States of rapid bone formation: osteopetrosis, renal bone disease (osteitis fibrosa cystica).
5. Other conditions: parental hyperalimentation.
6. Uncommonly associated with bone or soft tissue tumors (see Chapter 6, Oncogenic Osteomalacia).

Treatment

1. Treatment depends on the underlying cause and may include both medical and surgical approaches.
2. Medical therapy includes the following:
   a. Nutritional rickets: cholecalciferol or ergocalciferol.
   b. Vitamin D dependent rickets: Vitamin D and Vitamin D analogs, supplemental calcium.

c. Hypophosphatemia vitamin-D-resistant rickets: phosphate and vitamin D supplementation.

3. Surgical therapy includes the following:

a. Individualized treatment, depending on the type of fracture or deformity.

b. Protected weight-bearing for painful stress fractures.

c. Closed versus open treatment for fracture.

d. Removal of tumor in those rare cases of oncogenic osteomalacia.

References

Bingham CT, Fitzpatrick LA: Noninvasive testing in the diagnosis of osteomalacia. *Am J Med* 95:519–523, 1993.

Chazan JA, Libbey NP, London MR, et al: The clinical spectrum of renal osteodystrophy in 57 chronic hemodialysis patients: a correlation between biochemical parameters and bone pathology findings. *Clin Nephrol* 35(2):78–85, 1991.

Cooper KL: Radiology of metabolic bone disease. *Endocrinol Metab Clin North Am* 18:955–976, 1989.

Llach F: Renal bone disease. *Transplant Proc* 23(2):1818–1822, 1991.

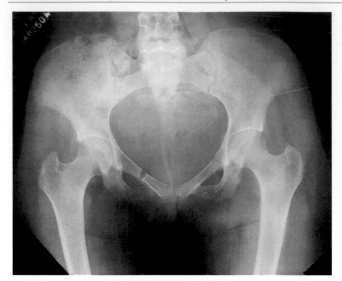

Figure 5–1 Pelvic radiograph of a patient with osteomalacia showing generalized osteopenia. Pelvic fracture is also evident. Similar fractures may occur in the small bones of the feet; however, the axial skeleton is more commonly involved than the appendicular skeleton. Pseudofractures represent zones of nonmineralized osteoid commonly found in regions where vessels cross near the bone.

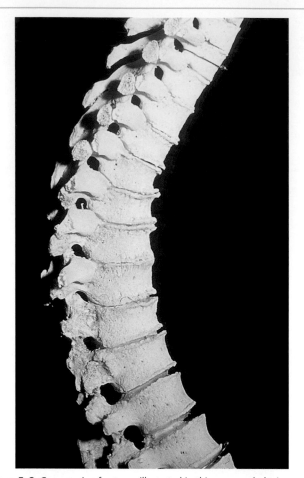

Figure 5–3 Compression fractures, illustrated in this gross pathologic specimen, are commonly identified in patients with longstanding osteomalacia. Radiographically, the osteomalacic vertebrae may bear a superficial resemblance to vertebrae affected by Paget's disease of bone.

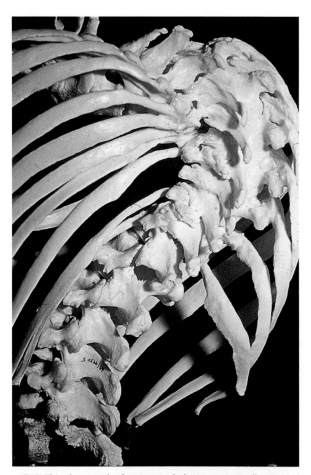

Figure 5–2 This photograph of a gross pathologic specimen illustrates the deformation associated with longstanding osteomalacia. Such bowing is commonly seen in long bones.

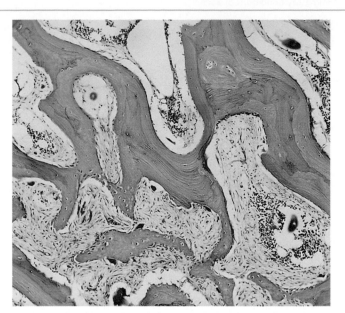

Figure 5–4 This photomicrograph illustrates the histologic features of osteomalacia in a patient suffering from sprue. The biopsy specimen is from the ilium and shows apparent irregular mineralization of the bony trabeculae reflective of poor mineralization of the osteoid. Osteomalacia is difficult to diagnose without the use of nondecalcified specimens or tetracycline labeling prior to bone biopsy.

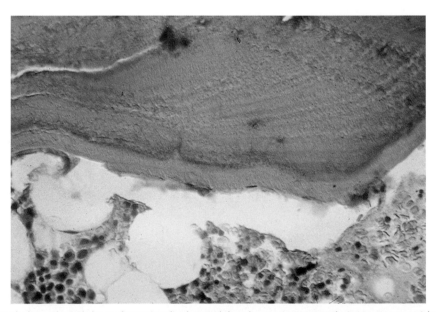

Figure 5–5 This photomicrograph shows the wide layer of nonmineralized osteoid that characterizes osteomalacia. Von Kossa or trichrome stains (see Figs. 5–6 and 5–7) more dramatically demonstrate the absence of calcification; however, the same feature is subtly noticeable in well-developed cases of osteomalacia when evaluated with hematoxylin and eosin–stained sections.

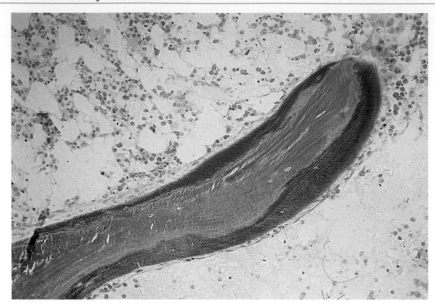

Figure 5–6 This trichrome stain dramatically demonstrates the increased nonmineralized bone in patients with osteomalacia. Morphometric analysis typically reveals that such nonmineralized bony matrix represents more than 10% of the bone mass.

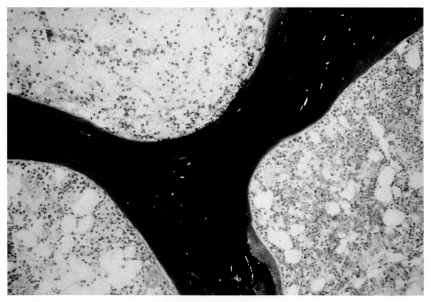

Figure 5–7 This von Kossa stain also illustrates the thick layer of osteoid covering mineralized bone in a patient with osteomalacia. The black staining corresponds to regions of calcified matrix in the biopsy specimen.

Oncogenic Osteomalacia (Phosphaturic Mesenchymal Tumor)

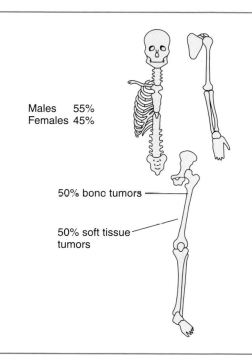

Males 55%
Females 45%

50% bone tumors

50% soft tissue tumors

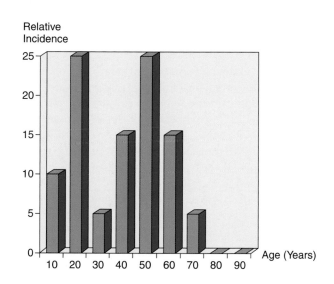

Clinical Signs

1. Generalized muscle weakness may be present.
2. Hypophosphatemia is the major biochemical abnormality.
3. Serum calcium concentrations are normal to slightly decreased.
4. Serum alkaline phosphatase concentrations are variably elevated.
5. Serum concentrations of 1,25-dihydroxyvitamin D are decreased or undetectable.
6. Parathyroid hormone concentrations may be increased in approximately half the patients.

Clinical Symptoms

1. There is a gradual onset of pain in the lower back, lower legs, hips, and/or ankles.
2. Pain is frequently accompanied by generalized muscular weakness and easy fatigability.
3. Patients may be so debilitated as to be bedridden.
4. Symptoms may precede the identification of the tumor by months to years (approximately 60% of patients have had symptoms for 1–5 years, and 20% have had symptoms for 5–10 years).
5. Joint pain may be present.
6. An affected bone may fracture with minor trauma.

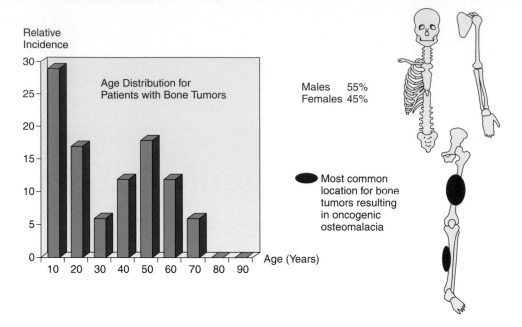

Major Radiographic Features

Bone Findings Apart from Tumor

1. Bone findings almost always are unremarkable.
2. Pseudofractures or cortical lucent areas may show increased uptake on isotope bone scan (in approximately 20% of cases), particularly of the long bones and wrists.
3. Bone scan may be more sensitive in identifying multiple abnormal areas of increased isotope uptake.
4. In children, signs of rickets may be present.

Tumor

1. The radiographic features of the bone tumor are as follows:
   a. Fibrous dysplasia.
   b. Osteosarcoma.
   c. Chondroblastoma.
   d. Chondromyxoid fibroma.
   e. Giant cell tumor.
   f. Metaphyseal fibrous defect.
   g. Hemangioma.
   h. Other.
2. Tumors associated with osteomalacia may also be of soft tissue origin.

Radiographic Differential Diagnosis

1. Rickets not associated with a tumor.
2. Osteomalacia not associated with a tumor.
3. Hypophosphatemic rickets and osteomalacia associated with ifosfamide chemotherapy.
4. X-linked hypophosphatemic rickets/osteomalacia.

Major Pathologic Features

1. Tumors associated with oncogenic osteomalacia (approximately half are primary soft tissue tumors, and half are primary bone tumors) include the following:
   a. Vascular tumors (approximately half of all tumors show a vascular histologic pattern):
      i. Hemangiopericytoma.
      ii. Hemangioma.
      iii. "Fibrovascular" lesions.
   b. Giant cell lesions:
      i. Giant cell tumor of bone.
      ii. Soft tissue giant cell tumors.
      iii. Other (e.g., pigmented villonodular synovitis [PVNS], malignant fibrous histiocytoma [MFH]).
   c. Metaphyseal fibrous defect.
   d. Osteoblastoma.
   e. Fibrous dysplasia.
   f. Phosphaturic mesenchymal tumor.
   g. Other.
2. The pathologic features of the osteomalacia are identical to those of osteomalacia not associated with a tumor.

Pathologic Differential Diagnosis

1. Osteomalacia (apart from the tumor that is causing the osteomalacia, the histologic features are identical to those of osteomalacia not associated with a tumor).
2. Rickets not associated with a tumor.
3. Histologic features of fibrous dysplasia, osteosarcoma, chondroblastoma, chondromyxoid fibroma, malignant fibrous histiocytoma, giant cell tumor, metaphyseal fibrous defect, hemangioma, or a soft tissue tumor—revealed by biopsy of the lesion causing the osteomalacia.

Treatment

1. Any patient with nondietary hypophosphatemic osteomalacia or rickets should be evaluated for a tumor.
2. If no tumor is found, then the patient should be treated with phosphorous supplementation and 1, 25(OH)$_2$ D or can use "calcitriol".
3. If the urinary phosphate concentration does not decrease and the serum phosphate concentration increases after tumor removal, then incomplete tumor removal should be suspected.

References

Cotton GE, Van Puffelen P: Hypophosphatemic osteomalacia secondary to neoplasia. *J Bone Joint Surg (Am)* 68(1):129–133, 1986.

Folpe AL, Fanburg-Smith JC, Billings SD et al: Most osteomalacia-associated mesenchymal tumors are a single histopathologic entity; an analysis of 32 cases and a comprehensive review of the literature. *Am J Surg Pathol* 28(1):30, 2004.

McClure J, Smith PS: Oncogenic osteomalacia. *J Clin Pathol* 40(4): 446–453, 1987.

Nuovo MA, Dorfman HD, Sun CC, et al: Tumor-induced osteomalacia and rickets. *Am J Surg Pathol* 13(7):588–599, 1989.

Park YK, Unni KK, Beabout JW, et al: Oncogenic osteomalacia: a clinico-pathologic study of 17 bone lesions. *J Korean Med Sci* 9(4):289–298, 1994.

Salassa RM, Jowsey J, Arnaud CD: Hypophosphatemic osteomalacia associated with "non-endocrine" tumors. *N Engl J Med* 283(2):65–70, 1970.

Sundaram M, McCarthy EF: Oncogenic osteomalacia. *Skeletal Radiol* 29(3):117–124, 2000.

Weidner N, Santa Cruz D: Phosphaturic mesenchymal tumors: a polymorphous group causing osteomalacia or rickets. *Cancer* 59(8): 1442–1454, 1987.

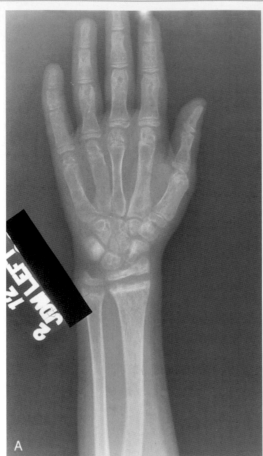

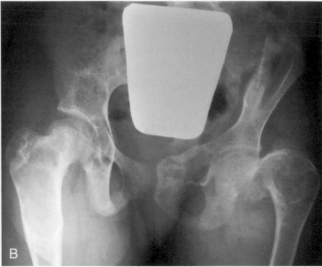

Figure 6–1 *A*: This radiograph illustrates changes of polyostotic fibrous dysplasia in the small bones. The growth plates of the distal radius and ulna are widened, showing radiographic features of osteomalacia. *B*: Characteristic radiographic features of fibrous dysplasia are evident in this pelvic radiograph of the 7-year-old female patient whose fibrous dysplasia was associated with osteomalacia *(A)*.

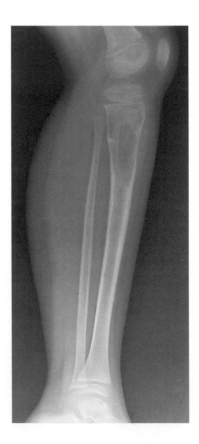

Figure 6–2 This radiograph shows a case of oncogenic osteomalacia associated with an osteosarcoma of the proximal tibia. The physes are widened, and flaring of the metaphyseal region of the distal tibia is also evident.

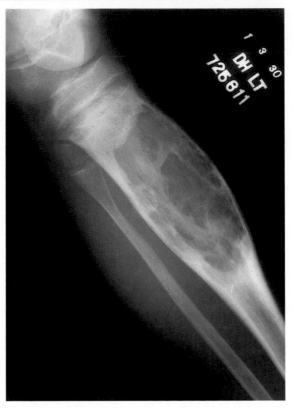

Figure 6–3 This radiograph illustrates a case of tumor-associated osteomalacia. The proximal tibial tumor is a chondromyxoid fibroma that occurred in a 13-year-old patient.

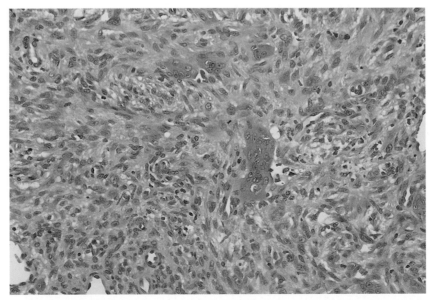

Figure 6–4 This photomicrograph illustrates the histologic features of a phosphaturic mesenchymal tumor. Lesions such as this may be of bone or soft tissue origin. This tumor was a soft tissue tumor in the leg. The tumors may be very small and difficult to localize clinically.

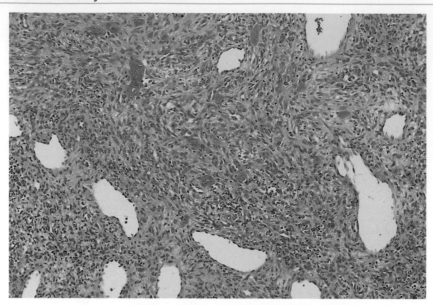

Figure 6–5 This photomicrograph demonstrates a tumor with hemangiopericytomatous histology that was associated with osteomalacia. Many of the neoplasms associated with osteomalacia have a prominent vascular pattern.

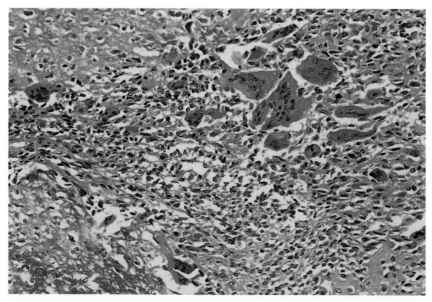

Figure 6–6 Phosphaturic mesenchymal tumors may show diffuse, fine, lacelike calcification. Multinucleated giant cells also may be present, as illustrated in this tumor involving the navicular bone.

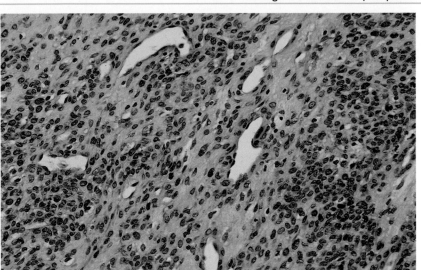

Figure 6–7 This tumor from the humerus was associated with osteomalacia. A hemangiopericytomatous pattern of growth is evident. Excision of the tumor resulted in resolution of the osteomalacia.

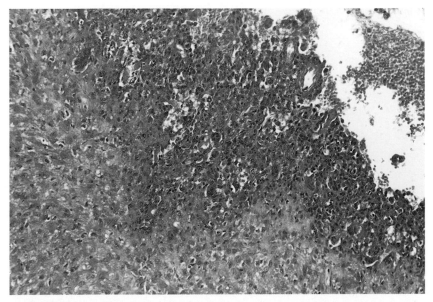

Figure 6–8 This photomicrograph illustrates the histologic pattern of giant cell tumor with secondary aneurysmal bone cyst changes. This tumor of the ilium in a 41-year-old woman was associated with osteomalacia.

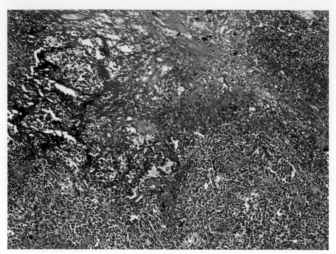

Figure 6–9 Phosphaturic mesenchymal tumors can produce a myxoid to myxochondroid matrix, which often is associated with a distinctive pattern of calcification, as shown in this photomicrograph.

Paget's Disease

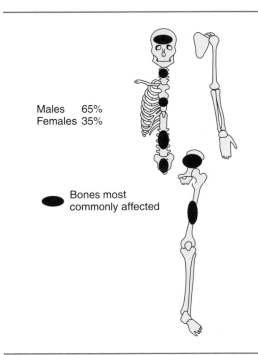

Males 65%
Females 35%

⬤ Bones most commonly affected

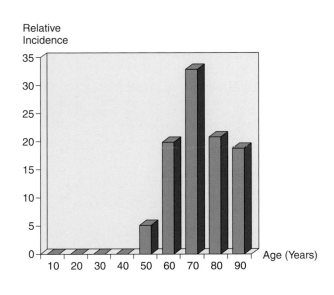

Incidence

1. Paget's disease is most common in individuals of Northern European origin (approximately 33% of the European population).
2. The male-to-female ratio is approximately 2:1.
3. The most common locations are the innominate bone and femur.
4. Based on routine radiographic evaluation of the pelvis and lumbar vertebrae, the incidence has been estimated to increase from approximately 3.5 per 1000 to greater than 90 per 1000 between the fourth and ninth decades of life in Northern European countries.

However, recent epidemiologic studies demonstrate a declining incidence.
5. Autopsy studies indicate an incidence of approximately 3.5% in patients older than 40 years of age. (Approximately 90% of symptomatic patients are older than 40 years of age.)

Clinical Signs

1. Fracture may occur.
2. Arthritis may be present.
3. Heart failure may occur.

4. The serum alkaline phosphatase concentration is elevated.
5. Serum calcium and phosphorus concentrations are within normal limits.
6. The serum calcium concentration increases with prolonged bed rest.
7. Bone deformity is present in approximately 25% of patients (e.g., forehead prominence, bowing of long bones).
8. Bone pain or periosteal tenderness may be present.
9. An extremity may show increased warmth.
10. Paget's sarcoma is characterized by the following:
    a. A painful mass felt in the region of the affected bone.
    b. Rapidly progressive symptoms.

Clinical Symptoms

1. Pain—constant, aching, and diffuse in nature—is felt in the affected region and is the presenting complaint in approximately half the patients. Increased pain in one bone in a patient with Paget's disease should arouse suspicion of the development of a sarcoma.
2. Hearing impairment may be present.
3. Dentures may be ill-fitting.
4. There may be difficulties with mastication.

Note: Approximately only one third of the sites of pagetic bone disease result in clinical symptoms.

Major Imaging Features

1. There is a propensity to involve the lumbar spine, pelvis, skull, femur, and tibia.
2. The skull shows the following features:
   a. Early changes: well-marginated radiolucent defects (osteoporosis circumscripta).
   b. Late changes: bone thickened and of increased density (radiodense foci with a cotton-wool appearance).
3. The vertebral bodies have a "picture frame" appearance, showing increased width.
4. In long bones the lucent defect extends to the end of the affected bone, with sharp demarcation from uninvolved bone; the junction between affected and unaffected bone is wedge-shaped ("flame" sign or "blade of grass" sign).
5. Fractures that occur through pagetoid long bones are characteristically transverse ("banana" fracture).
6. Fractures are frequently associated with excessive callus formation.
7. The bone scan shows more pagetic sites of osseous involvement than are identified using routine radiographic evaluation; however, once the disease is in the inactive sclerotic phase, the bone scan may not yield positive findings.

8. The magnetic resonance imaging (MRI) is particularly helpful in excluding the possibility of sarcomatous transformation in Paget's disease.
9. There is a high incidence of arthritis and joint narrowing adjacent to the involved bone or bones.
10. Uncomplicated Paget's disease is perhaps the only known lesion to have extensive radiographic abnormality with marrow fat preserved on T1-weighted MR imaging.
11. Paget's sarcoma is characterized by the following:
    a. The bone of origin usually showing the changes of Paget's disease.
    b. Extension of the tumor into the surrounding soft tissue (MRI may show this best).
    c. A pattern of geographic bone destruction.
    d. A predilection for the humerus, the tumor only rarely arising in the spine (in comparison with the location of uncomplicated Paget's disease).

Note: Although most cases of Paget's disease progress through the active osteolytic phase to the osteosclerotic stage and remain relatively stable, reversion from the sclerotic to the osteolytic phase can occur. In general, however, if a lytic region is identified within a region of pagetoid bone that has previously been osteosclerotic radiographically, then sarcomatous degeneration should be excluded by MRI.

Radiographic Differential Diagnosis

1. Metastatic carcinoma.
2. Malignant lymphoma.
3. Hyperparathyroidism (if vertebral disease presents in a "rugger jersey" pattern).
4. Vertebral hemangioma.
5. Malignant lymphoma (when the spine is involved).

Major Pathologic Features

1. The disease is arbitrarily divided into three phases:
   a. Osteolytic phase: marrow space replaced by highly vascular fibrous connective tissue; active osteoclastic resorption; prominent osteoblastic new bone formation.
   b. Osteoblastic phase: trabecular plates widened but in a haphazard manner, leading to the mosaic pattern (increased number of cement lines).
   c. "Burnt-out" phase: less cellularity and reduced vascularity of the marrow space.
2. Histologic features include the following:
   a. Mosaic bone with accentuation of cement lines.
   b. Active bone remodeling early and quiescence late.
   c. Cancellous bone replaced by a network of disorganized-appearing thick bone trabeculae.
   d. Extremely vascular fibrous connective tissue occupying the intertrabecular space.

3. Paget's sarcoma is characterized by the following:
   a. Gross:
      i. A destructive lesion involves the bone and extends into the soft tissue.
      ii. The soft, fleshy tumor generally is whitish to brown.
   b. Microscopic:
      i. At low magnification, the tumor is highly cellular.
      ii. The tumor generally is composed of spindle cells.
      iii. At higher magnification, the spindle cells show significant pleomorphism and cytologic atypia.
      iv. The specific diagnosis may be that of osteosarcoma, fibrosarcoma, or malignant fibrous histiocytoma.

Pathologic Differential Diagnosis

1. Hyperparathyroidism.
2. Fibrous dysplasia.
3. Osteofibrous dysplasia.
4. Paget's sarcoma (if the lesion is in the florid lytic phase).

Treatment

Medical

1. Zoledronate is the most effective agent for treatment of Paget's disease. Risedronate and alendronate are also used.
2. Calcitonin can be used for patients who cannot tolerate bisphosphonates.

Surgical

1. Pathologic fracture is treated with closed versus open reduction.
2. Osteotomy is performed to correct deformity.
3. Arthroplasty is performed for advanced joint disease.

References

Bone HG, Kleerekoper M: Clinical review 39: Paget's disease of bone [review]. *J Clin Endocrinol Metab* 75(5):1179–1182, 1992.

Cundy T: Is Paget's disease of bone disappearing? *Skeletal Radiol* 35(6):350–351, 2006.

Chapman GK: The diagnosis of Paget's disease of bone [review]. *Aust N Z J Surg* 62(1):24–32, 1992.

Gallacher SJ: Paget's disease of bone [review]. *Curr Opin Rheumatol* 5(3):351–356, 1993.

Greenspan A: A review of Paget's disease: radiologic imaging, differential diagnosis, and treatment [review]. *Bull Hosp Jt Dis Orthop Inst* 51(1):22–33, 1991.

Hadjipavlou AG, Gaitanis IN, Kontakis GM: Paget's disease of the bone and its management. *J Bone Joint Surg (Br)* 84(2):160–169, 2002.

Haibach H, Farrell C, Dittrich FJ: Neoplasms arising in Paget's disease of bone: a study of 82 cases. *Am J Clin Pathol* 83:596–600, 1985.

Kaufmann GA, Sundaram M, McDonald DJ: Magnetic resonance imaging in symptomatic Paget's disease. *Skeletal Radiol* 20(6):413–418, 1991.

Mirra JM, Brien EW, Tehranzadeh J: Paget's disease of bone: review with emphasis on radiologic features, Parts I and II. *Skeletal Radiol* 24(3):173–184, 1995.

Roodman GD, Windle JJ: Paget disease of bone. *J Clin Invest* 115(2): 200–208, 2005.

Sundaram M, Khanna G, El-Khoury GY: T1 weighted MR imaging for distinguishing large osteolysis of Paget's disease from sarcomatous degeneration. *Skeletal Radiol* 30(7):378–383, 2001.

Tins BJ, Davies AM, Mangham DC: MR imaging of pseudosarcoma in Paget's disease of bone; a report of two cases. *Skeletal Radiol* 30(3):161–165, 2001.

Wick MR, Siegal GP, McLeod RA, et al: Sarcomas of bone-complicating osteitis deformans (Paget's disease): fifty years' experience. *Am J Surg Pathol* 5:47–59, 1981.

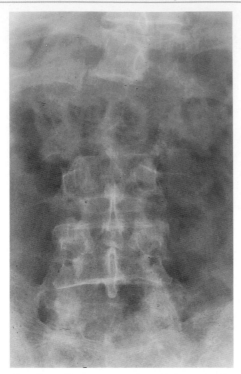

Figure 7–1 The radiographic appearance of Paget's disease involving a vertebra may simulate malignancy, as illustrated in this case. The florid lytic phase of the disease may radiographically simulate sarcoma or metastatic carcinoma. Other vertebral changes associated with Paget's disease include enlargement of the vertebra and peripheral sclerosis, resulting in a "picture frame" appearance of the vertebra.

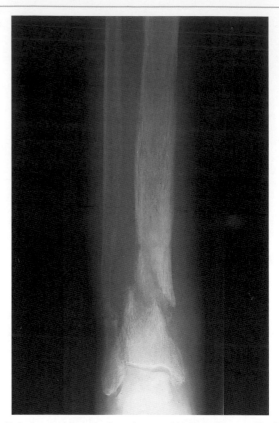

Figure 7–3 A typical fracture through pagetoid bone is illustrated in this radiograph. This "banana"-type transverse fracture most commonly involves the femur or tibia and is often associated with minimal or no trauma.

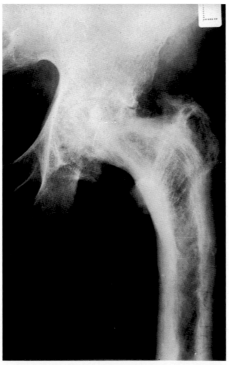

Figure 7–2 This radiograph of the proximal femur demonstrates Paget's disease involving a long bone. Paget's disease always extends to the end of the bone, as illustrated in this example. Other common features include thickening of the cortex, expansion of the bone, and thickened bony trabeculae.

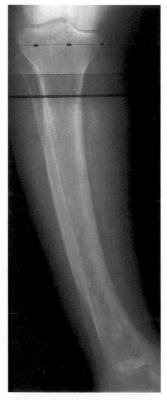

Figure 7–4 This radiograph shows the bowing bony deformity of Paget's disease involving the tibia.

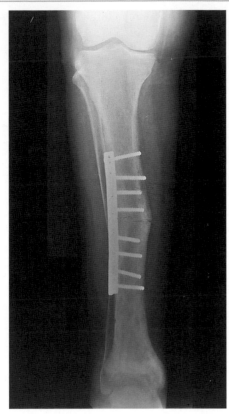

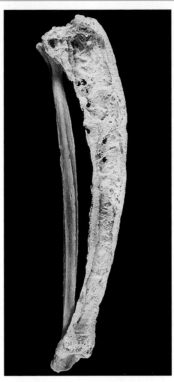

Figure 7–7 This gross specimen of the tibia and fibula shows the changes of Paget's disease involving the proximal tibia. Bowing related to the altered mechanical properties of the pagetoid bone has occurred.

Figure 7–5 This radiograph shows the surgical approach to the correction of the bony deformity in Figure 7-4. Treatment of such bony deformities or fractures is complicated by the altered mechanical properties of pagetoid bone.

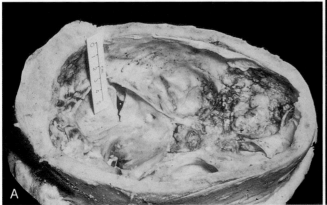

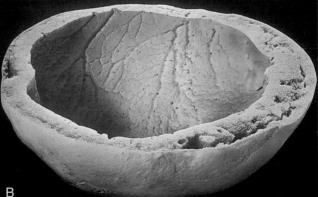

Figure 7–6 *A* and *B*: These two gross specimens illustrate the changes of Paget's disease involving the skull. Thickening of the skull as shown in these examples may compromise the foramina of cranial nerves, resulting in nerve loss. The thickened trabeculae eventually distort the normal diploetic architecture, as illustrated.

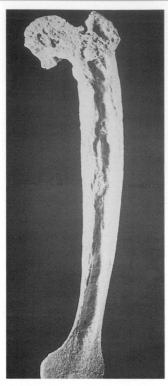

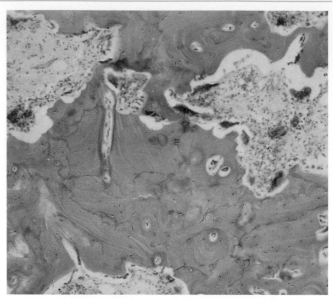

Figure 7–10 This photomicrograph illustrates the thickened bony trabeculae with prominent cement lines characteristic of Paget's disease. Numerous osteoclasts and increased osteoblastic activity are seen in this example as well. The irregular cement lines may be better appreciated in nondecalcified specimens.

Figure 7–8 Paget's disease of the proximal femur is illustrated in this photograph of a gross specimen. Cortical thickening is evident, and the process extends to the proximal end of the femur. Transition from pagetoid bone to normal bone is usually abrupt unless the disease has been complicated by the development of a sarcoma.

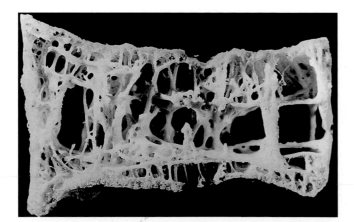

Figure 7–9 This vertebral specimen dramatically illustrates widening of the medullary bony trabeculae from a 72-year-old man with longstanding Paget's disease.

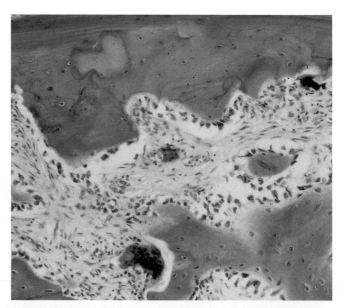

Figure 7–11 Higher magnification of the histologic features of pagetoid bone reveals increased osteoclastic and osteoblastic activity. Osteoclasts may be larger than normal in such cases. The medullary bone also is filled with a loose fibrovascular connective tissue that is frequently seen in Paget's disease.

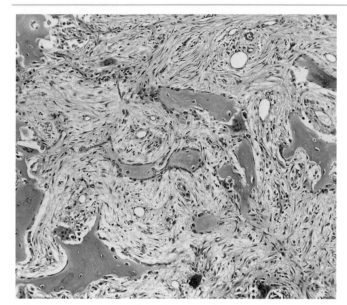

Figure 7–12 This example of well-developed Paget's disease shows the histologic features that can simulate those of fibrous dysplasia. The irregular pattern of pagetoid bone in association with the fibrous tissue replacement of the medullary contents can result in a confusing histologic pattern for the pathologist.

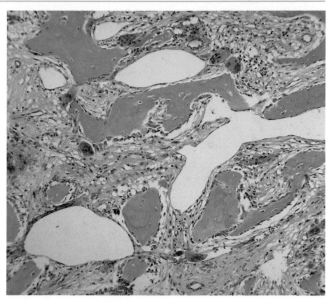

Figure 7–14 Increased vascularity of pagetoid bone is illustrated in this photomicrograph. Such vascularity may become so pronounced as to cause significant changes in the cardiovascular function of the affected patient. When the biopsy shows prominent vascularity in pagetoid bone, the differential diagnosis entertained by the pathologist may even include a vascular tumor.

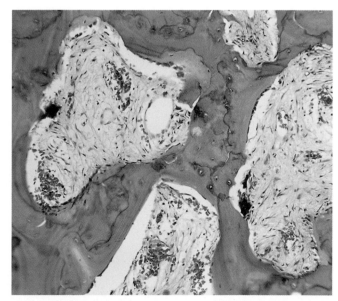

Figure 7–13 Irregular cement lines are often visible in pagetoid bone, even in decalcified specimens such as this one.

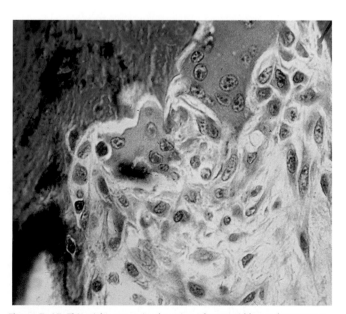

Figure 7–15 This trichrome stained section of pagetoid bone shows osteoclastic resorption of the trabecular bone. Osteoblastic deposition of osteoid is also evident.

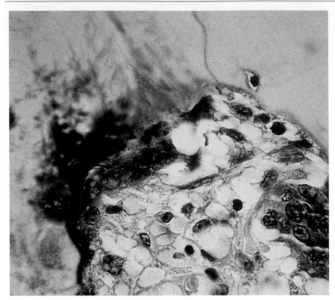

Figure 7–16 This acid phosphatase stain of pagetoid bone illustrates the enzymatic activity of osteoclasts.

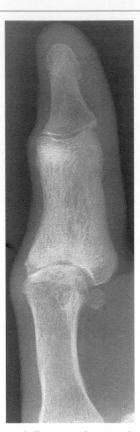

Figure 7–18 This radiograph illustrates sclerosis and expansion of the proximal phalanx of the thumb as a result of Paget's disease.

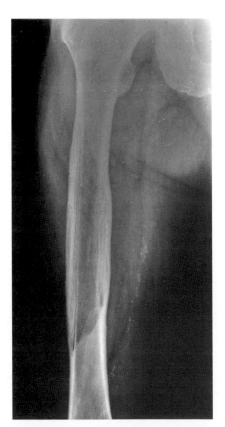

Figure 7–17 This radiograph illustrates the lytic phase of Paget's disease involving the proximal femur. The "blade of grass" appearance is evident in the proximal extent of the lesion.

Camurati-Engelmann Disease (Progressive Diaphyseal Dysplasia)

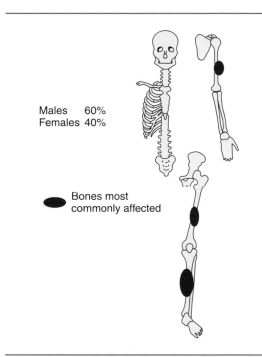

Males 60%
Females 40%

Bones most commonly affected

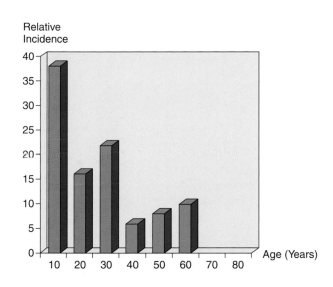

Clinical Signs

1. Waddling gait may become evident early in life (before 10 years of age).
2. Limb pain and deformity may be present.
3. Lumbar lordosis may be seen.
4. Flat feet may occur.
5. Muscle wasting may occur early in life (before 10 years of age).
6. If the medullary cavity is narrowed sufficiently to compromise medullary hematopoiesis, splenomegaly may result.

7. Proptosis may be present.
8. Serum chemistries generally are normal, but the alkaline phosphatase concentration of bone origin may be increased.
9. Failure to thrive may occur.
10. There is a dominant pattern of inheritance with variability in the clinical severity of expression.
11. Laboratory studies are usually within normal limits; however, elevated serum alkaline phosphatase activity and elevated urinary hydroxyproline concentrations have been reported.

Clinical Symptoms

1. Painful limbs may be experienced. The pain, usually described as aching or stabbing, is intermittent and worse with exercise.
2. Easy fatigability may occur.
3. Deafness associated with sclerosis of the ossicles may be present.

Major Radiographic Features

1. Symmetric sclerosis may be seen.
2. Fusiform enlargement of the diaphysis of the long bones (tibiae and femora particularly) may be evident.
3. The pelvis, mandible, ribs, clavicle, vertebrae, and small bones are relatively spared.
4. The base of the skull is usually involved.

Radiographic Differential Diagnosis

1. Hyperostosis generalisata with pachyderma (involves epiphysis or metaphysis as well as diaphysis).
2. Periosteal new bone formation similar to that seen as a result of the following:
   a. Trauma.
   b. Infection.
   c. Osteoid osteoma.
   d. Fluorosis.
   e. Vitamin D intoxication.
3. Hereditary multiple diaphyseal dysplasia.
4. Erdheim-Chester disease.
5. Hypertrophic pulmonary osteoarthropathy.

Major Pathologic Features

1. Cortical bone is thickened secondary to endosteal new bone formation.
2. Occasionally, periosteal new bone formation may be seen.
3. In children the medullary cavity may be narrowed.

4. Deposition of woven bone, in addition to cancellous and cortical bone, may occur.
5. Thick-walled blood vessels may be described in the periosteum and endosteum.

Pathologic Differential Diagnosis

1. Hypertrophic osteoarthropathy.
2. Trauma with exuberant periosteal new bone formation.
3. Infection.
4. Fluorosis.
5. Osteoid osteoma.

Treatment

1. Physical therapy modalities can be used.
2. Symptomatic measures (e.g., nonsteroidal anti-inflammatory drugs [NSAIDs]) can be used for painful legs. Short term glucocorticoid therapy has also been proposed.

References

Clybouw C, Desmyttere S, Bonduelle M: Camurati-Engelmann disease: contribution of bone scintigraphy to genetic counseling. *Genet Couns* 5(2):195–198, 1994.

De Vits A, Keymeulen B, Bossuyt A, et al: Progressive diaphyseal dysplasia (Camurati-Engelmann's disease). Improvement of clinical signs and of bone scintigraphy during pregnancy. *Clin Nucl Med* 19(2):104–107, 1994.

Fallon MD, Whyte MP, Murphy WA: Progressive diaphyseal dysplasia (Engelmann's disease). *J Bone Joint Surg (Am)* 62:465–472, 1980.

Janssens K, Vanhoenacker F, Bonduelle M, et al: Camurati-Engelmann disease: review of the clinical, radiological, and molecular data of 24 families and implications for diagnosis and treatment. *J Med Genet* 43(1):1–11, 2006.

Kumar B, Murphy WA, Whyte MP: Progressive diaphyseal dysplasia (Engelmann's disease): scintigraphic-radiographic-clinical correlations. *Radiology* 140(1):87–92, 1981.

Lennon EA, Schechter MD, Hornabrook RW: Engelmann disease: report of a case and review of the literature. *J Bone Joint Surg (Br)* 43-B: 273–284, 1961.

Wirth CR, Kay J, Bourke R: Diaphyseal dysplasia (Engelmann's syndrome). *Clin Orthop* 171:186–195, 1982.

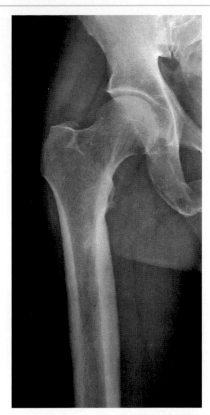

Figure 8–1 This radiograph illustrates the diffuse diaphyseal cortical thickening characteristic of Camurati-Engelmann disease. The patient was a 58-year-old man who presented with bilateral leg pain.

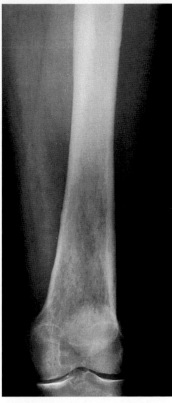

Figure 8–2 Sparing of the epiphyseal region, as shown in this radiograph, is characteristic of Camurati-Engelmann disease.

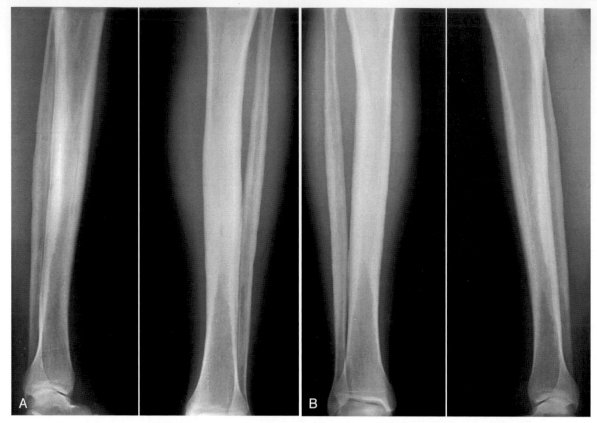

Figure 8–3 The bilateral symmetric nature of progressive diaphyseal dysplasia (Camurati-Engelmann disease) is evident in these radiographs of the right *(A)* and left *(B)* lower extremity.

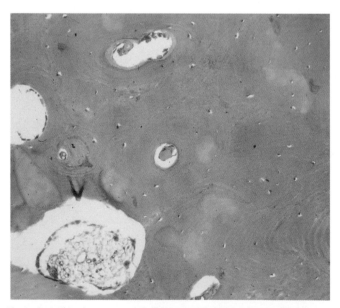

Figure 8–4 This photomicrograph illustrates the thickened cortical bone characteristic of Camurati-Engelmann disease. Increased osteoid may be seen.

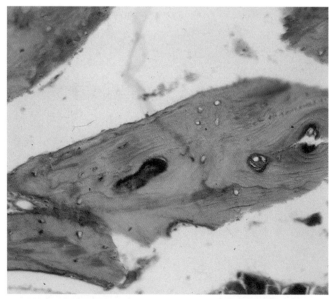

Figure 8–5 Although the bone of Camurati-Engelmann disease lacks the prominent cement lines associated with Paget's disease, this differentiation may be subtle, as shown in this photomicrograph of a specimen from the tibia in a patient with Camurati-Engelmann disease.

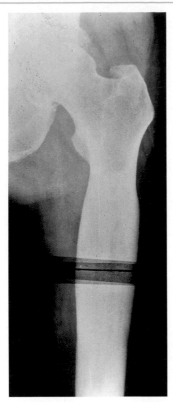

Figure 8–6 This radiograph illustrates the diaphyseal thickening of cortical bone seen in patients with Camurati-Engelmann disease. Although the disease begins early in life, sporadic cases with onset late in adult life have been reported.

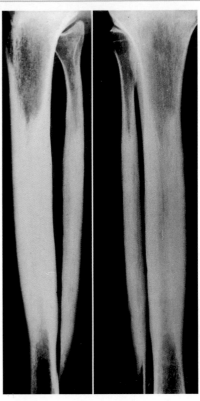

Figure 8–7 This radiograph of the lower extremities illustrates Camurati-Engelmann disease in a 67-year-old man. The skull and, rarely, vertebrae, small bones, clavicle, mandible, and pelvis also can be affected.

Hypertrophic Osteoarthropathy

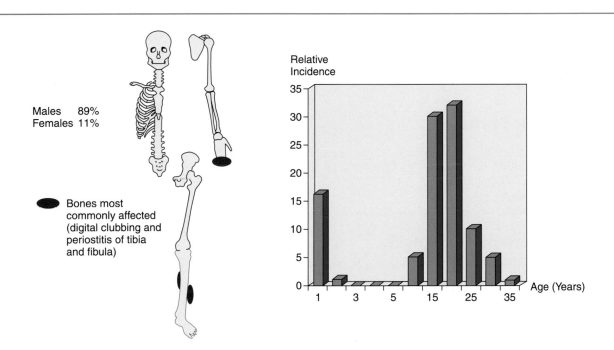

Males 89%
Females 11%

Bones most commonly affected (digital clubbing and periostitis of tibia and fibula)

Relative Incidence

Age (Years)

Classification

1. Primary.
2. Secondary:
   a. Generalized: related to pulmonary, cardiac, hepatic, intestinal, mediastinal, or miscellaneous conditions.
   b. Localized: related to hemiplegia, aneurysm, infective arteritis, or patent ductus arteriosus.

Clinical Signs

1. Fingers and toes may show clubbing.
2. Painful joint effusions are present in approximately 40% of patients with primary disease; knees, ankles, and wrists are most commonly affected.

3. Pachyderma is present in approximately 90% of patients with primary hypertrophic osteoarthropathy.

Clinical Symptoms

1. Arthralgia occurs and usually is relieved by aspirin.
2. Aching bone pain may be experienced.
3. Local hyperemia may be present.
4. Sweating is increased in approximately 25% of patients with primary disease.
5. Seborrhea is found in approximately 25% of patients with primary disease.
6. Acne may be present (seen in 10% of patients with primary disease).

Major Radiographic Features

1. Symmetric periosteal diaphyseal new bone formation can be seen and is particularly prominent in the appendicular skeleton (so-called onion skin periostitis), affecting the radius and ulna, tibia and fibula, humerus and femur, metacarpals, metatarsals, and proximal middle phalanges (in that order of frequency).
2. Radiographic densities may be evident at the sites of insertion of tendons and ligaments.
3. Bone scan may show increased uptake in various bones, even in asymptomatic cases.
4. Arthritic changes may be present in cases of secondary hypertrophic osteoarthropathy but are rare in primary disease.
5. MRI may show periostitis without marrow changes.

Radiographic Differential Diagnosis

1. Inflammatory arthritis (however, in hypertrophic osteoarthropathy, the adjacent bone is also involved).
2. Osteomyelitis.

Major Pathologic Features

1. Periosteal new bone formation is marked.
2. Mononuclear cell infiltration of the outer layers of periosteal new bone can be seen.
3. No endosteal new bone is formed.

Pathologic Differential Diagnosis

1. Callus.
2. Osteomyelitis with reactive new bone formation.

Treatment

1. Underlying illness—e.g., cardiovascular malformation or bronchogenic carcinoma—should be carefully identified and corrected.
2. Nonsteroidal anti-inflammatory agents can be administered for painful osteoarthropathy.

References

Epstein O, Ajdukiewicz AB, Dick R, et al: Hypertrophic hepatic osteoarthropathy: clinical, roentgenologic, biochemical, hormonal and cardiorespiratory studies, and review of the literature. *Am J Med* 67(1):88–97, 1979.

Jajic I: Epidemiology of hypertrophic osteoarthropathy [review]. *Clin Exp Rheumatol* 10(Suppl 7):13, 1992.

Johnson S, Knox AJ: Arthropathy in cystic fibrosis [review]. *Respir Med* 88(8):567–570, 1994.

Martinez-Lavin M: Pathogenesis of hypertrophic osteoarthropathy. *Clin Exp Rheumatol* 10(Suppl 7):49–50, 1992.

Martinez-Lavin M, Matucci-Cerinic M, Jajic I, et al: Hypertrophic osteoarthropathy: consensus on its definition, classification, assessment and diagnostic criteria. *J Rheumatol* 20(8):1386–1387, 1993.

Martinez-Lavin M: Hypertrophic osteoarthropathy. *Curr Opin Rheumatol* 9(1):83–86, 1997.

Matucci-Cerinic M, Lotti T, Calvieri S, et al: The spectrum of dermatological symptoms of pachydermoperiostosis (primary hypertrophic osteoarthropathy): a genetic, cytogenetic and ultrastructural study. *Clin Exp Rheumatol* 10(Suppl 7):45–48, 1992.

Oppenheimer DA, Jones HH: Hypertrophic osteoarthropathy of chronic inflammatory bowel disease. *Skeletal Radiol* 9(2):109–113, 1982.

Pineda C: Diagnostic imaging in hypertrophic osteoarthropathy. *Clin Exp Rheumatol* 10(Suppl 7):27–33, 1992.

Pineda CJ, Martinez-Lavin M, Goobar JE, et al: Periostitis in hypertrophic osteoarthropathy: relationship to disease duration. *Am J Rheumatol* 148:773–778, 1987.

Schumacher HR Jr: Hypertrophic osteoarthropathy: rheumatologic manifestations. *Clin Exp Rheumatol* 10(Suppl 7):35–40, 1992.

Simpson EL, Dalinka MK: Association of hypertrophic osteoarthropathy with gastrointestinal polyposis. *Am J Roentgenol* 144:983–984, 1985.

Spencer RP: Hepatic hypertrophic osteodystrophy detected on bone imaging. *Clin Nucl Med* 13:611–612, 1988.

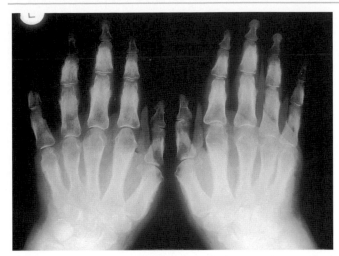

Figure 9–1 This radiograph shows the hands of a 62-year-old man with pulmonary hypertrophic osteoarthropathy. Clubbing of the fingers results in part from thickening of the subungual soft tissues. Other changes that may be seen involving the small bones include periosteal new bone formation.

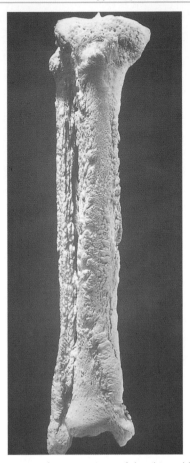

Figure 9–3 This macerated gross specimen of the tibia and fibula from a 58-year-old woman with pulmonary osteoarthropathy illustrates the dramatic thickening and irregularity of the cortical new bone characteristic of the condition.

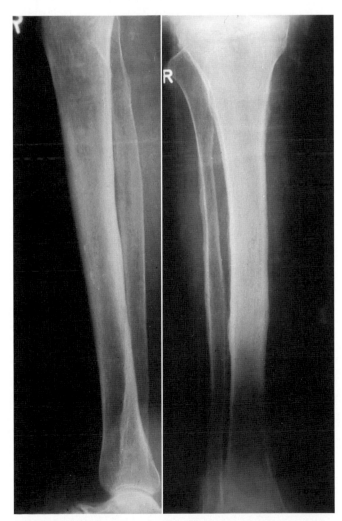

Figure 9–2 Thick periosteal new bone is often seen in the region of painful, swollen joints in pulmonary hypertrophic osteoarthropathy. These features are similar to those in patients with rheumatoid arthritis. This radiograph illustrates periosteal new bone formation in a 77-year-old woman with pulmonary hypertrophic osteoarthropathy.

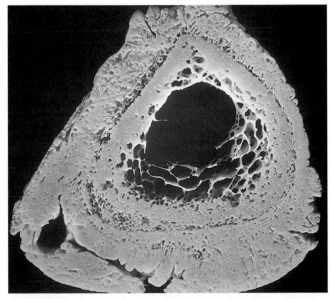

Figure 9–4 This cross-section of macerated tibia is from the specimen illustrated in Figure 9–3. It shows that the new bone is entirely on the periosteal surface, whereas the endosteal surface and medullary bone are relatively preserved.

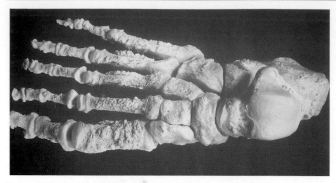

Figure 9–5 This macerated gross specimen illustrates changes in the small bones of the foot. Marked periosteal new bone formation and resultant distortion of the affected bones are evident.

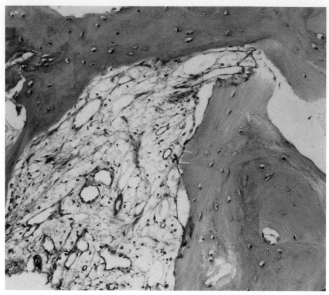

Figure 9–6 This histologic section is from the mature periosteal new bone seen in pulmonary hypertrophic osteoarthropathy. No characteristics of this new bone distinguish it from other conditions that result in periosteal new bone deposition. On occasion, a mononuclear cell infiltrate may also be present, suggesting that the new bone formed is related to inflammation in the adjacent joint.

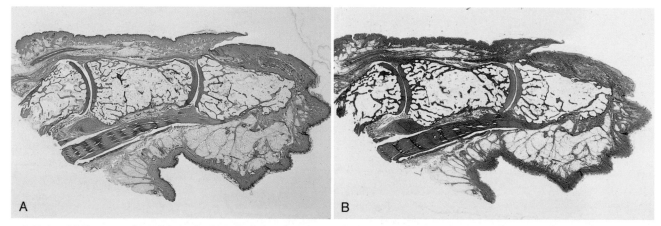

A   B

Figure 9–7 *A* and *B*: These two photomicrographs show the finger of a patient with idiopathic pulmonary fibrosis. Clubbing of the fingers related to soft tissue swelling is evident. The joints are unaffected.

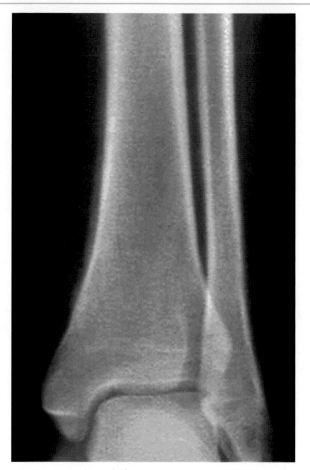

Figure 9–8 Anteroposterior (AP) roentgenogram of the distal tibia and ankle in a patient with pulmonary hypertrophic osteoarthropathy. Note the benign-appearing, laminated periosteal new bone formation of the distal tibial metaphysis. In most instances, bilateral changes are apparent.

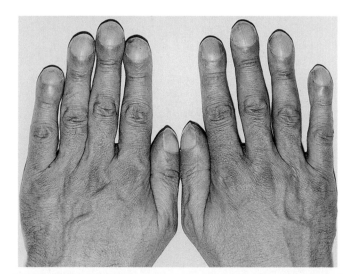

Figure 9–9 This photograph illustrates the clinical appearance of clubbing of the fingers associated with pulmonary hypertrophic osteoarthropathy in a patient with carcinoma of the lung.

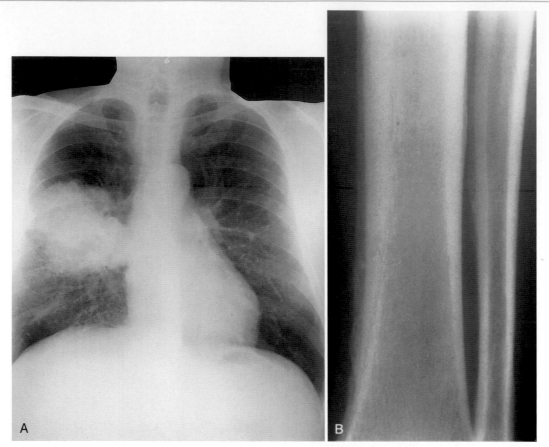

Figure 9–10 The chest radiograph (*A*) reveals a large carcinoma of the lung. The patient had leg pain and radiographic evidence of pulmonary hypertrophic osteoarthropathy involving the tibia and fibula (*B*).

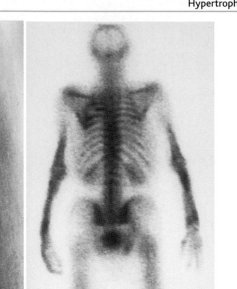

Figure 9–11 *A*: The diaphyseal periosteal new bone formation associated with pulmonary hypertrophic osteoarthropathy is illustrated in this radiograph. *B*: Such regions of periosteal new bone formation are hot on bone scan.

Melorheostosis

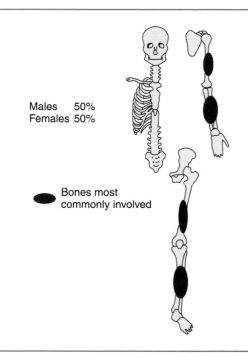

Males 50%
Females 50%

Bones most
commonly involved

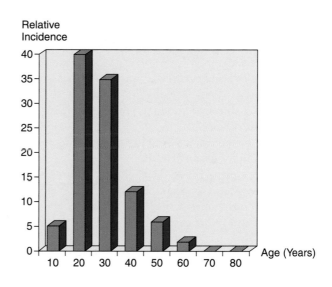

Clinical Signs

1. The long bones may exhibit deformity. (The lower limb is more commonly affected than the upper limb.)
2. Joint motion may be limited owing to contracture and fibrosis of the soft tissue in the region of the affected bone or bones.
3. The affected extremity may appear larger in circumference than normal.
4. The affected bone is usually shorter than normal.
5. The skin over the affected bone may be tense or erythematous.
6. Laboratory tests are usually within normal limits.

7. Fibromas, fibrolipomas, and capillary hemangiomas may be seen.

Clinical Symptoms

1. Angular joint deviation may be present.
2. Limb-length discrepancy may be exhibited.
3. Dull joint pain may be experienced. (Pain may be described as constant and low grade.)
4. Joint contractures may occur.
5. Paraarticular ossifications may be seen.
6. Muscle atrophy and patellar dislocation may occur.

7. Patients are often asymptomatic and the finding is often incidental on radiographs.

Major Radiographic Features

1. Cortical hyperostosis may be seen in a linear or segmental distribution, with sharp demarcation from the unaffected bone.
2. The characteristic appearance is that of melted wax dripping down the side of a candle.
3. The process may be monostotic or polyostotic or, rarely, may involve multiple limbs and the trunk.
4. The process may involve the shoulder or hip as well as the adjacent long bone.
5. When multiple bones are involved, the linear hyperostosis extends from one bone to the next in a nearly continuous manner.
6. If the process involves the lower portion of the leg or the forearm, then usually only one of the two bones is involved in keeping with the sclerotomal distribution of this disease.
7. Periarticular soft tissue may also show ossification. (When present, it is usually in association with extensive bony disease.)
8. Dense islands of bone can occur in the epiphysis of the affected bone.
9. Bone scan may show increased uptake in the involved bones and soft tissue.
10. Sites of involvement include the lower limb, upper limb, skull, spine, ribs, and pelvis.
11. In children, the primary radiographic feature is endosteal hyperostosis, as compared with the well-developed features noted previously.
12. Extraosseous soft tissue masses and ossification may be present.

Radiographic Differential Diagnosis

1. Myositis ossificans (heterotopic ossification).
2. Periosteal hematoma.

Major Pathologic Features

1. Hyperostotic bone is densely sclerotic.
2. Thickened lamellar bone may obliterate the haversian system.

3. New bone and cartilage may be present in the cartilage surrounding the affected joints.
4. Osteoclastic activity is not a prominent feature.
5. The marrow space may show some fibrous tissue proliferation.
6. Grossly, the cortex of the affected bone is thickened, with narrowing of the medullary canal.
7. Islands of dense bone may be present in the epiphyses of long bones and in the small bones of the hands and feet.

Pathologic Differential Diagnosis

1. Periostitis ossificans.
2. Myositis ossificans.
3. Periosteal hematoma.

Treatment

Medical

1. Pain can be controlled with analgesics.
2. Bracing can be used to prevent progressive joint contractures.

Surgical

1. Release of contractures can be accomplished.
2. Leg-length inequality can be corrected.
3. Ilizarov gradual distraction may be more effective than traditional osteotomies because of neurovascular stretch injury.

References

Campbell CJ, Papademetriou T, Bonfiglio M: Melorheostosis. A report of clinical, roentgenographic, and pathological findings in 14 cases. *J Bone Joint Surg Am* 50(7):1281–1304, 1968.

Dimar JR, Campion TS: Melorheostosis: two case presentations and review of the literature. *Orthop Rev* 16(9):615–621, 1987.

Murray RO, McCredie J: Melorheostosis and the sclerotomes. A radiological correlation. *Skeletal Radiol* 4(2):57–71, 1979.

Wynne-Davies R, Gormley J: The prevalence of skeletal dysplasias: an estimate of their minimum frequency and the number of patients requiring orthopaedic care. *J Bone Joint Surg* Br 67B:133–137, 1985.

Yu JS, Resnick D, Vaughan LM, et al: Melorheostosis with an ossified soft tissue mass: MR features. *Skeletal Radiol* 24(5):367–370, 1995.

Osteopetrosis

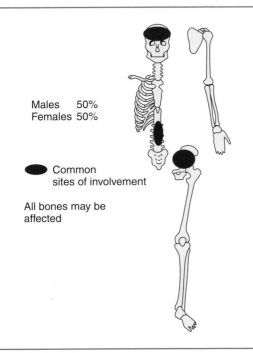

Males 50%
Females 50%

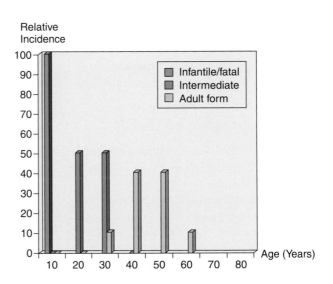 Common
sites of involvement

All bones may be
affected

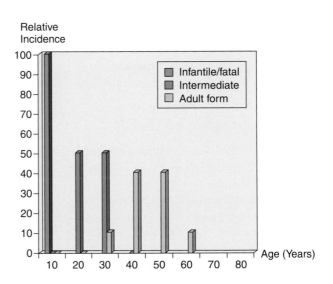

Synonyms: Osteopetrosis is also called marble bone disease, congenital osteosclerosis, and Albers-Schönberg disease.

Clinical Signs

1. Clinical signs depend on the type of disease (mode of inheritance). Autosomal recessive disease may result in intrauterine or early childhood death.

In the Newborn or Infant

1. Anemia or pancytopenia may be present.
2. Hepatosplenomegaly may be seen.

3. Failure to thrive and infections may occur.
4. Early death may occur.

In Childhood (Autosomal Recessive Inheritance)

1. Physical growth may be retarded.
2. Multiple fractures may occur.
3. Osteomyelitis may complicate up to 10% of cases.
4. Cranial nerve palsies are present in approximately 15% of cases, with particular propensity to involve cranial nerves II, III, and VII.

In Adulthood (Autosomal Dominant)

1. Approximately 45% of patients in this group may be asymptomatic.
2. Bone pain is present in approximately 20% of patients in this group.
3. Carpal tunnel syndrome may be seen.
4. Multiple fractures are present in approximately 40% of patients in this group; more than 30 fractures have been seen in a single patient.
5. Osteomyelitis is present in approximately 10% of patients in this group.
6. Cranial nerve palsies are present in approximately 5% of patients in this group.
7. The serum acid phosphatase concentration is elevated in the majority of patients.

Clinical Symptoms

1. Loss of hearing may occur.
2. Loss of vision may occur.
3. Multiple fractures are the major symptom in 40% of adult patients.
4. Bone pain is reported in approximately 25% of adults, particularly in the lumbar region.
5. Recurrent infections may be experienced.
6. Spontaneous bruising and bleeding may be seen.

Major Radiographic Features

1. The entire skeleton shows a diffuse marked increase in density.
2. Bones are shortened.
3. Metaphyses may be wider than normal.
4. Loss of corticomedullary differentiation may be seen.
5. In less severe cases, there are alternating areas of affected and apparently normal bone, resulting in a somewhat "striped" appearance.
6. A "bone within a bone" appearance may be seen (particularly in the tarsals, vertebral bodies, phalanges, and iliac wings).
7. In the adult autosomal dominant form of the disease, a "rugger jersey" spine appearance may be present owing to radiodensity of the superior and inferior portions of the vertebral body.
8. Computed tomography scan is helpful in assessing the diameter of the auditory and optic canals.
9. Magnetic resonance imaging is helpful in assessing the degree of marrow activity in the patient with osteopetrosis. (In the infantile autosomal recessive form of the disease, there is a lack of marrow signal from the vertebral bodies.)
10. Bone scan is helpful in identifying cases complicated by osteomyelitis. (Osteomyelitis in this condition has a propensity to involve the mandible.)

Radiographic Finding	Type I	Type II	Type III
Generalized	+	+	+
Calvarial sclerosis	+	−	+
Skull base sclerosis	−	+	−
"Rugger jersey" spine	−	+	−
Pelvic "endobones"	−	+	+

Modified from Kovacs CS, Lambert RG, Lavoie GJ, et al: Centrifugal osteopetrosis: appendicular sclerosis with relative sparing of the vertebrae. *Skeletal Radiol* 24(1):27–29, 1995.

11. Autosomal dominant osteopetrosis may be classified into at least three subtypes based on radiographic appearance. The following table summarizes the major features of each type.

Radiographic Differential Diagnosis

1. Widespread osteoblastic metastases.
2. Chronic fluorosis.
3. Myelosclerosis.
4. Idiopathic osteosclerosis.
5. Melorheostosis.
6. Mastocytosis.

Major Pathologic Features

Gross

1. The metadiaphyseal bone is widened, resulting in an Erlenmeyer flask–like appearance.
2. Bone has increased mass per unit volume.
3. Bone tends to be smaller than normal.
4. Bone is dense when cut in cross-section.

Histologic

1. Irregular bone surrounding a cartilage core may be seen.
2. Osteoclasts may be reduced in number.
3. Marrow space may be diminished or absent.
4. Epiphyseal microfractures may be present.
5. Prominent cement lines may be seen.

Pathologic Differential Diagnosis

1. Fracture callus (if the biopsy specimen is from the region of a healing fracture).
2. Other sclerosing bone dysplasias.

Treatment

Medical

1. Bone marrow transplantation may be performed.
2. Back pain is treated conservatively (rest, bracing, nonsteroidal anti-inflammatory drugs [NSAIDs]).

Surgical

1. Fractures are treated conventionally. (Healing may be delayed.)
2. Osteotomy is for long bone deformity and coxa vara.

References

Andersen PE Jr, Bollerslev J: Heterogeneity of autosomal dominant osteopetrosis. *Radiology* 164(1):223–225, 1987.

Bollerslev J, Mosekilde L: Autosomal dominant osteopetrosis. *Clin Orthop Relat Res* 294:45–51, 1993.

Coccia P, Krivit W, Cervenka J, et al: Successful bone-marrow transplantation for infantile malignant osteopetrosis. *N Engl J Med* 302(13):701–708, 1980.

El-Tawil T, Stoker DJ: Benign osteopetrosis: a review of 42 cases showing two different patterns. *Skeletal Radiol* 22(8):587–593, 1993.

Greenspan A: Sclerosing bone dysplasias—a target-site approach. *Skeletal Radiol* 20(8):561–583, 1991.

Helfrich MH, Aronson DC, Everts V, et al: Morphologic features of bone in human osteopetrosis. *Bone* 12(6):411–419, 1991.

Kolawole TM, Hawass ND, Patel PJ, et al: Osteopetrosis: some unusual radiological features with a short review. *Eur J Radiol* 8(2):89–95, 1988.

Kovacs CS, Lambert RGW, Lavoie GJ, et al: Centrifugal osteopetrosis: appendicular sclerosis with relative sparing of the vertebrae. *Skeletal Radiol* 24(1):27–29, 1995.

Milgram JW, Jasty M: Osteopetrosis: a morphologic study of twenty-one cases. *J Bone Joint Surg Am* 64(6):912–929, 1982.

Shapiro F: Osteopetrosis. Current clinical considerations [review]. *Clin Orthop Rel Res* 294:34–44, 1993.

Silvestrini G, Ferraccioli GF, Quaini F, et al: Adult osteopetrosis: study of two brothers. *Appl Pathol* 5(3):184–189, 1987.

Singer FR, Chang SS: Osteopetrosis [review]. *Semin Nephrol* 12(2):191–199, 1992.

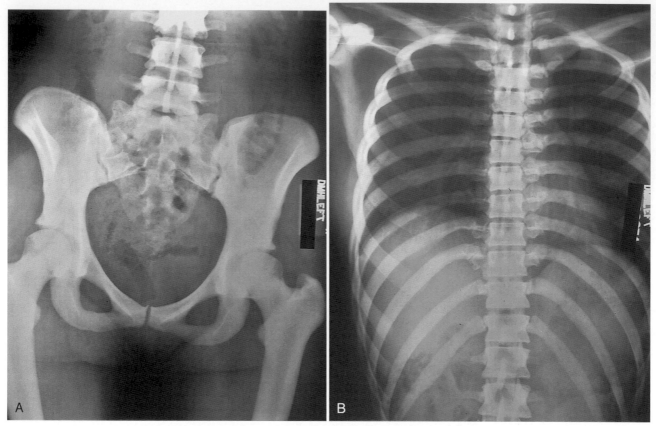

Figure 11–1 *A*: Anteroposterior (AP) roentgenogram of the pelvis and proximal femora in a patient with osteopetrosis. *B*: AP roentgenogram of the chest and thoracic spine. Note the focal cortical thickening of the glenoid and right shoulder.

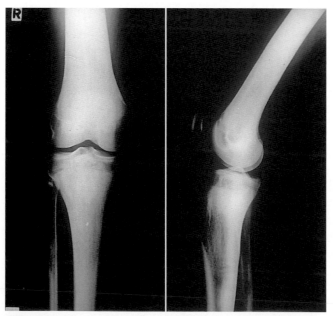

Figure 11–2 This radiograph illustrates the case of a 26-year-old man with osteopetrosis. The distal femur and proximal tibia are densely sclerotic, and some lack of metaphyseal remodeling is evident in the distal femur. Normal corticomedullary differentiation is not seen.

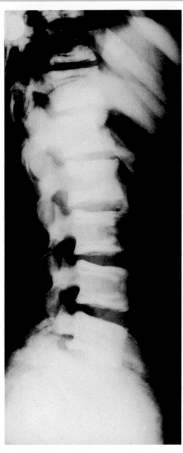

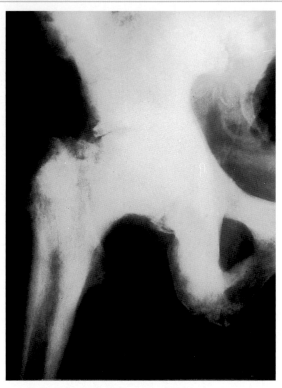

Figure 11–4 This radiograph of the proximal femur shows osteopetrosis in a 65-year-old man. Patients with less severe forms of this disease most commonly present with axial bony lesions or fractures through the mechanically inferior dense bone.

Figure 11–3 Osteopetrotic bone changes are evident in the vertebrae of this 21-year-old man. Increased density of the proximal and distal thirds of the vertebrae results in a striped pattern.

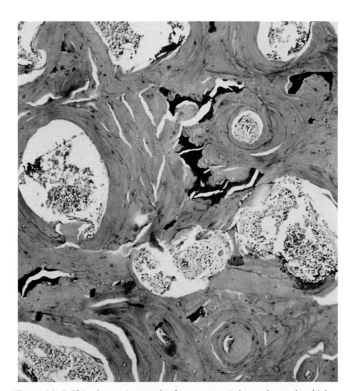

Figure 11–5 This photomicrograph of osteopetrotic bone shows the thickened and disorganized arrangement of the medullary bone. Frequently, within the bony trabeculae there are islands of calcified cartilage.

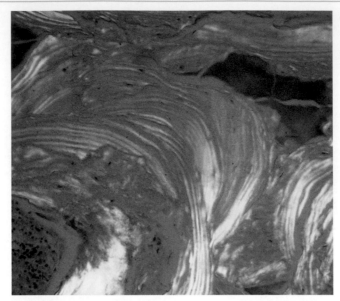

Figure 11–6 As shown in this photomicrograph, osteopetrotic bone, whether formed by endochondral ossification or from membranous bone, is abnormal. In the latter, primitive bone persists and cartilage cores are not seen.

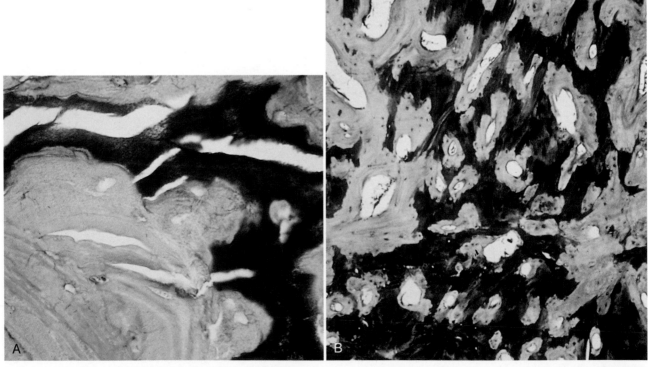

Figure 11–7 *A* and *B*: These two photomicrographs illustrate the histologic features of osteopetrotic bone formed by endochondral ossification. The heavily mineralized cartilage cores are evident in the deep purple–stained regions.

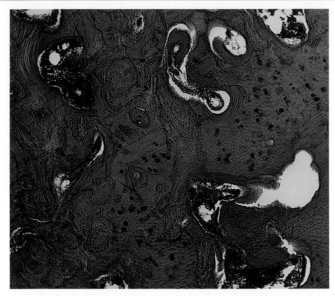

Figure 11–8 This photomicrograph illustrates densely ossified osteopetrotic bone with fewer cartilaginous islands. The histologic pattern of the disease is variable.

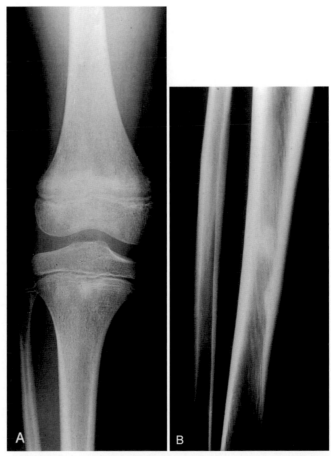

Figure 11–9 *A* and *B*: Densely sclerotic foci may also be radiographically identified in patients with lead poisoning, as shown in these radiographs of the tibia in an 8-year-old male patient.

Osteogenesis Imperfecta

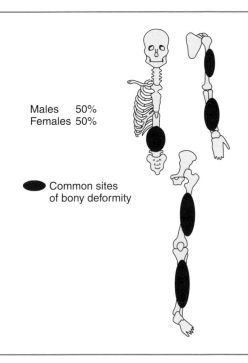

Males 50%
Females 50%

Common sites of bony deformity

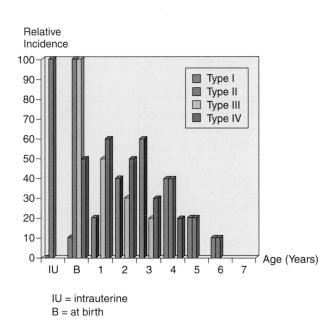

IU = intrauterine
B = at birth

Classification

1. Type I has an autosomal dominant inheritance (approximately 40% of cases). *Synonyms*: Dominantly inherited osteogenesis imperfecta with distinctly blue sclerae, van der Hoeve's syndrome, Eddowes' syndrome.
2. Type II has an autosomal recessive inheritance (approximately 25% of cases). *Synonyms*: lethal perinatal osteogenesis imperfecta, lethal osteogenesis imperfecta congenita, osteogenesis imperfecta letalis type Vrolik.
3. Type III has an autosomal recessive inheritance (approximately 3% of cases). *Synonyms*: progressively deforming osteogenesis imperfecta with normal sclerae, osteogenesis imperfecta congenita, osteogenesis imperfecta congenita type Vrolik, osteopsathyrosis idiopathica of Lobstein.
4. Type IV has an autosomal dominant inheritance (approximately 32% of cases). *Synonyms*: dominantly inherited osteogenesis imperfecta with normal sclera, osteopsathyrosis idiopathica of Lobstein, Ekman-Lobstein disease.
5. Type V has marked hypertrophic callus formation, calcification of the interosseous membrane of the forearm and white sclera.
6. Type VI has recently been identified.

Clinical Signs: General

1. There is an increased propensity to fracture. (Fractures may be present at birth.)
2. Immobilization of the fracture results in diffuse osteoporosis.
3. Blue sclerae are present in some patients.
4. Poorly formed dentition or early loss of multiple teeth may be seen in some patients.
5. Ligamentous laxity may occur.
6. Short stature may be present.
7. Scoliosis may be present.

Clinical Signs: Type Specific

Type I

1. Distinctly blue sclerae are present throughout life.
2. Presenile conductive hearing loss occurs in 20% of patients by 20 years of age and nearly 100% by 60 years of age.
3. Kyphoscoliosis occurs in approximately 20% of adults.
4. Joint hyperlaxity is found in approximately 50% of patients.
5. Premature arcus senilis may occur.
6. Dentinogenesis imperfecta may be present. (It occurs in approximately 40% of patients.)
7. Approximately 10% of patients have fractures at birth, but fractures may not commence until infancy or childhood.
8. The majority of patients are two to three standard deviations below the population mean for height.
9. The frequency of fractures decreases at adolescence and increases again in postmenopausal women.
10. Easy bruising may occur in approximately 80% of patients.

Type II

1. Intrauterine death occurs in approximately 50% of cases, and death in early infancy occurs in approximately 50%.
2. The tissues exhibit extreme fragility. (Limbs or head may be macerated during delivery.)
3. The facial and skull bones show extremely poor mineralization.
4. Micrognathia and a small, narrow nose may be present.
5. Girls outnumber boys by approximately 1.4:1.0.

Type III

1. Marked bone fragility leads to progressive deformity of the long bones, skull, and spine.
2. Approximately 50% of patients have fractures at birth, and all have fractures by 2 years of age.
3. Sclerae may be blue at birth but become progressively less so as the patient ages.

4. Growth failure is marked and mortality is high owing to complications of kyphoscoliosis.
5. The skull may be hypoplastic but is not as poorly ossified as in type II.

Type IV

1. Sclerae are normal at birth or become so by adulthood.
2. Approximately 25% of patients have fractures at birth or in the neonatal period.
3. The frequency of fracture peaks in childhood and markedly decreases at adolescence.
4. The opalescent dentin of dentinogenesis imperfecta is often present (approximately 70% of patients).
5. Short stature is common owing to progressive kyphoscoliosis.
6. Approximately 30% of patients older than 30 years of age have hearing impairment.
7. Easy bruising is present in approximately 40% of patients.

Type V

1. Clinically similar to Type IV.
2. A radiographically dense band is seen adjacent to the growth plate of long bones.
3. Hypertrophic calluses are present at the sites of fractures or surgical procedures.
4. Calcification of the interosseous membrane of the forearm may lead to restricted forearm motion.
5. Patients have white sclera and normal teeth.

Type VI

1. Teeth are not affected.
2. Show features similar to other types of osteogenesis imperfecta and the rare cases are best diagnosed by the distinctive histologic appearance of the bone ("fish scale") appearance.

Note: Babies with osteogenesis imperfecta frequently are delivered by cesarean section owing to a breech presentation.

Clinical Symptoms

1. Fractures occur frequently.
2. Hyperplastic callus formation may occur.

Major Radiographic Features

1. Osteopenia may be seen.
2. Fractures may be present. (Occasionally, exuberant callus formation may be confused with osteosarcoma.)
3. Bone deformities, primarily bowing, may be seen.
4. The long bones are small and slender compared with normal bones.

5. Vertebrae may show scoliosis, secondary compression fractures, and wedging of vertebral bodies. Expansion of the intervertebral discs causes so-called codfish vertebrae, characterized by their biconcave shape.

6. The skull exhibits multiple centers of ossification (so-called wormian bone).

7. Scalloped radiolucent areas with sclerotic margins at the epiphyseal end of the bone may be evident; such areas are more common in the lower extremities.

Radiographic Differential Diagnosis

1. Battered-child syndrome.
2. Multiple fractures.
3. Steroid-induced osteoporosis.
4. Osteosarcoma in cases with hyperplastic callus formation.

Major Pathologic Features

Gross

1. Eggshell-like thinning of the cortical bone may be seen.
2. Little medullary spongy bone is present.
3. Recent or healed fractures may be seen.
4. The long bones may show angulation and bowing.
5. Epiphyseal changes include the following:
   a. Cartilaginous nodules within secondary centers of ossification.
   b. One or more "indentations" into the metaphysis or complete disruption of the growth plate (corresponding to radiographic epiphyseal lucencies).

Microscopic

1. The growth plate shows disorganization.
2. The mineralized zone of the growth plate cartilage exhibits decreased thickness.
3. Fragments of growth plate may be seen.
4. Persistence of calcified cartilage into the diaphysis may be present.
5. Metaphyseal microfractures may be evident.
6. Abnormal bony callus formation may be seen.

Treatment

Medical

1. Recent studies have shown some benefits of treatment with bisphosphonates, though longer term follow-up is needed.
2. Gene therapy is promising.
3. Supportive care includes exercises, ambulation with bracing, and wheelchair use as necessary.

Surgical

1. Fractures are treated with closed reduction.
2. Intramedullary rod fixation (standard versus elongating rods) is used for recurrent fractures or deformities.
3. Scoliosis is managed with segmental instrumentation and fusion.

References

Byers PH, Wallis GA, Willing MC: Osteogenesis imperfecta: translation of mutation to phenotype [review]. *Am J Med Genet* 28(7):433–442, 1991.

Cassella JP, Barber P, Catterall AC, et al: A morphometric analysis of osteoid collagen fibril diameter in osteogenesis imperfecta. *Bone* 15(3):329–334, 1994.

Cole WG: Advances in osteogenesis imperfecta. *Clin Orthop Relat Res* 401:6–16, 2002.

Deak SB, Scholz PM, Amenta PS, et al: The substitution of arginine for glycine 85 of the alpha 1(I) procollagen chain results in mild osteogenesis imperfecta. The mutation provides direct evidence for three discrete domains of cooperative melting of intact type I collagen. *J Biol Chem* 266(32):21827–21832, 1991.

Glorieux FH. Experience with bisphosphonates in osteogenesis imperfecta. *Pediatrics* 2007 Mar; 119 Suppl 2:S163-5.

Glorieux FH, Rauch F, Plotkin H, Ward L, et al: Type V osteogenesis imperfecta: a new form of brittle bone disease. *J Bone Min Res* 15(9):1650–1658, 2000.

Löwing K, Aström E, Oscarsson KA, Söderhäll S, Eliasson AC. Effect of intravenous pamidronate therapy on everyday activities in children with osteogenesis imperfecta. *Acta Paediatr.* 2007 Aug; 96(8):1180-3. Epub 2007 Jun 18.

Marion MJ, Gannon FH, Fallon MD, et al: Skeletal dysplasia in perinatal lethal osteogenesis imperfecta. A complex disorder of endochondral and intramembranous ossification. *Clin Orthop Rel Res* 293:327–337, 1993.

Nerlich AG, Brenner RE, Wiest I, et al: Immunohistochemical localization of interstitial collagens in bone tissue from patients with various forms of osteogenesis imperfecta. *Am J Med Genet* 45(2):258–259, 1993.

Sillence D, Butler B, Latham M, et al: Natural history of blue sclerae in osteogenesis imperfecta. *Am J Med Genet* 45(2):183–186, 1993.

Steinmann B, Westerhausen A, Constantinou CD, et al: Substitution of cysteine for glycine-alpha 1-691 in the pro alpha 1(I) chain of type I procollagen in a proband with lethal osteogenesis imperfecta destabilizes the triple helix at a site C-terminal to the substitution. *Biochem J* 279(Pt 3):747–752, 1991.

Stoss H, Pontz B, Vetter U, et al: Osteogenesis imperfecta and hyperplastic callus formation: light- and electron-microscopic findings. *Am J Med Genet* 45(2):260, 1993.

Sztrolovics R, Glorieux FH, Travers R, et al: Osteogenesis imperfecta: comparison of molecular defects with bone histological changes. *Bone* 15(3):321–328, 1994.

Sztrolovics R, Glorieux FH, van der Rest M, et al: Identification of type I collagen gene (COL1A2) mutations in nonlethal osteogenesis imperfecta. *Hum Mol Genet* 2(8):1319–1321, 1993.

Vetter U, Pontz B, Zauner E, et al: Osteogenesis imperfecta: a clinical study of the first ten years of life. *Calcif Tissue Int* 50(1):36–41, 1992.

Zeitlin L, Fassier F, Glorieux FH: Modern approach to children with osteogenesis imperfecta. *J Ped Orthop B* 12(2):77–87, 2003.

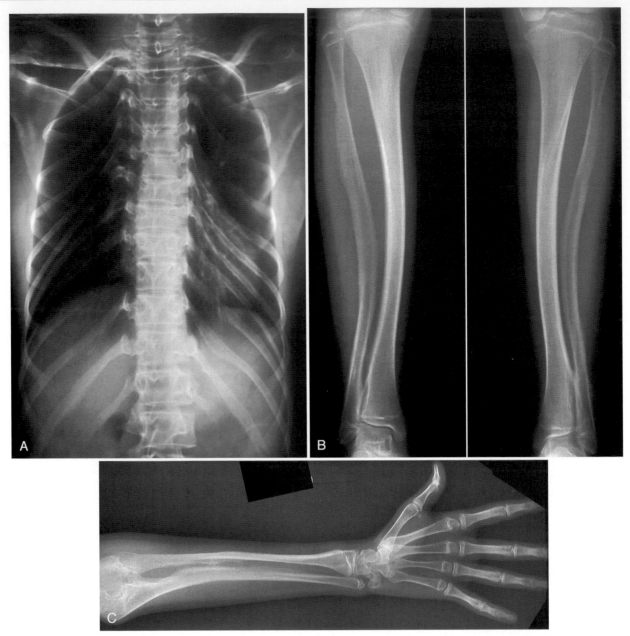

Figure 12–1 *A*: Anteroposterior (AP) roentgenogram of the thoracic spine in a patient with osteogenesis imperfecta. Note the diffuse demineralization of the bones. *B*: AP roentgenogram of both tibiae, showing similar findings. C: AP roentgenogram of the forearm and hand. The bones are overconstricted, with a thin, gracile appearance and bowing deformity.

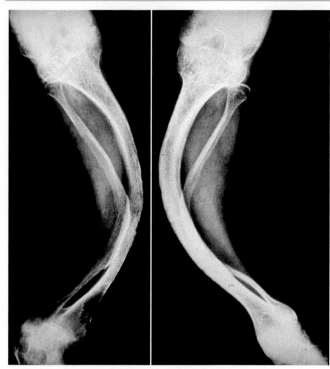

Figure 12–2 Marked deformity of the tibia and fibula is evident in this patient with osteogenesis imperfecta tarda. Such patients are less severely affected than patients who show evidence of the disease at birth, osteogenesis imperfecta congenita. Generalized osteoporosis, multiple fractures, and micromelia may be present at birth in such cases.

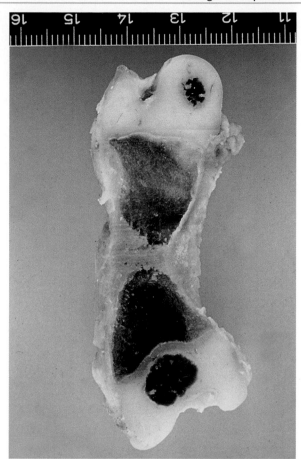

Figure 12–4 This gross pathologic specimen is from a patient who suffered from osteogenesis imperfecta. Fractures treated by immobilization lead to osteoporotic changes that predispose to additional fractures in these patients. This cycle results in marked bony deformity.

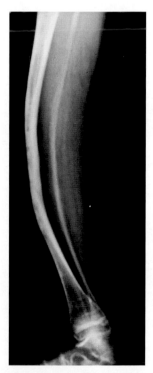

Figure 12–3 This radiograph illustrates the anterior bowing of the tibia seen in a patient with osteogenesis imperfecta tarda. Such bony deformity is more common in the tarda I subgroup of patients, who have deformities usually confined to the lower extremities.

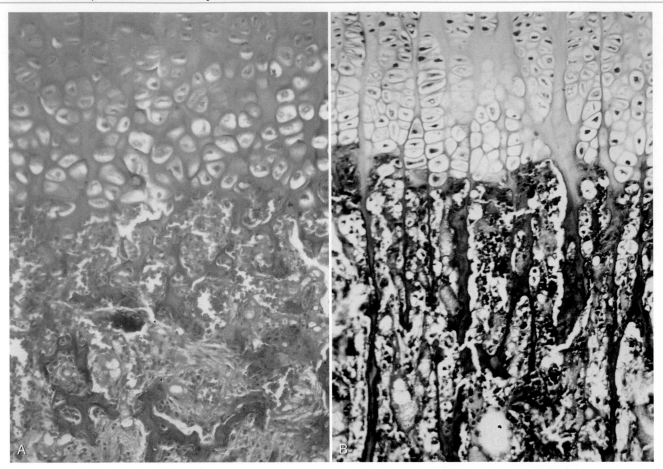

Figure 12–5 *A* and *B*: These two photomicrographs illustrate the histologic features of osteogenesis imperfecta in the region of endochondral ossification. The growth plates are variable in appearance. There is relative preservation of the columns of chondrocytes. Extension of the cartilage into the metaphyseal portion of the bone may be seen. Fragmentation of the growth plate may occur, possibly related to trauma. Islands of cartilage may be seen in the epiphysis and metaphysis when the growth plate has been disrupted.

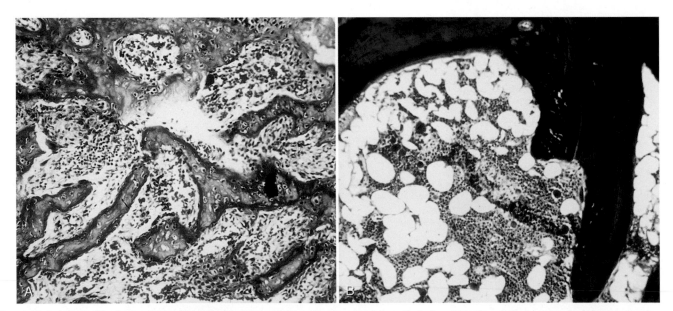

Figure 12–6 *A–C*: The histologic pattern of medullary bone in patients with osteogenesis imperfecta is variable. Bony trabeculae may be fine, as in *C*, or more normal in thickness, as in *A*. Osteoblasts may be increased in number, as may osteoclasts. The histologic appearance may be altered by the healing reaction related to pathologic fractures.

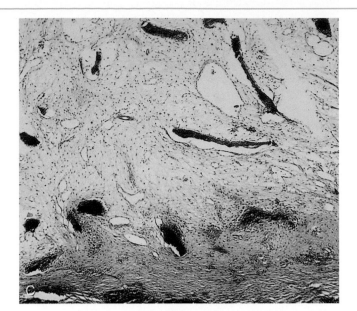

Figure 12–6 cont'd.

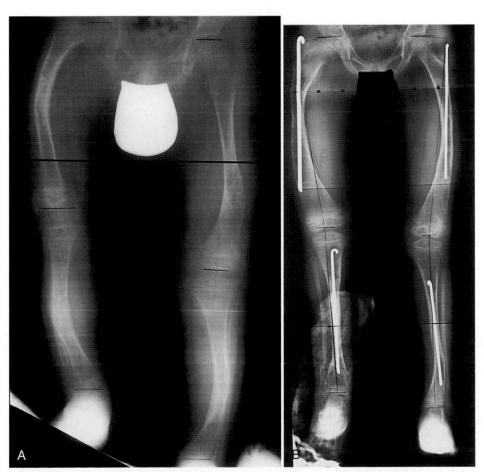

Figure 12–7 Surgical correction of the bony deformities related to multiple fractures in patients with osteogenesis imperfecta can be challenging. One approach is illustrated in *A* and *B*.

Fluorosis

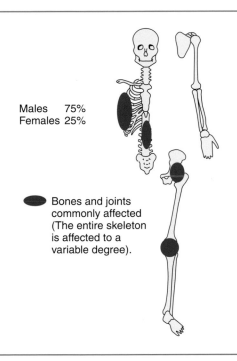

Males   75%
Females 25%

Bones and joints commonly affected (The entire skeleton is affected to a variable degree).

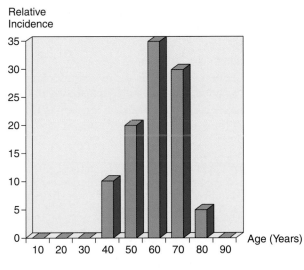

Relative Incidence

Age (Years)

Note: Radiographic evidence of dental changes may be documented in childhood.

Clinical Signs

1. Signs depend on duration and level of exposure to fluoride.
2. Longstanding exposure results in mottling of teeth and anemia.
3. Painful limbs may be present.
4. Joint deformities (knock-knee, limitation of motion) may occur.
5. Kyphosis may be seen.
6. Flexion deformity at the hips may occur.
7. Neurologic symptoms related to compression of the spinal cord and nerve roots may be present.

Clinical Symptoms

1. The spinal column may be stiff.
2. Symptoms related to cord compression or compression of nerve roots may be present.
3. Low back pain occurs in 70% of patients.
4. Leg or arm pain occurs in 70% of patients.
5. Loss of appetite occurs in 20% of patients.
6. Joint dysfunction occurs in 50% of patients.
7. Joint deformity occurs in 30% of patients.

Major Radiographic Features

1. Features are variable; osteosclerosis most commonly is present (in approximately 45% of patients), but osteopenia may also be seen (with approximately 20% showing an osteoporotic pattern and 20% showing an osteomalacic pattern).
2. Fluorosis preferentially involves the axial skeleton.
3. Bony osteophytes, particularly vertebral, may be seen.
4. Periosteal new bone formation may be present.
5. Calcifications may be seen in the soft tissues (interosseous membranes, muscle, ligaments, and tendon attachments) with longstanding exposure. Of patients in endemic areas, 90% show ligamentous calcification.
6. The skull is thickened and dense in adults (particularly prominent at skull base).
7. Generalized skeletal sclerosis (particularly prominent in the vertebrae) may be exhibited.
8. Coarse bony trabeculae may be seen.
9. Calcification of the costal cartilages may be present.
10. Calcification of the falx cerebri may be evident.
11. "Growth lines" (linear shadows of mineralization) are present in approximately 70% of patients with fluorosis in endemic areas.
12. Diaphyseal widening may be seen.
13. Bone scan in patients with fluorosis reveals increased uptake in the axial and appendicular skeleton, reduced soft tissue uptake, and poor or absent renal imaging. Costochondral junctions are often prominent.

Radiographic Differential Diagnosis

1. Metastatic carcinoma with osteoblastic metastases.
2. Myelosclerosis.
3. Paget's disease.
4. Osteosclerotic myeloma.
5. X-linked hypophosphatemic osteomalacia.
6. Mastocytosis.

Major Pathologic Features

Gross

1. The bones are heavy.
2. The bones have an irregular and dull surface.
3. Sites of muscular attachment are abnormally prominent.
4. Calcification of ligaments may be identified (particularly ligamentum flavum).
5. The vertebrae are enlarged and show bony osteophytes.
6. The vertebrae may be fused after longstanding exposure.
7. Skull bones lack a normal diploic pattern, and the sella turcica may be fused.

8. The ribs are large and the cortical surface is rough in the regions of muscular attachment.
9. Ossification may be present in the interosseous membranes.

Microscopic

1. Increased osteocytes, irregularly arranged, may be seen.
2. Prominent cement lines are present in irregularly deposited osteoid.
3. The cortical haversian system shows increased diameter.
4. Osteoid extends into skeletal muscle.

Pathologic Differential Diagnosis

1. Paget's disease.
2. Osteopetrosis.

Treatment

1. The source of exposure to fluoride must be identified and reduced.
2. After cessation of overexposure and treatment of fluorosis, hypercalciuria and nephrolithiasis can be expected. This risk can be minimized with prophylactic hydration and diuretics.
3. Musculoskeletal pain must be relieved.
4. Deformities must be corrected.

References

Augenstein WL, Spoerke DG, Kulig KW, et al: Fluoride ingestion in children: a review of 87 cases. *Pediatrics* 88(5):907–912, 1991.

Christie DP: The spectrum of radiographic bone changes in children with fluorosis. *Radiology* 136:85–90, 1980.

Gilbaugh JH Jr, Thompson GJ: Fluoride osteosclerosis simulating carcinoma of the prostate with widespread bony metastasis: a case report. *J Urol* 96:944–946, 1966.

Gupta SK, Gambhir S, Mithal A, et al: Skeletal scintigraphic findings in endemic skeletal fluorosis. *Nucl Med Commun* 14(5):384–390, 1993.

Kurland ES, Schulman RC, Zerwekh JE, Reinus WR, Dempster DW, Whyte MP. Recovery from skeletal fluorosis (an enigmatic, American case). *J Bone Miner Res* 2007 Jan; 22(1):163-70.

Leone NC, Stevenson CA, Hilbish TF, et al: A roentgenologic study of a human population exposed to high-fluoride domestic water; a ten-year study. *Am J Roentgenol Radium Ther Nucl Med* 74(5):874–875, 1955.

Mithal A, Trivedi N, Gupta SK, et al: Radiological spectrum of endemic fluorosis: relationship with calcium intake. *Skeletal Radiol* 22(4): 257–261, 1993.

Reddy DR, Prasad VS, Reddy JJ, et al: Neuro-radiology of skeletal fluorosis. *Ann Acad Med Singapore* 22(3 Suppl):493–500, 1993.

Wang Y, Yin Y, Gilula LA, et al: Endemic fluorosis of the skeleton: radiographic features in 127 patients. *Am J Radiol* 162(1):93–98, 1994.

Whitford GM: Acute and chronic fluoride toxicity [review]. *J Dent Res* 71(5):1249–1254, 1992.

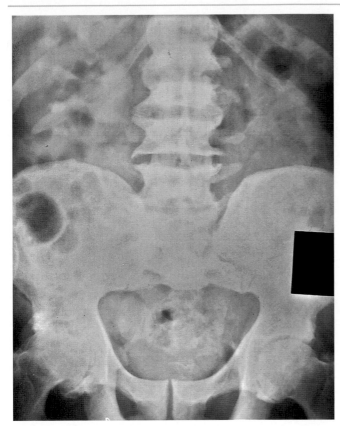

Figure 13–1 Diffuse bony sclerosis is evident in this pelvic radiograph of a 73-year-old man with chronic fluorosis.

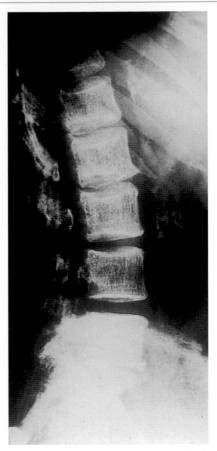

Figure 13–3 This radiograph illustrates bony changes in the lumbar vertebrae in fluorosis. Increased radiodensity of vertebrae may be seen in patients with osteoporosis treated with sodium fluoride. Although the bone mass of such patients increases, clinical trials have not shown that the increased bone mass is associated with a reduced risk of fracture.

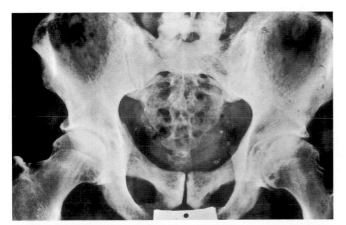

Figure 13–2 Radiographic evidence of bony sclerosis is seen in this case of fluorosis. Coarse thickening of the bony trabeculae more pronounced in the axial skeleton is a common feature in such cases. In longstanding cases, a generalized increase in bone density is evident and periosteal new bone formation may be seen.

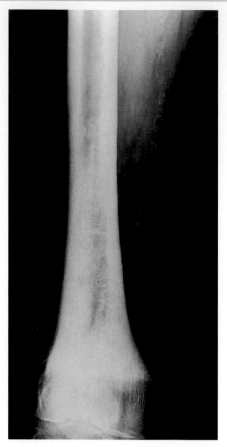

Figure 13–4 Increased bone density is seen in this case of fluorosis involving the femur. The most common radiographic abnormality in patients with endemic fluorosis is calcification or ossification of ligaments, tendons, or soft tissues. Such changes are present in more than 80% of patients with endemic fluorosis. Osteosclerosis and osteopenia are seen with about equal frequency in endemic fluorosis.

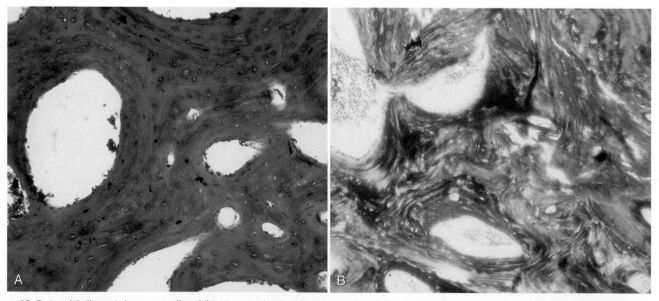

Figure 13–5 *A* and *B*: Fluorotic bone generally exhibits increased trabecular volume. The new bone associated with fluorotic bony trabeculae may show increased osteocytes and altered tinctorial characteristics. Increased osteoblastic and osteoclastic activity may also be present.

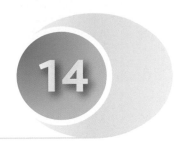

Gaucher's Disease

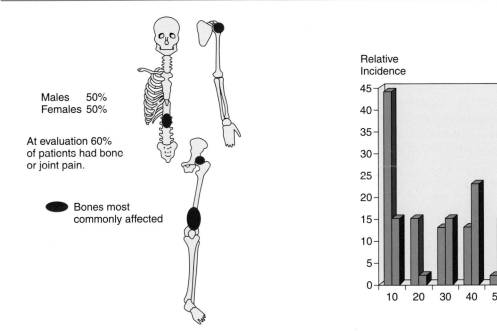

Males   50%
Females 50%

At evaluation 60% of patients had bone or joint pain.

⬤ Bones most commonly affected

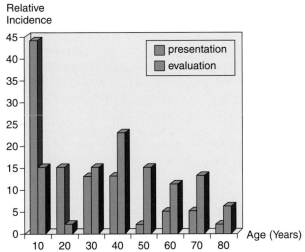

Inheritance Pattern and Types

1. Inheritance is autosomal recessive.
2. Types are as follows:
   a. Type I: most common (lacks central nervous system involvement).
   b. Type II: rare (involves central nervous system).
   c. Type III: rare (involves central nervous system).

Clinical Signs

1. Splenomegaly (secondary to accumulation of glucosyl ceramides) may cause abdominal discomfort. Patients with a positive family history of disease may first manifest disease with splenomegaly.
2. Frequency is high in the Ashkenazi Jewish population.
3. The majority of symptomatic patients present with splenomegaly and thrombocytopenia.
4. In children, short stature may be associated with splenomegaly.
5. Cytopenias include the following:
   a. Thrombocytopenia, the most common, present in approximately 50% of patients.
   b. Anemia, mostly of a mild nature, present in approximately 40% of patients.

6. Liver function tests are abnormal.
7. The serum acid phosphatase concentration is elevated.

Clinical Symptoms

1. Most patients have a chronic form of the disease with a benign course and may present with fatigue.
2. Abdominal pain (related to splenomegaly) may be present.
3. Weight loss may occur.
4. Rarely, young patients present at younger than 3 years of age with an acute neuropathic form of the disease.
5. Bony fractures and cord compression related to the associated bone disease can occur.
6. Bone pain is common and may be severe and episodic in nature.
7. The most common presenting symptom is a manifestation of bleeding such as epistaxis, bruising easily, or prolonged bleeding after a superficial wound.
8. Pulmonary involvement may lead to shortness of breath.

Major Imaging Features

1. Long bones show irregular cortical thinning.
2. The metadiaphyseal region may expand, producing an Erlenmeyer flask–like deformity particularly of the distal femur, proximal tibia, and proximal humerus.
3. Avascular necrosis of the femoral head is present in approximately 20% of patients.
4. Avascular necrosis of the humeral head is present in approximately 10% of patients.
5. Compression fractures of the thoracic or lumbar vertebrae or both are present in approximately 10% of patients.
6. Endosteal scalloping in the humeri and, less commonly, tibiae is present in approximately 10% of patients.
7. Widening of the humeri, particularly proximally, may be seen.
8. Lytic lesions of the long bones or pelvic bones or both may be evident.
9. Joint space narrowing may be seen.
10. Bone scan may show increased uptake in the region of the proximal humeri, distal femora, and proximal tibiae.
11. Positive bone scan is present in approximately 60% of patients with Gaucher's disease overall. (Bone scan is the most sensitive method for assessing bony involvement in Gaucher's disease.)
12. Magnetic resonance imaging can be used to monitor treatment response.

Radiographic Differential Diagnosis

1. Niemann-Pick disease.

Major Pathologic Features

1. The marrow space is replaced by histiocytes that have abundant crumpled- or wrinkled-appearing cytoplasm.
2. Periodic acid–Schiff (PAS) stains show abundant cytoplasmic positivity in the histiocytes.
3. Infarction may be seen as a secondary change.

Pathologic Differential Diagnosis

1. Other storage diseases.
2. Xanthoma.
3. Degenerative change in fibrous dysplasia.

Treatment

Medical

1. Enzyme replacement therapy shows promising results.
2. Supportive care is given during an acute crisis (rest and administration of narcotics).
3. Osteomyelitis (often a result of anaerobic agents) should be recognized and treated.
4. Back pain may be treated nonoperatively.

Surgical

1. Pathological fractures are treated by closed versus open reduction.
2. Arthroplasty is performed for advanced avascular necrosis and arthritis.

References

Beutler E: Modern diagnosis and treatment of Gaucher's disease [review]. *Am J Dis Child* 147(11):1175–1183, 1993.

Carrington PA, Stevens RF, Lendon M: Pseudo-Gaucher cells. *J Clin Pathol* 45(4):360, 1992.

Chan AC, Wu PC, Ormiston IW, et al: Periosteal Gaucher-like cells in beta-thalassemia major. *J Oral Pathol Med* 22(7):331–333, 1993.

Charrow J, Esplin JA, Gribble TJ, et al: Gaucher disease: recommendations on diagnosis, evaluation, and monitoring. *Arch Int Med* 158(16):1754–1760, 1998.

Hainaux B, Christophe C, Hanquinet S, et al: Gaucher's disease. Plain radiography, US, CT and MR diagnosis of lungs, bone and liver lesions. *Pediatr Radiol* 22(1):78–79, 1992.

Hermann G, Shapiro RS, Abdelwahab IF, et al: MR imaging in adults with Gaucher's disease type I: evaluation of marrow involvement and disease activity. *Skeletal Radiol* 22(4):247–251, 1993.

Hermann G, Shapiro R, Abdelwahab IF, et al: Extraosseous extension of Gaucher's cell deposits mimicking malignancy. *Skeletal Radiol* 23(4):253–256, 1994.

Hill SC, Damaska BM, Ling A, et al: Gaucher's disease: abdominal MR imaging findings in 46 patients. *Radiology* 184(2):561–566, 1992.

Horev G, Kornreich L, Hadar H, et al: Hemorrhage associated with "bone crisis" in Gaucher's disease identified by magnetic resonance imaging. *Skeletal Radiol* 20(7):479–482, 1991.

Horowitz M, Zimran A: Mutations causing Gaucher's disease [review]. *Hum Mutat* 3(1):1–11, 1994.

Mankin HJ, Rosenthal DI, Xavier R: Gaucher disease. New approaches to an ancient disease. *J Bone Joint Surg Am* 83-A(5):748–762, 2001.

Mistry PK, Smith SJ, Ali M, et al: Genetic diagnosis of Gaucher's disease. *Lancet* 339(8798):889–892, 1992.

Rosenthal DI, Barton NW, McKusick KA, et al: Quantitative imaging of Gaucher's disease. *Radiology* 185(3):841–845, 1992.

Schindelmeiser J, Radzun HJ, Munstermann D: Tartrate-resistant, purple acid phosphatase in Gaucher's cells of the spleen. Immuno- and cytochemical analysis. *Pathol Res Pract* 187(2–3):209–213, 1991.

Zimran A, Kay A, Gelbart T, et al: Gaucher's disease. Clinical, laboratory, radiologic, and genetic features of 53 patients. *Medicine* 71(6):337–353, 1992.

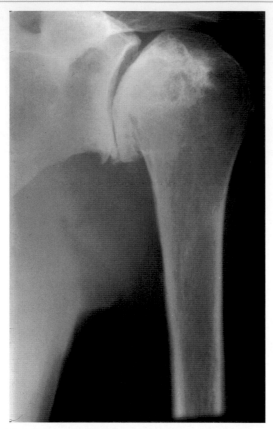

Figure 14–1 This radiograph of the proximal humerus illustrates a common sequela of Gaucher's disease. The accumulation of lipid within histiocytes in the medullary bone interferes with the local circulation, resulting in aseptic necrosis. Other radiographic clues to the diagnosis include abnormal tubulation of the bone, particularly the distal femora.

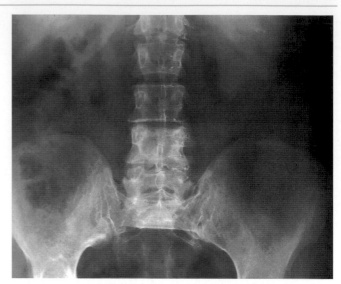

Figure 14–3 Bony sclerosis may be a sign of Gaucher's disease, as illustrated in this case involving the fourth and fifth lumbar vertebrae.

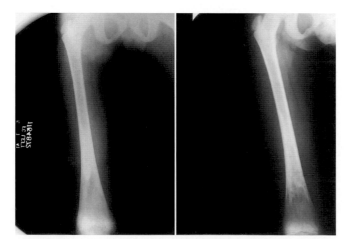

Figure 14–2 This radiograph of the distal femur shows some abnormality of tubulation and associated mineralization of infarcted bone. The characteristic Erlenmeyer flask–type change may also be seen in some cases and is particularly common in the distal femur.

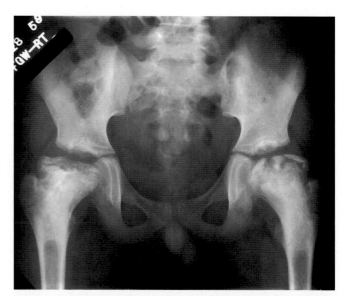

Figure 14–4 In longstanding cases of aseptic necrosis in Gaucher's disease, there may be significant associated bony deformity, as in this case involving the femoral heads bilaterally.

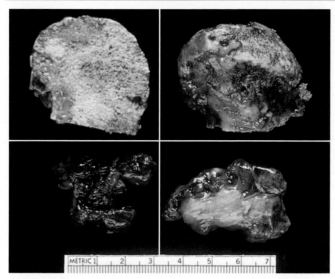

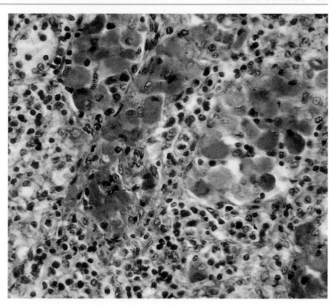

Figure 14–5 Grossly, the femoral head may show only regions of avascular necrosis, as in this example of Gaucher's disease. Areas of yellow discoloration correspond to avascular necrosis and to regions with numerous lipid-laden histiocytes. The synovium shown in the lower portion of the photograph is diffusely thickened owing to infiltration by lipid-laden histiocytes.

Figure 14–7 This photomicrograph illustrates the periodic acid–Schiff (PAS) positivity of the lipid within the foamy histiocytes in Gaucher's disease involving the marrow. Residual hematopoietic elements are present.

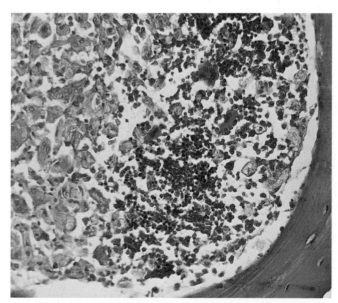

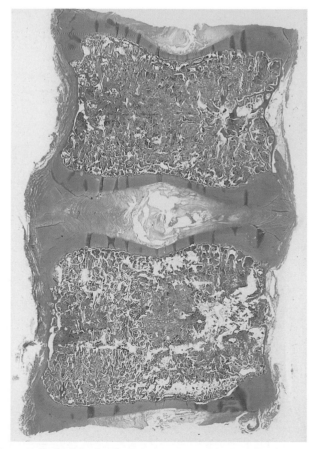

Figure 14–6 This photomicrograph illustrates the abundant cytoplasm of lipid-laden Gaucher's cells. These histiocytes may totally replace the normal fatty and hematopoietic marrow elements.

Figure 14–8 This low-magnification photomicrograph of two vertebrae shows multifocal collections of histiocytes in a patient with Gaucher's disease.

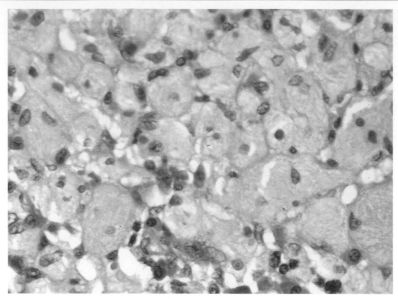

Figure 14–9 The histologic features of the lipid-laden histiocytes of Gaucher's disease involving the rib are illustrated in this photomicrograph. Other storage diseases may show a similar histologic pattern of histiocytes with abundant, clear cytoplasm.

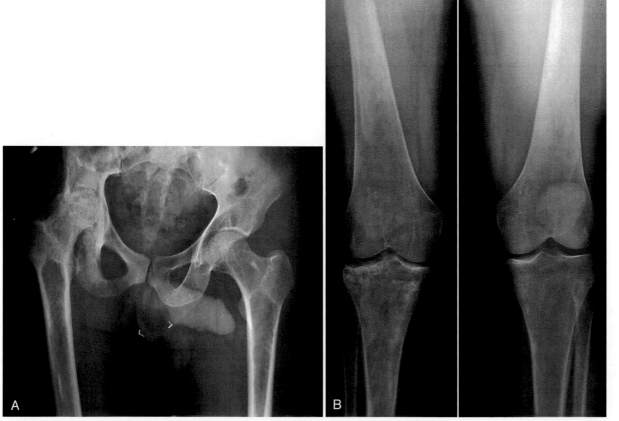

Figure 14–10 *A:* Anteroposterior (AP) roentgenogram of the pelvis and proximal femora in a patient with Gaucher's disease. There is demineralization with cortical thinning and coarse trabeculae. Both medullary canals are expanded in the femoral metaphysis. Note the avascular necrosis with collapse of the right femoral head. *B:* AP roentgenogram of the distal femora and proximal tibiae showing a similar pattern with mixed sclerotic and lucent changes in the medullary canals. On the right, there also appear to be changes of avascular necrosis, with collapse of the lateral tibial plateau.

Osteoarthritis

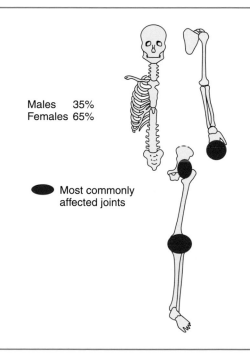

Males   35%
Females   65%

● Most commonly affected joints

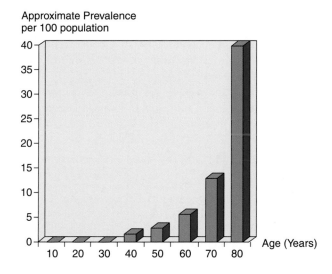

Approximate Prevalence per 100 population

Age (Years)

Classification

Approximately 20% of patients have an antecedent condition that predisposes to degenerative joint disease. Conditions associated with such secondary osteoarthritis include the following:

1. Congenital dislocation or subluxation of the hip.
2. Joint space infection.
3. Late-stage avascular necrosis.
4. Hip dysplasia.
5. Slipped capital femoral epiphysis.
6. Legg-Perthes disease.
7. Intraarticular fracture.
8. Radiation damage.

Clinical Signs

1. Pain may occur with motion of the affected joint and is worse at night.
2. Motion may be limited, with lack of full flexion or extension.
3. Heberden's nodes may be seen, mainly in women.
4. Pain subsides later in the course of the disease.
5. Swelling about the affected joint may occur.

6. Crepitus may be present.
7. The affected joint may exhibit instability.
8. The joint may be tender.
9. The erythrocyte sedimentation rate is normal.
10. Synovial fluid analysis shows a noninflammatory pattern.
11. Tests for rheumatoid factor are negative.

Clinical Symptoms

1. Pain may occur in the affected joint.
2. Joint dysfunction—e.g., limitation of motion (often of limited duration)—may be experienced.
3. Malalignment and deformity may be present.

Major Radiographic Features

1. The joint space narrows.
2. Osteophytes may be seen at the periphery of the joint.
3. The bone shows increased density.
4. Subchondral cystic change may be evident.
5. In primary generalized osteoarthritis, Heberden's nodes (distal interphalangeal joint) may cause flexion deformities and lateral deviation (index and middle fingers most commonly affected).
6. In magnetic resonance imaging studies, the hyaline cartilage shows uniform thinning and varying degrees of signal loss, and osteophytes show a central high signal intensity as a result of the marrow within the central portion of the osteophyte.

Radiographic Differential Diagnosis

1. Posttraumatic or postinflammatory conditions with development of secondary osteoarthritis.

Major Pathologic Features

Gross

1. The shape of the articular surface of the affected joint may be altered.
2. Cartilage may be absent in the weight-bearing regions of the affected joint.
3. Subchondral bone is polished or eburnated when the articular cartilage is absent.
4. Cystic change is evident; cysts are filled with loose fibromyxoid tissue.
5. Osteophytes are particularly common on the medial surface of the femoral head.

Microscopic

1. Vertical clefting of the articular cartilage may be seen.
2. Villous hyperplasia of the synovium with mild lymphoplasmacytic infiltration may be present.

3. Osteocartilaginous loose body formation may be evident.
4. The articular cartilage may show overgrowth of cells, producing "growth centers."
5. Pannus, although more common in rheumatoid arthritis, may be seen in osteoarthritis.

Pathologic Differential Diagnosis

1. Rheumatoid arthritis (although there is generally more inflammation associated with rheumatoid arthritis than with osteoarthritis, there is considerable overlap between the two conditions).
2. Other inflammatory arthritides.

Treatment

1. Treatment must be individualized depending on the extent of disease and amount of disability.
2. Medical approaches include the following:
   a. Analgesic agents (e.g., acetaminophen, nonsteroidal anti-inflammatory drugs) (NSAIDs).
   b. Relief of joint overstress (i.e., use of walking aid, weight reduction in patients who are obese, use of compartment uploading braces, and modification of activities).
   c. Physical therapy to relieve pain and maintain range of motion and strength.
   d. Intra-articular injections, including corticosteroids or viscosupplementation (i.e., Synvisc, Hyalgan, Supartz, Euflexa, and others) can provide symptomatic relief, though their effects are generally temporary.
3. Surgical therapy is individualized depending on location, extent of disease, associated deformity, age, and expectations of the patient:
   a. Arthroscopic techniques for lavage and debridement.
   b. Osteotomy for malalignment of the knee with unicompartmental disease.
   c. Arthrodesis.
   d. Joint arthroplasty for unicompartmental or total joint replacement.

References

Bullough PG: Pathologic changes associated with the common arthritides and their treatment [review]. *Pathol Annu* 14(2):69–105, 1979.

Gold RH, Bassett LW, Seeger LL: The other arthritides. Roentgenologic features of osteoarthritis, erosive osteoarthritis, ankylosing spondylitis, psoriatic arthritis, Reiter's disease, multicentric reticulohistiocytosis, and progressive systemic sclerosis. *Radiol Clin North Am* 26(6):1195–1212, 1988.

Hamerman D: Osteoarthritis [review]. *Orthop Rev* 17(4):353–360, 1988.

Lane NE, Kremer LB: Radiographic indices for osteoarthritis. *Rheum Dis Clin North Am* 21(2):379–394, 1995.

Martel W, Adler RS, Chan K, et al: Overview: new methods in imaging osteoarthritis. *J Rheumatol (Suppl)* 27:32–37, 1991.

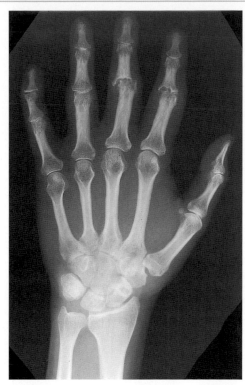

Figure 15–1 This radiograph illustrates osteoarthritic changes in the hand. The interphalangeal joints are commonly involved, with the formation of osteophytes that correspond to clinically identified Heberden's nodes.

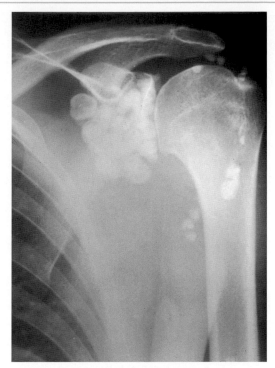

Figure 15–3 This radiograph illustrates degenerative joint disease involving the shoulder joint. Numerous osteocartilaginous loose bodies are present in the joint. Calcification of the cartilaginous component of these bodies, when they are numerous, may even raise a suspicion of chondrosarcoma.

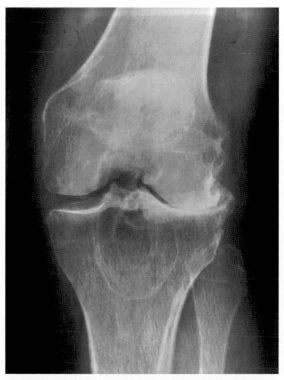

Figure 15–2 This radiograph reveals longstanding changes of osteoarthritis. A subchondral degenerative cyst is present in the proximal tibia. Subchondral sclerosis is identifiable as well. Osteophyte formation also commonly accompanies these two changes.

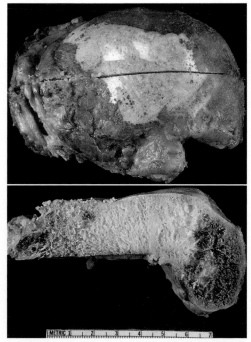

Figure 15–4 This gross specimen of the femoral head is from a patient who suffered from congenital hip dysplasia and subsequent degenerative joint disease. The whitish glistening surface of the femoral head in the upper portion of the photograph corresponds to the region of articular cartilage loss and eburnation of the underlying subchondral bone.

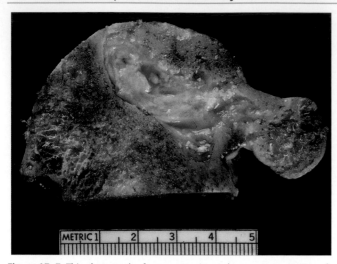

Figure 15–5 This photograph of a gross specimen shows a cross-section of a femoral head with advanced osteoarthritis. A degenerative cyst is present in the subchondral bone to the left of the large osteophyte.

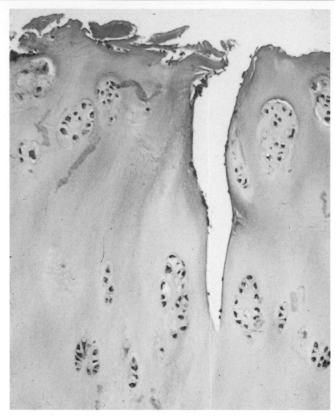

Figure 15–7 This photomicrograph illustrates the first morphologic changes seen in osteoarthritis. Such vertical clefting has been termed "fibrilization." Subsequent softening of the cartilage leads to further degeneration. The process does not uniformly affect the entire articular cartilage surface but is variable from region to region.

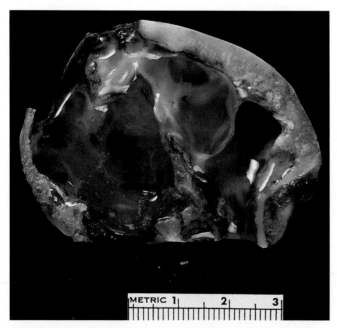

Figure 15–6 This photograph of a gross specimen illustrates advanced degenerative cyst formation nearly replacing the entire femoral head. Clear, glistening synovial fluid is present within the cyst.

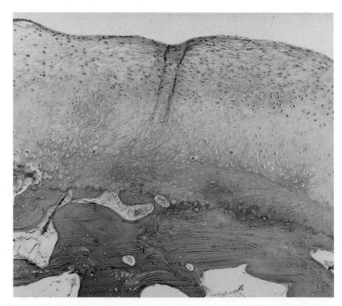

Figure 15–8 Early in the course of the disease, regions of the articular cartilage may be relatively normal histologically, as in this specimen from the femoral head.

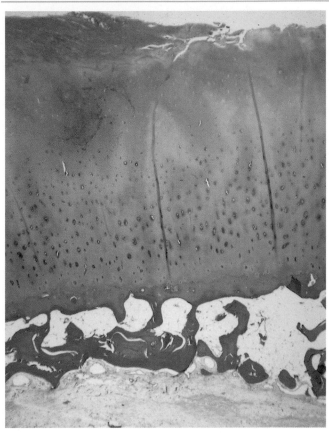

Figure 15–9 This photomicrograph illustrates degenerative clefting of the articular cartilage. In addition, a degenerative cyst is identified in the lower portion of the photomicrograph.

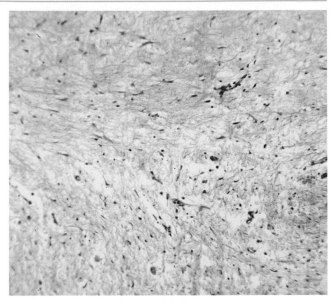

Figure 15–11 This photomicrograph illustrates the histologic appearance of a degenerative cyst of the tibia that contains hypocellular myxoid connective tissue. Radiographically, the appearance of this cyst simulated that of a neoplasm.

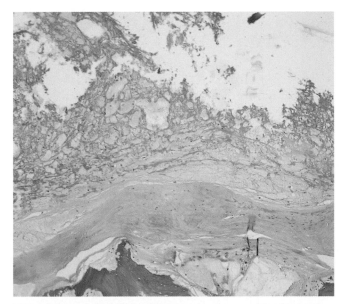

Figure 15–10 This photomicrograph shows the contents of the degenerative cyst at higher magnification. Such cysts are filled with amorphous eosinophilic debris. The cyst wall is generally a hypocellular fibrotic connective tissue.

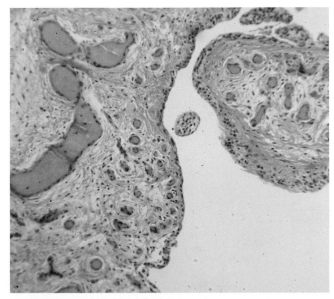

Figure 15–12 This photomicrograph illustrates villous hyperplasia of the synovium from a patient with osteoarthritis. In advanced cases of osteoarthritis, villous hypertrophy of the synovium may be marked and associated with fibrous thickening of the joint capsule.

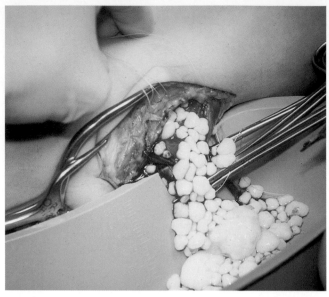

Figure 15–13 This photomicrograph demonstrates the histologic features of an osteocartilaginous loose body from a patient with osteoarthritis of the knee. Such loose bodies may become embedded in the hypertrophic synovium.

Figure 15–15 Numerous loose bodies may be associated with osteoarthritis, as shown in this intraoperative photograph.

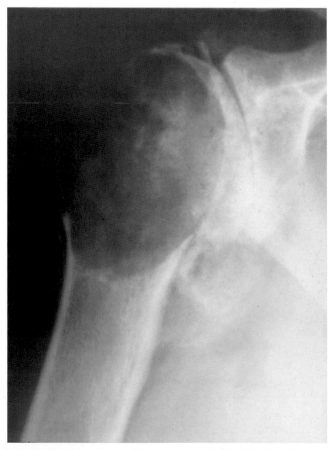

Figure 15–14 This radiograph illustrates osteoarthritis of the shoulder with an associated large degenerative cyst occupying the proximal humerus. Although large, the cyst is well circumscribed with mild peripheral sclerosis.

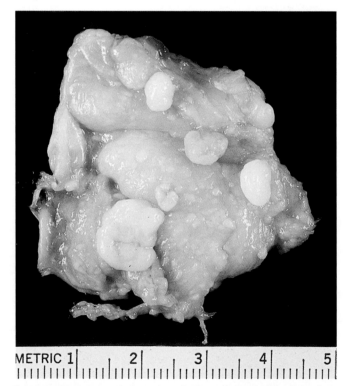

Figure 15–16 Osteocartilaginous loose bodies associated with osteoarthritis may become embedded in the synovium, as shown in this photograph. Such cases may be indistinguishable from synovial chondromatosis.

Neuropathic Joint (Charcot's Joint)

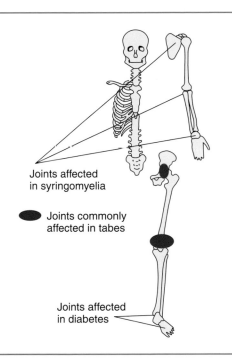

Joints affected
in syringomyelia

● Joints commonly
affected in tabes

Joints affected
in diabetes

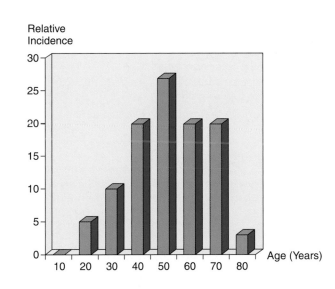

Incidence

The incidence of Charcot's joint in patients with diabetes is approximately 0.4% but increases to 16% in patients with diabetic neuropathy.

Clinical Signs

1. Charcot's joint is characterized by rapidly destructive arthritis of a single joint in the absence of pain or a history of trauma.
2. Charcot's joint is associated with peripheral neuropathies and spinal cord degenerative diseases, including the following:
   a. Tabes dorsalis.
   b. Syringomyelia.
   c. Advanced diabetes mellitus with peripheral neuropathy.
   d. Congenital insensitivity to pain.
   e. Amyloidosis.
   f. Leprosy.
   g. Residual effect from repeated glucocorticoid injection in the joint.
   h. Transverse myelitis.
   i. Traumatic paralysis.
   j. Spinal dysraphism.

3. Joint crepitation may be present.
4. Loose bodies may be palpated in the joint cavity.
5. The joint changes may precede the identification of a neurologic deficit.
6. Although classically the process is painless, some patients (up to one third in some series) have pain early in the course of the disease.
7. Deep tendon reflexes are absent.
8. Large knee effusions may be seen and may rupture into the surrounding soft tissues and present as Baker's cyst.
9. The affected joint may be swollen and warm, mimicking the appearance of an infected joint.
10. Scoliosis may be seen in patients with spinal causes. (Approximately 50% of patients with syringomyelia have scoliosis.)
11. Synovial fluid analysis shows a clear, straw-colored fluid with a normal white blood cell count.

Clinical Symptoms

1. The process is painless.
2. Joint instability may occur.
3. Crepitation in the joint may be present.
4. There is rapid progression of joint abnormality. (It may evolve in a period of weeks.)
5. The ability to ambulate progressively decreases.

Major Radiographic Features

1. Extensive destruction of the joint space may be seen.
2. Extensive destruction of the bone adjacent to the joint may be evident.
3. Osteopenia may be present.
4. The destructive process may show sharp cortical margins.
5. There may be considerable bony debris about the joint (hypertrophic neuroarthropathy) or none to minimal bony debris (atrophic neuroarthropathy).

Radiographic Differential Diagnosis

1. Osteoarthritis.

Major Pathologic Features

Gross

1. Synovium may appear rusty brown.
2. Synovium may be hyperplastic.
3. Marked destruction of the normal bony contour may be present.
4. Bony and cartilaginous debris may be embedded in synovium and soft tissue.

Microscopic

1. Bone and cartilaginous detritus.
2. Synovial hyperplasia.
3. Inflammatory reaction in the synovium and adjacent soft tissues.
4. Giant cell reaction to debris.

Pathologic Differential Diagnosis

1. Posttraumatic osteoarthritis.
2. Rheumatoid arthritis (in general, the inflammatory reaction is much less pronounced in Charcot joints than in rapidly destructive rheumatoid arthritis).

Treatment

Medical

1. The underlying disorder must be promptly recognized and treated.
2. Decreased weightbearing and walking aids can be used.
3. Bracing and orthosis can be used to decrease stress and retard progression of destruction.

Surgical

1. Arthrodesis is difficult to achieve but may be effective in the knee or ankle.
2. Below-knee amputation may become necessary for distal joints or if concomitant infection complicates the clinical course.
3. Resection arthroplasty may be performed.
4. Total joint arthroplasty is generally not recommended because of its high failure rate.

References

Allman RM, Brower AC, Kotlyarov EB: Neuropathic bone and joint disease. *Radiol Clin North Am* 26(6):1373–1381, 1988.

Helms CA, Chapman S, Wild JH: Charcot-like joints in calcium pyrophosphate dihydrate deposition disease. *Skeletal Radiol* 7(1): 55–58, 1981.

Kovacs JP, Bowen JR: Neurotrophic arthropathy. *Contemp Orthop* 23(4):359–361, 1991.

Park YH, Taylor JA, Szollar SM, et al: Imaging findings in spinal neuroarthropathy. *Spine* 19(13):1499–1504, 1994.

Peh WC, Brockwell J, Chau MT, et al: Imaging features of dissecting neuropathic joints. *Australas Radiol* 39(3):249–253, 1995.

Resnick D: Neuropathic osteoarthropathy. In Resnick D (ed): *Diagnosis of Bone and Joint Disorders*, 4th ed. Philadelphia: WB Saunders, 2002.

Soudry M, Binazzi R, Johanson NA, et al: Total knee arthroplasty in Charcot and Charcot-like joints. *Clin Orthop Relat Res* 208: 199–204, 1986.

Rheumatoid Arthritis

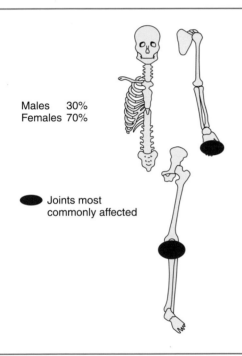

Males 30%
Females 70%

● Joints most
commonly affected

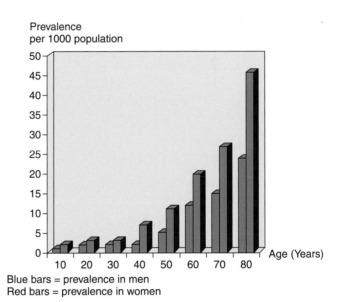

Prevalence
per 1000 population

Age (Years)

Blue bars = prevalence in men
Red bars = prevalence in women

Prevalence

Approximately 1% of the adult population (approximately 6 per 1000 men and 14 per 1000 women) suffers from rheumatoid arthritis; the prevalence increases with age in both men and women (see prevalence graph).

Clinical Signs

1. Symmetric polyarthritis results in hot, swollen, tender joints.
2. The synovial fluid is milky.
3. Rheumatoid nodules in the skin are present in about one fourth of patients, particularly over the extensor surface of the forearm.
4. Synovial fluid analysis generally shows 20,000 to 50,000 inflammatory cells, with approximately 50% polymorphonuclear leukocytes.
5. Carpal tunnel syndrome may be present.
6. Trigger finger may be present.
7. Tests are positive for rheumatoid factor. (*Note:* Rheumatoid factor is not specific and may be seen in systemic lupus erythematosus, chronic liver disease, Sjögren's syndrome, and other conditions.)

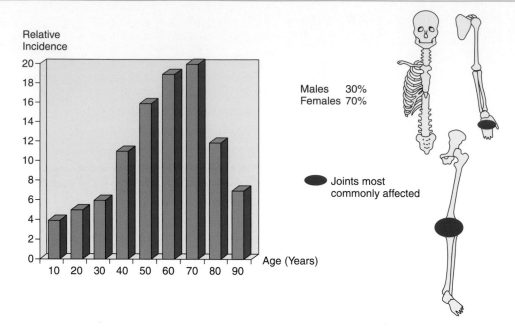

Males   30%
Females 70%

Joints most commonly affected

8. The erythrocyte sedimentation rate is elevated.
9. Anemia of chronic disease may be present.
10. Of patients who are positive for rheumatoid factor, 70% are positive for HLA-DR4.

Clinical Symptoms

1. The course of the disease is characterized by remissions and exacerbations:
  a. Fatigue.
  b. Weight loss.
  c. Fever.
  d. Morning stiffness.
2. Joint pain is present.
3. Skin nodules (rheumatoid nodules) may be seen.
4. Epidemiologic studies show that 50% of patients have symptoms 2 months to 3 years prior to diagnosis (similar for both men and women).

Major Radiographic Features

1. Osteopenia of the juxta-articular bone may be seen.
2. The joint space may show narrowing.
3. Juxta-articular bony erosions may be present.
4. Periarticular soft tissue swelling may be evident.
5. Subluxation of the joint may be seen.
6. Marginal bony erosions may be seen.
7. Subchondral cyst formation may be present.
8. Joint effusion may be evident.

Radiographic Differential Diagnosis

1. Psoriatic arthritis.
2. Atrophic osteoarthritis.
3. Septic arthritis, if monoarticular.

Major Pathologic Features

1. The synovium may show the following features:
  a. Synovial papillary hyperplasia with thickening of the villi.
  b. Lymphoplasmacytic infiltration of the synovium.
  c. Subsynovial multinucleated giant cells.
  d. Lymphoid follicle formation in the synovium.
  e. Fibrinous exudate on the surface of the synovium.
  f. Hyperplastic synovium extending over the articular surface (pannus formation).
  g. Fibrinous exudate on the surface and in the substance of the synovium.
  h. Inflamed synovium invading the bone at the articular margin.
2. Bony changes include the following:
  a. Destruction of the articular cartilage by hyperplastic synovium, resulting in "fraying" of the cartilage.
  b. Lymphoplasmacytic infiltration of subchondral bone and even follicle formation.
  c. Infiltration of pannus-like tissue into the articular cartilage from the synovium and subchondral bone.

Pathologic Differential Diagnosis

1. Psoriatic arthritis.
2. Arthritis associated with systemic lupus erythematosus.
3. Arthritis associated with ulcerative colitis.

Treatment

Medical

Treatment must be individualized. The goal is to relieve pain and inflammation while maintaining joint function and preventing joint deformity.

1. Supportive care (e.g., education, rest, and nutrition) should be instituted.
2. Physical and occupational therapy may be undertaken.
3. Aspirin and other nonsteroidal anti-inflammatory drugs (NSAIDs) may be taken.
4. Corticosteroids may be beneficial in selected patients.
5. Disease-modifying anti-rheumatic drugs (DMARDs) often play a central role in treatment. These medications include methotrexate, etanercept (Enbrel), adalimumab (Humira), anakinra (Kineret), and infliximab (Remicade).

Surgical

1. Arthroscopic synovectomy is occasionally indicated in selected cases.
2. Usually, reconstructive joint surgery (i.e., total joint arthroplasty) is performed for advanced destruction.

References

Hunter DJ, Conaghan PG: Imaging outcomes and their role in determining outcomes in osteoarthritis and rheumatoid arthritis. *Curr Opin Rheumatol* 18(2):157–162, 2006.

Linos A, Worthington JW, O'Fallon WM, et al: The epidemiology of rheumatoid arthritis in Rochester, Minnesota: a study of incidence, prevalence and mortality. *Am J Epidemiol* 111(1):87–98, 1980.

Peterfy CG: New developments in imaging in rheumatoid arthritis. *Curr Opin Rheumatol* 15(3):288–295, 2003.

Sommer OJ, Kladosek A, Weiler V, et al: Rheumatoid arthritis: a practical guide to state-of-the-art imaging, image interpretation, and clinical implications. *Radiographics* 25(2):381–398, 2005.

Wakefield RJ, Conaghan PG, Jarrett S, et al: Noninvasive techniques for assessing skeletal changes in inflammatory arthritis: imaging technique. *Curr Opin Rheumatol* 16(4):435–442, 2004.

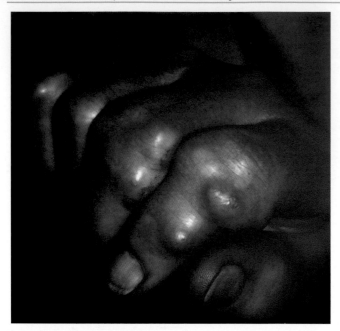

Figure 17–1 This photograph illustrates rheumatoid nodules in the soft tissues of the fingers.

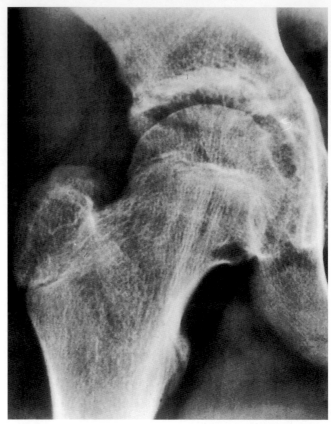

Figure 17–3 This radiograph illustrates juvenile rheumatoid arthritis involving the hip. Patients with juvenile rheumatoid arthritis may have systemic symptoms.

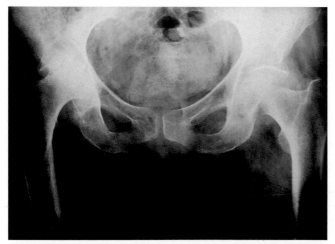

Figure 17–2 This radiograph shows rheumatoid disease with marked degenerative change.

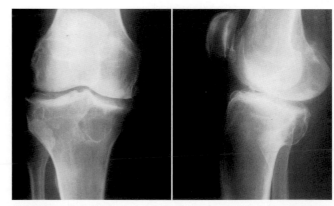

Figure 17–4 This radiograph of the knee shows joint space narrowing related to rheumatoid arthritis. In addition, a degenerative cyst is present in the proximal tibia.

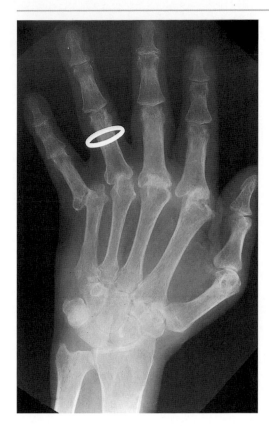

Figure 17–5 This radiograph of the hand shows subluxation of the metacarpophalangeal joints secondary to rheumatoid disease. Joint laxity related to the underlying process contributes to the subluxation. Joint space narrowing and osteopenia are also present.

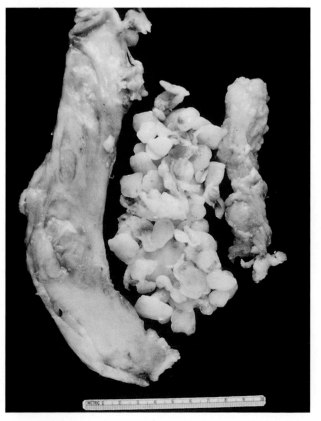

Figure 17–6 This photograph of a gross specimen illustrates the features of hyperplastic synovium and multiple "rice bodies" from the knee of a patient with rheumatoid arthritis.

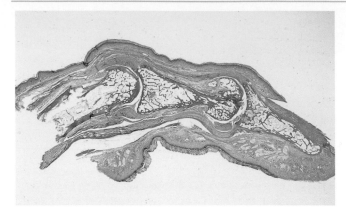

Figure 17–7 This photograph demonstrates the gross pathologic changes associated with rheumatoid arthritis of the finger. Periarticular bony erosion and ligamentous laxity are present. Ligamentous laxity leads to subluxation, as shown in Figure 17–5.

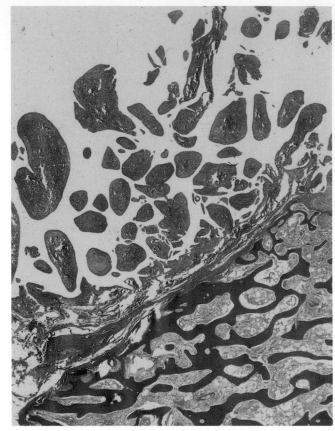

Figure 17–9 This photomicrograph illustrates the dramatic villous hyperplasia of the synovium present in rheumatoid arthritis. Lymphoid nodules are identifiable within the hyperplastic synovial villi.

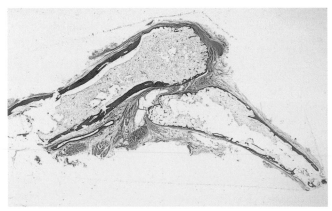

Figure 17–8 This photograph illustrates subluxation of the metacarpophalangeal joint in a patient with rheumatoid arthritis.

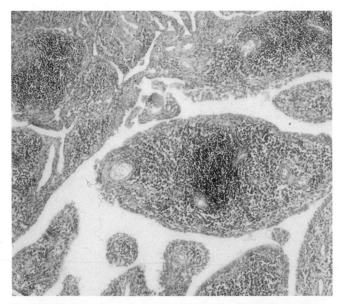

Figure 17–10 This photomicrograph reveals the lymphoid hyperplasia of rheumatoid disease at higher magnification. Plasma cells may form a significant proportion of the lymphoplasmacytic synovial infiltrate.

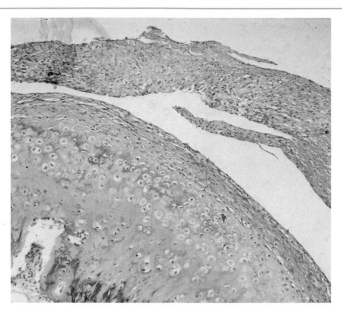

Figure 17–11 This photomicrograph illustrates hyperplastic synovial proliferation extending over the articular surface of the femoral head. Such pannus proliferation results in destruction of the articular cartilage.

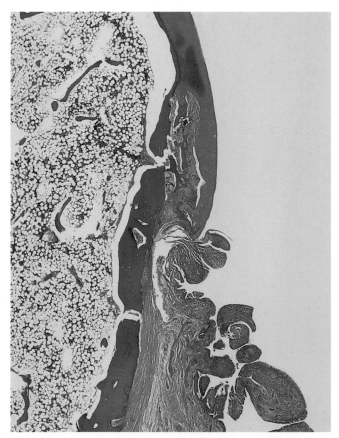

Figure 17–12 Further encroachment of the proliferative synovium onto the articular surface of the femoral head is illustrated in this photomicrograph. Erosion of the articular cartilage may result in eburnation of the underlying bone in longstanding rheumatoid disease.

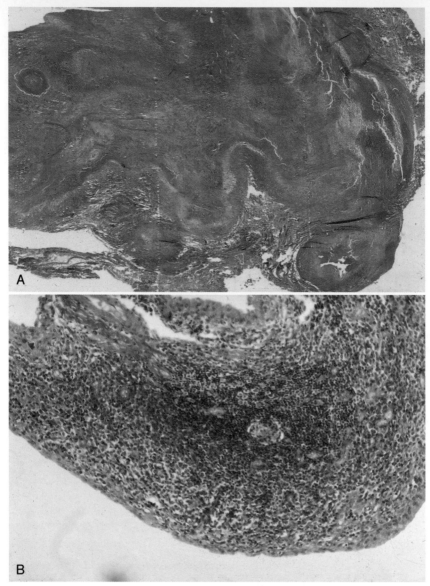

Figure 17–13 *A* and *B*: These two photomicrographs reveal the histologic features of rheumatoid granulomas. Such rheumatoid nodules may simulate infectious granulomas. Central necrosis and surrounding histiocytic and giant cell reaction are present in the necrotic region.

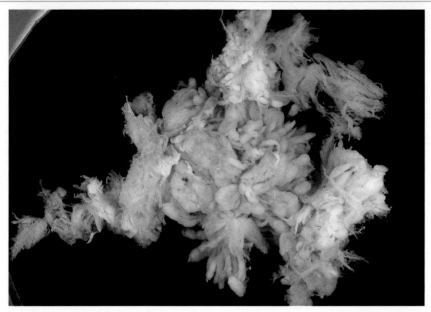

Figure 17–14 This photograph of a gross specimen illustrates villous hyperplasia of the synovium in rheumatoid arthritis. Similar features would be evident at arthroscopy.

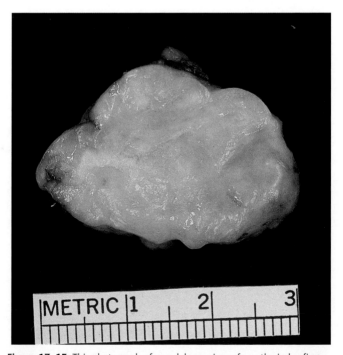

Figure 17–15 This photograph of a nodule specimen from the index finger exemplifies the appearance of a rheumatoid nodule. Rheumatoid nodules are variable in color and may show foci of necrosis grossly.

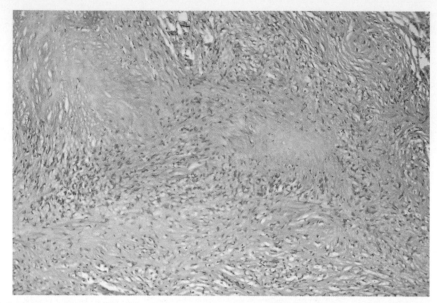

Figure 17–16 The histologic features of a rheumatoid nodule are shown in this photomicrograph. The central necrosis with peripheral histiocytic palisading may mimic the appearance of an infectious granuloma. Special stains for fungi and mycobacteria are negative in such rheumatoid nodules.

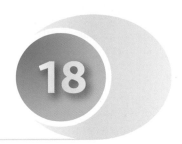

Ochronosis—Disorder of Tyrosine and Phenylalanine Catabolism Secondary to Homogentisic Acid and Related Compounds

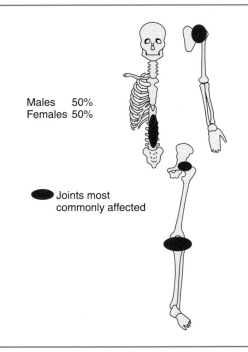

Males   50%
Females 50%

⬤ Joints most commonly affected

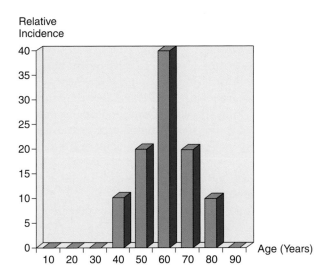

Note: males tend to be affected by joint disease earlier than females and have more severe manifestations

Inheritance

Inheritance is autosomal recessive (related to deficiency of homogentisic acid oxidase).

Clinical Signs

1. Alkaptonuria (homogentisic acid in the urine) is present.
2. Sclerae may be darkened (from deposition of homogentisic acid in collagen in this tissue).
3. The earlobes may be discolored (from deposition of homogentisic acid in collagen in this tissue).

4. Black discoloration of other tissues related to the accumulation of homogentisic acid (e.g., cardiovascular, genitourinary, and respiratory tissues, as well as sclerae and skin) may be exhibited.

Clinical Symptoms

1. The urine turns dark after exposure to air (alkaptonuria); this may first appear as dark staining of the diapers in childhood.
2. Clinical symptoms of ochronosis are usually present by 40 years of age.

121

3. Arthritis—a "premature osteoarthritis"—may be present, most commonly involving the knees, shoulders, and hips. (Small joints of the hands and feet are rarely involved.)
4. Spinal involvement results in dull back pain, limited motion, and loss of height. (The earliest manifestation of the bony disease involves the spine.)
5. Acute disc herniation may be the initial presentation (almost exclusively occurs in male patients).
6. The Achilles tendon may rupture secondary to weakness caused by deposition of homogentisic acid within the tissue.
7. Most patients are asymptomatic until adulthood.

Major Radiographic Features

1. Calcification of the intervertebral disc may be seen. Deposition of homogentisic acid in the disc leads to brittleness and degeneration of the disc.
2. The disc space may show narrowing.
3. The disc may be collapsed, with resultant fusion of vertebrae.
4. Kyphosis may be present.
5. Subchondral sclerosis similar to that seen in osteoarthritis may be present.
6. Osteophyte formation tends to be relatively modest.
7. Peripheral joint disease follows spinal disease by years. Knees are most frequently involved, followed by shoulders and hips. Joint space narrowing and calcific deposits are the most common features of large joint disease.
8. Shoulder joints may exhibit extreme joint space narrowing.
9. Calcification within tendons, particularly in the knees and pelvis, may be seen.
10. Irregular sclerosis of the pubic symphysis may be evident.
11. Calculi may be identified within the prostate on pelvic radiographs.

Radiographic Differential Diagnosis

1. Osteoarthritis.

Major Pathologic Features

1. Gross examination shows black discoloration of the articular cartilage.
2. Histologic study reveals the following:
   a. Irregular fragments of pigmented cartilage lie embedded in a hyperplastic synovium.
   b. Fragmented articular cartilage is embedded in a proliferative synovium and shows the characteristic black color associated with the disease. Foreign body giant cell reaction to the cartilage fragments is common.

Pathologic Differential Diagnosis

1. There is no differential diagnosis. Although other pigments may be identified in histologic sections, the features of ochronosis are sufficiently unique as to be diagnostic.

Treatment

1. There is no cure for alkaptonuria, although diets low in protein, phenylalanine, and tyrosine may reduce the excretion of homogentisic acid in the urine.
2. The arthropathy and disc disease associated with ochronosis should be treated as symptoms arise, with a conservative approach to associated arthropathies and disc disease.
3. Total joint replacement can have good results, but overall patient satisfaction is often limited due to concurrent disease in other joints and/or the spine.
4. Early studies of nitisinone have shown some potential. Nitisinone is a triketone herbicide that inhibits 4-hydrophenylpyruvate dioxygenase, which causes direct pharmacological reduction of homogentisic acid (HGA) production by inhibiting the tyrosine degradation pathway. This helps prevent HGA accumulation.

References

Bayindir P, Yilmaz Ovali G, Pabucu Y, et al: Radiologic features of lumbar spine in ochronosis in late stages. *Clin Rheumatol* 25(4):588–590, 2006.

Linduskova M, Hrba J, Vykydal M, et al: Needle biopsy of joints—its contribution to the diagnosis of ochronotic arthropathy (alcaptonuria). *Clin Rheumatol* 11(4):569–570, 1992.

Martin RF, Sanchez JL, Gonzalez A, et al: Exogenous ochronosis [review]. *Puerto Rico Health Sci J* 11(1):23–26, 1992.

Melis M, Onori P, Aliberti G, et al: Ochronotic arthropathy: structural and ultrastructural features. *Ultrastruct Pathol* 18(5):467–471, 1994.

Paul R, Ylinen SL: The "whisker sign" as an indicator of ochronosis in skeletal scintigraphy. *Eur J Nucl Med* 18(3):222–224, 1991.

Perrone A, Impara L, Bruni A, et al: Radiographic and MRI findings in ochronosis. *Radiologia Medica* 110(4):349–358, 2005.

Rooney PJ: Hyperlipidemias, lipid storage disorders, metal storage disorders, and ochronosis [review]. *Curr Opin Rheumatol* 3(1):166–171, 1991.

Ryan SJ, Smith CD, Slevin JT: Magnetic resonance imaging in ochronosis, a rare cause of back pain [abstract]. *J Neuroimaging* 4(1):41–42, 1994.

Snider RL, Thiers BH: Exogenous ochronosis. *J Am Acad Dermatol* 28(4):662–664, 1993.

Suwannarat P, O'Brien K, Perry MB, Sebring N, Bernardini I, Kaiser-Kupfer MI, Rubin BI, Tsilou E, Gerber LH, Gahl WA. Use of nitisinone in patients with alkaptonuria. *Metabolism* 54(6):719–728, 2005.

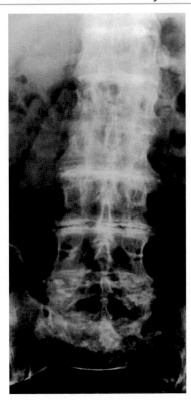

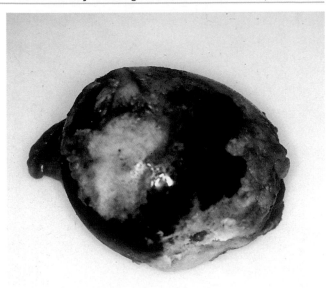

Figure 18–1 This radiograph of the vertebrae illustrates the changes in ochronosis. There is narrowing of the disc spaces and deposition of calcium in the degenerated disc material.

Figure 18–3 This gross specimen of the femoral head from a patient with ochronosis illustrates the black discoloration of the cartilage. In addition, there is degeneration of the articular cartilage and eburnation of the underlying bone.

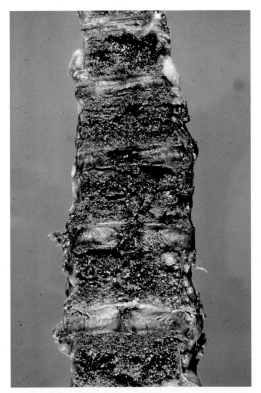

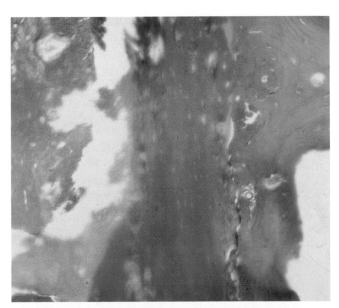

Figure 18–2 This gross specimen of the vertebrae shows the characteristic appearance of degenerated disc material in patients with ochronosis. The black discoloration is present in disc material and in cartilage.

Figure 18–4 This photomicrograph illustrates the appearance of articular cartilage in a patient with ochronosis. Hematoxylin and eosin–stained sections are brown to black, depending on the extent of homogentisic acid deposition in the tissue. The articular cartilage may be frayed.

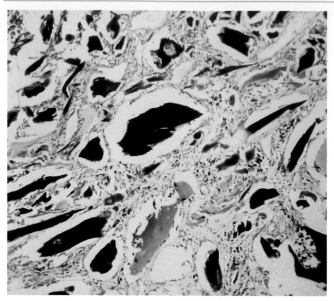

Figure 18–5 The deposition of homogentisic acid leads to altered mechanical properties and degeneration of the cartilage. Flaking of the cartilage into the synovium results in mild inflammatory changes and fibrosis as shown on this photomicrograph.

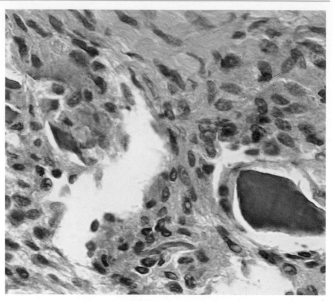

Figure 18–7 Fragments of ochronotic cartilage embedded in the synovium of the knee are illustrated in this photomicrograph. Histiocytic and giant cell reaction surrounds the brownish discolored cartilage.

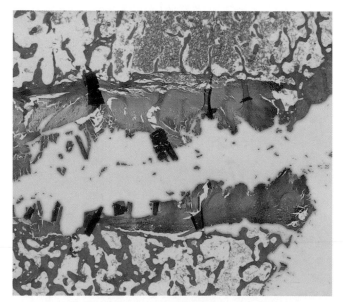

Figure 18–6 This low-power photomicrograph shows the discoloration of an intervertebral disc as a result of ochronosis. The mechanical properties of the disc tissue are altered and thus subject to degeneration.

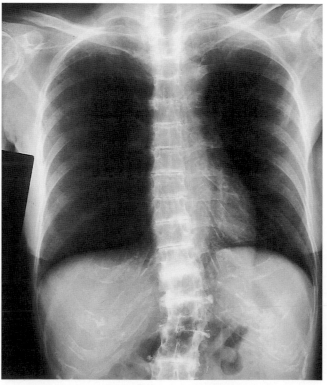

Figure 18–8 The chest radiograph of this 56-year-old woman shows mineralization of the intervertebral disc secondary to ochronosis.

Gout

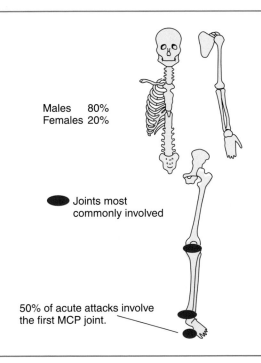

Males   80%
Females 20%

Joints most
commonly involved

50% of acute attacks involve
the first MCP joint.

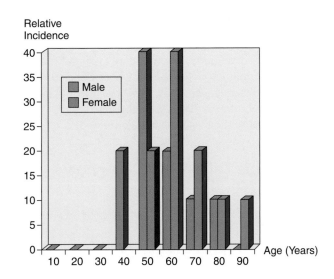

Clinical Signs

1. Hyperuricemia is present. (Although hyperuricemia is present in 2% to 18% of the population, the prevalence of gout is between 0.1% and 0.4%.)
2. Leukocytosis may be found.
3. Joint fluid analysis reveals inflammatory exudate, negatively birefringent needle-like crystals.
4. Gouty tophi may appear in the chronic stage of disease and are present in approximately 7% of the population with gouty arthritis.
5. Renal stones occur almost exclusively in male patients with gouty arthritis.
6. Patients are more often overweight.
7. The average age of the first attack for men is 45 years of age and for women it is 50 years of age.

Clinical Symptoms

1. Monoarticular arthritis of the lower extremities occurs, with peculiar propensity to involve the first metatarsophalangeal joint. (Approximately 80% of patients with gouty arthritis have involvement of the metatarsophalangeal joint with their first attack. The remaining patients usually experience ankle or knee involvement

with the acute attack. The incidence of attacks is variable, but in the gouty population overall it may be a high as one every other year.)
2. Severe swelling of affected joint may be seen.
3. Low-grade fever may be present.
4. Polyarticular disease at onset is seen in approximately 30% of cases.
5. Acute attacks last from a few days to 2 weeks and then resolve, followed by symptom-free intervals.
6. Symptoms respond to colchicine therapy.

Major Imaging Features

1. Punched-out areas of lytic bony destruction involving multiple joints can be seen.
2. Little bony reaction to the lytic destruction is evident.
3. The metatarsophalangeal joint of the first toe is classically involved.
4. No regional osteoporosis is present (helpful in distinguishing gout from rheumatoid arthritis).
5. Swelling of soft tissues may be seen.
6. Eccentric soft tissue swelling with or without calcification of the tophus may be seen.
7. On magnetic resonance imaging gout is one of the few entities that may show low signal (short T2) on T2-weighted sequences. This, however, is not always the case, and intermediate or bright signal on T2-weighted sequences is also encountered.

Radiographic Differential Diagnosis

1. Seronegative arthritides.
2. Chronic low-grade infection, if monoarticular.

Major Pathologic Features

1. The acute phase is characterized by the following:
   a. Inflammatory reaction in the synovium.
   b. Crystals in the synovium that are negatively birefringent under polarized light.
   c. Crystals present in the neutrophils.
2. The chronic phase is characterized by the following:
   a. Gouty tophi, which grossly are white, chalky masses.
   b. A microscopic appearance of the tophi consisting of crystal deposits surrounded by histiocytes, multinucleated giant cells, and fibrous connective tissue.

Pathologic Differential Diagnosis

1. Pseudogout.
2. Infection.

Treatment

1. Adherence to proper management guidelines provides predictable relief of symptoms and prevention of disabling complications.
2. Treatment for an acute gouty attack may include the following:
   a. Nonsteroidal anti-inflammatory drugs (NSAIDs) such as indomethacin, 50 mg every 8 hours, until symptoms resolve (usually 5 to 10 days).
   b. Colchicine, which is effective during the first 24 to 48 hours of the attack.
   c. Corticosteroids, which may be useful in patients who are unable to tolerate NSAIDs:
      i. Monoarticular attack may be treated with intraarticular injection of the steroid.
      ii. Polyarticular disease may be treated with oral prednisone, 40 to 60 mg tapered over 7 days.
3. Prevention of acute exacerbations may include the following:
   a. Avoidance of food and alcoholic beverages that may precipitate the attacks.
   b. Colchicine prophylaxis (0.6 mg, twice a day).
   c. Decrease in serum uric acid concentration with the following:
      i. Uricosuric agents.
      ii. Interval use of allopurinol.

References

Agarwal AK: Gout and pseudogout [review]. *Prim Care* 20(4):839–855, 1993.
Agudelo CA, Wise CM: Gout: diagnosis, pathogenesis, and clinical manifestations. *Curr Opin Rheumatol* 13(3):234–239, 2001.
Barthelemy CR, Nakayama DA, Carrera GF, et al: Gouty arthritis: a prospective radiographic evaluation of sixty patients. *Skeletal Radiol* 11(1):1–8, 1984.
Cobby MJ, Martel W: Some commonly unrecognized manifestations of metabolic arthropathies [review]. *Clin Imaging* 16(1):1–14, 1992.
Cohen PR, Schmidt WA, Rapini RP: Chronic tophaceous gout with severely deforming arthritis: a case report with emphasis on histopathologic considerations. *Cutis* 48(6):445–451, 1991.
Pennes DR, Martel W: Hyperuricemia and gout. *Semin Roentgenol* 21(4):245–255, 1986.
Pritzker KP: Calcium pyrophosphate dihydrate crystal deposition and other crystal deposition diseases [review]. *Curr Opin Rheumatol* 6(4):442–447, 1994.
Underwood M: Diagnosis and management of gout. *BMJ* 332(7553):1315–1319, 2006.
Watt I, Middlemiss H: The radiology of gout. *Clin Radiol* 26(1):27–36, 1975.

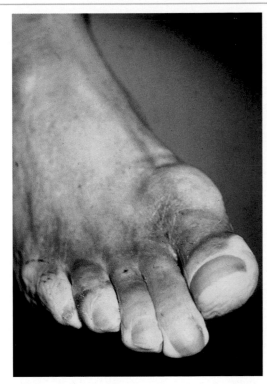

Figure 19–1 The first metatarsophalangeal joint of the foot is the most common location for an acute gouty attack. Such attacks are frequently associated with an extremely painful, red, and swollen joint. Aspiration of the joint yields synovial fluid containing negatively birefringent urate crystals.

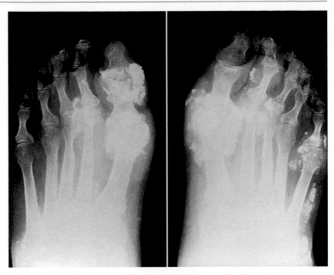

Figure 19–3 A later stage of the disease with associated tophaceous gouty deposits is shown in this radiograph. Destruction of multiple joints in a distribution atypical of rheumatoid disease is often evident at this late stage of the process.

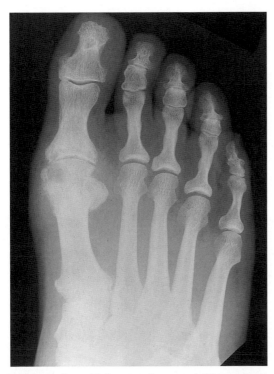

Figure 19–2 The radiographic features of gouty arthritis involving the first metatarsophalangeal joint are illustrated in this radiograph. Soft tissue swelling is seen early in the course of the disease. Later the characteristic punched-out bony erosion without adjacent bony reaction is evident, as shown in this radiograph.

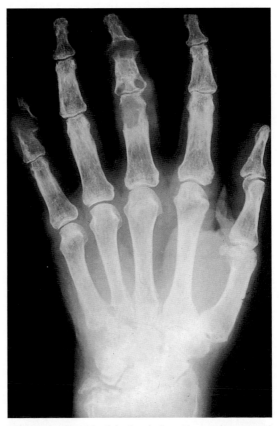

Figure 19–4 This radiograph of the hand of a patient with gouty arthropathy demonstrates periarticular punched-out lytic lesions similar to those commonly seen in the foot.

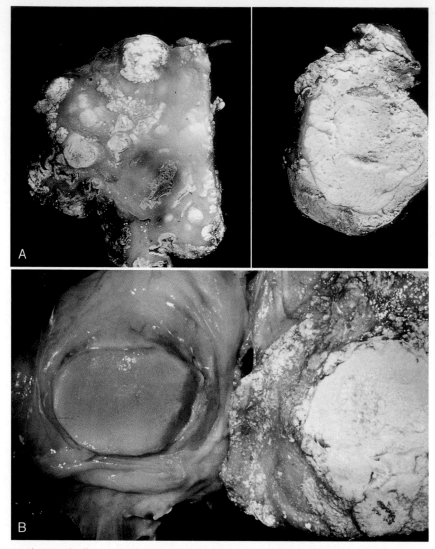

Figure 19–5 *A* and *B*: These gross photographs illustrate tophaceous deposits of urate crystals in the soft tissues about the knee. The white crystals can be spread on a slide and viewed under polarized light to confirm the diagnosis of gout.

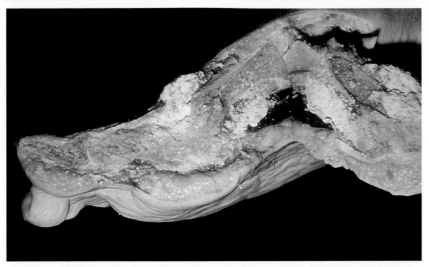

Figure 19–6 This photograph of a soft tissue gross specimen from the foot also shows the appearance of gouty tophi. Urate crystal deposition may occur in tendons, bone, and even articular cartilage.

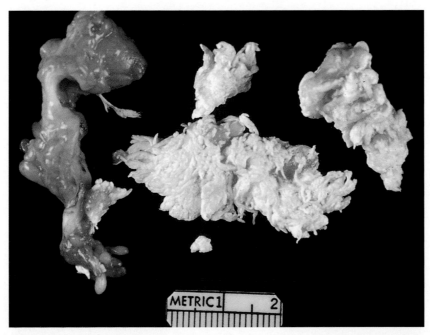

Figure 19–7 Crystalline material from other sources may mimic the gross appearance of gouty tophi. This gross specimen illustrates the appearance of crystalline debris in the soft tissues related to a steroid injection. Such crystalline debris does not show the characteristic birefringence of urates.

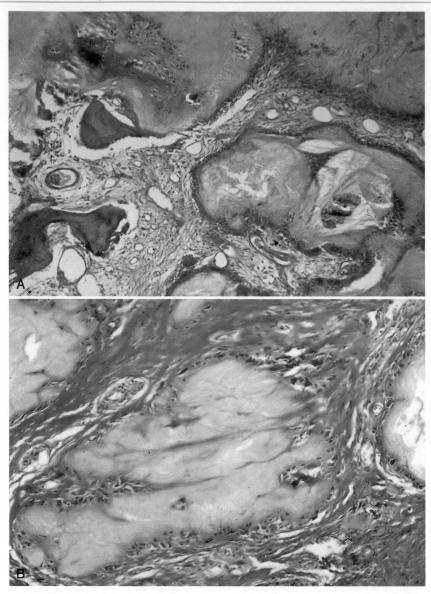

Figure 19–8 *A* and *B*: These two photomicrographs illustrate the histologic appearance of urate in tissue sections stained with hematoxylin and eosin. The urate crystals may be dissolved in processing through water-based solutions, but if present in significant quantities, the crystals will frequently be found even after routine processing.

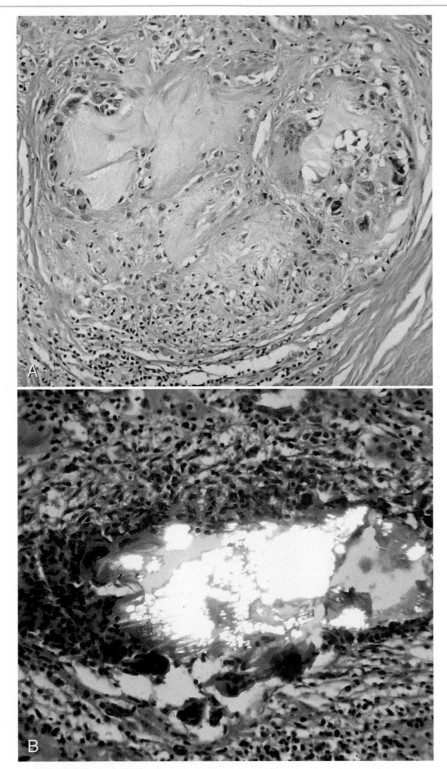

Figure 19–9 *A* and *B*: These two photomicrographs illustrate a histiocytic and giant cell reaction to urate deposits that is common in the soft tissues surrounding gouty tophi. Processing of tissue in alcohol and staining with the De Galantha technique may aid in the identification of these deposits.

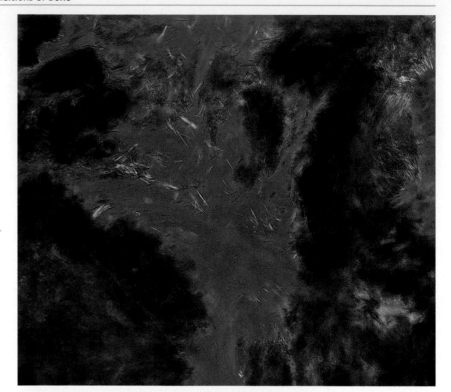

Figure 19–10 This photomicrograph demonstrates the appearance of urate crystals in a frozen section stained with toluidine blue. With this technique the crystals appear brown.

Figure 19–11 This photomicrograph reveals a lytic defect in the calcaneus of a 25-year-old female patient. The characteristic punched-out pattern of lytic bone destruction without the reaction of gout is present. This patient was asymptomatic (see Fig. 19–12).

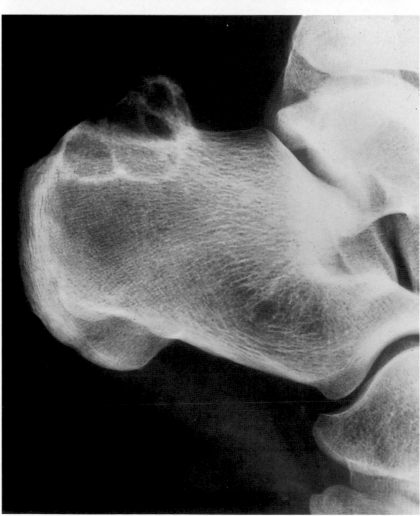

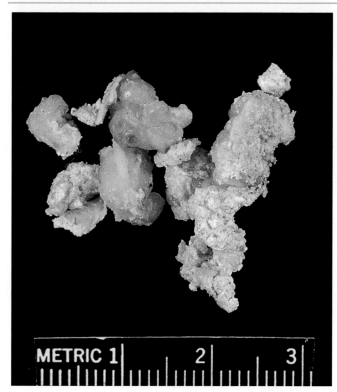

Figure 19–12 This photograph of a gross specimen illustrates the appearance of the curetted material from the calcaneal lytic lesion shown in Figure 19–11. Whitish urate crystalline islands are identifiable within reactive connective tissue.

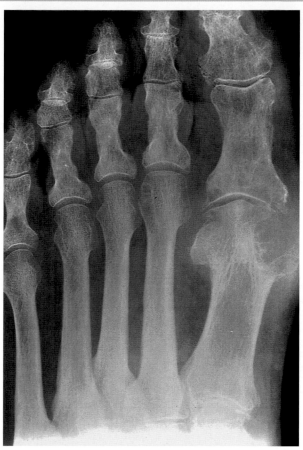

Figure 19–14 This radiograph of the foot of a 75-year-old man demonstrates the punched-out lytic lesions typical of gout involving the metacarpophalangeal joint of the great toe.

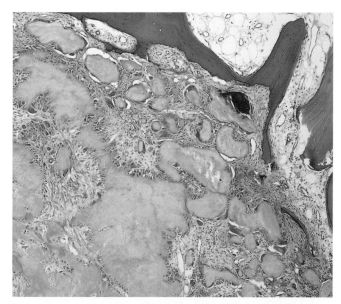

Figure 19–13 Histologically, urate crystals within the bony lytic defects of gout are frequently surrounded by a giant cell reaction. At low magnification, the pattern may mimic that of a caseating granulomatous infectious disease.

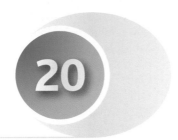

Chondrocalcinosis (Pseudogout, Calcium Pyrophosphate Dihydrate Crystal Deposition Disease)

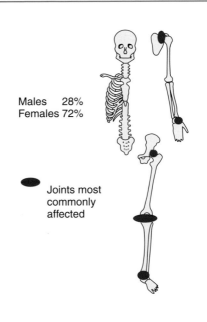

Males   28%
Females 72%

Joints most commonly affected

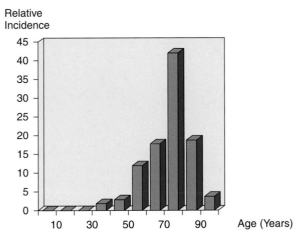

Note: Acute arthritic complaints involve knee, wrist, ankle and hand in decreasing order of frequency.
Prevalence: increases in the population with age up to 30% of those older than 75 years

Clinical Signs

1. The earliest signs are most commonly related to the knee joint. (Although the lower limb joints are most commonly involved in both men and women, the predilection is more marked in men.)
2. Multiple joints commonly affected, in order of frequency, are knees, ankles, wrists, elbows, hips, and shoulders.
3. Hyperuricemia may be present (gout must be ruled out).
4. Effusion of the knee joint is seen in patients with chronic disease.
5. Heberden's nodes may be seen.

6. Diseases associated with calcium pyrophosphate deposition disease include the following:
   a. Hemochromatosis.
   b. Hypophosphatasia.
   c. Hypomagnesemia.
   d. Hyperparathyroidism.
   e. Hypothyroidism.

Clinical Symptoms

1. Acute swelling (goutlike symptoms) can occur and may be associated with trauma, surgery, or other illness.

2. The majority of patients are asymptomatic.
3. Onset is in the sixth or seventh decade of life.
4. Multiple joints may be symmetrically affected, simulating rheumatoid disease.
5. Rapid joint destruction simulates Charcot's arthropathy.
6. Stiffening of the spine, usually familial, may occur.
7. Although patients may present with acute attacks, the mean duration of symptoms prior to diagnosis is approximately 10 years.

Major Radiographic Features

1. Punctate or linear mineralization is evident in fibrocartilage and possibly in hyaline cartilage, usually bilaterally.
2. Fibrocartilage is most intensely mineralized in the knee menisci, triangular ligament of the wrist, and pubic symphysis.
3. Capsular mineralization involving the hips and shoulders, as well as the metacarpophalangeal and metatarsophalangeal joints, may be seen. Capsular calcification is often the result of hydroxyapatite deposition (HADD).
4. Subchondral linear mineralization parallel to the end plate may be evident.
5. The joint space may show narrowing.
6. Calcification of the interspinous and supraspinous ligaments and the ligamentum flavum may be seen.
7. Spinal canal narrowing may occur related to massive crystal deposition ("tophaceous pseudogout") and osteophyte formation.
8. Large, weightbearing joints tend to show the greatest probability for progressive degenerative changes.

Radiographic Differential Diagnosis

1. Osteoarthritis.
2. Hyperparathyroidism.
3. Hemochromatosis.
4. Wilson's disease.

Major Pathologic Features

1. Grossly, deposits are chalky white and may be either crystalline or amorphous.
2. Deposits are usually surrounded by a cuff of histiocytes and multinucleated giant cells.
3. The crystals are more rhomboid than needle-like (as in gout) and are weakly positively birefringent.
4. The cartilaginous lacunae become enlarged and may coalesce.
5. The cartilage matrix adjacent to the lacunae undergoes a mucoid degenerative change.

Pathologic Differential Diagnosis

1. Gout.
2. Residual effect from prior steroid injection.

Treatment

1. Primary disease, if present (e.g., hemochromatosis, hyperparathyroidism, diabetes, ochronosis) must be identified and treated.
2. For acute attacks, the following may be used:
   a. Nonsteroidal anti-inflammatory agents (NSAIDs) (e.g., indomethacin, naproxen).
   b. Aspiration and intraarticular injection of steroids (e.g., triamcinolone, 10 to 40 mg).
3. Prophylaxis may be accomplished with colchicine (0.6 mg by mouth twice a day).

References

Agarwal AK: Gout and pseudogout [review]. *Prim Care* 20(4):839–855, 1993.

Doherty M: Calcium pyrophosphate in joint disease [review]. *Hosp Pract (Off Ed)* 29(11):93–96, 99–100, 103–104, 1994.

Elborn JS, Kelly J, Roberts SD: Pseudogout, chondrocalcinosis and the early recognition of haemochromatosis. *Ulster Med J* 61(1):119–123, 1992.

Keen CE, Crocker PR, Brady K, et al: Calcium pyrophosphate dihydrate deposition disease: morphological and microanalytical features. *Histopathology* 19(6):529–536, 1991.

Masuda I, Ishikawa K, Usuku G: A histologic and immunohistochemical study of calcium pyrophosphate dihydrate crystal deposition disease. *Clin Orthop Rel Res* (263):272–287, 1991.

Pritzker KP: Calcium pyrophosphate dihydrate crystal deposition and other crystal deposition diseases [review]. *Curr Opin Rheumatol* 6(4):442–447, 1994.

Ryan LM: Calcium pyrophosphate dihydrate crystal deposition and other crystal deposition diseases [review]. *Curr Opin Rheumatol* 5(4):517–521, 1993.

Timms AE, Zhang Y, Russell RG, Brown MA: Genetic studies of disorders of calcium crystal deposition. *Rheumatology* 41(7):725–729, 2002.

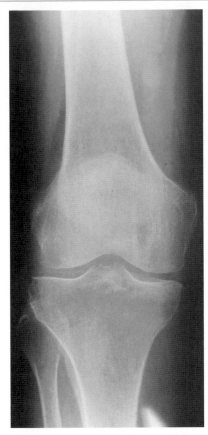

Figure 20–1 This radiograph illustrates the features of chondrocalcinosis of the knee in a 94-year-old woman. Calcification of the menisci and articular cartilage is common in this condition.

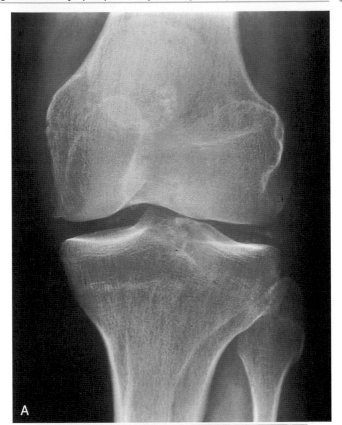

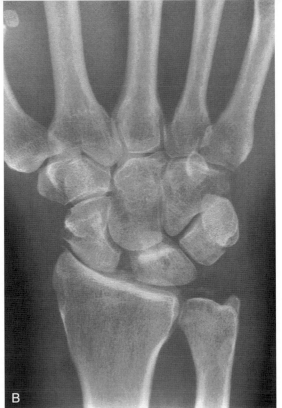

Figure 20–3 Radiographs of the knee (*A*) and wrist (*B*) illustrate chondrocalcinosis involving the joints of a 64-year-old female patient.

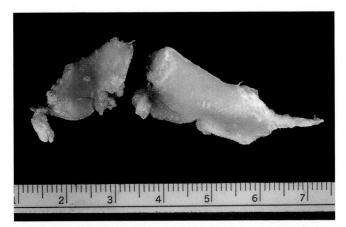

Figure 20–2 The gross appearance of chondrocalcinosis is demonstrated in this specimen from a meniscus. Grossly, the whitish crystalline deposition of calcium pyrophosphate can mimic the appearance of urate tophi.

Amyloidosis

Clinical Signs

1. Clinically evident masses of amyloid are uncommon.
2. Generally, amyloidosis involves multiple joints bilaterally because it is a systemic process.
3. Patients with hemodialysis-related amyloidosis may present with trigger finger, flexor tendon contracture, spontaneous tendon rupture, or pathologic fracture.
4. Carpal tunnel syndrome, most often bilateral, may be seen.
5. Findings related to other organ malfunction (e.g., chronic renal failure or cardiomyopathy) may be present.

Clinical Symptoms

1. The patient may be asymptomatic.
2. Symptoms of carpal tunnel syndrome may be present.
3. Pain secondary to compression fracture may be experienced.
4. Joint pain is the most common presenting complaint of patients with hemodialysis-related amyloidosis.
5. Joint stiffness may be present.

Major Imaging Features

1. Juxta-articular osteoporosis may be seen.
2. Soft tissue swelling may be present.
3. Subchondral bone cysts may be evident.
4. The joint spaces appear relatively preserved.
5. Vertebral compression fractures may be seen.
6. The localized lytic form of the disease tends to affect the long bones, skull, and ribs, resulting in well-marginated lytic lesions.
7. Pathologic fracture may be present.
8. Amyloid deposits in soft tissue and especially synovium usually have a distinctive short T2-signal appearance on magnetic resonance imaging.

Radiographic Differential Diagnosis

1. Metastases.
2. Lymphoma.
3. Myeloma.

Major Pathologic Features

1. Deposits of eosinophilic amorphous material may be seen in soft tissues or bone.
2. Congo red stains reveal apple-green birefringent masses when viewed with polarized light.
3. Deposits tend to occur in vessel walls.
4. When tumefactive deposits are present, histiocytic and giant cell reactions are commonly seen.
5. Dialysis-associated amyloid bone disease likely shows the histologic changes associated with chronic renal failure because patients who develop amyloid bone disease in this setting have almost invariably been receiving dialysis for longer than 10 years.

Pathologic Differential Diagnosis

1. Dense fibrosis.
2. Amyloid deposition associated with plasma cellular proliferative disorders.

Treatment

Medical

1. The predisposing disease must be treated. Most cases at this time are related to an underlying plasma cell dyscrasia, which may require chemotherapy.

Surgical

1. Localized amyloid deposits (amyloidomas) may be excised.
2. Symptoms resulting from carpal tunnel syndrome may be treated with carpal tunnel decompression.

References

Boccalatte M, Pratesi G, Calabrese G, et al: Amyloid bone disease and highly permeable synthetic membranes. *Int J Artif Organs* 17(4): 203–208, 1994.

Georgiades CS, Neyman EG, Barish MA, et al: Amyloidosis: review and CT manifestations. *Radiographics* 24(2):405–416, 2004.

Gravallese EM, Baker N, Lester S, et al: Musculoskeletal manifestations in beta 2-microglobulin amyloidosis. Case discussion [clinical conference]. *Arthritis Rheum* 35(5):592–602, 1992.

Kurer MH, Baillod RA, Madgwick JC: Musculoskeletal manifestations of amyloidosis. A review of 83 patients on haemodialysis for at least 10 years. *J Bone Joint Surg Br* 73(2):271–276, 1991.

Ross LV, Ross GJ, Mesgarzadeh M, et al: Hemodialysis-related amyloidomas of bone. *Radiology* 178(I):263–265, 1991.

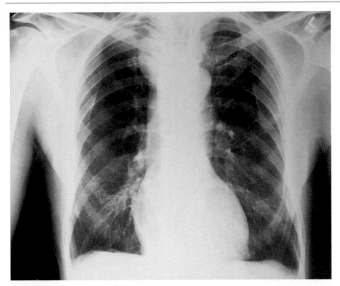

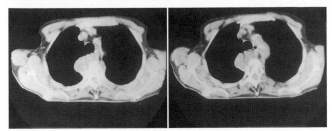

Figure 21–2 The lesion of Figure 21–1 is better seen in this computed tomographic (CT) scan. The patient had an amyloid tumor destroying the vertebra and had no evidence of myeloma at the time of diagnosis.

Figure 21–1 This radiograph of the chest of a 78-year-old man demonstrates a lytic lesion in the fourth thoracic vertebra.

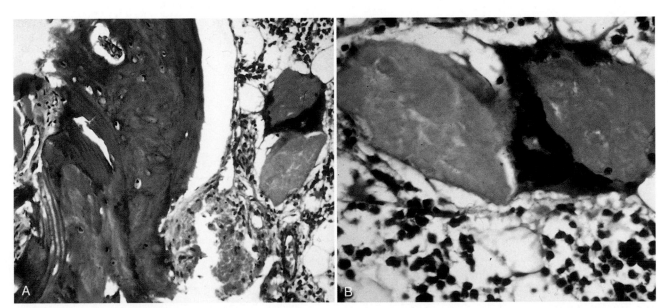

Figure 21–3 *A* and *B*: A region of calcified amyloid is identified adjacent to a bony trabecula in this biopsy specimen from a 55-year-old woman. The surrounding marrow does not show evidence of a plasmacytosis.

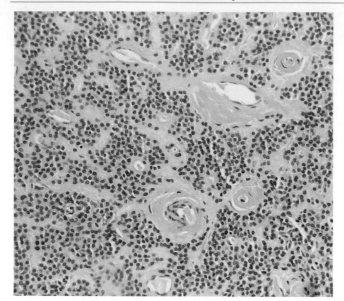

Figure 21–4 This photomicrograph illustrates amyloid deposition in the region of a plasmacellular proliferation from the 12th thoracic vertebra of a 51-year-old man. This was a solitary lesion at the time of diagnosis. The condition is best diagnosed as a solitary plasmacytoma rather than an amyloid tumor because of the presence of a plasmacellular proliferation in the region of the amyloid.

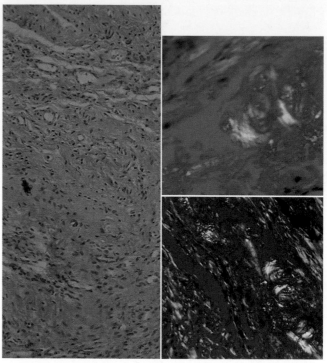

Figure 21–6 This set of photomicrographs shows specimens from the carpal tunnel of an elderly patient who presented with signs of carpal tunnel syndrome. A dense eosinophilic amorphous deposit of amyloid is visible in the tissue from the carpal ligament. When the specimen is viewed under polarized light, Congo red stains show the congophilic material to have the apple-green birefringent characteristic of amyloid.

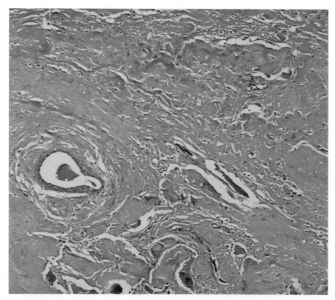

Figure 21–5 At times the amyloid deposited in regions of myeloma may be so dense as to almost totally replace any plasmacellular proliferation, as shown in this example of myeloma involving the scapula. Any plasmacellular proliferation associated with amyloid deposition should raise doubts about a diagnosis of any amyloid tumor.

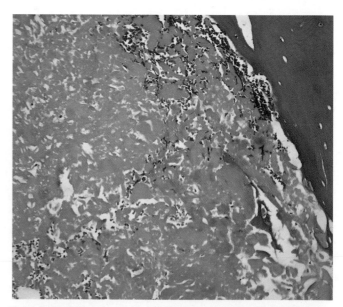

Figure 21–7 This photomicrograph illustrates a nodule of amyloid in the femur. Only when there are no identifiable plasma cells in the region of the amyloid, as in this case, is it reasonable to make a diagnosis of an amyloid tumor of bone. The majority of such lesions are associated with myeloma.

Figure 21–8 Amyloid deposition associated with long-term renal dialysis complicates the changes seen in the small bones of the hand in this 50-year-old patient who receives dialysis.

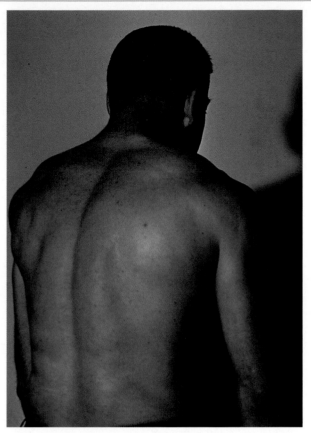

Figure 21–9 Amyloid deposition in skeletal muscle may result in striking changes, as illustrated in this clinical photograph. There is a great disparity between the clinical appearance of well-formed muscle masses and the deterioration of strength associated with amyloid deposition.

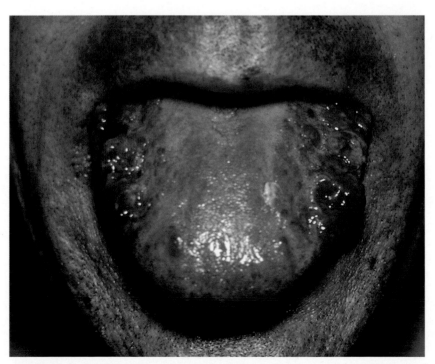

Figure 21–10 Masses of amyloid involve the tongue in this patient. Macroglossia may be associated with amyloidosis.

Xanthomatosis

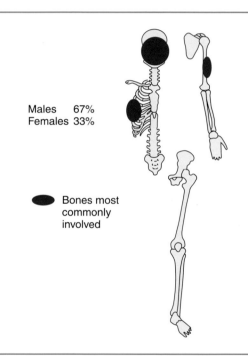

Males   67%
Females   33%

⬤ Bones most commonly involved

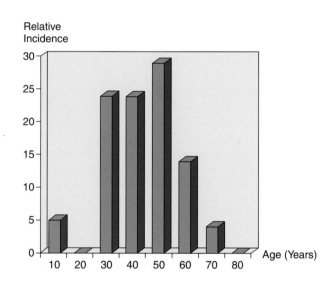

Clinical Signs

1. Lipid may accumulate in histiocytes, forming skin nodules (particularly over the extensor tendons of the fingers and the Achilles tendon).
2. Hypercholesterolemia may be present.

Clinical Symptoms

1. Pain may be experienced.
2. There may be incidental skeletal findings.
3. Involvement of the orbital bones may result in proptosis or diplopia or both.

Major Imaging Features

1. Xanthomatosis rarely results in skeletal abnormalities; when it does, patchy sclerosis and focal lytic destruction can be seen.
2. Lesions tend to be round to oval and less than 4 cm.
3. Lesions are sharply marginated, with a rim of surrounding sclerosis.
4. Cortical expansion may be present.
5. Ultrasound and magnetic resonance imaging (MRI) will demonstrate thickening of affected tendons.

6. On MRI the axial images show a diffuse reticulated pattern, and on T1-weighted sequences foci of high signal are attributed to triglyceride deposition.

Imaging Differential Diagnosis

1. Giant cell tumor.
2. Sinus histiocytosis with massive lymphadenopathy.
3. Fibrous dysplasia.
4. Metaphyseal fibrous defect.
5. Unicameral bone cyst.
6. Osteoblastoma.
7. Langerhans' cell histiocytosis.
8. Radiographic differential diagnosis is broad because of nonspecific osseous findings.
9. MRI: differential diagnoses; traumatic or degenerative Achilles tendinopathy when the process involves tendon.

Major Pathologic Features

1. Grossly, the lesional tissue is yellowish.
2. Histologically, the marrow is replaced by foamy histiocytes and shows varying degrees of fibrosis and inflammation.
3. Cleftlike spaces are present amid the lipid-laden histiocytes, and these spaces represent cholesterol crystals that have been dissolved during tissue processing.
4. Multinucleated giant cells are commonly present.
5. Hemosiderin pigment is present in approximately 60% of lesions.
6. Fibrosis is commonly seen.
7. Scattered foci of calcification may be evident.

Pathologic Differential Diagnosis

1. Erdheim-Chester disease.
2. Langerhans' cell histiocytosis.
3. Sinus histiocytosis with massive lymphadenopathy (Rosai-Dorfman disease).

4. Osteomyelitis.
5. Metastatic clear cell carcinoma (particularly if the biopsy is a needle biopsy or aspiration cytology).
6. Benign fibrous histiocytoma.

Treatment

Medical

1. Underlying hyperlipoproteinemias must be recognized and treated.
2. Articular, tendinous, and periarticular manifestations are treated symptomatically (e.g., nonsteroidal anti-inflammatory drugs [NSAIDs]).

Surgical

1. Symptomatic xanthomas are excised.

References

Bertoni F, Capanna R, Calderoni P, et al: Case report 223. Benign fibrous histiocytoma. *Skeletal Radiol* 9(3):215–217, 1983.

Eble JN, Rosenberg AE, Young RH: Retroperitoneal xanthogranuloma in a patient with Erdheim-Chester disease [review]. *Am J Surg Pathol* 18(8):843–848, 1994.

Fink MG, Levinson DJ, Brown NL, et al: Erdheim-Chester disease. Case report with autopsy findings. *Arch Pathol Lab Med* 115(6):619–623, 1991.

Hamilton WC, Ramsey PL, Hanson SM, et al: Osseous xanthoma and multiple hand tumors as a complication of hyperlipidemia. Report of a case. *J Bone Joint Surg Am* 57(4):551–553, 1975.

Liem MSL, Leuven JAG, Bloem JL, et al: Magnetic resonance imaging of Achilles tendon xanthomas in familial hypercholesterolemia. *Skeletal Radiol* 21(7):453–457, 1992.

Yaghmai I: Intra- and extraosseous xanthomata associated with hyperlipidemia. *Radiology* 128(1):49–54, 1978.

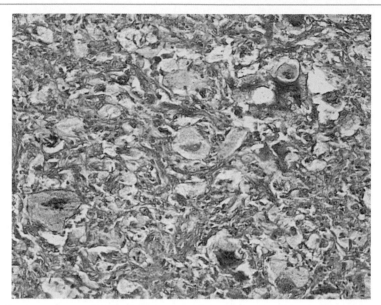

Figure 22–1 This photomicrograph illustrates numerous lipid-laden histiocytes and scattered giant cells in a xanthoma. Many benign bone tumors may undergo degenerative changes and show a similar xanthomatous morphology.

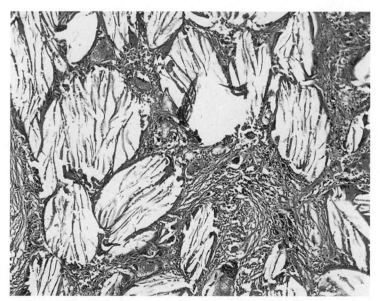

Figure 22–2 Numerous cholesterol clefts, the result of cholesterol crystal formation that is subsequently removed by tissue processing, are present in this lesion from the ilium. If no residual identifiable benign tumor is present in such a lesion, then xanthoma may be used as a descriptive diagnosis.

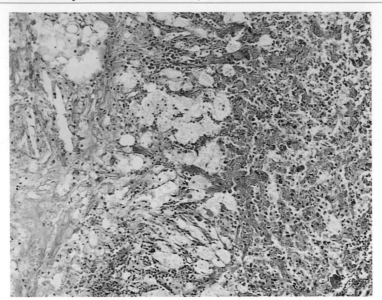

Figure 22–3 This photomicrograph illustrates xanthomatous degenerative changes in a giant cell tumor of the proximal tibia. Hemorrhage and necrosis frequently precede the xanthomatous degeneration in giant cell tumors. If the lesion involves the epiphysis of a long bone in a patient older than 20 years of age, then such histologic features most likely represent degenerative change in a preexisting giant cell tumor.

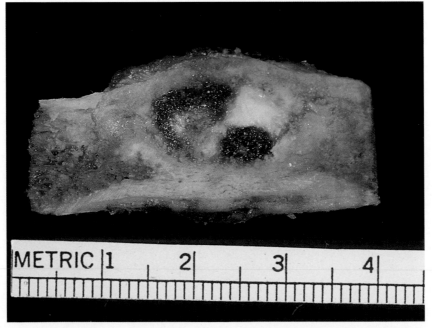

Figure 22–4 This photograph of a gross specimen shows a portion of resected rib with a well-circumscribed defect. The yellow portion of the lesion represents a region of lipid-laden histiocytes, which microscopically have a xanthomatous appearance. Such xanthomatous degeneration of fibrous dysplasia, a lesion commonly found in the ribs, may be mistaken for other tumors when sampled with fine-needle aspiration.

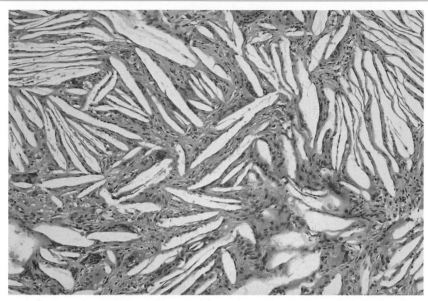

Figure 22–5 This photomicrograph illustrates the degenerative pattern that can be seen in giant cell tumors. Cholesterol clefts and multinucleated giant cells are present. This pattern may simulate that seen in a xanthoma of bone.

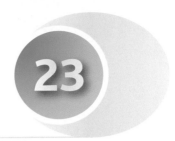

Fibrous Dysplasia

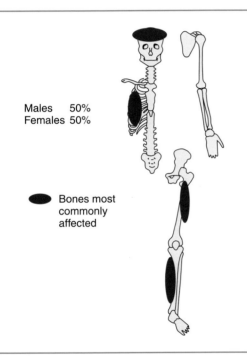

Males   50%
Females 50%

⬤ Bones most
commonly
affected

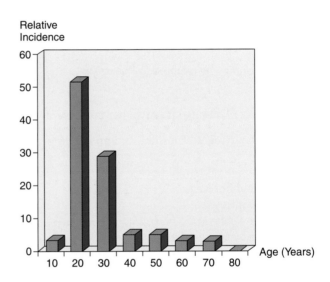

Clinical Symptoms

1. Most patients are asymptomatic.
2. Abnormal bone growth may result in deformity.
3. Pain may be present.
4. Swelling may be noted; when the process involves the skull bones, the patient may present with exophthalmos.
5. Involvement of the femoral neck may result in weakening and resultant pathologic fracture.

Clinical Signs

1. A localized swelling may be found.
2. Exophthalmos may be present if skull bones are involved.

3. Cutaneous pigmentation may be seen in association with polyostotic disease (Albright's syndrome).
4. Precocious puberty in girls may be associated with polyostotic disease (Albright's syndrome).
5. Soft tissue myxomas have been reported in association with fibrous dysplasia (Mazabraud's syndrome).

Major Radiographic Features

1. The location of the lesion is metaphyseal or diaphyseal.
2. The lesion is usually lytic or ground glass–like in density.
3. The affected bone shows expansion and sharp margination of the lesion.

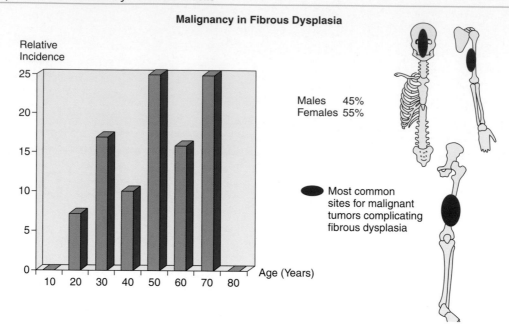

Malignancy in Fibrous Dysplasia

Males   45%
Females 55%

Most common sites for malignant tumors complicating fibrous dysplasia

4. Bowing and pathologic fracture may be seen.
5. The lesion may be surrounded by a thick rind of sclerotic bone.
6. Multiple bones may be affected (polyostotic).

Radiographic Differential Diagnosis

1. Fibroma (metaphyseal fibrous defect, nonossifying fibroma).
2. Unicameral bone cyst (simple cyst).
3. Chondromyxoid fibroma.
4. Aneurysmal bone cyst.
5. Malignancy, if a soft tissue myxoma (Mazabraud's syndrome) is adjacent to the bony lesion.

Major Pathologic Features

Gross

1. Lesional tissue is usually dense and fibrous.
2. Osteoid trabeculae within the fibrous tissue impart a gritty quality to the lesion when it is cut.
3. Prominent cyst formation may be present; such cysts are most commonly filled with a clear, yellowish fluid.
4. Dense ossification may also occur within the lesional tissue.

Microscopic

1. At low magnification, the lesion is composed of proliferating fibroblasts that produce a dense, collagenous matrix.

2. Osteoid trabeculae course irregularly through the connective tissue.
3. The trabeculae are arranged in a haphazard, nonfunctional manner, and they may contain reversal lines mimicking the appearance of Paget's disease.
4. A metaplastic chondroid component may be present and rarely is so prominent as to raise the question of whether the lesion represents a hyaline cartilage neoplasm.
5. Cystic degeneration may be identified. These regions of degeneration may also show numerous lipophages and benign multinucleated giant cells. Rarely, the lesion shows marked myxoid change.
6. At higher magnification, no cytologic atypia is seen.

Pathologic Differential Diagnosis

Benign lesions

1. Paget's disease.
2. Giant cell reparative granuloma.

Malignant lesions

1. Low-grade central osteosarcoma.
2. Parosteal osteosarcoma (if the location is not known).

Treatment

1. **Primary modality**: observation if the lesion is asymptomatic.
2. **Other possible approaches**: curettage and grafting or resection.

References

Azouz EM: Magnetic resonance imaging of benign bone lesions: cysts and tumors. *Topics in Magnetic Resonance Imaging* 13(4):219–229, 2002.

Campanacci M, Laus M: Osteofibrous dysplasia of the tibia and fibula. *J Bone Joint Surg Am* 63(3):367–375, 1981.

DiCaprio MR, Enneking WF: Fibrous dysplasia. Pathophysiology, evaluation, and treatment. *J Bone Joint Surg Am* 87(8):1848–1864, 2005.

Huvos AG, Higinbotham NL, Miller TR: Bone sarcoma arising in fibrous dysplasia. *J Bone Joint Surg Am* 54(5):1047–1056, 1972.

Nager GT, Kennedy DW, Kopstein E: Fibrous dysplasia: a review of the disease and its manifestations in the temporal bone. *Ann Otol Rhinol Laryngol* 92:1–52, 1982.

Nakashima Y, Yamamuro T, Fumiwara Y, et al: Osteofibrous dysplasia (ossifying fibroma of long bones): a study of 12 cases. *Cancer* 52(5):909–914, 1983.

Ruggieri P, Sim FH, Bond JR, et al: Malignancies in fibrous dysplasia. *Cancer* 73(5):1411–1424, 1994.

Weatherby RP, Dahlin DC, Ivins JC: Postradiation sarcoma of bone: review of 78 Mayo Clinic cases. *Mayo Clin Proc* 56(5):294–306, 1981.

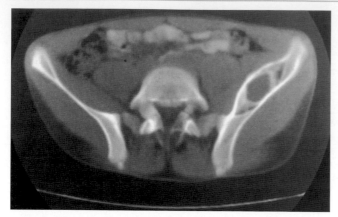

Figure 23–1 This computed tomographic (CT) scan illustrates a sharply marginated lesion of fibrous dysplasia expanding the left iliac bone.

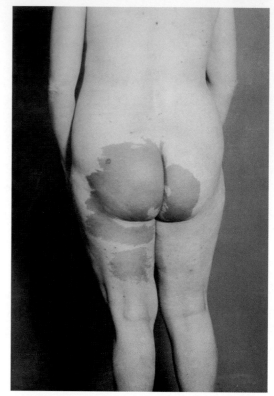

Figure 23–3 Pigmentation, as shown in this photograph, may be seen in cases of Albright's syndrome (polyostotic fibrous dysplasia).

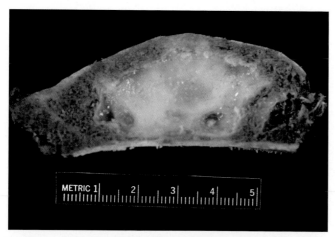

Figure 23–2 The gross pathologic features of the case shown in Figure 23–1 are seen in this photograph. The lesional tissue is whitish. Cystic degeneration is common in old fibrous dysplasia; such degeneration may be accompanied by the presence of numerous lipid-laden histiocytes seen on histologic examination.

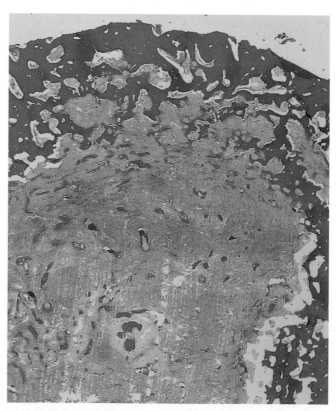

Figure 23–4 At low magnification, fibrous dysplasia is relatively hypocellular and composed of a spindle cell stroma, within which numerous irregular trabeculae of osteoid are present.

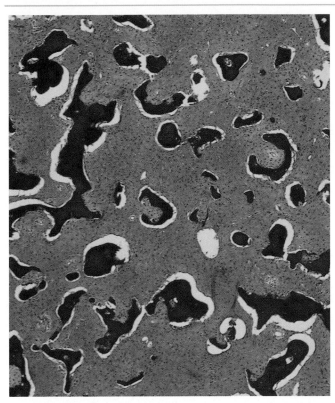

Figure 23–5 At higher magnification, the osteoid is seen to be arranged in a nonfunctional manner. The shape of the osteoid may be irregular or round to oval, as in this case of fibrous dysplasia involving the rib.

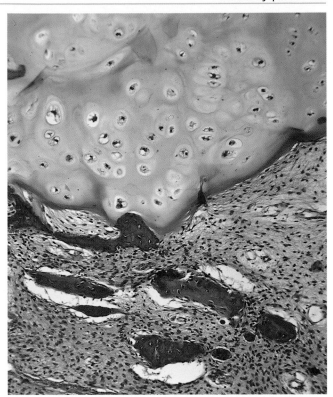

Figure 23–7 Fibrous dysplasia may also have a cartilaginous component; in such cases, the designation of "fibrocartilaginous dysplasia" is appropriate. This example of such a lesion was taken from the femur of a patient with Albright's syndrome.

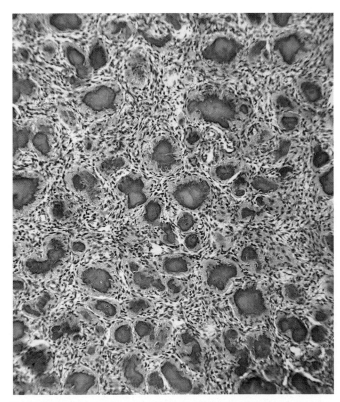

Figure 23–6 Occasionally, the osteoid produced in fibrous dysplasia may mimic the appearance of cementum or even psammomatous calcification, as seen in a meningioma. Such is the case in this lesion of the ilium.

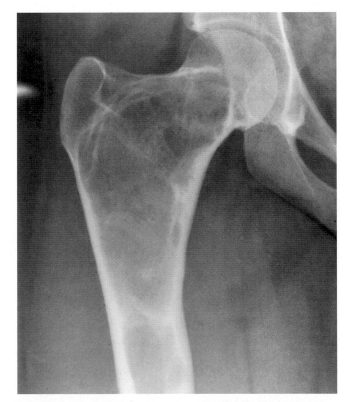

Figure 23–8 The proximal femur is a common location for fibrous dysplasia. This lesion, which has resulted in extensive expansion of the proximal femur, shows the sharp margination and sclerotic rim associated with a benign process.

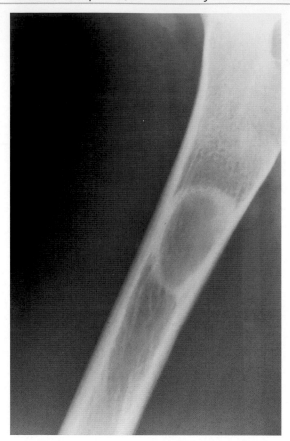

Figure 23–9 The "ground glass" density of fibrous dysplasia is evident in this radiograph of a lesion involving the medulla of the femur. Note the thick rind of surrounding sclerosis.

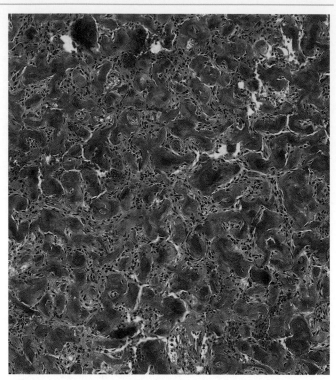

Figure 23–11 Fibrous dysplasia may involve the flat bones of the skull, as in this case. In such cases, the irregular psammoma body–like ossification of the lesion may result in a pattern simulating that of a meningioma secondarily involving the affected bone.

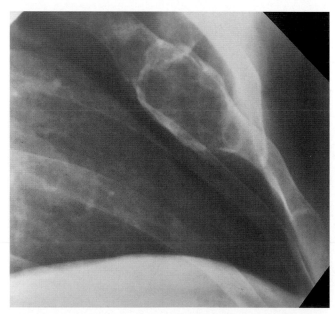

Figure 23–10 The ribs are a common location for fibrous dysplasia. This example shows expansion of the affected rib, frequently seen in such cases, and sclerosis of the surrounding bone.

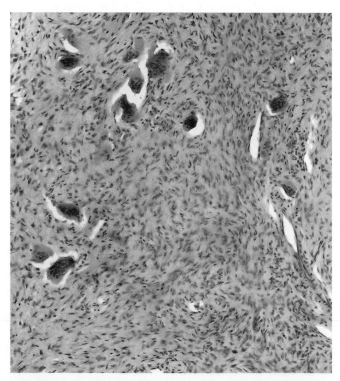

Figure 23–12 Benign multinucleated giant cells may be seen in fibrous dysplasia, as in this case involving the humerus. Like other lesions that contain numerous giant cells, this lesion may be confused with giant cell tumor and other giant cell–containing bone lesions.

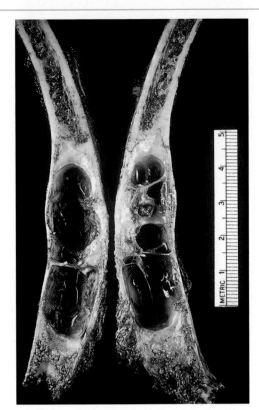

Figure 23–13 Cystic degeneration is most commonly associated with fibrous dysplasia of the rib, as in this case.

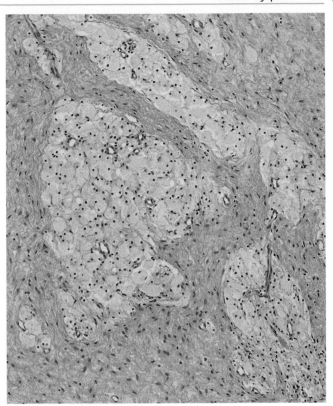

Figure 23–14 Foam cells, or lipid-laden macrophages, also indicate a degenerative process. Such foci are evident in this example of fibrous dysplasia involving the proximal femur.

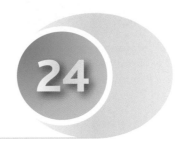

Osteofibrous Dysplasia

Clinical Signs

1. Bowing of the lower extremity may be seen.
2. Abnormal gait (limp) may be present.
3. Leg-length discrepancy may be seen.
4. Pathologic fracture may occur through the lesion.

Clinical Symptoms

1. A painless or, less commonly, painful mass is usually associated with minor trauma.
2. An enlarging mass may be present.
3. Bowing of the lower extremity may be seen.

Major Radiographic Features

1. Osteofibrous dysplasia almost exclusively involves the tibia. (The adjacent fibula may be involved in up to 20% of cases.)
2. Multiple eccentric lytic defects may be seen, most commonly affecting the cortex anteriorly.
3. A diaphyseal location is most common, but the dysplasia may extend to involve the metaphysis.
4. Some cases show a "ground-glass" appearance similar to that of fibrous dysplasia.
5. The cortex is thinned or, rarely, absent in areas of involvement. (Generally, a thin rim of cortex separates the lesion from the medullary bone.)
6. The tibia may be bowed anteriorly.
7. The lesion may have a multiloculated appearance.
8. The periosteum is preserved.
9. Calcifications may be identified within the lesion.
10. Computed tomographic (CT) scans demonstrate cortical involvement without extension to involve the medullary bone.

11. Increased signal on both T1- and T2-weighted magnetic resonance images may be seen.
12. Isotopic bone scan shows increased uptake by the lesional tissue.

Radiographic Differential Diagnosis

1. Adamantinoma.
2. Fibrous dysplasia.
3. Infection.

Major Pathologic Features

Gross

1. Lesional tissue is gray–white and firm.
2. Bony sclerosis may surround the lesional tissue.
3. Lesional tissue is identified within the cortex, which is commonly expanded.

Microscopic

1. Lesional tissue is composed of irregularly shaped trabecular bone lying in fibrous connective tissue.
2. In contrast to typical fibrous dysplasia, the trabecular bone is characteristically surrounded by prominent osteoblastic "rimming."
3. Foci of hemorrhage may be present.
4. Foamy macrophages, presumably degenerative in origin, may be present.
5. In contrast to adamantinoma, epithelial islands are absent.
6. Isolated, scattered individual keratin-positive cells may be identified immunohistochemically within the fibrous connective tissue.

Pathologic Differential Diagnosis

1. Adamantinoma.
2. Fibrous dysplasia.
3. Paget's disease.

Treatment

1. Observation is essential because the process "involutes" with skeletal maturity.
2. Biopsy should be performed if the diagnosis is in question.
3. Resection may be necessary.

References

Campanacci M, Laus M: Osteofibrous dysplasia of the tibia and fibula. *J Bone Joint Surg Am* 63(3):367–375, 1981.

Castellote A, Garcia-Pena P, Lucaya J, et al: Osteofibrous dysplasia. *Skeletal Radiol* 17(7):483–486, 1988.

Park YK, Unni KK, McLeod RA, et al: Osteofibrous dysplasia: clinico-pathologic study of 80 cases. *Hum Pathol* 24(12):1339–1347, 1993.

Wang JW, Shih CH, Chen WJ: Osteofibrous dysplasia (ossifying fibroma of long bones). *Clin Orthop* 278:235–243, 1992.

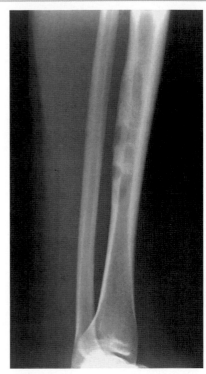

Figure 24–1 This radiograph illustrates the typical appearance of osteofibrous dysplasia involving the tibial cortex. Multiple areas of lucency are surrounded by bony sclerosis. The corresponding gross pathologic appearance of the lesion is shown in Figure 24–2.

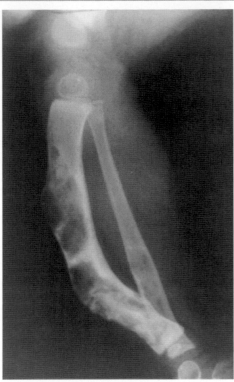

Figure 24–3 This radiograph of the tibia from a 3-year-old girl shows marked bowing of the tibia as a result of its involvement by osteofibrous dysplasia. Although osteofibrous dysplasia is likely a "developmental" condition, congenital cases only rarely have been documented.

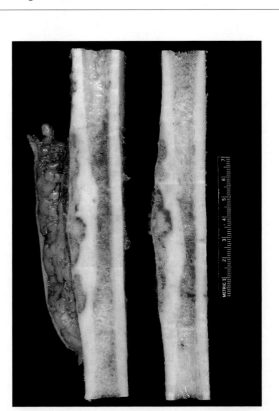

Figure 24–2 This gross specimen is from a case of osteofibrous dysplasia treated with resection. The gray–white lesional tissue involving the cortex is clearly distinct from the surrounding sclerotic reactive bone. Note that the process does not involve the underlying medullary bone.

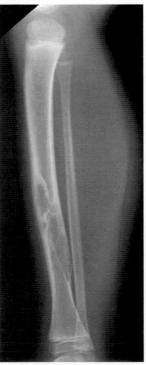

Figure 24–4 Figures 24–4 and 24–5 show the radiographic and CT appearance, respectively, of osteofibrous dysplasia in a 5-year-old male patient. Note the bony sclerosis surrounding the regions of osteolysis and the lack of periosteal reaction.

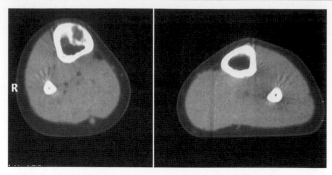

Figure 24–5 This CT scan of the patient in Figure 24–4 shows that the cortex is expanded and deformed by the process of osteofibrous dysplasia, and the underlying medullary bone is uninvolved.

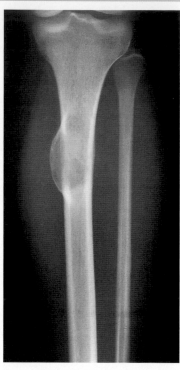

Figure 24–7 This 17-year-old girl presented with a mass lesion involving the anterior aspect of her lower extremity. The radiograph illustrates a more "aneurysmal" expansion of the tibia than is commonly seen in osteofibrous dysplasia. No significant periosteal reaction is evident. Aneurysmal bone cyst change can be seen in a wide variety of bone lesions.

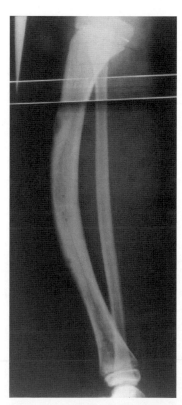

Figure 24–6 This radiograph illustrates osteofibrous dysplasia involving the tibia. Significant bowing is present. This case of a 10-year-old girl had been followed since birth, and the process appeared to be resolving radiographically. Osteofibrous dysplasia generally "involutes" with skeletal maturity.

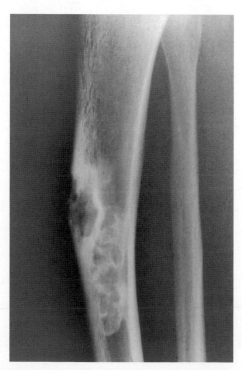

Figure 24–8 This 15-year-old boy has osteofibrous dysplasia of the tibia. The cortex is partially absent, but no significant periosteal reaction is evident. The differential diagnosis for such a lesion most commonly includes adamantinoma.

Ankylosing Spondylitis

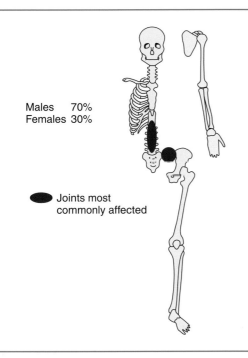

Males 70%
Females 30%

Joints most
commonly affected

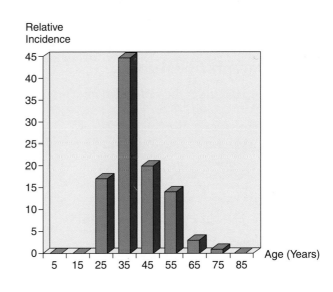

Incidence

The incidence of ankylosing spondylitis is approximately 6.6 per 100,000 population, with a peak incidence in the third and fourth decades. An association exists between the presence of HLA-B27 and a high incidence of ankylosing spondylitis.

Prevalence

The prevalence of ankylosing spondylitis is approximately 400 per 100,000 population. The peak prevalence is in the fifth and sixth decades.

Clinical Signs

1. Males are affected more commonly than females (ratio approximately 9:1 in some studies).
2. Movement of the spine is restricted in all three planes (anterior flexion, lateral flexion, and extension).
3. Approximately 90% of patients have HLA-B27. (*Note:* HLA-B27 is associated with the other spondyloarthropathies as well.)
4. Expansion of the chest is limited, as measured at the level of the fourth intercostal space.
5. Morning stiffness may be present.
6. Symptoms may improve with exercise.

7. A family history of similar disease may be present.
8. Diagnostic criteria for ankylosing spondylitis include the following:
   a. Low back pain and stiffness of greater than 3 months' duration.
   b. Thoracic pain and stiffness.
   c. Limitation of motion of the lumbar vertebrae.
   d. Limitation of chest expansion.
   e. History of iritis or its sequelae.
   f. Bilateral sacroiliac changes on radiography that are characteristic of ankylosing spondylitis.

Clinical Symptoms

1. Low back pain is usually present.
2. Stiffness of the back is greater in the early morning.
3. Involvement of the peripheral joints with arthritic symptoms generally occurs late in the course of the disease.
4. Fatigue, weight loss, and low-grade fever may be present during periods of active disease.

Major Radiographic Features

1. Squaring of the margins of the vertebral bodies may be seen.
2. A "bamboo spine" appearance may be evident.
3. Sclerosis may be present on both sides of the sacroiliac joint.
4. The sacroiliac joint may show fusion.

Radiographic Differential Diagnosis

1. Psoriatic arthritis.
2. Reiter's syndrome.
3. Enteropathic spondylitis.
4. Diffuse idiopathic skeletal hyperostosis (DISH), sacroiliac joint not involved in this condition.

Major Pathologic Features

1. Active endochondral ossification across the intervertebral disc or articular cartilage may be apparent.
2. Inflammatory changes in the synovium are similar but less intense than those seen in rheumatoid arthritis.

Pathologic Differential Diagnosis

1. Rheumatoid arthritis.
2. Psoriatic arthritis.
3. Reiter's syndrome
4. Enteropathic spondylitis.

Treatment

Medical

1. Supportive care, education, and proper nutrition are mainstays of treatment.
2. Physical therapy, exercise to maintain motion, and prevention of spinal deformity are important.
3. Nonsteroidal anti-inflammatory drugs (NSAIDs) may be used. (Aspirin is not as effective as other agents.)
4. Common spine fractures must be recognized and subsequently braced.

Surgical

1. Vertebral wedge osteotomy may be used to correct severe kyphosis.
2. Total joint replacement may be performed in advanced disease.

References

Barozzi L, Olivieri I, De Matteis M, et al: Seronegative spondylarthropathies: imaging of spondylitis, enthesitis and dactylitis. *Eur J Radiol* 27 (Suppl 1):S12–S17, 1998.

Braun J, Bollow M, Sieper J: Radiologic diagnosis and pathology of the spondyloarthropathies. *Rheum Dis Clin North Am* 24(4):697–735, 1998.

Calin A: Differentiating the seronegative spondyloarthropathies: how to characterize and manage ankylosing spondylitis. *J Musculoskel Med* 3:14, 1986.

Gladman DD: Clinical aspects of the spondyloarthropathies. *Am J Med Sci* 316(4):234–238, 1998.

Gran JT, Husby G: Clinical, epidemiologic, and therapeutic aspects of ankylosing spondylitis. *Curr Opin Rheumatol* 10(4):292–298, 1998.

McVeigh CM, Cairns AP: Diagnosis and management of ankylosing spondylitis. *BMJ* 333(7568):581–585, 2006.

Olivieri I, Barozzi L, Padula A, et al: Clinical manifestations of seronegative spondylarthropathies. *Eur J Radiol* 27 (Suppl 1):S3–S6, 1998.

Van der Heijde D, Landewe R: Imaging in spondylitis. *Curr Opin Rheumatol* 17(4):413–417, 2005.

Van der Linden S, van der Heijde D: Ankylosing spondylitis. Clinical features. *Rheum Dis Clin North Am* 24(4):663–766, 1998.

Wordsworth P: Genes in the spondyloarthropathies. *Rheum Dis Clin North Am* 24(4):845–863, 1998.

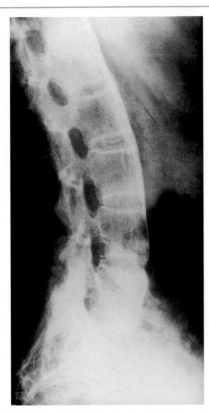

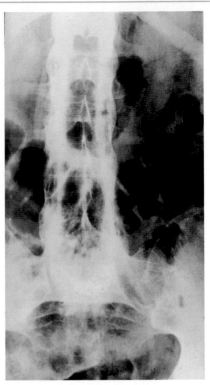

Figure 25–3 This radiograph illustrates the "bamboo spine" appearance of well-developed ankylosing spondylitis.

Figure 25–1 This radiograph illustrates the classic features of ankylosing spondylitis, including squaring of the vertebrae, ossification of the anterior ligament, and fusion of the facets.

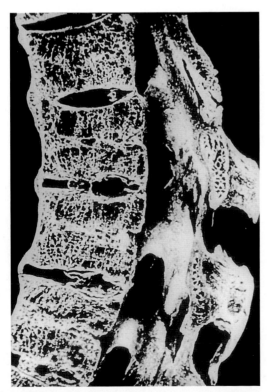

Figure 25–2 This photograph of a macerated specimen is from a patient with ankylosing spondylitis. Some squaring of the vertebrae is evident, but the major feature illustrated is ossification of the anterior ligament and fusion of the vertebral facets.

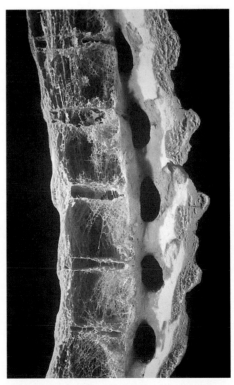

Figure 25–4 This photograph of a macerated specimen from a 71-year-old man who suffered from ankylosing spondylitis demonstrates squaring of the vertebrae and bony ankylosis.

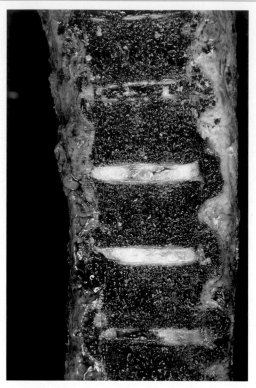

Figure 25–5 This photograph of a gross specimen shows a coronal cross-section of vertebrae in a patient who had well-developed ankylosing spondylitis. Bony ankylosis is evident, and hematopoietic marrow occupies the medullary space of the ankylosed bone.

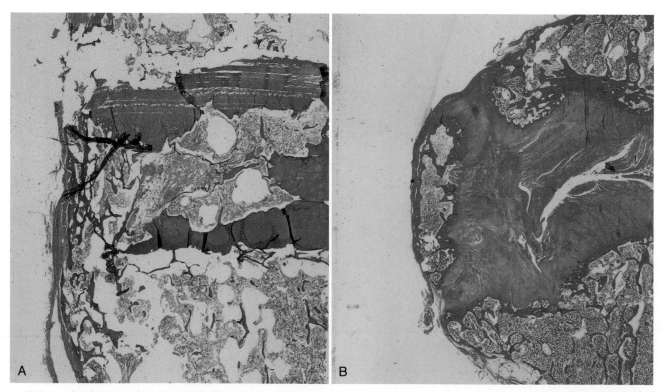

Figure 25–6 *A* and *B*: These two photomicrographs illustrate the histologic appearance of bony ankylosis of the vertebrae. Active endochondral ossification may be seen.

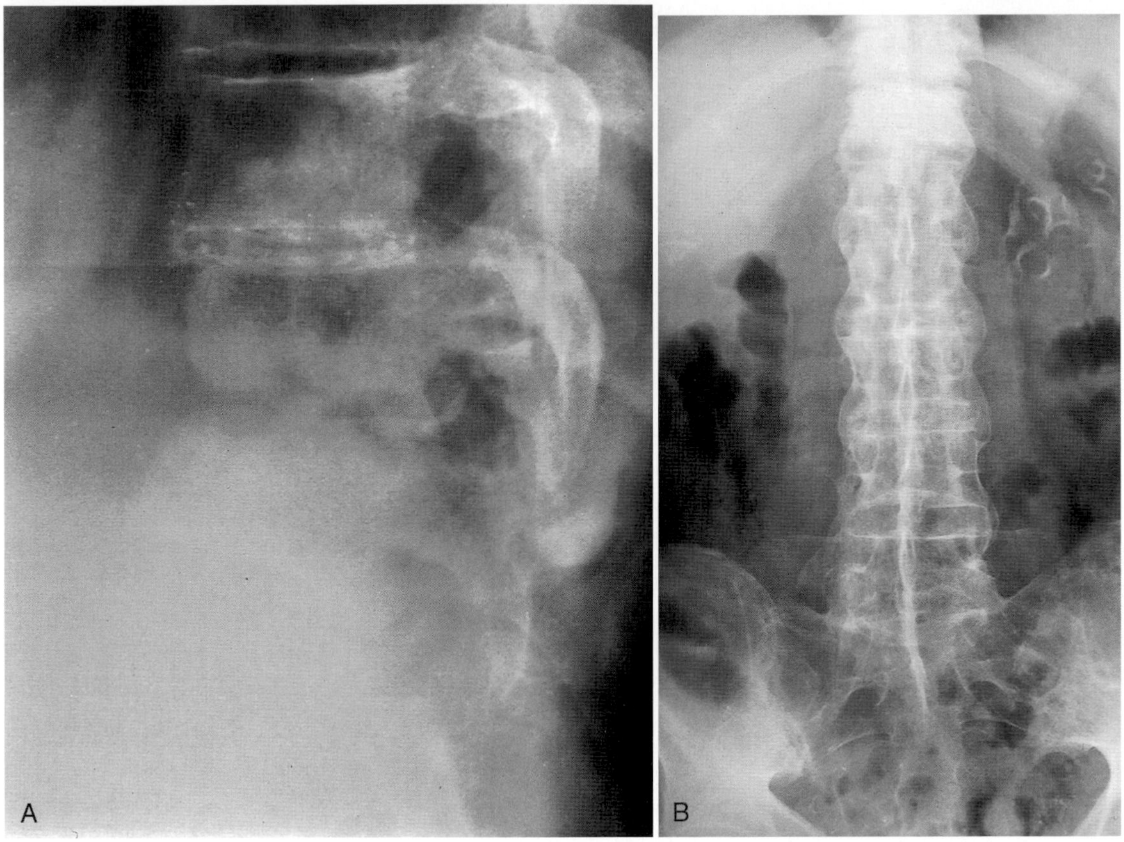

Figure 25–7 Ankylosing spondylitis is shown in these lateral (*A*) and anteroposterior (AP) (*B*) radiographs from a 71-year-old male patient. Bony ankylosis is particularly evident in the AP radiograph.

Synovial Chondromatosis

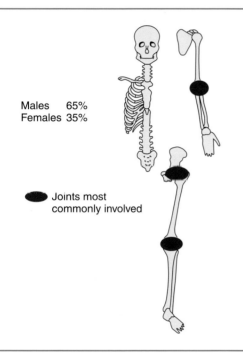

Males 65%
Females 35%

Joints most commonly involved

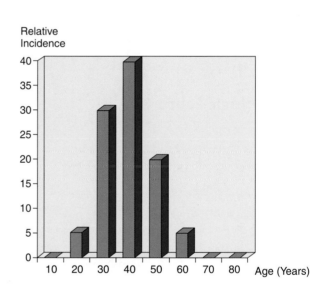

Clinical Signs

1. A monoarticular process is noted.
2. The knee, hip, and elbow are most commonly involved.
3. Joint effusion may be present.
4. Joint aspiration may reveal hemorrhagic fluid, but no crystals are identified.
5. Palpable loose bodies may be present.
6. Progressive arthropathy may occur.

Clinical Symptoms

1. Pain may be experienced in the affected joint. (An insidious course is common.)

2. The affected joint may show swelling.
3. Palpable loose bodies may be present.
4. The affected joint may exhibit loss of motion.
5. "Locking" of the joint may be seen.
6. The affected joint may show instability.

Major Radiographic Features

1. There are soft tissue masses with varying amounts of calcification in the region of the affected joint.
2. Bony erosion may be seen (particularly in joints with tight capsules).
3. Calcific bodies may be present in the soft tissues adjacent to the joint.

4. Joint effusion may be evident.
5. Secondary arthropathy may be present in advanced cases.
6. Arthrogram outlines space-occupying masses in the joint.
7. Bone scan is generally unremarkable.
8. The appearance on magnetic resonance imaging (MRI) is characterized by the following:
   a. Lobulated, homogeneous intra-articular signal isointense to slightly hyperintense to muscle on Tl-weighted images and hyperintense on T2-weighted images.
   b. Pattern **a** with foci of signal void on all pulse sequences (the majority).
   c. Patterns **a** and **b** with foci of peripheral low signal surrounding a central fatlike signal.

Radiographic Differential Diagnosis

1. Osteoarthritis.
2. Pigmented villonodular synovitis.
3. Lipoma arborescens.
4. Chondrosarcoma.
5. Xanthoma (localized nodular synovitis).
6. Popliteal cyst.
7. Gout.

Major Pathologic Features

Gross

1. The synovium is hyperplastic.
2. Nodular projections are present on the synovial surface.
3. Pedunculated masses may be present.
4. Loose bodies may be found in the joint.
5. Masses of cartilage with osseous metaplasia may "invade" the adjacent soft tissue.
6. Secondary osteoarthritic changes may occur, with bony erosion and extension of cartilaginous masses into the eroded bone.

Microscopic

1. Masses of hyaline cartilage are arranged in a nodular pattern.
2. The hyaline cartilage is relatively hypercellular.
3. Mild cytologic atypia may be present.
4. Osseous metaplasia may be seen (particularly at the periphery of the hyaline cartilage masses).
5. Myxoid stromal change of the chondroid matrix is generally absent.

Note: The histologic features resemble those of intramedullary low-grade chondrosarcoma.

Pathologic Differential Diagnosis

1. Chondrosarcoma.
2. Osteoarthritis.

Treatment

1. Total synovectomy (open or arthroscopic) with removal of loose bodies may be performed in patients with active disease.
2. Partial synovectomy (open or arthroscopic) with removal of loose bodies may be performed in patients with localized disease.
3. Loose bodies may be removed in the late phase of the disease.
4. Reconstructive surgery (i.e., total joint arthroplasty) may be performed in patients with advanced arthropathy.

References

Campeau NG, Lewis BD: Ultrasound appearance of synovial osteochondromatosis of the shoulder. *Mayo Clin Proc* 73(11):1079–1081, 1998.

Church JS, Breidahl WH, Janes GC: Recurrent synovial chondromatosis of the knee after radical synovectomy and arthrodesis. *J Bone Joint Surg Br* 88(5):673–675, 2006.

Hamilton A, Davis RI, Nixon JE: Synovial chondrosarcoma complicating synovial chondromatosis: report of a case and review of the literature. *J Bone Joint Surg Am* 69(7):1084–1088, 1987.

Kramer J, Recht M, Deely DM, et al: MR appearance of idiopathic synovial osteochondromatosis. *J Comput Assist Tomogr* 17(5):772–776, 1993.

Maurice H, Crone M, Watt I: Synovial chondromatosis. *J Bone Joint Surg Br* 70(5):807–811, 1988.

Milgram JW: Synovial osteochondromatosis: a histological study of thirty cases. *J Bone Joint Surg Am* 59(6):792–801, 1977.

Murphy FP, Dahlin DC, Sullivan CR: Articular synovial chondromatosis. *J Bone Joint Surg Am* 44:77, 1962.

Ogilvie-Harris DJ, Saleh K: Generalized synovial chondromatosis of the knee: a comparison of removal of the loose bodies alone with arthroscopic synovectomy. *Arthroscopy* 10(2):166–170, 1994.

Shpitzer T, Ganel A, Engelberg S: Surgery for synovial chondromatosis: 26 cases followed up for 6 years. *Acta Orthop Scand* 61(6):567–569, 1990.

Sim FH: Synovial proliferative disorders: role of synovectomy. *Arthroscopy* 1(3):198–204, 1985.

Sim FH, Dahlin DC, Ivins JC: Extra-articular synovial chondromatosis. *J Bone Joint Surg Am* 59(4):492–495, 1977.

Sundaram M, McGuire MH, Fletcher J, et al: Magnetic resonance imaging of lesions of synovial origin. *Skeletal Radiol* 15(2):110–116, 1986.

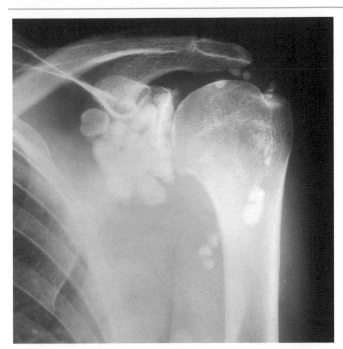

Figure 26–1 This radiograph illustrates synovial chondromatosis involving the shoulder joint. Multiple well-circumscribed calcific densities are noted. Extension into the soft tissues surrounding the joint can occur.

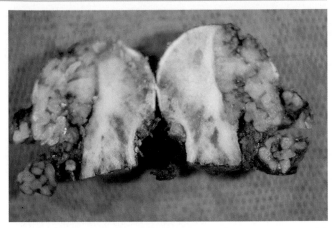

Figure 26–3 This photograph of a gross specimen shows recurrent synovial chondromatosis involving the hip joint. The recurrent lesion has eroded into the head and neck of the femur.

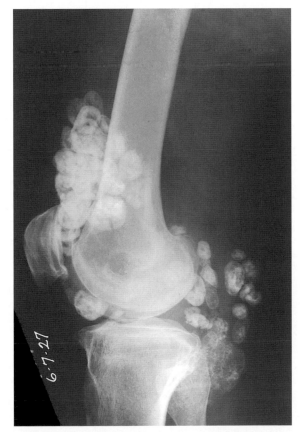

Figure 26–2 This radiograph illustrates synovial chondromatosis involving the knee. Well-circumscribed calcific densities are present both anteriorly and posteriorly. Bony destruction on either side of the joint may occur in such cases.

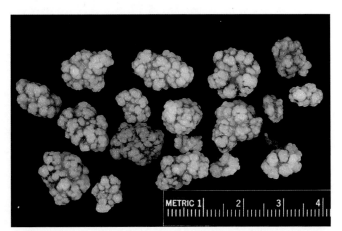

Figure 26–4 This photograph of a gross specimen illustrates the multilobulated nature of loose bodies in synovial chondromatosis. Such loose bodies may be large or small and may mimic the "rice bodies" of osteoarthritis.

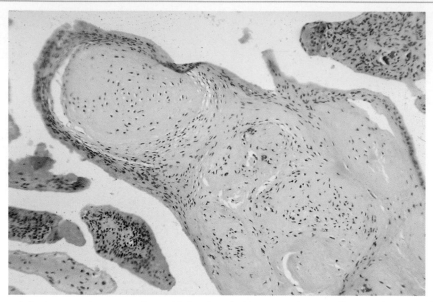

Figure 26–5 This photomicrograph demonstrates the pattern of synovial chondromatosis as seen at low magnification. The synovial lining is identified as overlying the cartilage.

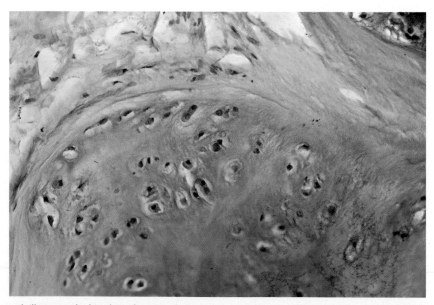

Figure 26–6 This photomicrograph illustrates the histologic features of synovial chondromatosis as seen at high magnification. The cartilage is characteristically relatively hypercellular and may show some nuclear enlargement. These features may mimic a low-grade chondrosarcoma. The lesion is usually lobulated, as shown in this example.

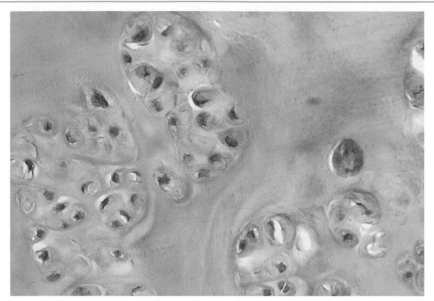

Figure 26–7 This photomicrograph shows the degree of nuclear pleomorphism that can be seen in synovial chondromatosis. The histologic criteria used to differentiate benign from malignant intraosseous cartilage tumors do not apply to cartilaginous lesions of the synovium.

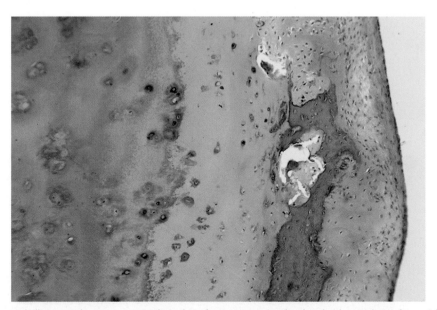

Figure 26–8 This photomicrograph illustrates the osseous metaplasia that often accompanies the chondroid metaplasia of synovial chondromatosis. The bone in such cases most frequently is at the periphery of the cartilage islands.

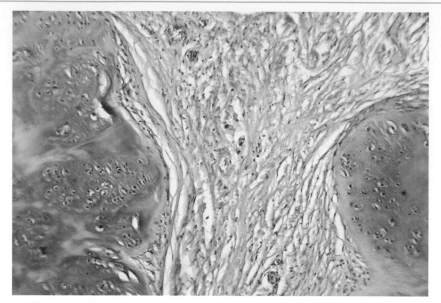

Figure 26–9 This photomicrograph illustrates soft tissue "invasion" in a case of synovial chondromatosis involving the hip. Such invasion is not indicative of malignant degeneration.

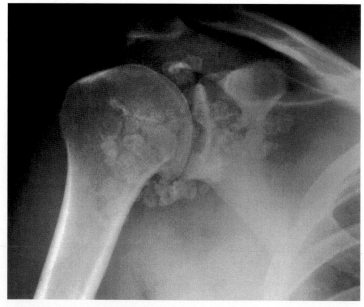

Figure 26–10 This radiograph reveals synovial chondromatosis in the shoulder of a 24-year-old man.

Pigmented Villonodular Synovitis

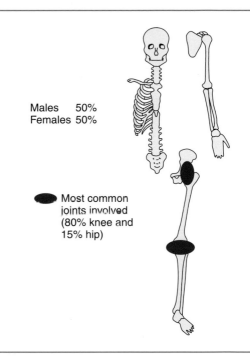

Males 50%
Females 50%

Most common joints involved (80% knee and 15% hip)

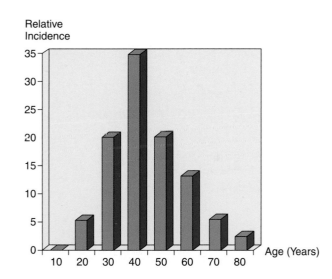

Relative Incidence

Age (Years)

Clinical Signs

1. Joint mobility is limited (in up to 90% of cases).
2. A palpable mass may be present (in approximately 10% of cases).
3. Skin temperature is increased.
4. The clinical examination is often nonspecific.
5. Laboratory tests are generally within normal limits.
6. Synovial fluid is variable in color (yellow to brown or bloody).
7. Recurrent bloody effusions may occur.

Clinical Symptoms

1. The process is monoarticular.
2. Pain may be experienced with motion of the affected joint.
3. Painful swelling of the affected joint may occur.
4. The motion of the affected joint may be limited. ("Locking" of the joint may be described.)
5. Symptoms are generally present for months (average is approximately 4 years).
6. A sudden exacerbation of pain because of torsion of nodules that result from the pathologic process.

Major Radiographic Features

1. Plain radiograph shows the following characteristics:
   a. Lucencies on either side of the affected joint. When present, these are generally multiple and have a thin, sclerotic margin.
   b. Joint space narrowing, particularly if the disease involves the hip.
   c. Associated osteoporosis.
   d. Associated osteosclerosis.
   e. Osteophytes, which are uncommonly present.
   f. Soft tissue swelling.
2. Magnetic resonance imaging (MRI) shows the following characteristics:
   a. Low signal on both T1- and T2-weighted images (as a result of hemosiderin deposition and fibrous connective tissue in the lesion).
   b. Presence of "fat" signal within the mass lesion.
   c. Erosion of bone (most common in the hips, tibiofibular joint, and lumbar facet joints and detected in approximately 60% of cases on MRI).
   d. Preservation of the joint space.
   e. Grapelike mass with a signal density approximately equal to that of muscle.
   f. Effusion, which is present in the majority of patients with knee involvement.

Radiographic Differential Diagnosis

1. Synovial chondromatosis.
2. Rheumatoid arthritis.
3. Synovial hemangioma.
4. Lipoma arborescens.
5. Osteoarthritis.
6. Hemophilia.

Major Pathologic Features

Gross

1. The synovium is characterized as the following:
   a. Nodular.
   b. Villous.
   c. Diffuse.
   d. Combination of the above.
2. The cut surface of the synovium is thickened and usually diffusely yellow and light brown, depending on whether regions rich in hemosiderin-laden macrophages or lipid-laden macrophages predominate.

Microscopic

1. There is proliferation of round to polygonal cells, with scant cytoplasm forming villous finger-like or rounded masses underlying the synovial lining.
2. Nuclei are small and round to oval.
3. Nuclear grooves may be identifiable.
4. Variable amounts of fibrous connective tissue are present.
5. Mitoses are generally inconspicuous.
6. Lipid-laden histiocytes are scattered throughout the lesion or gathered in clusters.
7. Multinucleated giant cells are scattered throughout the lesion.
8. Hemosiderin-laden macrophages are variable in number but may be present in large numbers, giving the synovium a dark-brown appearance.

Pathologic Differential Diagnosis

1. Changes associated with prior arthroplasty.
2. Synovial hyperplasia associated with degenerative joint disease.
3. Benign fibrous histiocytoma (if location is not known).
3. Giant cell tumor of tendon sheath (if location is not known).
4. Malignant fibrous histiocytoma.

Note: The histologic features of pigmented villonodular synovitis, metaphyseal fibrous defect (nonossifying fibroma), giant cell tumor of tendon sheath type, and benign fibrous histiocytoma overlap entirely. The location of the lesion is the differentiating feature of these conditions.

Treatment

1. Total synovectomy by open or arthroscopic techniques is necessary in the diffuse type of disease. Usually anterior and posterior synovectomy of the knee is required, and the recurrence rate is approximately 20% to 40%.
2. Intraarticular yttrium-90 radiation synovectomy is experimental.
3. Surgical excision (arthroscopic or open) is curative in patients with localized disease.
4. Reconstructive surgery is indicated for patients with extensive joint destruction (i.e., arthrodesis or joint replacement).

References

Bertoni F, Unni KK, Beabout JW, et al: Malignant giant cell tumor of the tendon sheaths and joints (malignant pigmented villonodular synovitis). *Am J Surg Pathol* 21(2):153–163, 1997.

Cotten A, Flipo RM, Chastanet P, et al: Pigmented villonodular synovitis of the hip: review of radiographic features in 58 patients. *Skeletal Radiol* 24(1):1–6, 1995.

Dorwart RH, Genant HK, Johnston WH, et al: Pigmented villonodular synovitis of synovial joints: clinical, pathologic and radiologic features. *Am J Roentgenol* 143(4):886–888, 1984.

Flandry F, Hughston JC: Pigmented villonodular synovitis. *J Bone Joint Surg Am* 69(6):942–949, 1987.

Giannini C, Scheithauer BW, Wenger, DE, et al: Pigmented villonodular synovitis of the spine: a clinical, radiological and morphological study of 12 cases. *J Neurosurg* 84(4):592–597, 1996.

Gitelis S, Heligman D, Morton T: The treatment of pigmented villonodular synovitis of the hip. *Clin Orthop* 239:154–160, 1989.

Goldman AB, DiCarlo EF: Pigmented villonodular synovitis. Diagnosis and differential diagnosis. *Radiol Clin North Am* 26(6):1327–1347, 1988.

Hughes TH, Sartoris DJ, Schweitzer ME, et al: Pigmented villonodular synovitis: MRI characteristics. *Skeletal Radiol* 24(1):7–12, 1995.

Ogilvie-Harris DJ, McLean J, Zarnett ME: Pigmented villonodular synovitis of the knee. The results of total arthroscopic synovectomy, partial, arthroscopic synovectomy, and arthroscopic local excision. *J Bone Joint Surg Am* 74(1):119–123, 1992.

Schwartz HS, Unni KK, Pritchard DJ: Pigmented villonodular synovitis. A retrospective review of affected large joints. *Clin Orthop* 247:243–255, 1989.

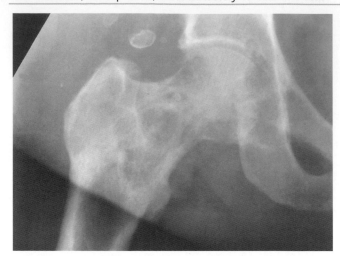

Figure 27–1 This radiograph illustrates bony destruction on either side of the hip joint in a 66-year-old woman with pigmented villonodular synovitis. Well-defined lytic defects with some adjacent sclerosis are identified.

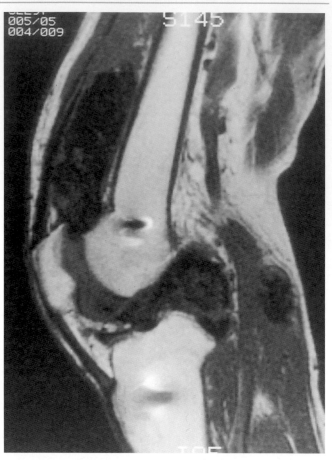

Figure 27–3 The magnetic resonance imaging (MRI) appearance of pigmented villonodular synovitis involving the knee is illustrated in this figure. The low–signal-intensity lesion extends posteriorly into the popliteal fossa and into the distal femur and proximal tibia.

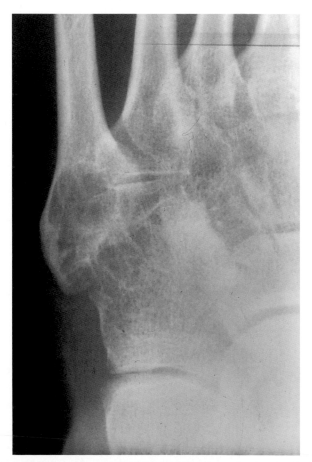

Figure 27–2 This radiograph illustrates the bony destruction associated with pigmented villonodular synovitis of the foot in a 50-year-old woman. Peripheral sclerosis adjacent to the bony lytic defects is well illustrated. Soft tissue masses may also be appreciated in such cases.

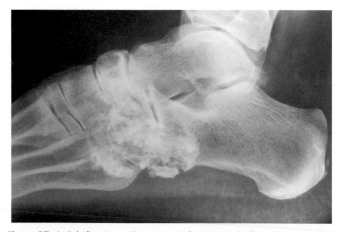

Figure 27–4 Calcification within masses of pigmented villonodular synovitis is uncommon. This example from a 64-year-old male patient with pigmented villonodular synovitis of the foot shows calcification (see Figure 27–5).

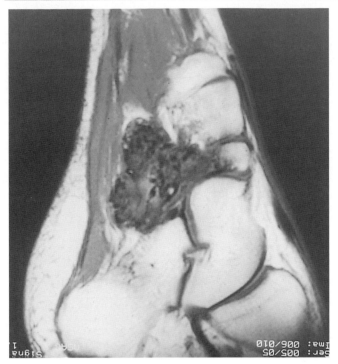

Figure 27–5 This MRI scan corresponds to the case illustrated in Figure 27–4. Foci of high-signal intensity within the low-signal mass correspond to regions with numerous lipid-laden histiocytes. Regions of proliferation with abundant hemosiderin show low signal on T1- and T2-weighted images.

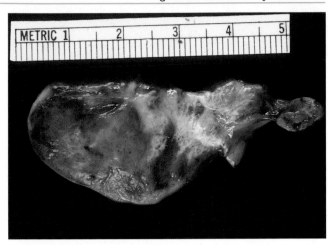

Figure 27–7 Pigmented villonodular synovitis may present grossly in a localized nodular pattern, as seen in this case.

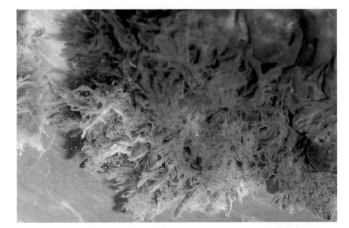

Figure 27–6 This photograph of a gross specimen of resected synovium placed in water illustrates the characteristic villous proliferation of the synovium in pigmented villonodular synovitis. Arthroscopically this same pattern may be seen.

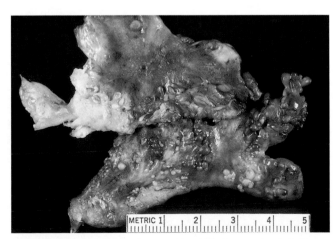

Figure 27–8 Other causes for pigmentation within the synovium include synovial hemorrhage, ochronosis, and metallic synovitis after total joint arthroplasty. This photograph illustrates the appearance of metallic synovitis.

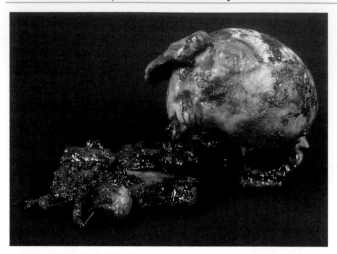

Figure 27–9 This femoral head was resected at the time of placement of a total hip prosthesis in a patient with pigmented villonodular synovitis. Bony erosion by the synovial proliferation is evident. The color of lesional tissue grossly varies, depending on the relative numbers of hemosiderin-laden and lipid-laden macrophages in the specimen.

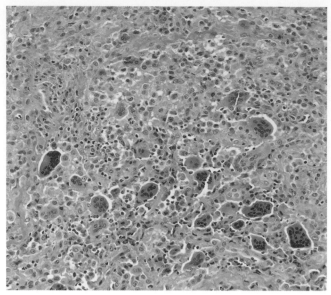

Figure 27–11 At low magnification, pigmented villonodular synovitis shows scattered multinucleated giant cells lying within a mononuclear cell background with varying degrees of fibrosis, as illustrated in this photomicrograph.

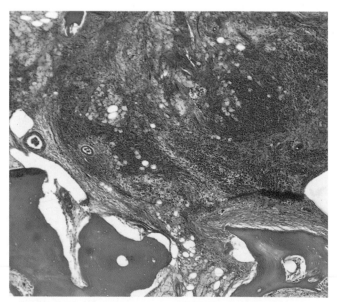

Figure 27–10 This photomicrograph shows the low-magnification pattern of pigmented villonodular synovitis invading the acetabulum. The defect is well circumscribed, mirroring the radiographic appearance.

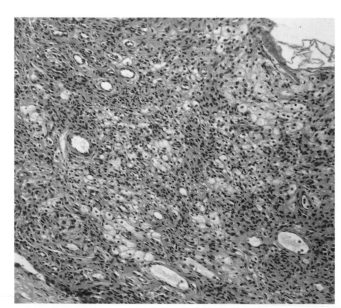

Figure 27–12 Regions of lipid-laden macrophages often form small clusters within the proliferation, as illustrated in this photomicrograph. Adjacent hemosiderin-laden macrophages show brownish discoloration of the cytoplasm.

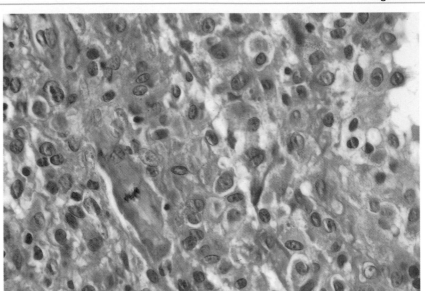

Figure 27–13 At high magnification, pigmented villonodular synovitis shows mononuclear cells with abundant cytoplasm and multinucleated giant cells. The mononuclear cells are eosinophilic, with clear or brown-staining cytoplasm.

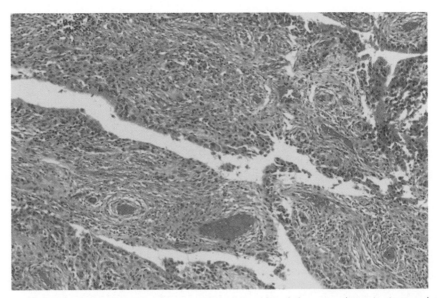

Figure 27–14 This photomicrograph shows a residual synovial cell layer overlying hemosiderin-laden macrophages in pigmented villonodular synovitis.

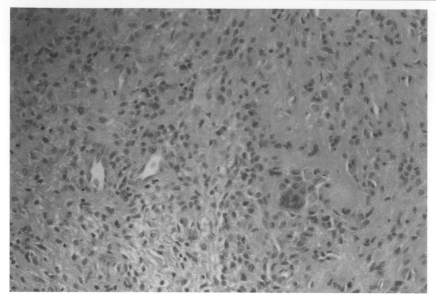

Figure 27–15 This photomicrograph illustrates the microscopic features of giant cell tumor of tendon sheath type. Histologically this entity is indistinguishable from pigmented villonodular synovitis. Giant cell tumors of tendon sheath type are well-circumscribed soft tissue masses, as illustrated in this photomicrograph.

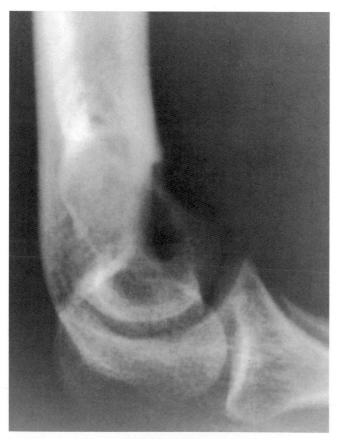

Figure 27–16 This radiograph illustrates pigmented villonodular synovitis of the elbow in a 13-year-old girl.

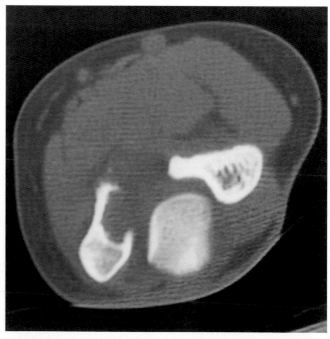

Figure 27–17 Computed tomographic (CT) scan of the patient in Figure 27–16.

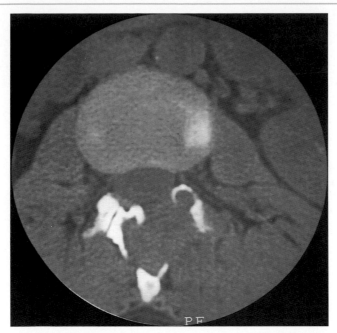

Figure 27–18 CT scan showing pigmented villonodular synovitis of the lumbar spine in a 47-year-old man.

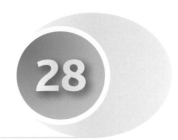

Arthroplasty Effect

Clinical Signs

1. Most patients are asymptomatic if the implant remains well fixed.

Clinical Symptoms

1. Pain is the most common symptom related to implant loosening.
2. Joint dysfunction is related to implant loosening.

Major Radiographic Features

1. Nonseptic periprosthetic osteolysis has two patterns:
   a. Diffuse benign pattern:
      i. Radiolucency surrounds the bone–prosthesis interface.
      ii. The affected area may be surrounded by radiodense lines.
   b. Focal aggressive pattern:
      i. Isolated lytic lesions, 0.5 to 2.0 cm, may be seen.
      ii. Little reactive bone is present.
      iii. The lesions may coalesce to form contiguous lytic zones of destruction.
2. With loosening, cement or implant fractures result in a position change of components.

Radiographic Differential Diagnosis

1. Infection.
2. Stress shielding resorption.
3. Osteoporosis.

Major Pathologic Features

1. There may be a foreign body granulomatous reaction to particulate implant materials (e.g., polyethylene, methacrylate, or metal).

2. Fibrovascular, villous membrane infiltrated with sheets of foamy macrophages and giant cells may be seen.
3. Patients with prostheses in which metal articulates on metal may show gray–black discoloration of the synovium as a result of metallic debris.
4. Polyethylene may engender a host reaction producing a pseudotumor.

Pathologic Differential Diagnosis

1. Sepsis.
2. Granulomatous infection.
3. Pigmented villonodular synovitis.

Treatment

1. Improvement in implant design and techniques should prevent this condition.
2. Medical treatment includes symptomatic measures and close follow-up for cases in which there is mild osteolysis.
3. Surgical treatment consists of revision arthroplasty for patients with the following:
   a. Symptomatic loosening and osteolysis.
   b. Significant osteolysis compromising bone stock even in asymptomatic patients.

References

Fehring TK, McAlister JA Jr: Frozen histologic section as a guide to sepsis in revision joint arthroplasty. *Clin Orthop* 304:229–237, 1994.

Mauerhan DR, Nelson CL, Smith DL, et al: Prophylaxis against infection in total joint arthroplasty. One day of cefuroxime compared with three days of cefazolin. *J Bone Joint Surg Am* 76(1):39–45, 1994.

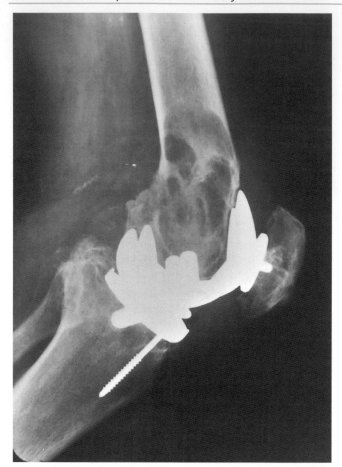

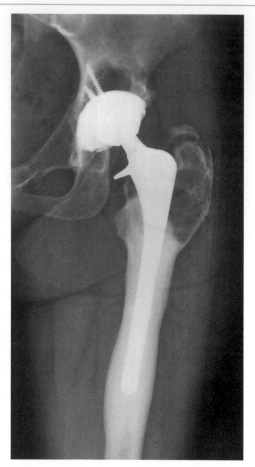

Figure 28–1 Radiograph of the knee in a 77-year-old man who presented with knee pain after total knee arthroplasty. Although infection was thought to be the most likely cause of the bony destruction adjacent to the prosthesis, cultures and histologic evaluation yielded negative findings, and the changes were thus ascribed to periprosthetic osteolysis.

Figure 28–2 Radiograph of the hip in a 40-year-old woman who had previously had a total hip arthroplasty after suffering avascular necrosis of the femoral head. She presented with a 3-month history of pain. Pathologic evaluation, including cultures, confirmed a diagnosis of aseptic periprosthetic osteolysis.

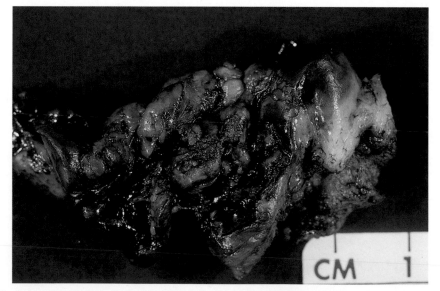

Figure 28–3 This photograph of a gross specimen illustrates the deeply stained appearance of synovium that can be seen in "metallic synovitis." Similar changes may be seen in the synovium in patients who suffer from aseptic periprosthetic osteolysis.

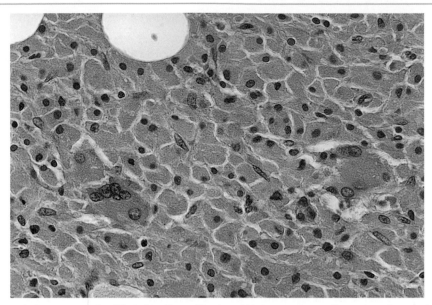

Figure 28–4 This photomicrograph demonstrates the diffuse sheetlike proliferation of histiocytes commonly seen in periprosthetic tissues. Careful examination for polymorphonuclear leukocytes and special stains for organisms, as well as cultures, are necessary to exclude an infectious cause in such cases.

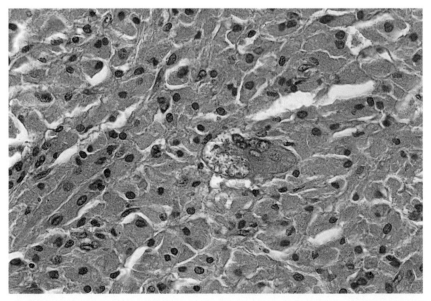

Figure 28–5 This photomicrograph illustrates the histiocytic proliferation associated with aseptic periprosthetic osteolysis. Immediately adjacent to the prosthesis, a zone of dense collagenous tissue may be present.

Bone Tumors and Tumorlike Conditions

Section 2A:
Bone-Forming Tumors

Section 2B:
Cartilage-Forming Tumors

Section 2C:
Fibrous and Fibrohistiocytic Tumors

Section 2D:
Hematopoietic Tumors

Section 2E:
Vascular Tumors

Section 2F:
Tumors of Unknown Origin

Section 2G:
Secondary Sarcomas

Section 2H:
Tumorlike Conditions

Section 2A: Bone-Forming Tumors

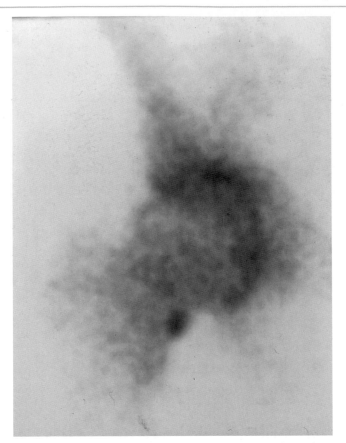

Figure 29–9 An isotope bone scan is also extremely useful in identifying small osteoid osteomas that are radiographically inapparent, as this bone scan illustrates.

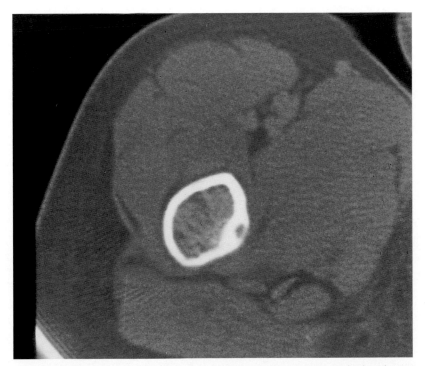

Figure 29–10 A computed tomographic (CT) scan may also be helpful in some instances. In this case, a cortical subtrochanteric osteoid osteoma of the femur was identified on a CT scan.

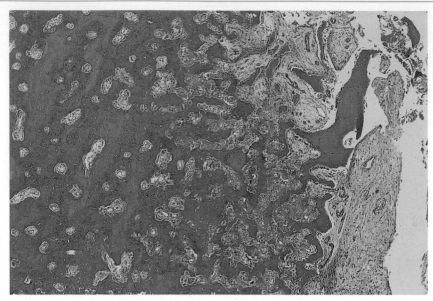

Figure 29–11 Some osteoid osteomas show extensive ossification of the nidus, as illustrated in this photomicrograph. Note the marked circumscription, which results in the lesion appearing to "break away" from the surrounding bone.

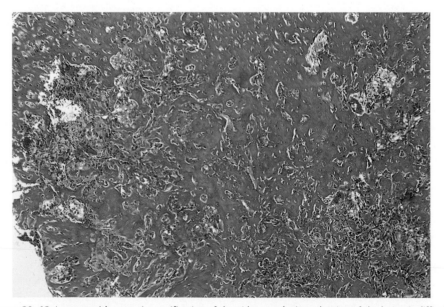

Figure 29–12 In cases with extensive ossification of the nidus, cytologic evaluation of the lesion is difficult.

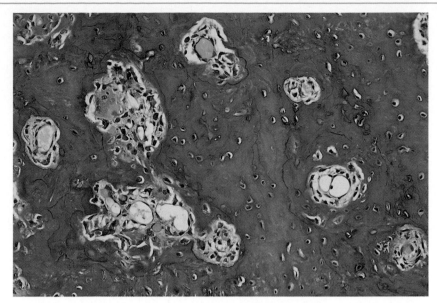

Figure 29–13 At higher magnification, the histologic features may resemble those of pagetoid bone. Attention to the radiographic features helps to avoid a misdiagnosis in such cases.

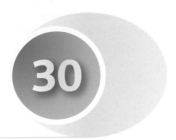

Osteoblastoma

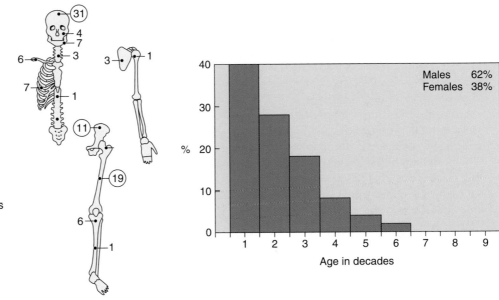

Numbers indicate percentage of cases involving the indicated bone.
The percentage of the three bones most commonly affected are circled.

Males 62%
Females 38%

% / Age in decades

Clinical Signs

1. A tender mass lesion may be found on physical examination.
2. Scoliosis or atrophy of muscle groups in the region of the tumor may be present.
3. Neurologic deficit may be appreciable owing to compression of the cord or nerve roots by vertebral tumors.

Clinical Symptoms

1. Local pain is generally the presenting complaint and is usually of long duration.
2. The pain may follow the characteristic pattern of osteoid osteoma but more commonly does not.

3. Patients with lesions in the lower extremity may present with a limp.
4. Rarely, patients (and all younger than age 10 years) have presented with severe systemic symptoms, which were ameliorated by surgical treatment of the tumor.

Major Radiographic Features

1. The radiographic features may be similar to those of osteoid osteoma.
2. The appearance is variable and may be nonspecific.
3. Of cases, 25% show features suggestive of a malignant neoplasm.

4. In the vertebra, osteoblastoma usually results in expansion and is located in the dorsal elements. Fifty percent show ossification radiographically.
5. Mandibular lesions (cementoblastomas) are "ossified," surrounded by a lucent halo, and located near a tooth root.

Radiographic Differential Diagnosis

1. Osteoid osteoma.
2. Osteosarcoma.
3. Aneurysmal bone cyst.
4. Vascular tumor, when multiple.

Major Pathologic Features

Gross

1. The lesional tissue is hemorrhagic and reddish.
2. The lesional tissue is granular and friable.
3. At its periphery, the tumor shows sharp circumscription.

Microscopic

1. At low magnification, the pattern of the tumor is that of irregular osteoid arranged haphazardly amid a loose fibrovascular connective tissue.
2. At low magnification, the vascular component is obvious, with the presence of wide lumina.
3. Prominent osteoblastic rimming of the osteoid is evident.
4. The periphery of the lesion is well circumscribed, but the osteoid may merge with the adjacent normal bone.
5. At higher magnification, the osteoblasts are uniform but do not totally fill the intertrabecular space.
6. Cartilage is rarely found in osteoblastoma, but it may be present.
7. The osteoid may be quite fine and lacelike, as is seen in osteosarcoma, but cartilaginous differentiation is not present.
8. Mitotic figures may be identified and may be numerous, but atypical mitoses are not present.

Pathologic Differential Diagnosis

Benign lesions

1. Osteoid osteoma.
2. Aneurysmal bone cyst.

Malignant lesions

1. Osteosarcoma.

Treatment

1. **Primary modality:** curettage and grafting.
2. **Other possible approaches:** en bloc resection with a marginal margin and grafting, depending on location. Spinal lesions may require complete removal by excision or curettage, with preservation of new roots. Bone grafting to stabilize the vertebral column is often necessary.

References

Bertoni F, Unni KK, McLeod RA, et al: Osteosarcoma resembling osteoblastoma. *Cancer* 55(2):416–426, 1985.

Cheung FM, Wu WC, Lam CK, et al: Diagnostic criteria for pseudomalignant osteoblastoma. *Histopathology* 31(2):196–200, 1997.

Della Rocca C, Huvos AG: Osteoblastoma: varied histological presentations with a benign clinical course. An analysis of 55 cases. *Am J Surg Pathol* 20(7):841–850, 1996.

Dorfman JD, Weiss SW: Borderline osteoblastic tumors: problems in the differential diagnosis of aggressive osteoblastoma and low-grade osteosarcoma. *Semin Diagn Pathol* 1(3):215–234, 1984.

Jackson RP, Reckling FW, Mants FA: Osteoid osteoma and osteoblastoma: similar histologic lesions with different natural histories. *Clin Orthop* 128:303–313, 1977.

Kyriakos M, El-Khoury GY, McDonald DJ, et al: Osteoblastomatosis of bone. A benign, multifocal osteoblastic lesion, distinct from osteoma and osteoblastoma, radiologically simulating a vascular tumor. *Skeletal Radiol* 36(3):237–246, 2007.

McLeod RA, Dahlin DC, Beabout JW: The spectrum of osteoblastoma. *Am J Roentgenol* 126(2):321–335, 1976.

Mirra JM, Theros E, Smasson J, et al: A case of osteoblastoma associated with severe systemic toxicity. *Am J Surg Pathol* 3(5):463–471, 1979.

Papagelopoulos PJ, Galanis EC, Sim FH, et al: Clinicopathologic features, diagnosis, and treatment of osteoblastoma. *Orthopedics* 22(2):244–247, 1999.

Shaikh MI, Saifuddin A, Pringle J, et al: Spinal osteoblastoma: CT and MR imaging with pathological correlation. *Skeletal Radiol* 28(1):33–40, 1999.

Theologis T, Ostlere S, Gibbons CLMH, et al: Toxic osteoblastoma of the scapula. *Skeletal Radiol* 36(3):253–257, 2007.

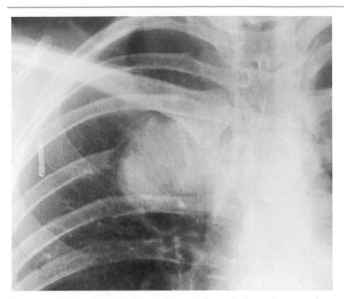

Figure 30–1 This radiograph illustrates a partially ossified mass lesion involving a rib posteriorly. There is associated bone destruction and a soft tissue mass indicative of an aggressive lesion.

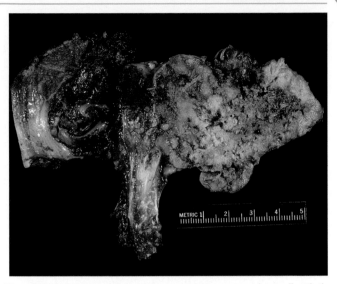

Figure 30–3 The gross pathologic features in this case correlate well with the plain radiographic and CT appearance of this lesion. The tumor was confirmed histologically to be an osteoblastoma.

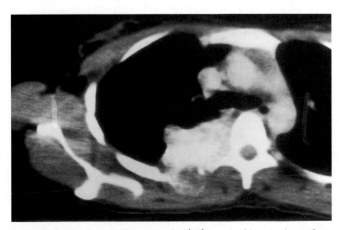

Figure 30–2 The computed tomographic (CT) scan in this case shows the same features that are evident in the plain radiograph.

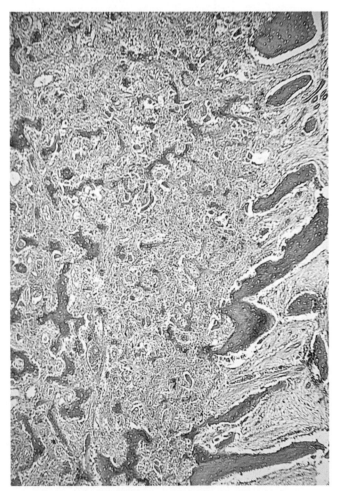

Figure 30–4 At low magnification, the periphery of an osteoblastoma is well circumscribed, as illustrated in this photomicrograph.

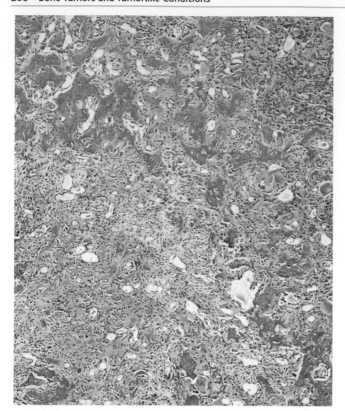

Figure 30–5 The tumor is composed of numerous irregularly shaped bony trabeculae between which there is hypocellular fibrovascular connective tissue.

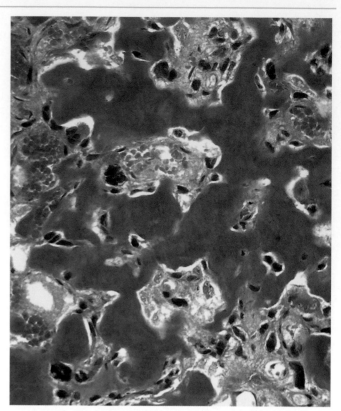

Figure 30–7 At high magnification, the lesion is not hypercellular and nuclear pleomorphism is generally not marked. However, some lesions can show cytologic changes that may simulate osteosarcoma, as demonstrated in this photomicrograph.

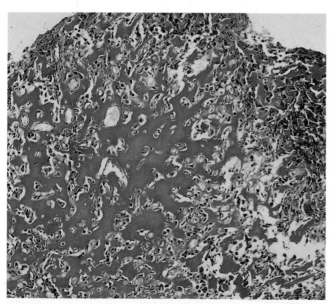

Figure 30–6 Numerous multinucleated giant cells and a prominent osteoblastic rimming of the bony trabeculae are evident. Vascular spaces are generally prominent.

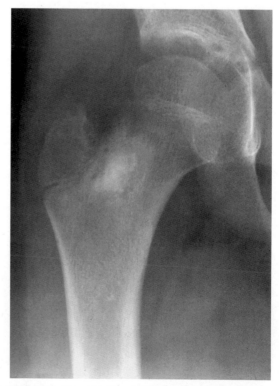

Figure 30–8 This radiograph of the proximal femur shows a heavily ossified oval osteoblastoma. A lucent halo surrounds the ossified lesion and is itself surrounded by a zone of sclerosis—features that support a benign diagnosis.

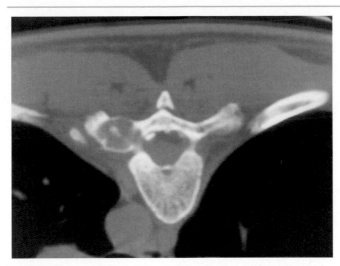

Figure 30–9 Osteoblastomas commonly involve the vertebrae; the dorsal elements are usually the location of such lesions, as illustrated in this case. The central ossification is also characteristic of this tumor.

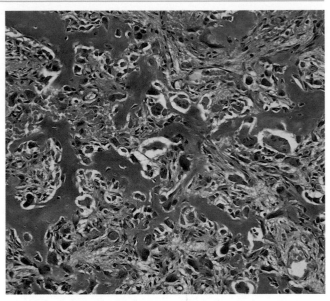

Figure 30–11 Although the irregular bony trabeculae of osteoblastoma may simulate the osteoid produced by osteosarcomas, the hypocellular nature of the fibrovascular connective tissue seen between such trabeculae supports a diagnosis of osteoblastoma.

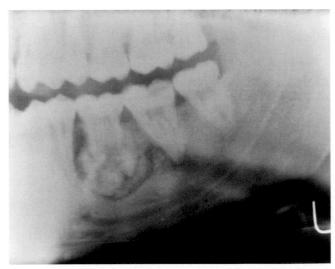

Figure 30–10 Lesions histologically indistinguishable from osteoblastoma also involve the maxilla and mandible, as shown here. Such lesions have been termed "cementoblastomas." Note the ossified tumor surrounding the tooth root with a lucent halo.

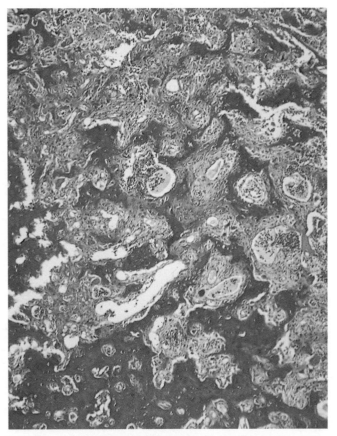

Figure 30–12 Ossification of osteoblastomas is variable from region to region in the tumor. This photomicrograph illustrates the transition from a more heavily ossified area to a less ossified region.

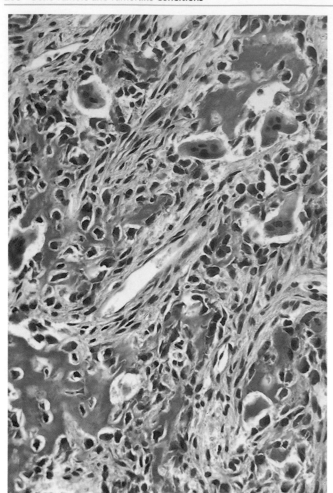

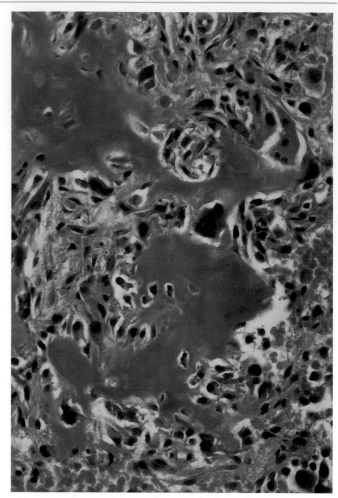

Figure 30–13 Careful attention should be paid to the appearance of the lesion at low magnification and to the radiographic features because overemphasis on the high-power appearance of a lesion may lead to a mistaken diagnosis of malignancy.

Figure 30–14 Although the nuclei in an osteoblastoma may be somewhat hyperchromatic, the cells do not lie "shoulder to shoulder" as in an osteosarcoma. Thus, the osteoblastoma has a looser appearance, as illustrated in this photomicrograph.

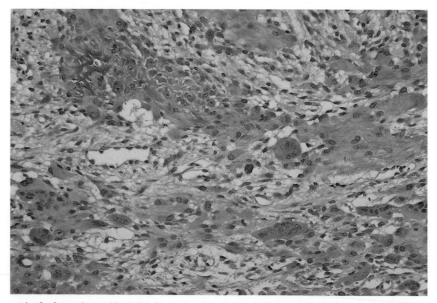

Figure 30–15 This photomicrograph of a femoral osteoblastoma shows the characteristic loose hypocellular fibrovascular connective tissue that helps differentiate osteoblastoma from osteoblastoma-like osteosarcomas.

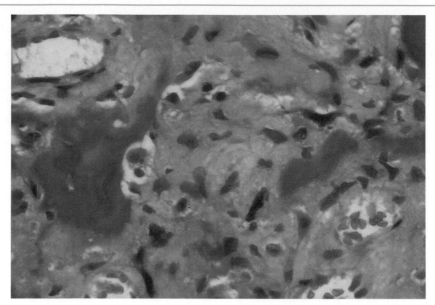

Figure 30–16 Cells showing degenerative cytologic atypia, resulting in irregularly shaped hyperchromatic nuclei, as seen in this photomicrograph, can be mistaken for malignant osteoblastomas. This photomicrograph of a femoral osteoblastoma shows these cytologic features.

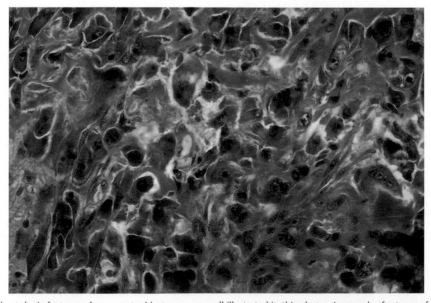

Figure 30–17 The epithelioid cytologic features of some osteoblastomas are well illustrated in this photomicrograph of a tumor from the clavicle. Regions that show prominent epithelioid cytologic features and the irregular osteoid seen here can be strikingly similar to the histologic features of some osteosarcomas.

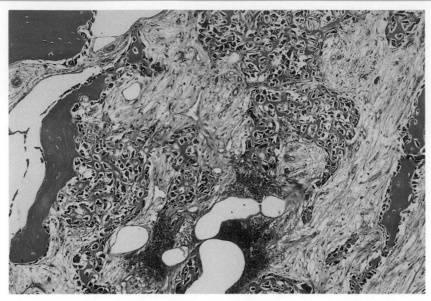

Figure 30–18 Although osteoblastomas form a solitary lesion radiographically, microscopically they may appear multicentric, as illustrated in this photomicrograph. Presumably, such "dangling lobules" of tumor may result in recurrence if the osteoblastoma is not thoroughly curetted.

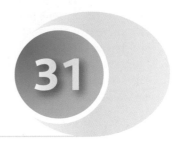

Osteosarcoma (Conventional)

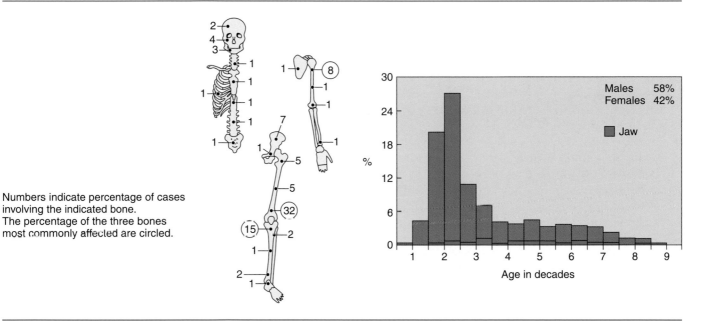

Numbers indicate percentage of cases involving the indicated bone.
The percentage of the three bones most commonly affected are circled.

Males 58%
Females 42%

■ Jaw

%

Age in decades

Clinical Signs

1. A tender mass generally is palpable on physical examination because soft tissue extension is common.
2. When the mass is very large, dilated, and engorged, veins may be seen overlying it.
3. Edema distal to the lesion resulting from blockage of lymphatics or venous compression occurs uncommonly.
4. Elevation of serum alkaline phosphatase concentrations occurs in about 50% of patients.

Clinical Symptoms

1. Pain, which may be intermittent initially, is universally present.

2. A swelling in the region of the affected bone is also a cardinal, although nonspecific, symptom.
3. Pathologic fracture is uncommon as the presenting complaint.
4. The duration of symptoms is generally short, varying from weeks to several months.

Major Radiographic Features

1. The favored site is the metaphysis of a long bone, especially the distal femur and proximal tibia.
2. There may be lytic, blastic, or mixed bone destruction and production.
3. Trabecular and cortical destruction is usually geographic and poorly marginated.

4. Periosteal new bone is frequent and often takes the form of spiculation or Codman's triangles.
5. Soft tissue extension is the rule in larger lesions.
6. Magnetic resonance imaging (MRI) and computed tomography (CT) are essential for pretreatment staging.

Radiographic Differential Diagnosis

1. Ewing's sarcoma.
2. Fibrosarcoma or malignant fibrous histiocytoma.
3. Chondrosarcoma.
4. Osteomyelitis.
5. Osteoblastoma.
6. Giant cell tumor.

Major Pathologic Features

Gross

1. The tumors generally have violated the cortex of the affected bone at the time of diagnosis.
2. An associated soft tissue mass is commonly found.
3. The tumor may extend within the medullary cavity beyond the abnormality defined by plane radiography. (MRI is particularly helpful in defining the extent of intramedullary disease.)
4. The tumor is variable in consistency and may be distinctly sclerotic; in general, however, soft areas are identifiable as well.
5. The tumor varies from yellow–brown to whitish, depending on whether the predominant differentiation is fibroblastic, chondroblastic, or osteoblastic.
6. Necrosis, cyst formation, and hemorrhage are most commonly seen in the softer portions of the tumor.

Microscopic

1. At low magnification, the tumor may show great variability. However, all tumors classified as osteosarcoma must show a frankly sarcomatous stroma that produces osteoid. (Frequently, the osteoid shows a fine, lacelike pattern.)
2. The tumor is hypercellular, and generally the stromal cells are spindled.
3. Zones of chondroid matrix may be identified.
4. Sclerotic zones of extensive ossification may appear hypocellular, having undergone degeneration.
5. The spindle cells may be arranged in a "herring bone" or storiform pattern.
6. At higher magnification, the spindle cells show marked pleomorphism. The nuclei are extremely variable in size and shape and are hyperchromic.
7. Mitotic figures are generally abundant.
8. The degree to which osteoid is produced is greatly variable, and a careful search may be needed to identify the eosinophilic matrix surrounding atypical cells.

9. Variable numbers of benign multinucleated giant cells are seen; when abundant, they may focally mimic the appearance of a giant cell tumor.

Pathologic Differential Diagnosis

Benign lesions

1. Osteoblastoma.
2. Osteoid osteoma.
3. Giant cell tumor.
4. Fracture callus.

Malignant lesions

1. Fibrosarcoma.
2. Chondrosarcoma.
3. Malignant fibrous histiocytoma.

Treatment

1. **Primary modality:** surgical ablation by amputation or limb-saving resection with a wide margin. If preoperative staging indicates that a successful limb-salvage procedure can be performed, the extremity can be reconstructed with a custom joint prosthesis, an osteochondral allograft, or a resection arthrodesis. The reconstructive procedure should be tailored to the needs of the individual. Protocols employing preoperative (neoadjuvant) chemotherapy use the extent of tumor "necrosis" at the time of definitive operation as a measure of effectiveness. Current advances in chemotherapy are making an important contribution to the improved survival of patients with osteosarcoma. An aggressive approach with thoracotomy is saving approximately one third of the patients who develop pulmonary metastases.
2. **Other possible approaches:** radiation therapy, possibly combined with neutron beam radiation for lesions of inaccessible sites such as the spine and sacrum.

References

Campanacci M, Bacci G, Bertoni F, et al: The treatment of osteosarcoma of the extremities: twenty years experience at the Istituto Ortopedico Rizzoli. *Cancer* 48(7):1569–1581, 1981.

Harvei S, Solheim O: The prognosis in osteosarcoma: Norwegian national data. *Cancer* 48(8):1719–1723, 1981.

Hoffer FA: Primary skeletal neoplasms: osteosarcoma and ewing sarcoma. *Topics in Magnetic Resonance Imaging* 13(4):231–239, 2002.

Marcove RC, Rosen G: En bloc resection for osteogenic sarcoma. *Cancer* 45(12):3040–3044, 1980.

Marina N, Gebhardt M, Teot L, et al: Biology and therapeutic advances for pediatric osteosarcoma. *Oncologist* 9(4):422–441, 2004.

Martin SE, Dwyer A, Kissane JM, et al: Small-cell osteosarcoma. *Cancer* 50(5):990–996, 1982.

Sanerkin NG: Definitions of osteosarcoma, chondrosarcoma and fibrosarcoma of bone. *Cancer* 46(7):178–185, 1980.

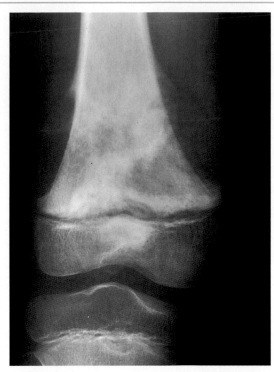

Figure 31–1 This anteroposterior (AP) radiograph demonstrates a mixed lytic and sclerotic lesion in the distal femur of a patient who is skeletally immature. Codman's triangle is present superiorly. The radiographic features are those of an osteosarcoma.

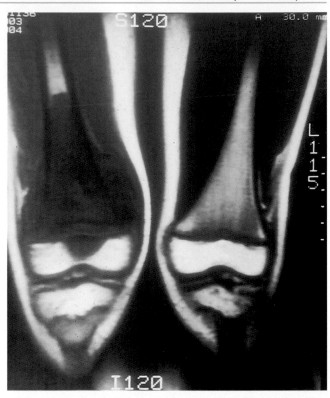

Figure 31–3 This coronal magnetic resonance imaging (MRI) scan of the same patient's distal femur demonstrates the extent of the low-signal tumor seen in contrast to the high-signal normal marrow. The extension of the tumor across the physis into the epiphysis is also readily demonstrated.

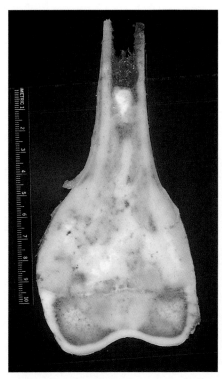

Figure 31–2 The gross pathologic features in this case correspond well to the plain x-ray film appearance shown in Figure 31–1. The tumor crosses the open physis, which often acts as a relative barrier to the intraosseous extension of osteosarcomas. The tumor is firm and gritty; however, soft areas are nearly always present.

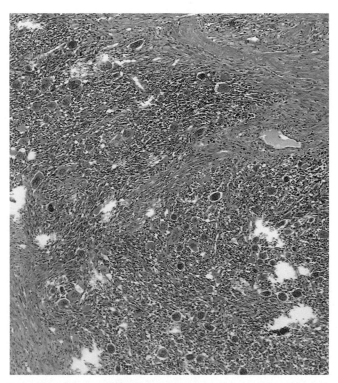

Figure 31–4 At low magnification, osteosarcomas show a variety of histologic patterns. This photomicrograph illustrates a tumor that is predominantly composed of spindle cells (fibroblastic) in which numerous benign multinucleated giant cells are present.

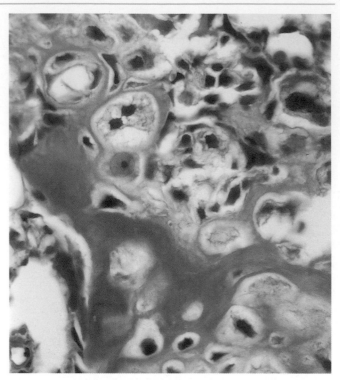

Figure 31–5 This photomicrograph illustrates the permeative growth of a chondroblastic osteosarcoma of the distal femur. Residual bony trabeculae are present. The chondroid portion of such a tumor may not show as significant a cytologic atypia as the spindle cell components of the lesion and thus, if taken out of context, may suggest the diagnosis of chondrosarcoma.

Figure 31–6 Osteoblastic osteosarcomas may be heavily ossified; however, the cytologic atypia of the proliferating cells is generally obvious in such cases, as is shown in this photomicrograph.

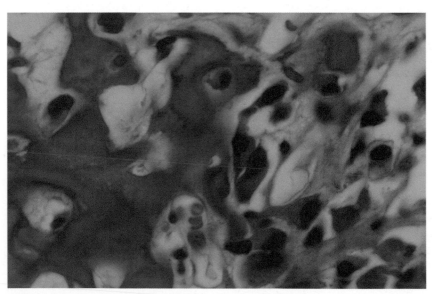

Figure 31–7 At high magnification, ordinary osteosarcomas are poorly differentiated or high-grade tumors. They show nuclear pleomorphism and anaplasia, and mitotic activity is generally brisk.

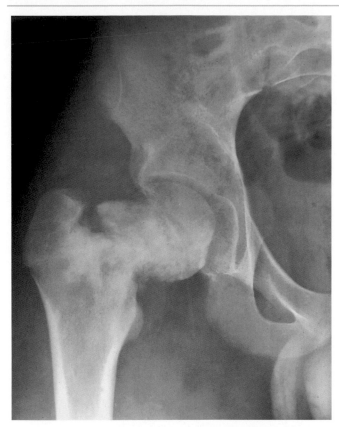

Figure 31–8 This radiograph of the proximal femur shows a sclerotic osteosarcoma that has resulted in a pathologic fracture.

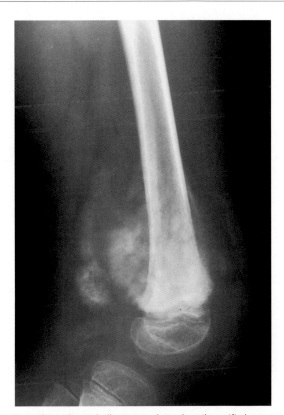

Figure 31–9 This radiograph illustrates a large, heavily ossified osteosarcoma of the lower femoral metaphysis, with a large soft tissue component.

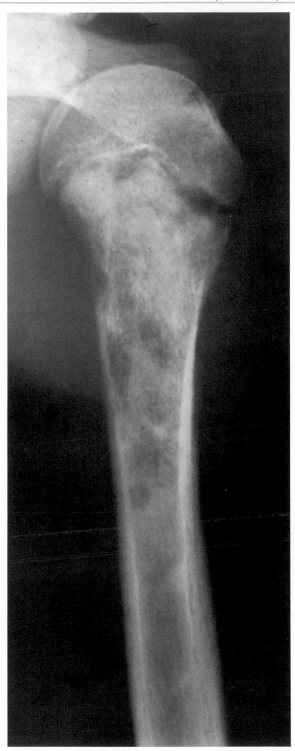

Figure 31–10 A mixed lytic and sclerotic radiographic appearance is common in osteosarcoma, as in this case involving the upper diametaphyseal region of the humerus.

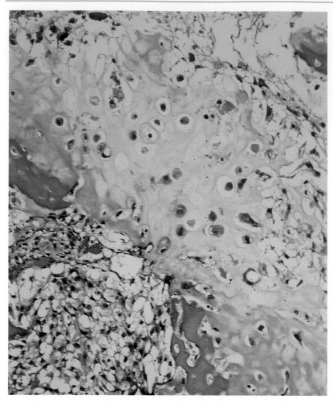

Figure 31–11 Ossification within a chondroblastic osteosarcoma may occur at the periphery of the cartilaginous masses, as illustrated in this photomicrograph, or within a spindle cell component of the lesion.

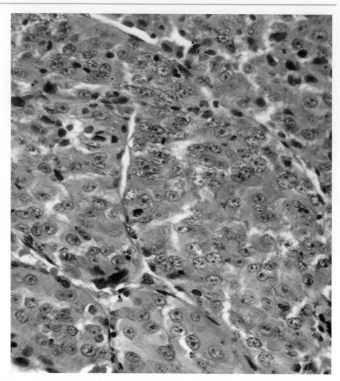

Figure 31–13 Some osteosarcomas show a distinctly epithelioid histologic pattern of growth, as illustrated in this photomicrograph of a tumor from the radius. Given the young age of most patients with osteosarcoma, such a pattern generally does not result in misdiagnosis.

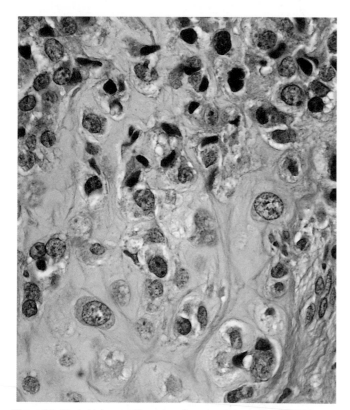

Figure 31–12 At high magnification, ordinary osteosarcomas show marked cytologic atypia. The "lacelike" osteoid that identifies the tumor as an osteosarcoma may be only focally present.

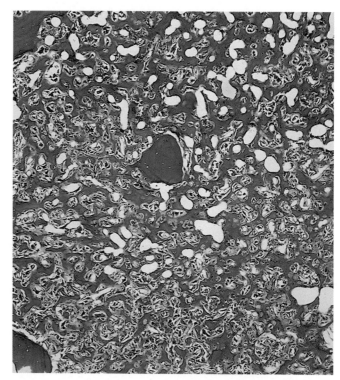

Figure 31–14 This photomicrograph illustrates the infiltrative pattern commonly seen in malignant bone tumors. Residual preexisting bony trabeculae are surrounded by the osteoblastic osteosarcoma.

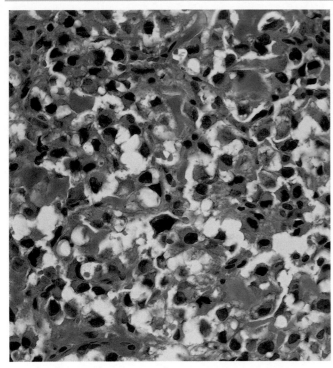

Figure 31–15 Conventional osteosarcomas may show epithelioid cytologic characteristics, as in this tumor from the distal femur. In elderly patients, such epithelioid differentiation may be sufficiently prominent to cause confusion with metastatic carcinoma.

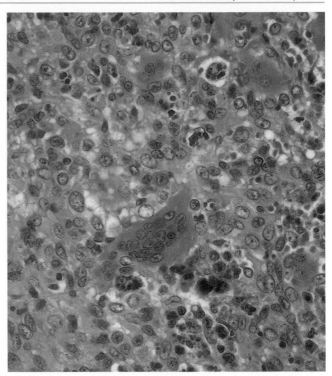

Figure 31–17 This photomicrograph illustrates the cytologic appearance of the giant cell–rich osteosarcoma depicted in Figure 31–16. The cytologic atypia of the mononuclear cells in such tumors is greater than that seen in benign giant cell tumors of bone.

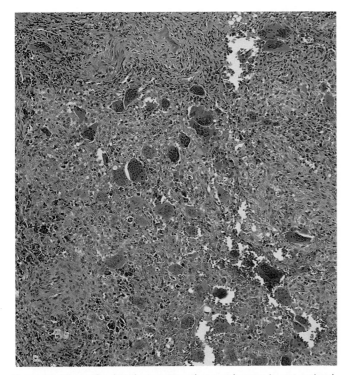

Figure 31–16 Another histologic pattern that may be seen in conventional osteosarcoma is a "giant cell–rich pattern," as illustrated in this photomicrograph. Such tumors may be easily confused with giant cell tumors of bone. This problem is further complicated by the fact that giant cell tumors may show a malignant appearance radiographically.

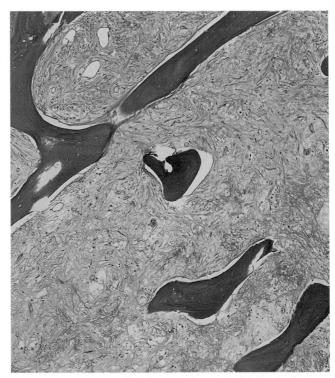

Figure 31–18 This photomicrograph illustrates a common pattern seen in postchemotherapy osteosarcoma. Regions such as this may be totally replaced by collagenized stroma devoid of malignant cells.

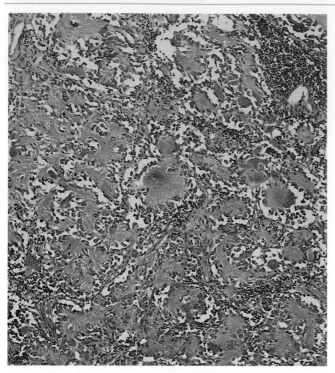

Figure 31–19 This photomicrograph demonstrates the histologic pattern seen in an osteoblastoma-like osteosarcoma. Such tumors are difficult to distinguish from osteoblastoma. The presence of cartilage in such a lesion favors the diagnosis of osteosarcoma.

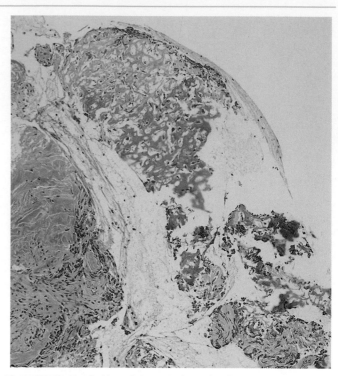

Figure 31–20 Needle biopsy is increasingly used to diagnose primary bone tumors. This photomicrograph illustrates the pattern seen in an osteosarcoma of the tibia. Careful correlation with the radiographic appearance of the lesion is even more critical when the amount of tissue sampled is limited, as in needle biopsy specimens.

Parosteal Osteosarcoma

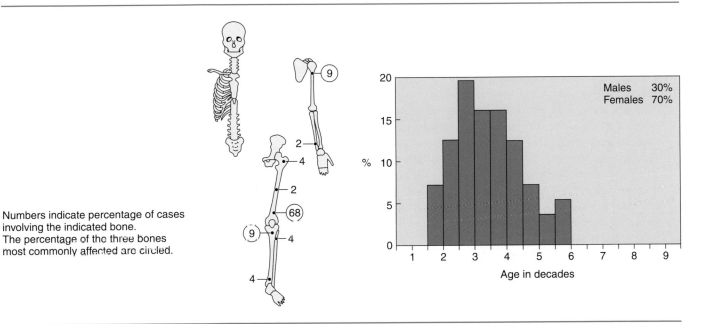

Numbers indicate percentage of cases involving the indicated bone.
The percentage of the three bones most commonly affected are circled.

Males 30%
Females 70%

%

Age in decades

Clinical Signs

1. A large mass lesion involves the affected bone.
2. The tumor may be tender to palpation.

Clinical Symptoms

1. A painless mass is present in the posterior distal thigh.
2. The mass is generally of long duration (up to several years).
3. If the mass is sufficiently large, some patients complain of an inability to bend the knee.
4. Pain is uncommon.

Major Radiographic Features

1. A lobulated and ossified mass arises on the metaphyseal surface of a long bone.
2. The posterior lower femur is a preferred site.
3. There is broad attachment to the adjacent cortex.
4. The cortex is thickened and deformed.
5. Larger tumors encircle the bone.

Radiographic Differential Diagnosis

1. Myositis ossificans.
2. Periosteal osteosarcoma.

3. Periosteal chondrosarcoma.
4. High-grade surface osteosarcoma.
5. Dedifferentiated parosteal osteosarcoma.
6. Ordinary (conventional) osteosarcoma.
7. Osteochondroma.

Major Pathologic Features

Gross

1. The tumor seems to be applied to the surface of the affected bone.
2. Medullary extension is absent unless the tumor is recurrent or has been present for many years.
3. The tumor is ossified and rock hard; if soft areas exist, they should be sampled because the tumor may have a higher-grade component in it.
4. Cartilaginous foci may be grossly evident and may form a "cap" over the tumor similar to an osteochondroma.

Microscopic

1. At low magnification, the pattern is that of a low-grade tumor. Osteoid trabeculae lie parallel to one another in a hypocellular fibroblastic stroma.
2. The fibroblastic component of the tumor shows minimal cytologic atypia, and only rarely are mitoses present.
3. At the surface of the tumor, a cartilaginous cap may be present, giving the tumor the appearance of an osteo-chondroma. However, between the bony trabeculae of an osteochondroma there is fatty or hematopoietic marrow, in contrast with the fibrous stroma of a paros-teal osteosarcoma. In addition, the chondrocytes show mild cytologic atypia and do not exhibit the columnar arrangement seen in an osteochondroma.

Pathologic Differential Diagnosis

Benign lesions

1. Osteochondroma.
2. Myositis ossificans (heterotopic ossification).

Malignant lesions

1. High-grade surface osteosarcoma.
2. Periosteal osteosarcoma.

Treatment

1. **Primary modality:** en bloc resection with a marginal margin and grafting, depending on location.
2. **Other possible approaches:** amputation if the tumor involves neurovascular structures and is not resectable.

References

Ahuja SC, Villacin AB, Smith J, et al: Juxtacortical (parosteal) osteogenic sarcoma: histological grading and prognosis. *J Bone Joint Surg Am* 59(5):632–647, 1977.

Chang CP, Chu YK, Chu LS, et al: Scintigraphic appearance of parosteal osteosarcoma. *Clin Nucl Med* 22(1):54–56, 1997.

Edeiken J, Farrell C, Ackerman LV, et al: Parosteal sarcoma. *Am J Roentgenol* 111(3):579–583, 1971.

Lin J, Yao L, Mirra JM, et al: Osteochondroma-like parosteal osteosar-coma: a report of six cases of a new entity. *Am J Roentgenol* 170(6): 1571–1577, 1998.

Meneses MF, Unni KK, Swee RG: Bizarre parosteal osteochondromatous proliferation of bone (Nora's lesion). *Am J Surg Pathol* 17(7):691–697, 1993.

Okada K, Frassica FJ, Sim FH, et al: Parosteal osteosarcoma. A clinico-pathological study. *J Bone Joint Surg Am* 76(3):366–378, 1994.

Raymond AK: Surface osteosarcoma. *Clin Orthop Relat Res* 270:140–148, 1991.

Unni KK, Dahlin DC, Beabout JW: Periosteal osteogenic sarcoma. *Cancer* 37(5):2476–2485, 1976.

Unni KK, Dahlin DC, Beabout JW, et al: Parosteal osteogenic sarcoma. *Cancer* 37(5):2466–2475, 1976.

Wold LE, Unni KK, Beabout JW, et al: Dedifferentiated parosteal osteosa-rcoma. *J Bone Joint Surg Am* 66(1):53–59, 1984.

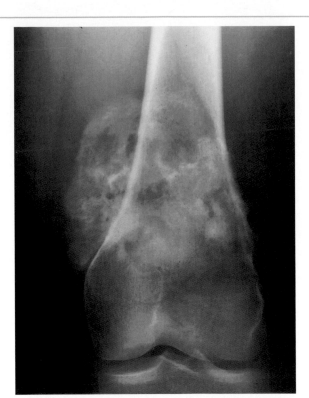

Figure 32–1 This anteroposterior (AP) radiograph illustrates the typical features of a parosteal osteosarcoma. The tumor is heavily ossified and broadly attached to the surface of the bone.

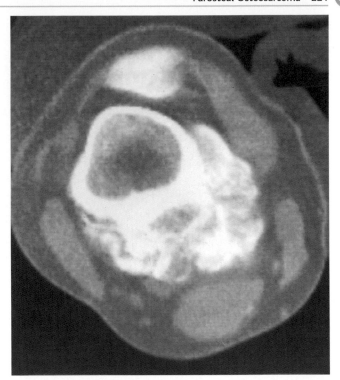

Figure 32–3 A computed tomographic (CT) scan of the tumor may be helpful in excluding medullary involvement. This scan shows the broad surface attachment of a parosteal osteosarcoma and the absence of medullary neoplasm.

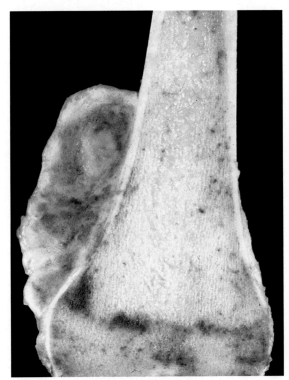

Figure 32–2 The gross pathologic features of the resected specimen correlate well with its radiographic appearance (see Fig. 32–1). The tumor is densely ossified, and no medullary involvement is present. Any soft areas of the tumor should be sampled because they may represent "transformation" of the tumor.

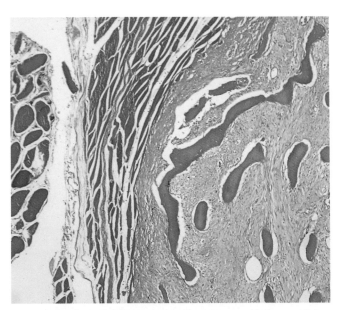

Figure 32–4 At low magnification, parosteal osteosarcoma shows an orderly appearance, with a hypocellular spindle cell component merging with mature-appearing, "normalized" bony trabeculae. The periphery of the lesion is generally well circumscribed, as shown in this photomicrograph.

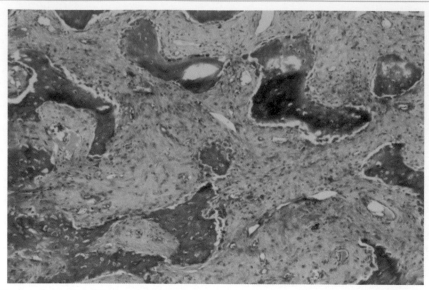

Figure 32–5 At higher magnification, the cytologic features of the spindle cell component of the tumor are more apparent. The juxtaposition of hypocellular spindle cells and mature bone may simulate the histologic features of fibrous dysplasia.

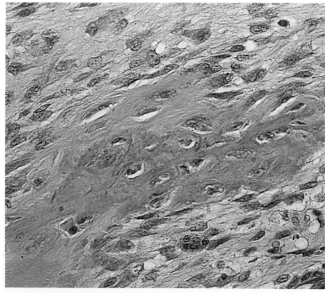

Figure 32–6 At high magnification, minimal cytologic atypia is apparent in the spindle cell component of the tumor.

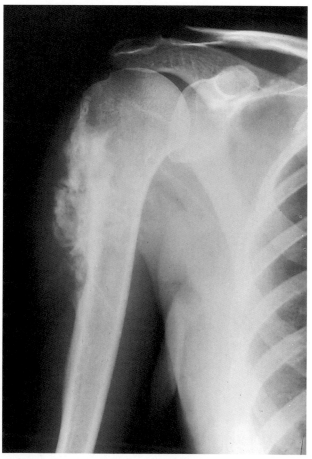

Figure 32–7 The proximal humerus is the second most common location for parosteal osteosarcoma. This tumor shows the characteristic broad-based bony attachment.

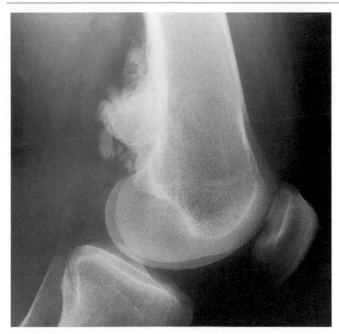

Figure 32–8 The distal posterior femur is the most common location for parosteal osteosarcoma. Medullary involvement is not identified in this lateral radiograph.

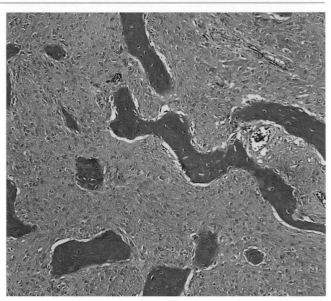

Figure 32–10 Irregular "matured" bony trabeculae of parosteal osteosarcoma may simulate the low-power pattern of fibrous dysplasia. However, the surface location of the lesion excludes the diagnosis of fibrous dysplasia.

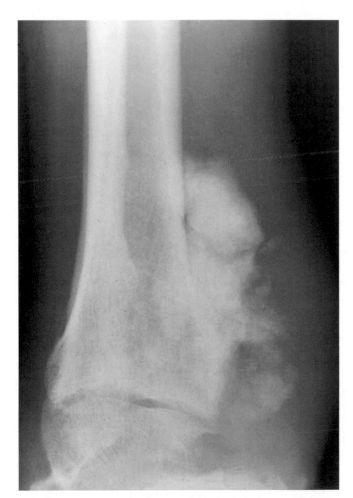

Figure 32–9 The radiographic features of this distal tibial parosteal osteosarcoma are identical with those of tumors in the more common location.

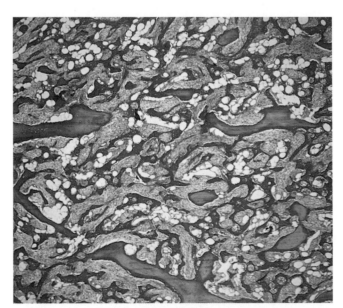

Figure 32–11 In recurrent or longstanding cases of parosteal osteosarcoma, the medullary cavity may be involved, as shown in this photomicrograph. The well-differentiated neoplasm is seen permeating the preexisting medullary bony trabeculae.

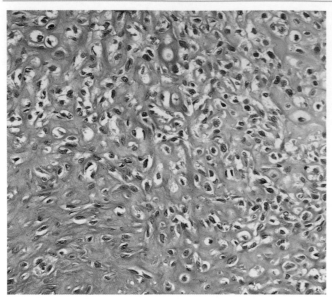

Figure 32–12 Any soft areas in a lesion that otherwise has the features of parosteal osteosarcoma should be histologically examined. This photomicrograph illustrates such a region in a recurrent tumor. The spindle cell proliferation shows much greater cytologic atypia than is seen in parosteal osteosarcoma. Such tumors have been termed "dedifferentiated parosteal osteosarcoma."

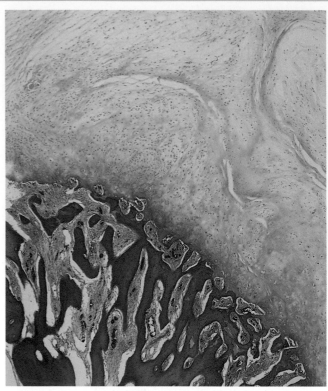

Figure 32–14 This photomicrograph illustrates the similarity between parosteal osteosarcoma and osteochondroma. Occasionally, as in this case, parosteal osteosarcomas have a well-developed cartilage cap.

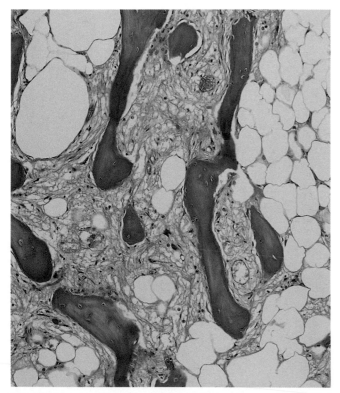

Figure 32–13 Minimal medullary invasion by low-grade parosteal osteosarcomas may be seen, as in this photomicrograph of a proximal humeral tumor. Such medullary invasion does not affect the patient's prognosis.

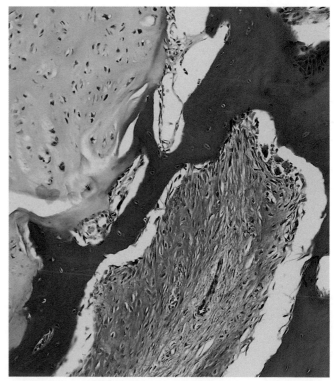

Figure 32–15 Parosteal osteosarcomas are generally composed of a bland fibroblastic proliferation lying between orderly trabecula-like bone. Occasionally, foci of cartilage differentiation may be present, as shown in this photomicrograph of a tumor from the distal posterior femur.

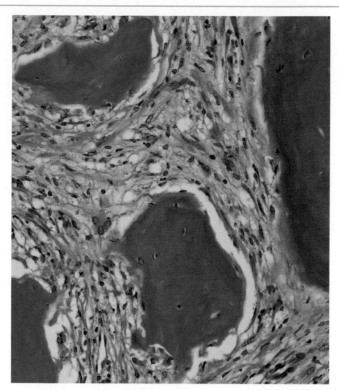

Figure 32–16 Parosteal osteosarcomas are low-grade tumors. The fibroblastic spindle cell portion of the neoplasm may show slight nuclear pleomorphism, as illustrated in this photomicrograph of a tumor from the distal posterior femur.

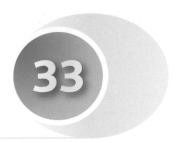

Periosteal Osteosarcoma

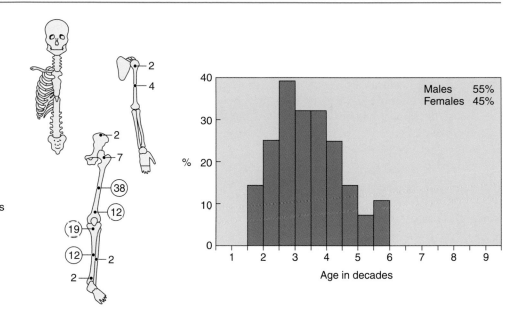

Numbers indicate percentage of cases involving the indicated bone.
The percentage of the three bones most commonly affected are circled.

Males 55%
Females 45%

%

Age in decades

Clinical Signs

1. A mass may be palpable on physical examination.
2. The lesion may be tender to palpation.

Clinical Symptoms

1. Pain is the most common presenting complaint.
2. A swelling may be noticed by the patient.

Major Radiographic Features

1. The lesion is diaphyseal in location, particularly in the tibia.

2. The lesion is located on the surface of the bone; the medullary canal is uninvolved.
3. Partial matrix mineralization may be seen.
4. The periphery of the soft tissue mass is free of mineral.
5. The adjacent cortex is thickened.
6. Periosteal reaction and Codman's triangle are common.

Radiographic Differential Diagnosis

1. Parosteal osteosarcoma.
2. High-grade surface osteosarcoma.
3. Periosteal chondrosarcoma.
4. Myositis ossificans (heterotopic ossification).

Major Pathologic Features

Gross

1. The tumor is lobulated, is situated on the surface of the bone, and may appear like a piece of putty applied to the periosteum.
2. The blue–gray color of a hyaline cartilage tumor is apparent.
3. Whitish spicules of bone may be seen to radiate through the tumor at right angles to the long axis of the underlying bone.
4. The medullary cavity is uninvolved.

Microscopic

1. At low magnification, the tumor exhibits abundant chondroid matrix production.
2. Traversing the chondroid matrix are spicules of osteoid.
3. The periphery is generally well circumscribed, and the tumor shows lobulation in these regions.
4. At the periphery of the lesion, the tumor exhibits a "condensation" of spindle-shaped cells.
5. At higher magnification, the cells lying within the chondroid matrix show mild cytologic atypia.
6. The spindled cells at the periphery also show cytologic atypia, and faint osteoid may be seen among them.
7. The cortical bone may be slightly eroded, but the medullary canal is free of tumor.
8. Mitotic activity is not brisk.

Pathologic Differential Diagnosis

Benign lesions

1. Periosteal chondroma.

Malignant lesions

1. Periosteal chondrosarcoma.
2. High-grade surface osteosarcoma.
3. Ordinary intramedullary osteosarcoma with a prominent surface component.

Treatment

1. **Primary modality:** This lesion lends itself to surgical resection with a wide margin, and the bone can be reconstructed with use of an intercalary allograft or a vascularized fibular graft.
2. **Other possible approaches:** When an adequate margin cannot be achieved by en bloc resection, amputation is indicated. Preoperative chemotherapy may improve the low risk for local recurrence after local resection.

References

Bertoni FB, Boriani S, Laus M, et al: Periosteal chondrosarcoma and periosteal osteosarcoma: two distinct entities. *J Bone Joint Surg Br* 64(3):370–376, 1982.

De Santos LA, Murray JA, Finklestein JB, et al: The radiographic spectrum of periosteal osteosarcoma. *Radiology* 127(1):123–129, 1978.

Grimer RJ, Bielack S, Flege S, et al: European Musculo Skeletal Oncology Society: Periosteal osteosarcoma—a European review of outcome. *Eur J Cancer* 41(18):2806–2811, 2005.

Murphey MD, Jelinek JS, Temple HT, et al: Imaging of periosteal osteosarcoma: radiologic-pathologic comparison. *Radiology* 233(1):129–138, 2004.

Ritts GD, Pritchard DJ, Unni KK, et al: Periosteal osteosarcoma. *Clin Orthop Relat Res* 219:299–307, 1987.

Unni KK, Dahlin DC, Beabout JW: Periosteal osteogenic sarcoma. *Cancer* 37(5):2476–2485, 1976.

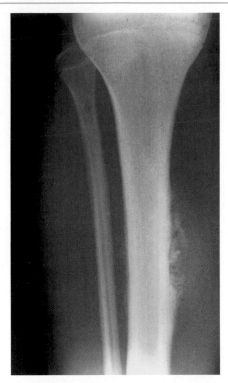

Figure 33–1 This radiograph illustrates the characteristic features of periosteal osteosarcoma. The tumor arises from the surface of the tibial diaphysis and is partially calcified.

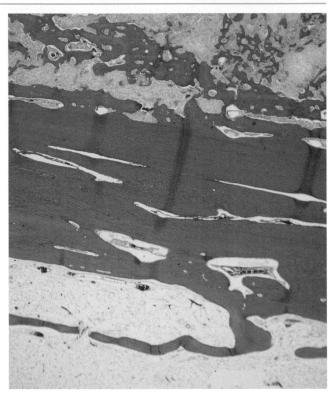

Figure 33–3 Periosteal osteosarcoma is a surface lesion of bone without medullary involvement. This photomicrograph at low magnification shows the uninvolved medullary region and the surface chondroblastic tumor.

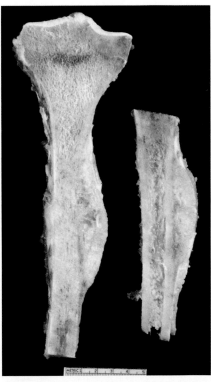

Figure 33–2 The bisected gross specimen of the tibial diaphysis shown in Figure 33–1 illustrates the surface nature of periosteal osteosarcoma as it affects the tibial diaphysis, the most commonly affected bone. Grossly, no visible tumor should be evident in the medullary portion of the affected bone.

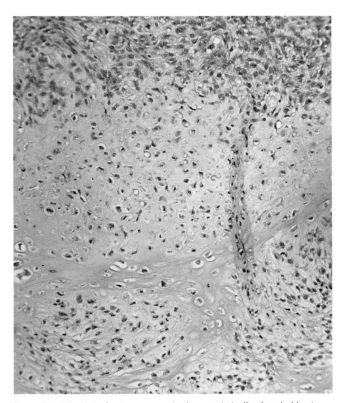

Figure 33–4 Periosteal osteosarcoma is characteristically chondroblastic, as shown in this photomicrograph. At the periphery of the chondroid islands a "condensation" of spindle cells is visible.

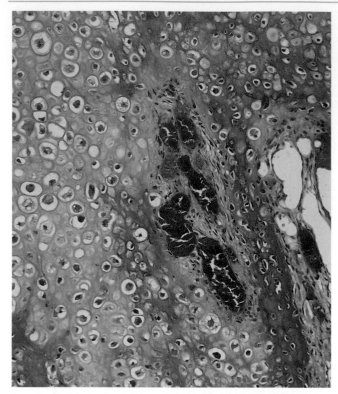

Figure 33–5 At higher magnification, osteoid is identified focally in the lesion. The focal nature of the osteoid production results in confusion of this tumor with periosteal chondrosarcoma and periosteal chondroma.

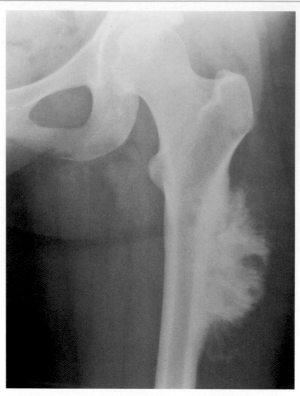

Figure 33–7 The femoral diaphysis is a common location for periosteal osteosarcoma, as shown in this radiograph. This tumor is large and shows the spiculated mineralization commonly identified in periosteal osteosarcoma.

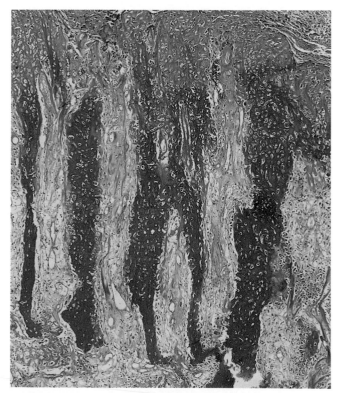

Figure 33–6 The radiating spicules of bone seen radiographically correspond to the bone seen at low magnification in the photomicrograph. Such osteoid frequently traverses the lesion perpendicularly to the underlying cortical bone.

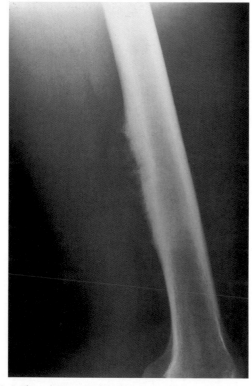

Figure 33–8 The radiating spicules of bone are seen centrally in this periosteal osteosarcoma of the lower femoral diaphysis. An unmineralized soft tissue mass is seen at the periphery of the tumor.

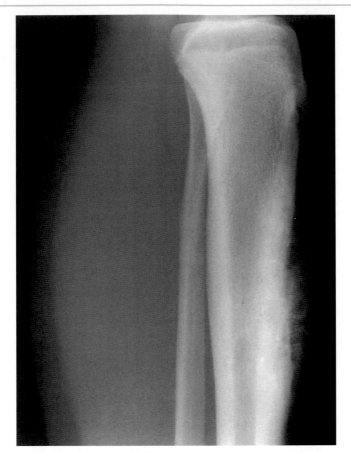

Figure 33–9 The most common location for periosteal osteosarcoma is the tibial diaphysis, as shown in this radiograph. The cortex in this case is thickened, but the underlying medulla is uninvolved.

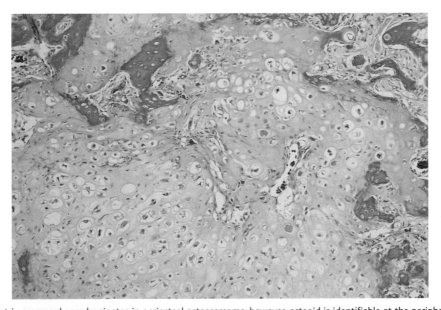

Figure 33–10 Chondroid matrix commonly predominates in periosteal osteosarcoma; however, osteoid is identifiable at the periphery of the chondroid zones in this photomicrograph.

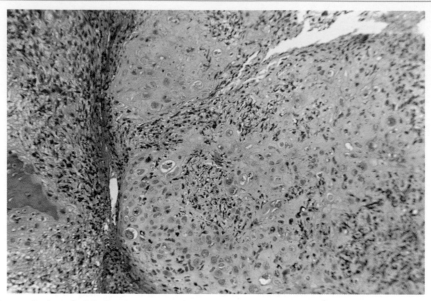

Figure 33–11 These tumors frequently show the lobulation that is commonly seen in cartilaginous tumors. However, at the periphery of the lobules, the tumor exhibits greater cellularity and atypia than is evident in chondrosarcomas.

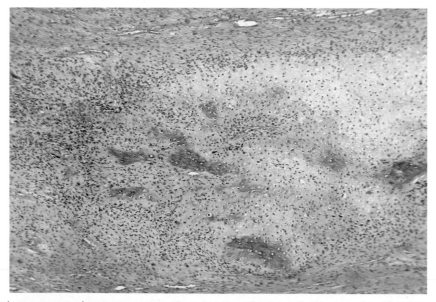

Figure 33–12 Some periosteal osteosarcomas show greater regions of spindle cell proliferation, as in this photomicrograph. With such lesions, the differential diagnosis is between high-grade surface osteosarcoma and periosteal osteosarcoma.

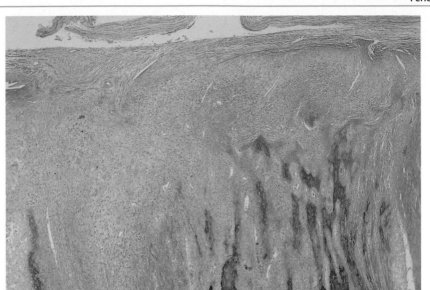

Figure 33–13 This low-power photomicrograph illustrates the classic histologic features of periosteal osteosarcoma. The chondroblastic tumor is transgressed by spiculated tumor osteoid that is arranged in a relatively orderly manner.

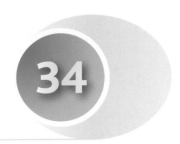

High-Grade Surface Osteosarcoma

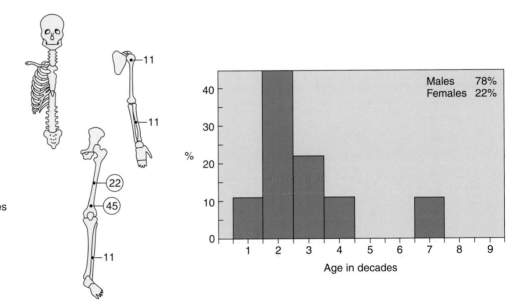

Numbers indicate percentage of cases
involving the indicated bone.
The percentage of the three bones
most commonly affected are circled.

Males 78%
Females 22%

Clinical Signs

1. A painful mass lesion is present.
2. The lesion may be warm.
3. Erythema may be present in the skin overlying the tumor.

Clinical Symptoms

1. Pain is present in the region of the tumor.
2. Swelling is noted in the region of the tumor.

Major Radiographic Features

1. A partially mineralized tumor is seen on the surface of a long bone, most commonly the femur.

2. Cortical destruction is usually apparent.
3. Periosteal new bone is often present.

Radiographic Differential Diagnosis

1. Periosteal osteosarcoma.
2. Parosteal osteosarcoma.
3. Periosteal chondrosarcoma.

Major Pathologic Features

Gross

1. The tumor is situated on the surface of the affected bone and may extend into the cortex, but it should lack significant medullary involvement.

2. Consistency of the lesional tissue varies from firm to soft and in general resembles that of ordinary osteosarcoma.
3. Chondroid differentiation consisting of bluish-white lobules of tissue may be grossly evident.

Microscopic

1. At low magnification, these tumors vary from region to region.
2. Zones of chondroid differentiation, zones of spindle cell proliferation, and zones containing dense osteoid may be identified.
3. At higher magnification, marked nuclear and cytologic pleomorphism—identical with that seen in conventional high-grade intramedullary osteosarcoma—is present.
4. Mitotic activity is usually brisk.
5. Lacelike osteoid production should be identifiable.
6. Minimal amounts of tumor may be present in the medullary cavity.

Pathologic Differential Diagnosis

Benign lesions

1. Myositis ossificans (heterotopic ossification).

Malignant lesions

1. Periosteal osteosarcoma.
2. Conventional osteosarcoma with prominent soft tissue extension.
3. Parosteal osteosarcoma.

Treatment

1. **Primary modality:** similar to that used for conventional osteosarcoma—limb-saving resection with a wide margin (if feasible) or amputation (if necessary) to obtain a wide margin. Neoadjuvant polychemotherapy protocols, similar to those for conventional osteosarcoma, are used.
2. **Other possible approaches:** radiotherapy for surgically inaccessible lesions and aggressive thoracotomy for pulmonary metastases.

References

Bertoni F, Bacchini P: Classification of bone tumors. *Eur J Radiol* 27 (Suppl 1):S74–S76, 1998.

Levine E, De Smet AA, Huntrakoon M: Juxtacortical osteosarcoma: a radiologic and histologic spectrum. *Skeletal Radiol* 14(1):38–46, 1985.

Okada K, Unni KK, Swee RG, et al: High grade surface osteosarcoma: a clinicopathologic study of 46 cases. *Cancer* 85(5):1044–1054, 1999.

Raymond AK: Surface osteosarcoma. *Clin Orthop Relat Res* 270: 140–148, 1991.

Schajowicz F, McGuire MH, Araujo ES, et al: Osteosarcomas arising on the surfaces of long bones. *J Bone Joint Surg Am* 70(4):555–564, 1988.

Unni KK: Osteosarcoma of bone. *J Orthop Sci* 3(5):287–294, 1998.

Wold LE, Unni KK, Beabout JW, et al: High-grade surface osteosarcomas. *Am J Surg Pathol* 8(3):181–186, 1984.

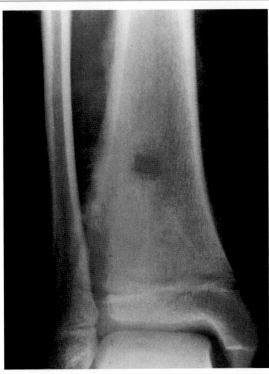

Figure 34–1 This radiograph illustrates the features of a high-grade surface osteosarcoma of the diametaphyseal region of the lower tibia. Note the matrix ossification projecting lateral to and over the tibia. The cortical defect evident is a result of prior biopsy.

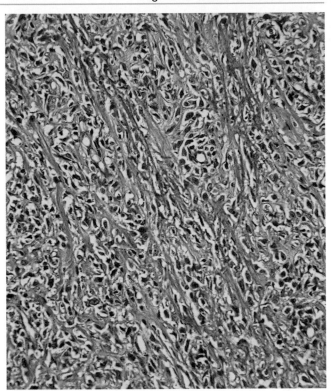

Figure 34–3 This low-power photomicrograph illustrates the cellular, anaplastic nature of high-grade surface osteosarcomas. The histologic spectrum of this subtype of osteosarcoma is identical with that of the usual intramedullary type of osteosarcoma.

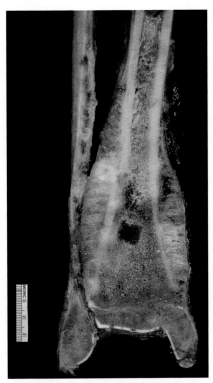

Figure 34–2 This photograph shows the gross appearance of a high-grade surface osteosarcoma involving the distal tibia. No medullary tumor is present; the defect at the center of the distal tibia represents a prior biopsy site.

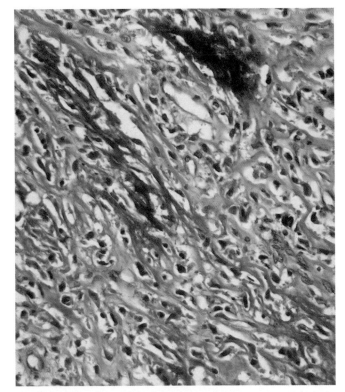

Figure 34–4 Examples of high-grade surface osteosarcoma may show little osteoid, as illustrated in this photomicrograph.

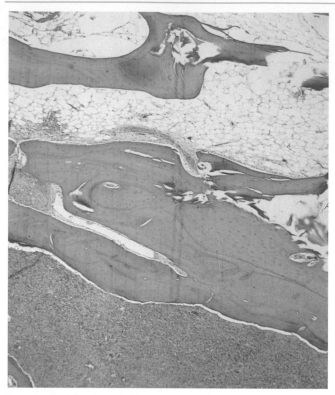

Figure 34–5 Although cortical bone may be eroded in the surface variants of osteosarcoma, medullary involvement is lacking, as illustrated in this example of a high-grade surface osteosarcoma of the tibia.

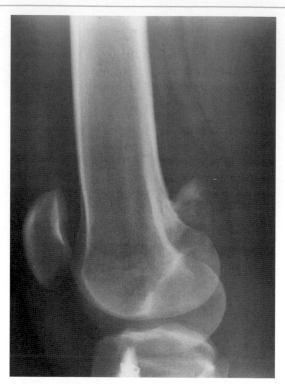

Figure 34–7 This radiograph illustrates a high-grade surface osteosarcoma arising from the posterior surface of the distal femoral metaphysis. Note the radiating bone spicules extending posteriorly into the sizable soft tissue mass. The medulla of the femur appears uninvolved.

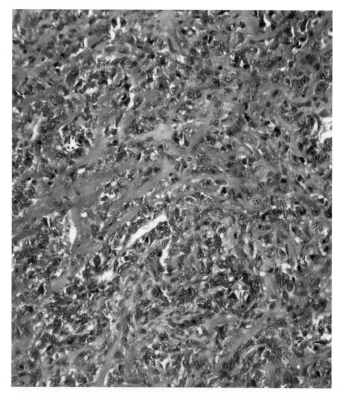

Figure 34–6 This photomicrograph demonstrates the histologic features of a high-grade surface osteosarcoma treated initially with limb salvage. The tumor metastasized to the pelvis, and the patient died of further metastatic disease.

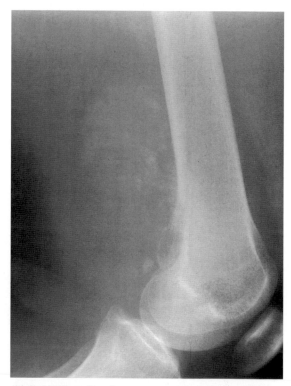

Figure 34–8 A high-grade surface osteosarcoma of the distal femur is shown in this radiograph. Note the large ossified soft tissue mass posterior to the femur. The tumor affects only the superficial cortical bone.

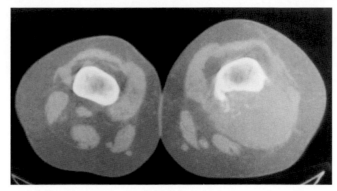

Figure 34–9 The computed tomographic (CT) scan of the same osteosarcoma shown in Figure 34–8 verifies the surface location of the tumor, delineating the soft tissue mass and confirming the absence of a medullary component of the lesion.

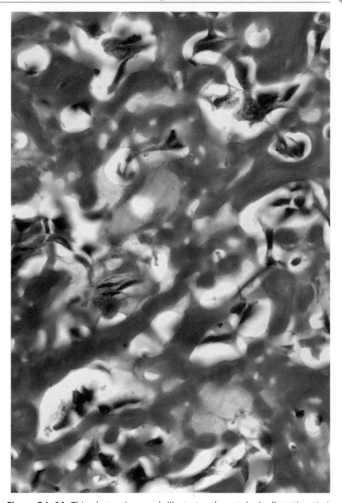

Figure 34–11 This photomicrograph illustrates the cytologic distortion that is commonly present in osteosclerotic osteosarcomas. This pattern may be seen in high-grade surface osteosarcomas or conventional high-grade intramedullary osteosarcomas.

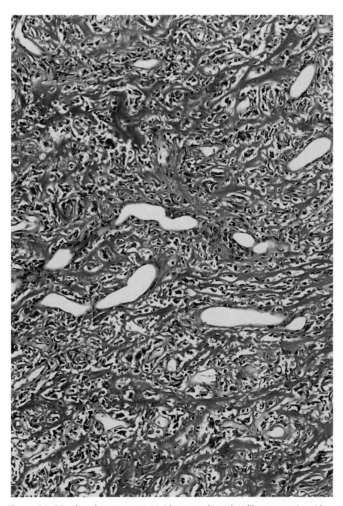

Figure 34–10 Abundant tumor osteoid arranged in a lacelike pattern is evident in this high-grade surface osteosarcoma of the femur.

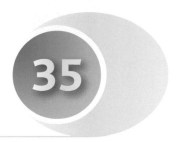

Telangiectatic Osteosarcoma

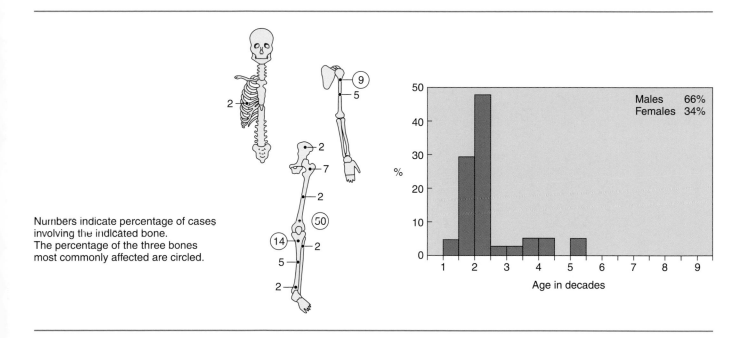

Numbers indicate percentage of cases involving the indicated bone.
The percentage of the three bones most commonly affected are circled.

Males 66%
Females 34%

% — (y-axis)

Age in decades — (x-axis)

Clinical Signs

1. A tender mass lesion is noted.
2. Occasional pathologic fracture may be seen.

Clinical Symptoms

1. Pain is present.
2. Swelling is noted in the region of the tumor.

Major Imaging Features

1. The tumor is large and metaphyseal.
2. Medullary and cortical bone destruction is considerable.

3. The lesion is purely lytic and poorly marginated.
4. Periosteal new bone and soft tissue mass are common.
5. Magnetic resonance imaging may show fluid–fluid levels with or without solid elements.

Radiographic Differential Diagnosis

1. Ordinary (conventional) osteosarcoma.
2. Fibrosarcoma.
3. Malignant fibrous histiocytoma.
4. Aneurysmal bone cyst.

Major Pathologic Features

Gross

1. Lesional tissue is hemorrhagic.
2. Firm, fleshy areas are not identifiable in tumor.
3. Lesional tissue is arranged in delicate strands coursing through the blood clot.

Microscopic

1. At low magnification, the features are similar to those of aneurysmal bone cyst.
2. Septa traverse and surround blood-filled spaces.
3. At higher magnification, the mononuclear cells are shown to be pleomorphic.
4. Benign multinucleated giant cells are almost uniformly present.
5. Osteoid production is generally focal and minimal.

Pathologic Differential Diagnosis

Benign lesions

1. Aneurysmal bone cyst.

Malignant lesions

1. Malignancy in giant cell tumor (malignant giant cell tumor).
2. Angiosarcoma.

Treatment

1. **Primary modality:** as in conventional osteosarcoma, surgical ablation by amputation or limb-saving resection. Multidrug chemotherapy in a neoadjuvant setting is most commonly used.
2. **Other possible approaches:** radiation therapy for lesions in inaccessible sites.

References

Bertoni F, Pignatti G, Bacchini P, et al: Telangiectatic or hemorrhagic osteosarcoma of bone: a clinicopathologic study of 41 patients at the Rizzoli Institute. *Prog Surg Pathol* 10:63–82, 1989.

Huvos AG, Rosen G, Bretsky SS, et al: Telangiectatic osteogenic sarcoma: a clinicopathologic study of 124 patients. *Cancer* 49(8):1679–1689, 1982.

Matsuno T, Unni KK, McLeod RA, et al: Telangiectatic osteogenic sarcoma. *Cancer* 38(6):2538–2547, 1976.

Mervak TR, Unni KK, Pritchard DJ, et al: Telangiectatic osteosarcoma. *Clin Orthop Relat Res* (270):135–139, 1991.

Murphey MD, wan Jaovisidha S, Temple HT, et al: Telangiectatic osteosarcoma: radiologic-pathologic comparison. *Radiology* 229(2):545–553, 2003.

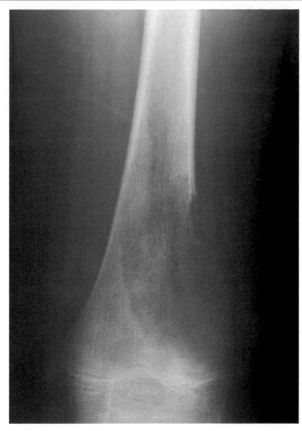

Figure 35–1 This radiograph illustrates a large, purely lytic, and poorly margin-ated tumor in the distal femoral metaphysis. Considerable destruction of the medullary and cortical bone is evident, with associated soft tissue extension. The purely lytic appearance is characteristic of telangiectatic osteosarcoma.

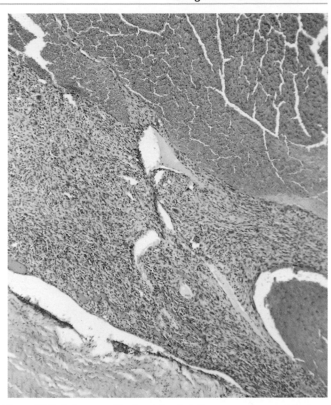

Figure 35–3 At low magnification, telangiectatic osteosarcoma contains large blood-filled spaces, similar to the pattern seen in an aneurysmal bone cyst.

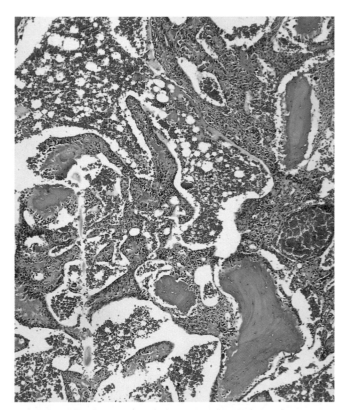

Figure 35–4 This photomicrograph shows the edge of a lesion demonstrating permeation of medullary bone. The bony trabeculae are normal and are not produced by the tumor.

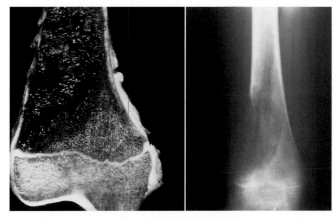

Figure 35–2 The gross pathologic features of telangiectatic osteosarcoma are illustrated in this photograph. The lesion is invariably hemorrhagic and may be quite cystic. Both grossly and microscopically, it may be mistaken for an aneurysmal bone cyst.

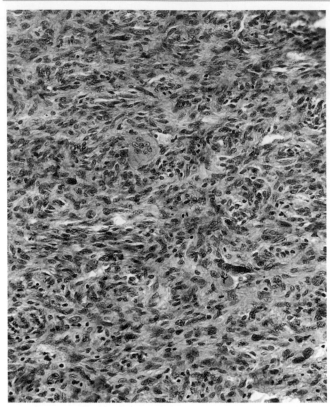

Figure 35–5 Solid areas of the tumor should be only a minor component of this tumor. Abnormal mitotic figures and benign giant cells are commonly found.

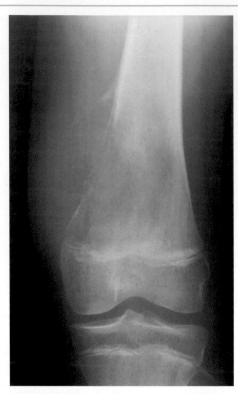

Figure 35–7 This lesion of the distal femur shows cortical destruction, Codman's triangle, and an associated soft tissue mass. These features support the diagnosis of a high-grade malignancy. The purely lytic nature of the lesion is compatible with the diagnosis of telangiectatic osteosarcoma, which it proved to be histologically.

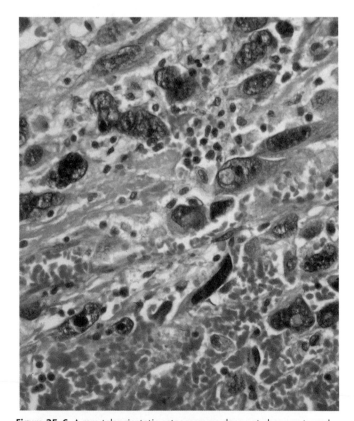

Figure 35–6 A rare telangiectatic osteosarcoma does not show septa and spaces but instead is composed of highly pleomorphic-appearing cells within a blood clot.

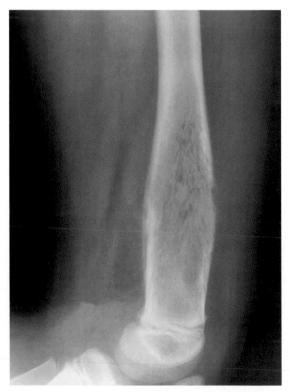

Figure 35–8 This diametaphyseal lytic lesion with poor margination and a permeative growth pattern also represents a telangiectatic osteosarcoma.

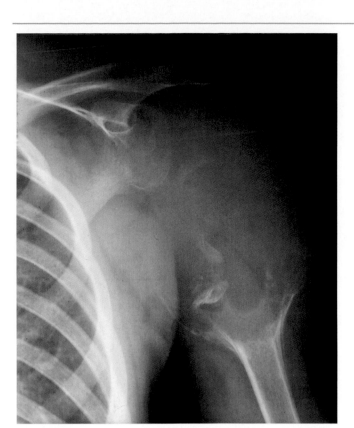

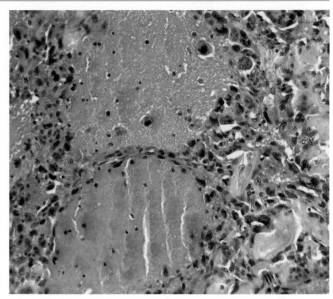

Figure 35–11 Careful examination of the septa is necessary to identify the cytologic atypia, shown in this photomicrograph, that distinguishes telangiectatic osteosarcoma from an aneurysmal bone cyst.

Figure 35–9 This proximal humeral lesion shows the "blown-out" appearance occasionally seen with an aneurysmal bone cyst. This lesion was confirmed histologically to be a telangiectatic osteosarcoma. The overlap of radiographic and histologic features of aneurysmal bone cyst and telangiectatic osteosarcoma presents particularly difficult diagnostic problems for the pathologist.

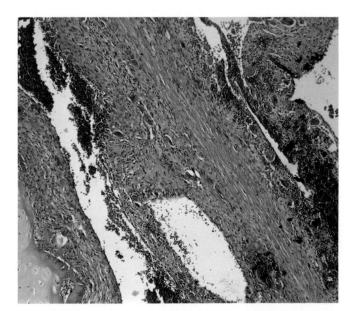

Figure 35–10 This photomicrograph illustrates a telangiectatic osteosarcoma that markedly simulates an aneurysmal bone cyst. Benign multinucleated giant cells are present, and some of the septa are fibrotic and hypocellular.

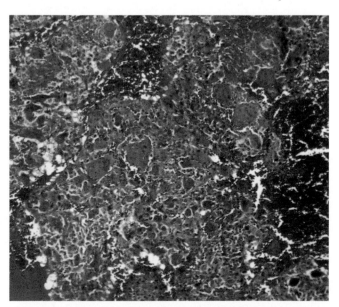

Figure 35–12 When multinucleated giant cells are numerous, as in this photomicrograph, a telangiectatic osteosarcoma may focally resemble a giant cell tumor.

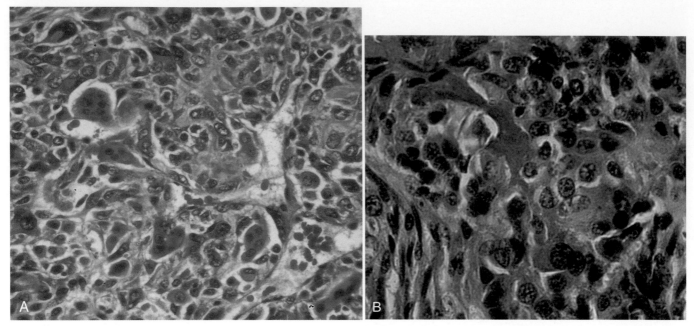

Figure 35–13 At high magnification, the cytologic atypia of the mononuclear cells illustrated in *A* and *B* distinguishes telangiectatic osteosarcoma from a giant cell tumor. Osteoid production *(B)* should be minimal.

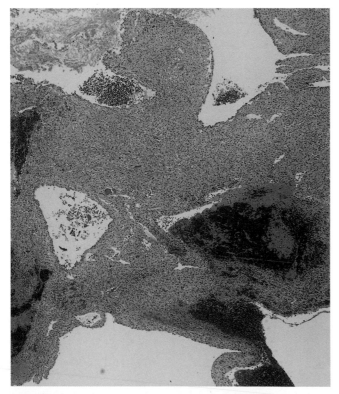

Figure 35–14 At low power, the histologic pattern of telangiectatic osteosarcoma, seen in this photomicrograph, mimics exactly the pattern of aneurysmal bone cyst.

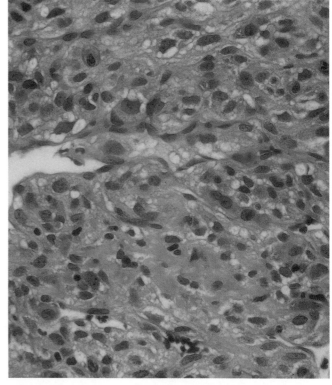

Figure 35–15 Moderate- to high-grade cytologic atypia is evident in the spindle cells of telangiectatic osteosarcoma. This photomicrograph shows the same tumor illustrated in Figure 35–14.

Low-Grade Central Osteosarcoma

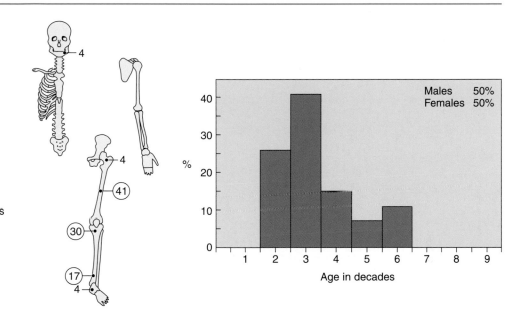

Numbers indicate percentage of cases involving the indicated bone.
The percentage of the three bones most commonly affected are circled.

Clinical Signs

1. Usually, no specific signs are elicited on physical examination.

Clinical Symptoms

1. Pain is a common presenting complaint.
2. A swelling is almost never noted.

Major Radiographic Features

1. Medullary lesions usually extend to the end of the bone.

2. The tumor is poorly marginated and large.
3. Most lesions are trabeculated or sclerotic.
4. Periosteal new bone and soft tissue mass are usually absent.
5. The overall appearance may suggest benignity, with only a small region showing features that suggest malignancy.

Radiographic Differential Diagnosis

1. Fibrous dysplasia.
2. Giant cell tumor.
3. Ordinary (conventional) osteosarcoma.
4. Fibrosarcoma.
5. Malignant fibrous histiocytoma.

Major Pathologic Features

Gross

1. These lesions are firm and fibrous, lacking the fleshy appearance of high-grade sarcomas.
2. A gritty quality, somewhat like that of fibrous dysplasia, may be noted.
3. The tumor is most commonly confined to the medullary cavity without an associated soft tissue mass; however, the cortex is destroyed, at least focally.

Microscopic

1. The low-magnification appearance of this tumor mimics that of fibrous dysplasia.
2. The lesional tissue is composed of disordered or irregular bony trabeculae, between which is a hypocellular spindle cell proliferation. (The pattern is essentially identical with that seen in parosteal osteosarcoma.)
3. At higher magnification, the spindle cells show little pleomorphism or anaplasia and mitotic activity is extremely low. The spindle cells may be arranged in a "herringbone" or a storiform pattern.
4. The osteoid appears "normalized" as in parosteal osteosarcoma.

Pathologic Differential Diagnosis

Benign lesions

1. Fibrous dysplasia.
2. Osteofibrous dysplasia.

Malignant lesions

1. Osteosarcoma, ordinary intramedullary type.
2. Parosteal osteosarcoma (if location is not considered).

Treatment

1. **Primary modality:** surgical resection with a wide margin and skeletal reconstruction with osteochondral allograft, custom prosthesis, or resection arthrodesis, depending on the location of the lesion and the patient's needs.
2. **Other possible approaches:** amputation if an adequately wide margin cannot be achieved by surgical resection. Chemotherapy is not indicated unless there has been recurrence and "dedifferentiation" of the tumor.

References

Andresen KJ, Sundaram M, Unni KK, et al: Imaging features of low grade central osteosarcoma of the long bones and pelvis. *Skeletal Radiol* 33(7):373–379, 2004.

Bertoni F, Bacchini P, Fabbri N, et al: Osteosarcoma. Low-grade intraosseous-type osteosarcoma, histologically resembling parosteal osteosarcoma, fibrous dysplasia and desmoplastic fibroma. *Cancer* 71(2):338–345, 1993.

Choong PF, Pritchard DJ, Rock MG, et al: Low grade central osteogenic sarcoma. A long-term follow up of 20 patients. *Clin Orthop Rel Res* 322:198–206, 1996.

Ellis JH, Siegel CL, Martel W, et al: Radiologic features of well-differentiated osteosarcoma. *Am J Roentgenol* 151(4):739–742, 1988.

Franceschina MJ, Hankin RC, Irwin RB: Low-grade central osteosarcoma resembling fibrous dysplasia. A report of two cases. *Am J Orthop* 26(6):432–440, 1997.

Franchi A, Bacchini P, Della Rocca C, et al: Central low-grade osteosarcoma with pagetoid bone formation: a potential diagnostic pitfall. *Mod Pathol* 17(3):288–291, 2004.

Iemoto Y, Ushigome S, Fukunaga M, et al: Case report 679. Central low-grade osteosarcoma with foci of dedifferentiation. *Skeletal Radiol* 20(5):379–382, 1991.

Kurt AM, Unni KK, McLeod RA, et al: Low-grade intraosseous osteosarcoma. *Cancer* 65(6):1418–1428, 1990.

Unni KK, Dahlin DC, McLeod RA, et al: Intraosseous well-differentiated osteosarcoma. *Cancer* 40(3):1337–1347, 1977.

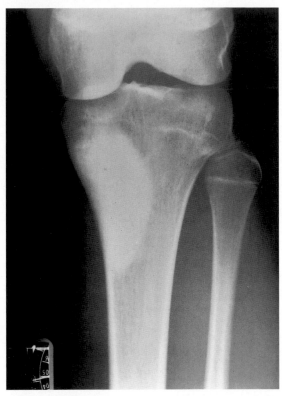

Figure 36–1 This radiograph illustrates a low-grade central osteosarcoma of the medulla of the upper tibia. The lesion is densely sclerotic.

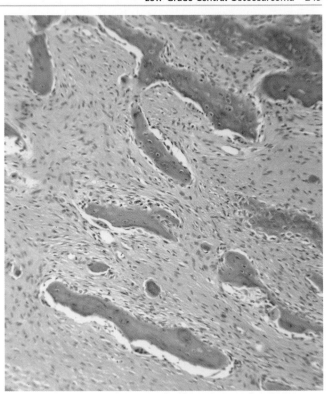

Figure 36–3 This low-power photomicrograph illustrates the parallel arrangements of bony trabeculae that can be seen in low-grade central osteosarcomas. This appearance is nearly identical with that of parosteal osteosarcoma.

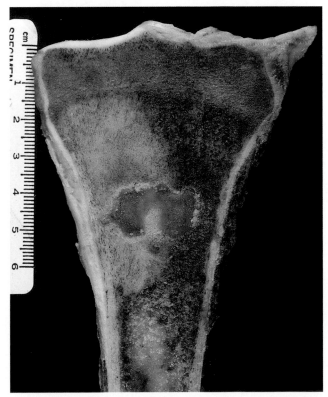

Figure 36–2 This photograph of a gross specimen of the proximal tibial lesion seen in Figure 36–1 shows the homogeneous nature of most low-grade central osteosarcomas. The central defect is the biopsy site. These tumors are frequently gritty when cut.

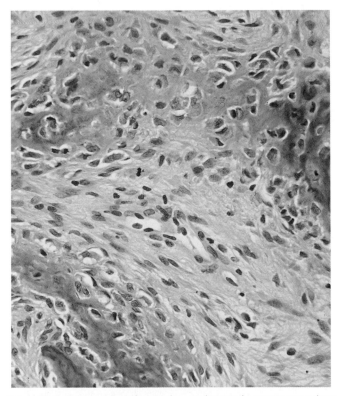

Figure 36–4 At higher magnification, low-grade central osteosarcomas show minimal cytologic atypia. The lesions are also less cellular than conventional osteosarcomas.

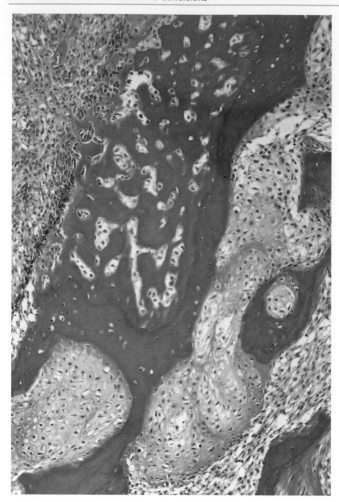

Figure 36–5 The osteoid produced by low-grade central osteosarcoma may grow in an appositional manner onto preexisting bony trabeculae.

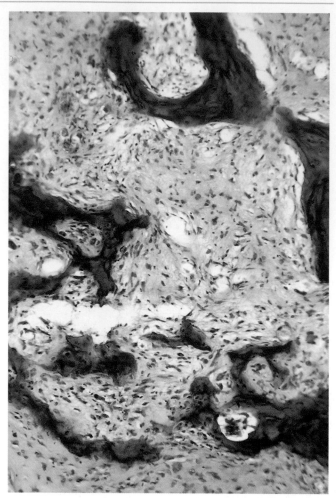

Figure 36–6 The histologic pattern of low-grade central osteosarcoma may also mimic that seen in fibrous dysplasia, as illustrated in this photomicrograph.

Small Cell Osteosarcoma

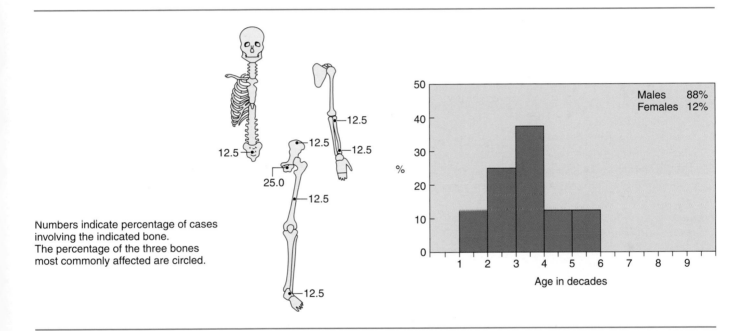

Numbers indicate percentage of cases involving the indicated bone.
The percentage of the three bones most commonly affected are circled.

Males 88%
Females 12%

%

Age in decades

Clinical Signs

1. A painful mass may be present.
2. A neurologic deficit may be seen if the tumor involves a vertebra.

Clinical Symptoms

1. Approximately two thirds of patients complain of pain in the region of the tumor.
2. Approximately 15% of patients complain of a mass or swelling in the region of the tumor, and 25% complain of both pain and swelling.
3. Neurologic symptoms may be present in patients with vertebral tumors.

4. Symptoms may be present from days to years before diagnosis of the tumor.

Major Radiographic Features

1. The tumor most commonly involves the metaphyseal region of long bones.
2. Epiphyseal extension is present in about one third of cases.
3. Approximately 15% of tumors are purely diaphyseal.
4. All tumors have a lytic component, and associated medullary sclerosis is present in approximately half the tumors.
5. Approximately 60% of tumors have an associated soft tissue mass.

6. Of tumors, 25% have an identifiable mineralized soft tissue mass.
7. All tumors have an indistinct margin, and periosteal reaction is present in approximately half the tumors.

Radiographic Differential Diagnosis

1. Conventional osteosarcoma.
2. Ewing's sarcoma.

Major Pathologic Features

Gross

1. Tumors are generally poorly circumscribed and infiltrative.
2. Soft tissue extension is ordinarily present.
3. The tumors are most commonly soft and gray–white.

Microscopic

1. Although the designation "small cell" is subjective, the nuclei are relatively uniform in shape (with a mean nuclear diameter of approximately 8.4 μm).
2. Nuclei are round to oval and generally hyperchromatic.
3. The shape of cells varies from round (most common) to short-spindled.
4. Osteoid is variably present but most commonly is scanty (approximately half the tumors).
5. The osteoid shows a lacelike pattern.
6. A hemangiopericytomatous pattern is present in about one third of tumors.
7. Glycogen is identified in approximately one third of tumors (periodic acid–Schiff [PAS] positivity).

Pathologic Differential Diagnosis

Benign lesions

1. None.

Malignant lesions

1. Ewing's sarcoma.
2. Hemangiopericytoma.
3. Osteosarcoma.
4. Metastatic small cell carcinoma.
5. Malignant lymphoma.

Treatment

1. **Primary modality:** limb-sparing surgery with adjuvant chemotherapy.
2. **Other possible approaches:** amputation.

References

Ayala AG, Ro JY, Raymond AK, et al: Small cell osteosarcoma. A clinicopathologic study of 27 cases. *Cancer* 64(10):2162–2173, 1989.

Bertoni F, Present D, Bacchini P, et al: The Istituto Rizzoli experience with small cell osteosarcoma. *Cancer* 64(12):2591–2599, 1989.

Nakajima H, Sim FH, Bond JR, et al: Small cell osteosarcoma of bone. Review of 72 cases. *Cancer* 79(11):2095–2106, 1997.

Park SH, Kim I: Small cell osteogenic sarcoma of the ribs: cytological, immunohistochemical, and ultrastructural study with literature review. *Ultrastruct Pathol* 23(2):133–140, 1999.

Sim FH, Unni KK, Beabout JW, et al: Osteosarcoma with small cells simulating Ewing's tumor. *J Bone Joint Surg Am* 61(2):207–215, 1979.

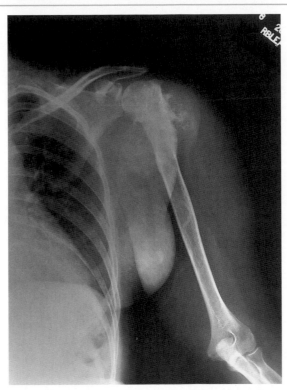

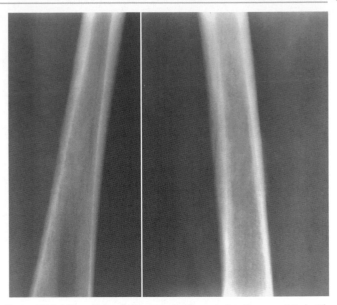

Figure 37–3 This radiograph illustrates the bony destruction associated with a small cell osteosarcoma involving the femoral diaphysis. Tumors such as this likely suggest a radiographic differential diagnosis of "small round cell tumor." Needle biopsy in such cases may be confusing because the cytologic features of small cell osteosarcoma overlap with those of Ewing's sarcoma.

Figure 37–1 This radiograph shows small cell osteosarcoma involving the proximal humerus. The metaphysis of long bones is the most common site of small cell osteosarcoma.

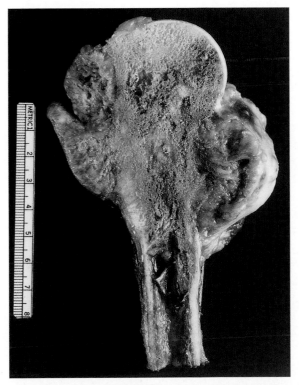

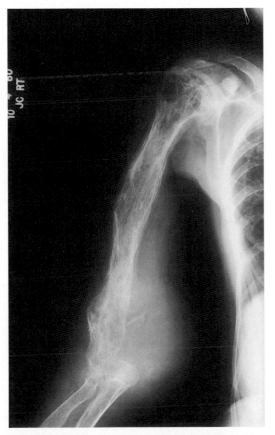

Figure 37–2 This photograph demonstrates the gross pathologic features of a small cell osteosarcoma (the specimen corresponds to the tumor illustrated in Fig. 37–1). There are no distinctive gross pathologic features of small cell osteosarcoma. Most tumors show a permeative destructive pattern of growth with soft tissue extension, as in this case.

Figure 37–4 This radiograph shows the humerus of a patient with Paget's disease. Small cell osteosarcoma has developed in the humerus affected by Paget's disease.

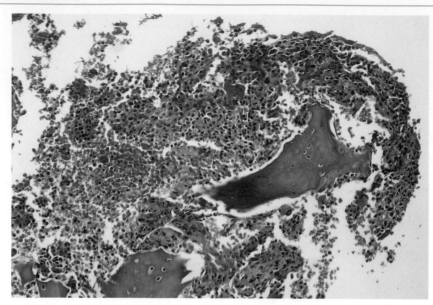

Figure 37–5 This photomicrograph of a small cell osteosarcoma involving a rib shows the permeative pattern of bony invasion commonly seen in malignant bony neoplasms. At low magnification, it may be difficult to determine whether such a small cell tumor is producing a matrix.

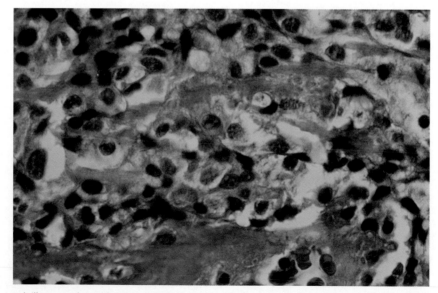

Figure 37–6 This photomicrograph illustrates the marked "crush artifact" that is commonly seen in needle biopsies of small cell tumors, including small cell osteosarcoma. Irregular fragments of osteoid are present, admixed with the small cell neoplasm, helping to identify this tumor as a small cell osteosarcoma.

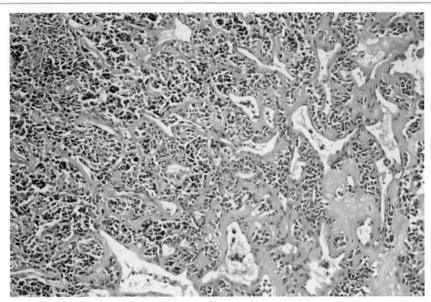

Figure 37–7 This photomicrograph illustrates the hemangiopericytomatous pattern that is commonly present in regions of small cell osteosarcoma. A similar pattern can be seen in the small cell areas of mesenchymal chondrosarcoma; therefore, these two tumors are usually in the same differential diagnosis.

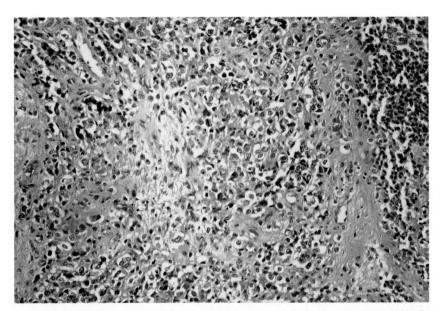

Figure 37–8 It may be necessary to search multiple sections to find tumor osteoid in cases of small cell osteosarcoma. When found, the bone produced by the tumor shows a lacelike pattern similar to that seen in conventional osteosarcoma.

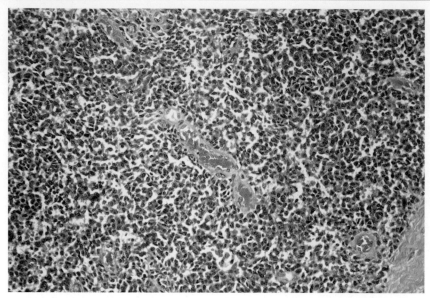

Figure 37–9 In this photomicrograph, this small cell osteosarcoma of the femur displays a low-power histologic pattern mimicking that of Ewing's sarcoma. The cytologic features of small cell osteosarcoma can also mimic those of Ewing's sarcoma (see Fig. 37–10).

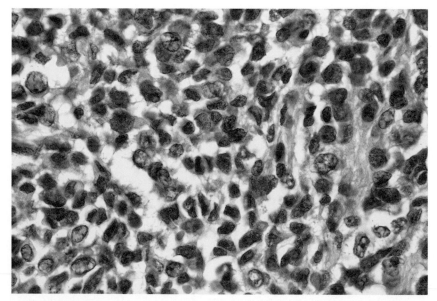

Figure 37–10 The cytologic features of small cell osteosarcoma, illustrated in this photomicrograph, mimic those of Ewing's sarcoma. Careful search for osteoid matrix is important to identify the tumor as an osteosarcoma.

Section 2B: Cartilage-Forming Tumors

Osteochondroma

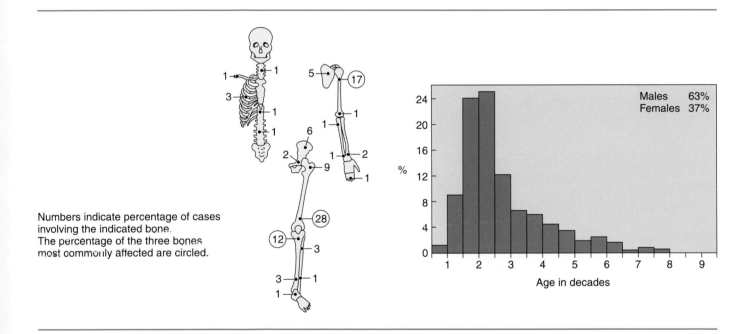

Numbers indicate percentage of cases involving the indicated bone.
The percentage of the three bones most commonly affected are circled.

Males	63%
Females	37%

Age in decades

Clinical Signs

1. A palpable mass is noted.

Clinical Symptoms

1. A mass lesion, usually of long duration, is present.
2. Pain may result secondary to impingement on an overlying structure or to bursa formation.
3. Rarely, pain may be related to fracture through the stalk of a pedunculated lesion.

Major Radiographic Features

1. Peripheral bone projection or growth is present.
2. The cortical and cancellous bone shows continuity from the underlying parent bone to the lesion.
3. There is flaring of the metaphysis of the affected bone.

Radiographic Differential Diagnosis

1. Bizarre parosteal osteochondromatous proliferation.
2. Parosteal osteosarcoma.

3. Myositis ossificans.
4. Chondrosarcoma, when a large bursa overlying an osteochondroma is mistaken for a malignant mass on magnetic resonance imaging.

Major Pathologic Features

Gross

1. The cut surface of the lesion shows a thin (usually less than 1 cm), smooth, translucent, bluish cartilaginous cap.
2. Cancellous bone underlies the cartilaginous cap.
3. Lesions may be pedunculated or sessile with a broad base.

Microscopic

1. The thin cartilaginous cap mimics the appearance of an epiphyseal plate with maturation via endochondral ossification to regular bony trabeculae.
2. At higher magnification, the chondrocytes are seen to be arranged in a linear fashion, and the nuclei lack pleomorphism, nuclear hyperchromasia, and binucleation.
3. The intertrabecular space is filled with fatty or hematopoietic marrow.

Pathologic Differential Diagnosis

Benign lesions

1. Bizarre parosteal osteocartilaginous proliferation.

Malignant lesions

1. Parosteal osteosarcoma.
2. Chondrosarcoma arising in an osteochondroma.

Treatment

1. **Primary modality:** Treatment is individualized depending on clinical circumstances. Most lesions, either solitary or multiple, are simply observed.
2. **Other possible approaches:** If the lesion is symptomatic or cosmetically disfiguring, surgical excision at the base of the exostosis is carried out to remove the entire cartilage cap.

References

Bandiera S, Bacchini P, Bertoni F: Bizarre parosteal osteochondromatous proliferation of bone. *Skeletal Radiol* 27(3):154–156, 1998.

Borges AM, Huvos AB, Smith J: Bursa formation and synovial chondrometaplasia associated with osteochondromas. *Am J Clin Pathol* 75(5):648–653, 1981.

Karasick D, Schweitzer ME, Eschelman DJ: Symptomatic osteochondromas: imaging features. *Am J Roentgenol* 168(6):1507–1512, 1997.

Landon GC, Johnson KA, Dahlin DC: Subungual exostoses. *J Bone Joint Surg Am* 61(2):256–259, 1979.

Mehta M, White LM, Knapp T, et al: MR imaging of symptomatic osteochondromas with pathological correlation. *Skeletal Radiol* 27(8): 427–433, 1998.

Murphey MD, Choi JJ, Kransdorf MJ, et al: Imaging of osteochondroma: variants and complications with radiologic-pathologic correlation. *Radiographics* 20(5):1407–1434, 2000.

Nora FE, Dahlin DC, Beabout JW: Bizarre parosteal osteochondromatous proliferations of the hands and feet. *Am J Surg Pathol* 7(3): 245–250, 1983.

Okada K, Terada K, Sashi R, et al: Large bursa formation associated with osteochondroma of the scapula: a case report and review of the literature. *Jpn J Clin Oncol* 29(7):356–360, 1999.

Shapiro F, Simon S, Glimcher MJ: Hereditary multiple exostoses: anthropometric, roentgenographic, and clinical aspects. *J Bone Joint Surg Am* 61(6A):815–824, 1979.

Solomon L: Hereditary multiple exostosis. *Am J Hum Genet* 16:351–363, 1964.

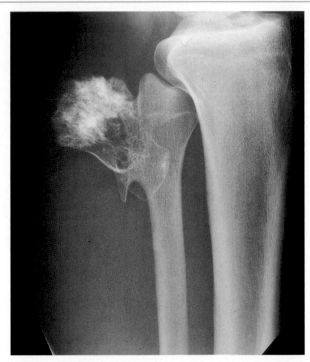

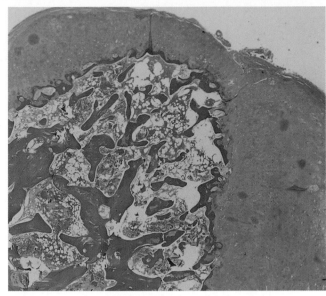

Figure 38–3 At low magnification, osteochondromas show a well-circumscribed periphery. The hyaline cartilage matures into the underlying trabecular bone.

Figure 38–1 This radiograph of the proximal tibia and fibula shows a heavily mineralized osteochondroma projecting posteriorly from the upper fibular metaphysis. The continuity of the cortical and cancellous bone of the fibula with the lesion is characteristic of osteochondroma.

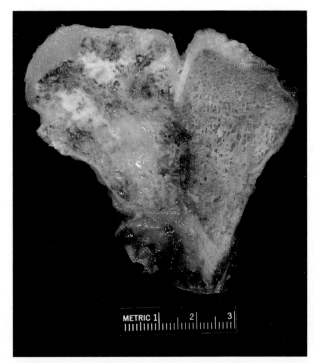

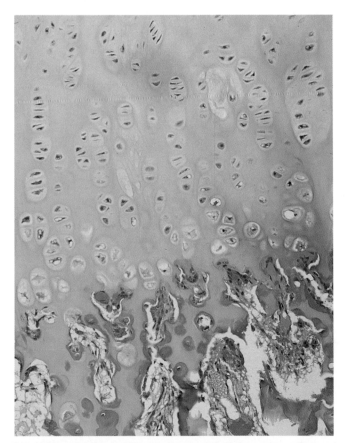

Figure 38–2 Grossly, the resected osteochondroma illustrated in Figure 38–1 shows a cartilaginous cap with regions of extensive calcification (white areas) corresponding to the heavily mineralized regions seen radiographically. The thickness of the cartilage cap is a gross pathologic feature that helps identify lesions that should be carefully assessed histologically for malignant transformation of the cartilage.

Figure 38–4 At higher magnification, the transition between the cartilage and the osseous trabeculae is identical with a normal growth plate, with columns of chondrocytes and ossification of the matrix material.

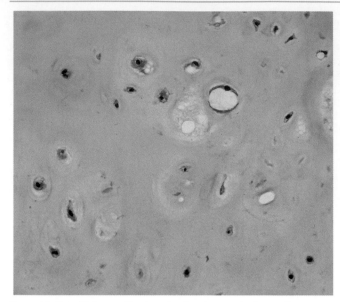

Figure 38–5 At high magnification, the chondrocytes in the cartilage cap have small, dark-staining nuclei that lack cytologic atypia.

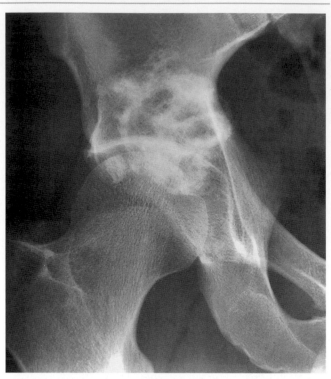

Figure 38–7 This radiograph of the pelvis demonstrates a mineralized lesion above the acetabulum. Flat bone osteochondromas such as this may be difficult to localize and characterize with plain radiographs. Computed tomographic (CT) scans are particularly helpful in this situation.

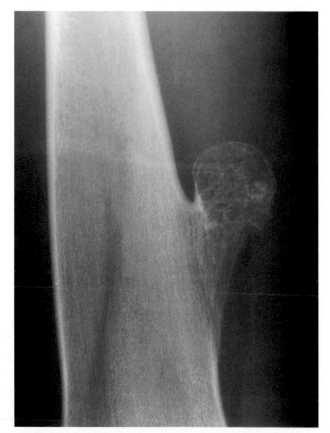

Figure 38–6 This radiograph shows an osteochondroma projecting from the lower femur. The continuity of cortical and cancellous bone is evident. In general, pedunculated osteochondromas point away from the closest joint.

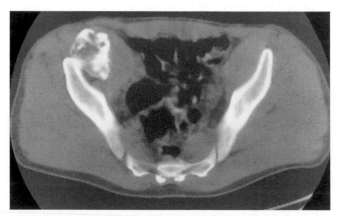

Figure 38–8 An axial CT scan of the patient in Figure 38–7 demonstrates the typical appearance of an osteochondroma projecting from the anterior iliac bone.

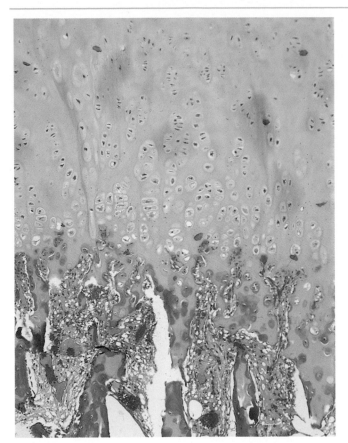

Figure 38–9 Between the osseous trabeculae of an osteochondroma is fatty or hematopoietic marrow, as shown in this photomicrograph. In contrast, parosteal osteosarcoma, which may also have a cartilaginous cap, has a spindle cell proliferation between the "normalized trabeculae" of bone.

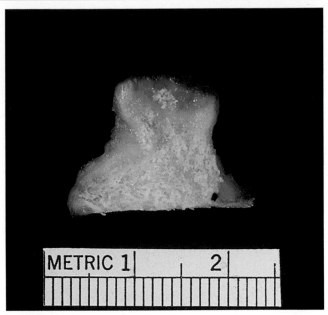

Figure 38–11 Subungual exostoses, as shown in this photograph, share some gross and microscopic features with osteochondromas.

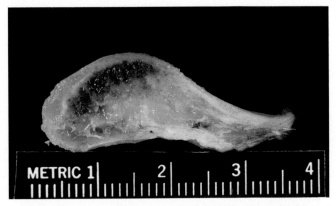

Figure 38–10 This osteochondroma of the distal femur shows the thin cartilage cap and the continuity of the cortical and cancellous bone that characterize these lesions.

Chondroma

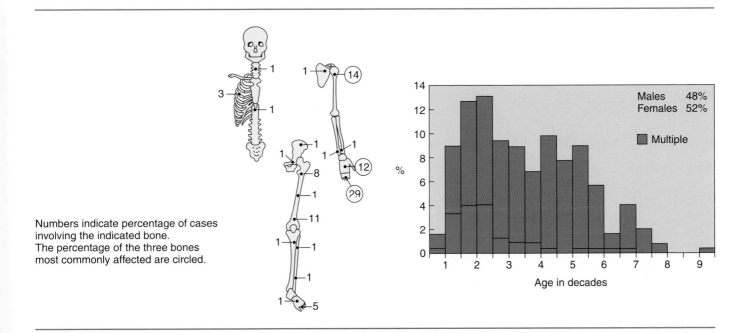

Numbers indicate percentage of cases involving the indicated bone.
The percentage of the three bones most commonly affected are circled.

Males 48%
Females 52%

■ Multiple

%

Age in decades

Clinical Signs

1. Frequently, chondromas are diagnosed incidentally on radiographic examination.
2. Chondromas are frequently "hot" on bone scan and may be incidentally identified in this way as well.

Clinical Symptoms

1. The majority of patients are asymptomatic.
2. Pain is rarely a presenting complaint but may occur in patients with pathologic fractures. This is commonly

the case with lesions of the small bones. If pain exists in the absence of pathologic fracture, a low-grade chondrosarcoma should be suspected.

Major Radiographic Features

1. The lesion has a medullary location.
2. The features are benign, showing sharp margination and expansion of the affected bone.
3. Punctate calcification frequently is present.
4. Multiple lesions may be seen.

Radiographic Differential Diagnosis

1. Bone infarct.
2. Chondrosarcoma.

Major Pathologic Features

Gross

1. Lesional tissue is characteristically translucent and blue–gray.
2. Whitish-yellow calcific foci may be scattered throughout the tissue.
3. The tumors vary in consistency, but most are relatively firm. Myxoid foci should arouse suspicion that the tumor is a low-grade chondrosarcoma.

Microscopic

1. At low magnification, the tumor is hypocellular, with a blue–gray aura to the cartilaginous matrix.
2. The nuclei are inconspicuous at low magnification.
3. At higher magnification, the nuclei are uniform in their cytologic characteristics. Each is small, regular, and darkly stained.
4. Binucleated cells are rare.

Pathologic Differential Diagnosis

Benign lesions

1. Fibrocartilaginous dysplasia with prominent chondroid regions.
2. The cartilage of a prominent costochondral junction.

Malignant lesions

1. Low-grade (well-differentiated) chondrosarcoma.
2. Chondroblastic osteosarcoma.

Treatment

1. **Primary modality:** A benign appearing, asymptomatic enchondroma that is not structurally weakening the bone warrants observation.
2. **Other possible approaches:** If the lesion is symptomatic, curettage and bone grafting usually are curative. If there is an associated pathologic fracture, curettage and grafting should be delayed until the fracture has healed and the continuity of the bone has been restored.

References

Bauer TW, Dorfman HD, Lathan JT Jr: Periosteal chondroma: a clinicopathologic study of 23 cases. *Am J Surg Pathol* 6(7):631–637, 1982.

Boriani S, Bacchini P, Bertoni F, et al: Periosteal chondroma: a review of twenty cases. *J Bone Joint Surg Am* 65(2):205–212, 1983.

DeSantos LA, Spjut HJ: Periosteal chondroma: a radiographic spectrum. *Skeletal Radiol* 6(1):15–20, 1981.

Kocher MS, Jupiter JB: Enchondroma versus chondrosarcoma of the phalanx. *Orthopedics* 23(5):493–494, 2000.

Ostrowski ML, Spjut HJ: Lesions of the bones of the hands and feet. *Am J Surg Pathol* 21(6):676–690, 1997.

Schreuder HW, Pruszczynski M, Veth RP, et al: Treatment of benign and low-grade malignant intramedullary chondroid tumours with curettage and cryosurgery. *Eur J Surg Oncol* 24(2):120–126, 1998.

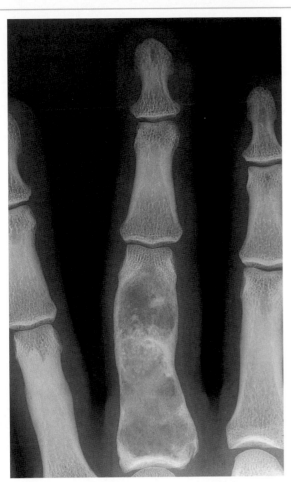

Figure 39–1 This radiograph shows an enchondroma in its most common location, a phalanx of the hand. The lesion is well marginated and expansile. The typical punctate calcification of a cartilaginous lesion is present.

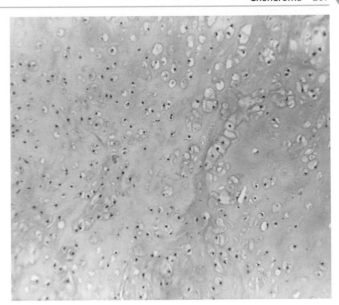

Figure 39–3 At low magnification, hyaline cartilage lesions are blue–gray. Benign lesions are hypocellular, as illustrated in this photomicrograph of a chondroma involving the femoral diaphysis.

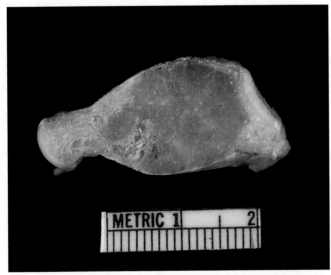

Figure 39–2 The gross appearance of hyaline cartilage lesions is shown in this photograph of a phalangeal chondroma. The lesion is well circumscribed, glistening, and gray–white. The small bones may be expanded by such a lesion, as in this case.

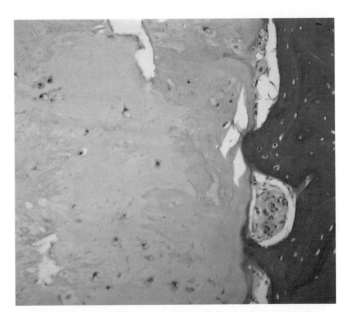

Figure 39–4 The periphery of a chondroma is well circumscribed, both grossly and microscopically, as seen in this photomicrograph of a fibular chondroma. The lesion does not show significant endosteal erosion.

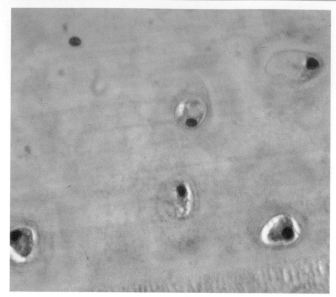

Figure 39–5 At higher magnification, the cytologic features of the chondrocytes are apparent. In a chondroma, the nuclei are uniformly small and darkly stained. Although binucleated cells may be seen occasionally, they are not common.

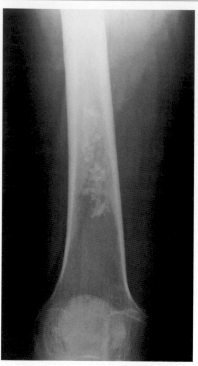

Figure 39–7 When chondromas involve the long bones, the lesions generally show an intramedullary collection of stippled calcification. Ringlike calcification may also be present. The endosteal surface of the affected bone does not show any irregularity. Endosteal erosion is a worrisome feature for a low-grade malignant cartilage tumor.

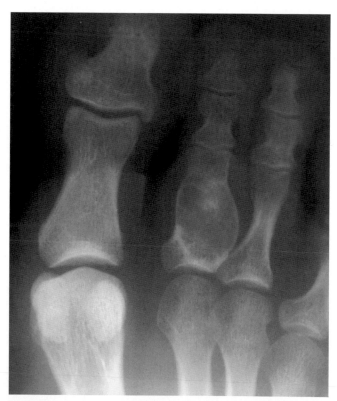

Figure 39–6 This radiograph illustrates a chondroma involving the proximal phalanx of the second toe. The lesion expands the affected bone, is calcified, and shows a sclerotic margin.

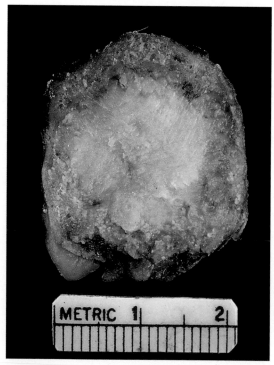

Figure 39–8 Grossly, chondromas in long bone locations are no different from those involving the small bones of the hands and feet. This chondroma of the upper fibular shows the well-marginated, glistening, gray–white aura of a hyaline cartilage tumor.

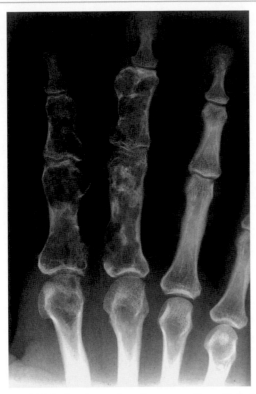

Figure 39–9 Multiple chondromas have the same radiographic features as solitary lesions, as in this case with multiple lesions involving the small bones of the hand.

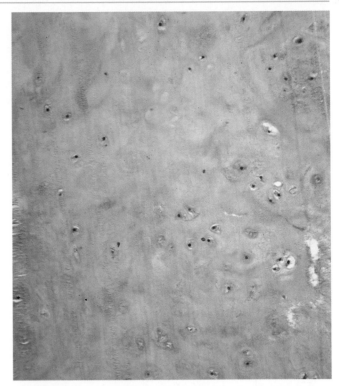

Figure 39–11 At low magnification, the nuclei of the chondrocytes are inconspicuous, appearing as small dark dots, as seen in this chondroma involving the distal femur in a male adult.

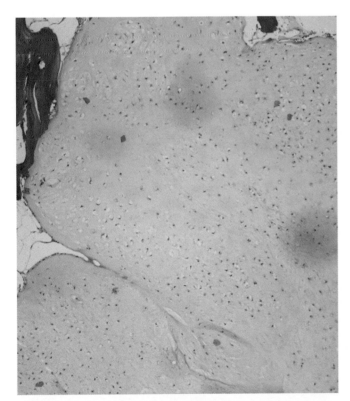

Figure 39–10 At low magnification, chondromas show a lobulated pattern, as illustrated in this photomicrograph. Many cartilage tumors share this low-power histologic feature.

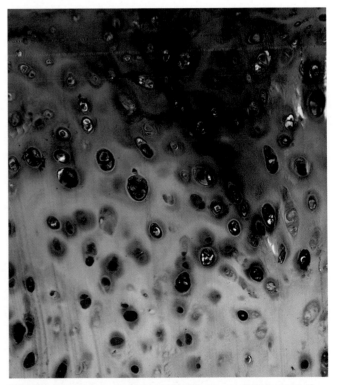

Figure 39–12 Prominent costochondral cartilage may clinically mimic the appearance of a neoplasm. If biopsy is performed, a mistaken diagnosis of a cartilage tumor may be made. However, the regular and orderly appearance of the chondrocytes is a clue that the tissue represents normal anatomy rather than neoplasm.

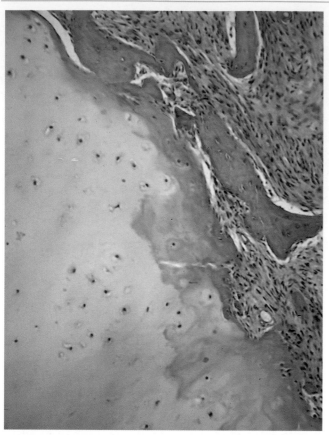

Figure 39–13 Some examples of fibrous dysplasia may demonstrate a chondroid component and thus be mistaken for a cartilage tumor. This case of fibrocartilaginous dysplasia involving the femur in a patient with Albright's syndrome shows such prominent chondroid differentiation.

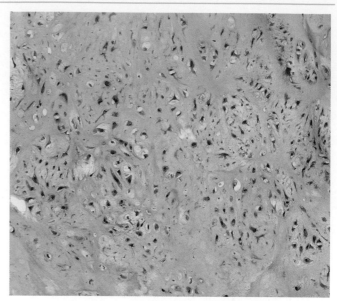

Figure 39–15 This photomicrograph illustrates the histologic features of a periosteal chondroma. The lesion is hypercellular, and the degree of cellularity is similar to that seen in small bone enchondromas. Periosteal chondromas are generally less than 5 cm in their greatest dimension.

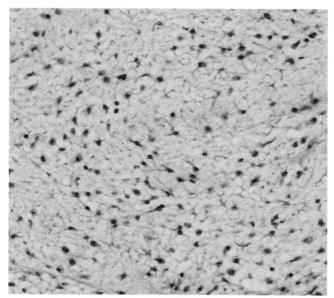

Figure 39–14 This photomicrograph shows a cartilage tumor in the thumb of a patient with Ollier's disease. Although the lesion is hypercellular and shows mild cytologic atypia, it is within the spectrum of a benign cartilage tumor of the small bones of the hands and feet.

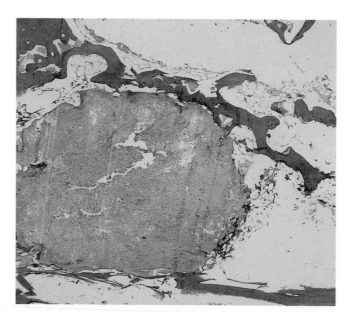

Figure 39–16 The chondroma represented in this photomicrograph involved the proximal fibula. Such lesions may show a more infiltrative pattern similar to that seen in small bone enchondromas.

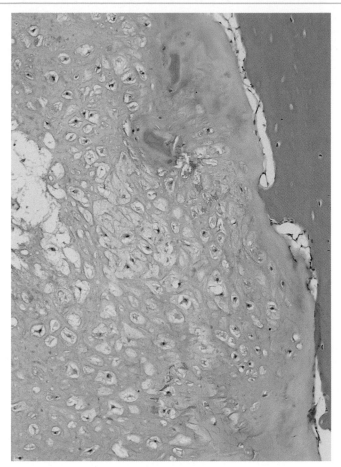

Figure 39–17 This low-power photomicrograph shows the sharp circumscription characteristic of benign hyaline cartilage tumors. A mild degree of endosteal scalloping may be allowed in enchondromas, but such lesions should be thoroughly curetted to ensure complete removal.

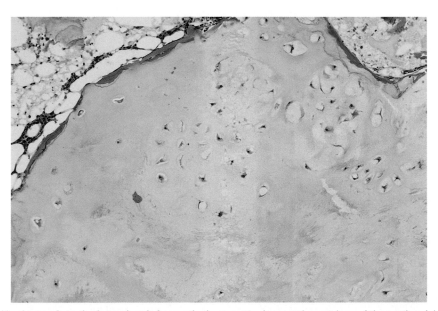

Figure 39–18 Chondromas, like this one from the femoral neck, frequently show reactive bone at the periphery of the cartilage lobules. This feature is helpful in distinguishing benign from low-grade malignant hyaline cartilage tumors.

Chondroblastoma

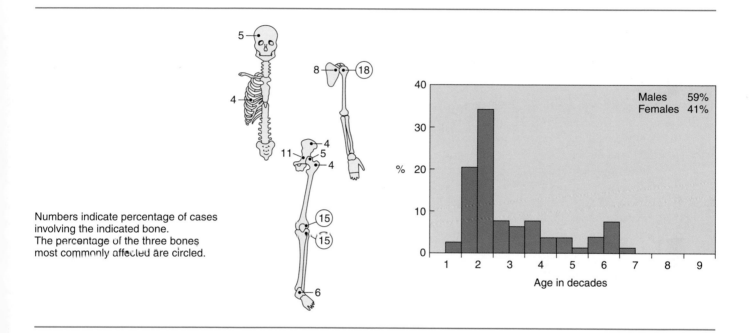

Numbers indicate percentage of cases
involving the indicated bone.
The percentage of the three bones
most commonly affected are circled.

Males 59%
Females 41%

%

Age in decades

Clinical Signs

1. Local tenderness is usually the only finding on physical examination.
2. Muscle wasting may be present in the region of the tumor.
3. Because approximately 30% of tumors occur around the knee joint, a limp may be noted.

Clinical Symptoms

1. Pain localized to the region of the tumor is the most common presenting complaint and is nearly universally present.

2. The pain usually is mild to moderate in severity and may have been present for months to years at the time of diagnosis.

Major Imaging Features

1. The lesion is located in the epiphysis or an apophysis.
2. The lesion is small and has sharp margins.
3. A sclerotic rim and expansion of the affected bone are commonly seen.
4. Matrix calcification is present in 25% of cases.
5. The lesion may cross an open physis.

6. Profound edema-like signal may be present on magnetic resonance imaging.
7. In vertebra, it has the appearance of a malignant lesion.

Radiographic Differential Diagnosis

1. Giant cell tumor.
2. Avascular necrosis.
3. Aneurysmal bone cyst.
4. Clear cell chondrosarcoma.

Major Pathologic Features

Gross

1. Lesional tissue is usually grayish-pink.
2. Only rarely is a grossly discernible chondroid matrix present.
3. Calcific foci may be present within curetted fragments of tissue.
4. Secondary aneurysmal bone cyst may be present, resulting in a grossly hemorrhagic or cystic specimen.

Microscopic

1. At low magnification, multinucleated giant cells are scattered randomly through a "sea" of mononuclear cells, resulting in an appearance superficially resembling that of giant cell tumor.
2. Pinkish-blue fibrochondroid islands are scattered randomly through the lesional tissue.
3. Calcification may take the form of a "chicken wire" pattern or may consist of larger masses.
4. At high magnification, the nuclei of the mononuclear (chondroblastic) component of the tumor are seen to be homogeneous and oval and to contain a longitudinal groove, resulting in a cytologic appearance similar to that of Langerhans' cell histiocytosis.
5. Mitotic figures, although not numerous, can be found in all cases.

Pathologic Differential Diagnosis

Benign lesions

1. Chondromyxoid fibroma.
2. Giant cell tumor.
3. Langerhans' cell histiocytosis.
4. Aneurysmal bone cyst.

Malignant lesions

1. Clear cell chondrosarcoma.
2. Chondroblastic osteosarcoma.

Treatment

1. **Primary modality:** Curettage and bone grafting are curative in more than 90% of cases.
2. **Other possible approaches:** En bloc excision with a marginal margin can be done if the location of the lesion permits it without significant compromise of the neighboring joint. Occasionally, in large lesions that compromise the joint with a pathologic fracture, resection with a wide margin and reconstruction with allograft, prosthesis, or arthrodesis may be necessary. Radiation therapy should be reserved for cases not amenable to surgical excision.

References

Dahlin DC, Ivins JC: Benign chondroblastoma: a study of 125 cases. *Cancer* 30(2):401–413, 1972.

de Silva MV, Reid R: Chondroblastoma: varied histologic appearance, potential diagnostic pitfalls, and clinicopathologic features associated with local recurrence. *Ann Diagn Pathol* 7(4):205–213, 2003.

Ilaslan H, Sundaram M, Unni KK: Vertebral chondroblastoma. *Skeletal Radiol* 32(2):66–71, 2003.

Huvos AG, Marcove RC: Chondroblastoma of bone: a critical review. *Clin Orthop Relat Res* 95:300–312, 1973.

Kurt AM, Turcotte RE, McLeod RA, et al: Chondroblastoma of bone. *Orthopedics* 13(7):787–790, 1990.

Kurt AM, Unni KK, Sim FH, et al: Chondroblastoma of bone. *Hum Pathol* 20(10):965–976, 1989.

Kyriakos M, Land VJ, Penning JL, et al: Metastatic chondroblastoma: report of a fatal case with a review of the literature on atypical, aggressive and malignant chondroblastoma. *Cancer* 55(8):1770–1789, 1985.

Lin PP, Thenappan A, Deavers MT, et al: Treatment and prognosis of chondroblastoma. *Clin Orthop Relat Res* 438:103–109, 2005.

McLeod RA, Beabout JW: The roentgenographic features of chondroblastoma. *Am J Roentgenol Radium Ther Nucl Med* 118(2):464–471, 1973.

Roberts PF, Taylor JG: Multifocal benign chondroblastomas: report of a case. *Hum Pathol* 11(3):296–298, 1980.

Suneja R, Grimer RJ, Belthur M, et al: Chondroblastoma of bone: long-term results and functional outcome after intralesional curettage. *J Bone Joint Surg Br* 87(7):974–978, 2005.

Turcotte RE, Kurt AM, Sim FH, et al: Chondroblastoma. *Hum Pathol* 24(9):944–949, 1993.

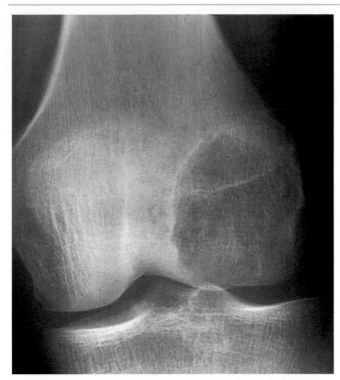

Figure 40–1 This radiograph shows a well-marginated lytic chondroblastoma located eccentrically in the distal femur. The knee region is the most common location for chondroblastoma, and this lesion involves the epiphysis, as is nearly always the case with chondroblastoma. The tumor also extends to involve the metaphysis.

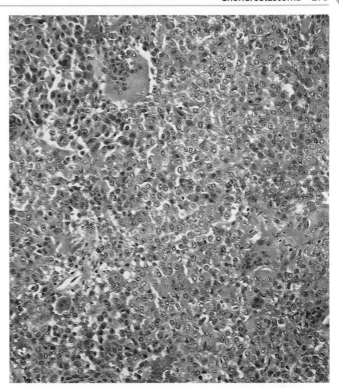

Figure 40–3 Chondroblastoma was originally thought to be a "calcifying giant cell tumor." The solid portion of the lesion may show numerous benign multinucleated giant cells, as illustrated in this photomicrograph.

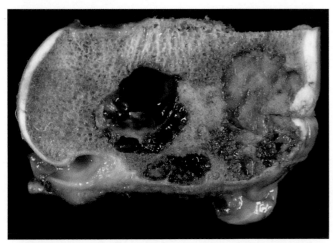

Figure 40–2 The gross characteristics of this chondroblastoma correlate well with its radiographic appearance in Figure 40–1. The lesion is fleshy and whitish in its solid regions. A hemorrhagic cystic region is also grossly evident. Secondary aneurysmal bone cyst frequently accompanies chondroblastoma.

Figure 40–4 In contrast to giant cell tumor, chondroblastoma contains zones of eosinophilic to amphophilic fibrochondroid matrix, as shown in this photomicrograph. These zones are typically hypocellular when compared with the surrounding regions.

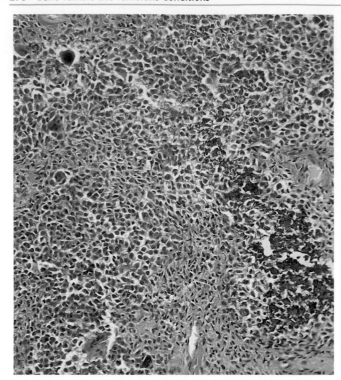

Figure 40–5 Calcification helps distinguish chondroblastoma from giant cell tumor. The calcification may be regional and identifiable radiographically, as in this tumor. At times, the calcification forms a "chicken wire" type of pattern.

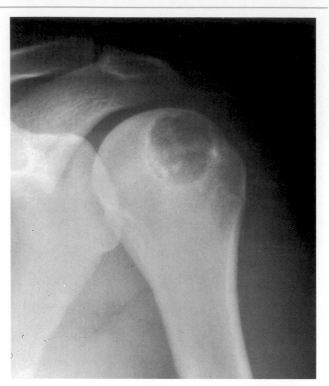

Figure 40–7 This radiograph illustrates a chondroblastoma involving the humeral head. In this region, the lesion may involve the epiphysis or apophysis. Chondroblastomas are characteristically lytic, but this tumor shows partial calcification. A thin rim of sclerosis at the periphery attests to the lesion's slow growth.

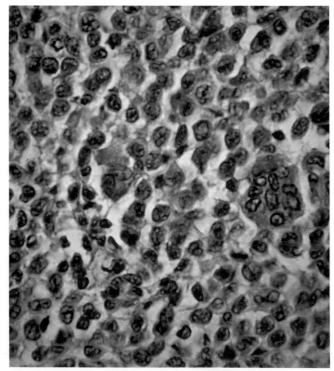

Figure 40–6 At high magnification, chondroblastoma is generally loosely organized, as seen in this photomicrograph. The nuclei are uniform and characteristically bean-shaped, with a central groove. This cytologic appearance is similar to that of the nuclei of Langerhans' cells in Langerhans' cell histiocytosis.

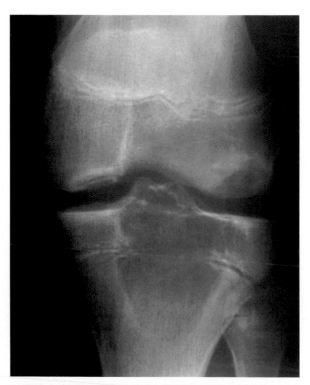

Figure 40–8 A sharply marginated chondroblastoma involving the proximal tibia is shown in this radiograph. The tumor crosses the open physis; this is a feature rarely seen in other tumors. Peripheral sclerosis is also present.

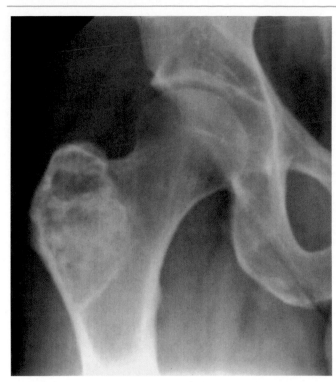

Figure 40–9 Chondroblastomas show mineralization to varying degrees. This example involving the greater trochanter (apophyseal location) is heavily mineralized.

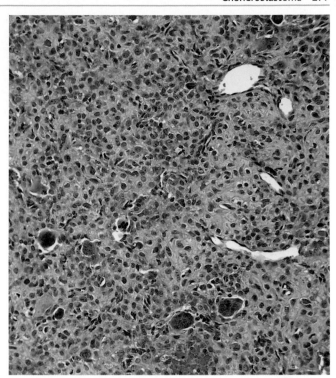

Figure 40–11 Although chondroblastoma most commonly involves the epiphyseal region of a long bone in a patient who is skeletally immature, some tumors occur in flat bones as well. This tumor involved the temporal bone in a 3-year-old girl. The temporal bone is the most common location for lesions involving the skull.

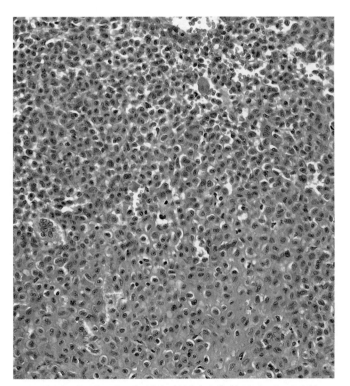

Figure 40–10 The fibrochondroid zones of chondroblastoma are variably scattered through the tumor and may not be a prominent component of the lesion, as in this photomicrograph.

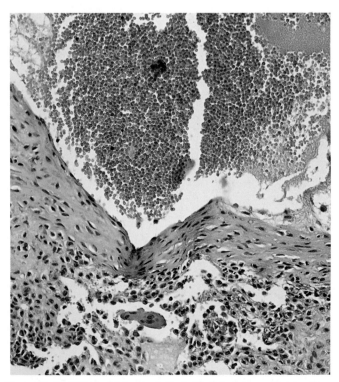

Figure 40–12 This photomicrograph illustrates the presence of a secondary aneurysmal bone cyst complicating a chondroblastoma. Such a secondary aneurysmal bone cyst may be so prominent as to mask the appearance of the chondroblastoma component and lead to a misdiagnosis.

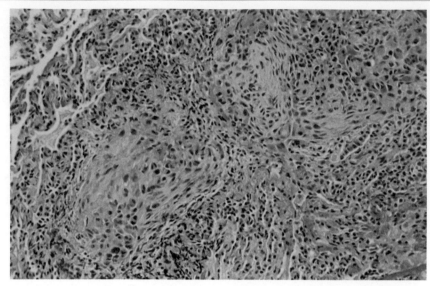

Figure 40–13 Chondroblastoma may recur within bone and soft tissue, and rarely such lesions may metastasize to the lungs. As this photomicrograph illustrates, such rare pulmonary metastases are histologically indistinguishable from their osseous primary lesions.

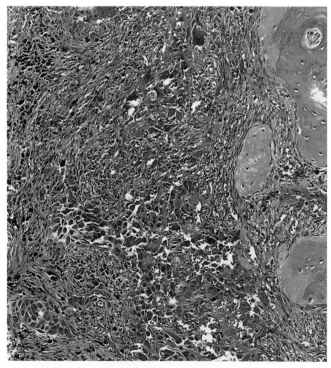

Figure 40–14 This pigmented lesion from the temporal bone contains multinucleated giant cells within a sea of mononuclear cells that have cytologic features similar to those of chondroblastoma. The differential diagnosis for such lesions includes pigmented villonodular synovitis of the temporomandibular joint and chondroblastoma.

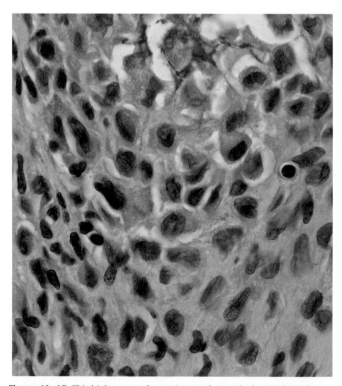

Figure 40–15 This high-power photomicrograph reveals the cytologic features of the mononuclear cells of chondroblastoma. These cells may appear epithelioid, with abundant eosinophilic cytoplasm and eccentric nuclei, as shown here.

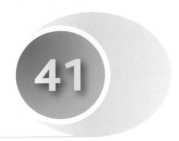

Chondromyxoid Fibroma

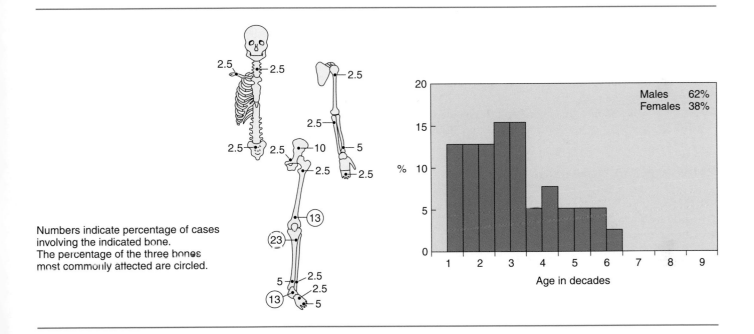

Numbers indicate percentage of cases involving the indicated bone.
The percentage of the three bones most commonly affected are circled.

Clinical Signs

1. Regional tenderness is usually the only finding on physical examination.
2. Tumefaction is more commonly found when the tumor involves bones of the hands or feet.

Clinical Symptoms

1. Pain is the most common presenting complaint.
2. Local swelling may be noted on rare occasions and is more frequently a presenting complaint when the tumor involves a small bone.

3. Occasionally, the lesion may be an asymptomatic, incidental radiographic abnormality.

Major Radiographic Features

1. The lesion has an eccentric metaphyseal location.
2. It shows sharp, sclerotic, and scalloped margins.
3. Matrix calcification is rare.

Radiographic Differential Diagnosis

1. Fibroma (metaphyseal fibrous defect).
2. Aneurysmal bone cyst.

3. Chondroblastoma.
4. Fibrous dysplasia.

Major Pathologic Features

Gross

1. Being translucent and bluish-gray, this tumor may grossly resemble hyaline cartilage; however, it is not soft and "runny" as in myxoid areas of chondrosarcoma.
2. The tumor is usually very well marginated and therefore may be lobulated grossly.
3. Bone surrounding the tumor usually shows sclerotic changes.

Microscopic

1. At low magnification, the tumor shows a distinctly lobulated pattern of growth, with peripheral hypercellularity of the lobules.
2. The tumor cells are spindled and stellate. Rarely, the nuclei may appear "bizarre." Benign giant cells are usually seen between the lobules of the tumor.
3. The stroma is myxoid, but only rarely is well-formed hyaline cartilage present.
4. More solidly cellular areas containing cells identical with those found in chondroblastoma may be seen.

Pathologic Differential Diagnosis

Benign lesions

1. Chondroblastoma.
2. Chondroma.

Malignant lesions

1. Chondrosarcoma.
2. Chondroblastic osteosarcoma.

Treatment

1. **Primary modality:** curettage and bone grafting.
2. **Other possible approaches:** en bloc resection with a marginal margin if the tumor's location makes it amenable to removal without significant loss of function.

References

Durr HR, Lienemann A, Nerlich A, et al: Chondromyxoid fibroma of bone. *Arch Orthop Trauma Surg* 120(1–2):42–47, 2000.

Gherlinzoni F, Rock M, Picci P: Chondromyxoid fibroma: the experience at the Istituto Ortopedico Rizzoli. *J Bone Joint Surg Am* 65(2):198–204, 1983.

Nielsen GP, Keel SB, Dickersin GR, et al: Chondromyxoid fibroma: a tumor showing myofibroblastic, myochondroblastic, and chondrocytic differentiation. *Mod Pathol* 12(5):514–517, 1999.

Kyriakos M: Soft tissue implantation of chondromyxoid fibroma. *Am J Surg Pathol* 3(4):363–372, 1979.

Rahimi A, Beabout JW, Ivins JC, et al: Chondromyxoid fibroma: a clinicopathologic study of 76 cases. *Cancer* 30(3):726–736, 1972.

Schajowicz F, Gallardo J: Chondromyxoid fibroma (fibromyxoid chondroma) of bone: a clinicopathological study of thirty-two cases. *J Bone Joint Surg Br* 53(2):198–216, 1971.

Wu CT, Inwards CY, O'Laughlin S, et al: Chondromyxoid fibroma of bone: a clinicopathologic review of 278 cases. *Hum Pathol* 29(5): 438–446, 1998.

Yamaguchi T, Dorfman HD: Radiographic and histologic patterns of calcification in chondromyxoid fibroma. *Skeletal Radiol* 27(10): 559–564, 1998.

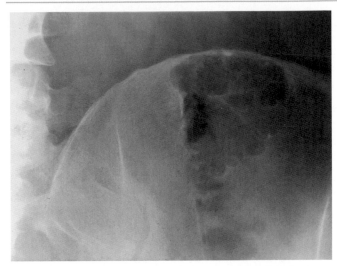

Figure 41–1 This radiograph shows a well-marginated lesion in the iliac bone. The periphery is scalloped and has a partially sclerotic rim. Although the majority of chondromyxoid fibromas are metaphyseal in long bones, approximately 10% occur in the ilium (as in this case).

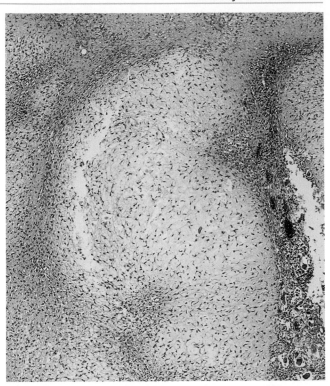

Figure 41–3 At low magnification, chondromyxoid fibromas are characteristically lobulated, as this photomicrograph illustrates. The lesion is relatively hypocellular toward the center of the lobules.

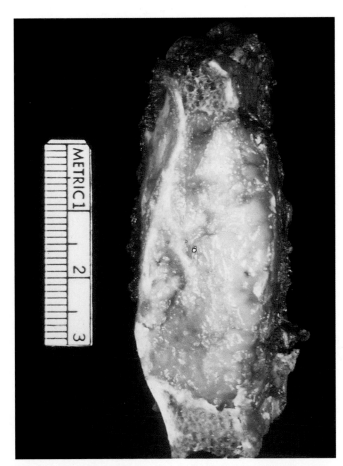

Figure 41–2 The gross features in this case correlate well with the radiograph shown in Figure 41–1. The lesion is whitish and well margined. The lesion may show myxoid change.

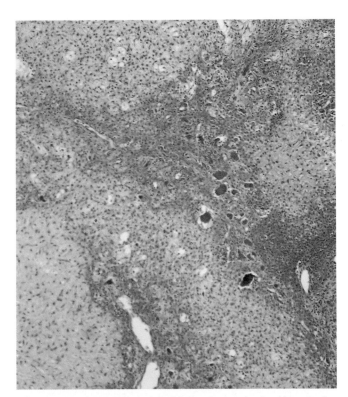

Figure 41–4 At the periphery of the lobules of tumor is a "condensation" of cellularity. In these regions, the tumor tends to show more spindling, and benign multinucleated giant cells are present. These foci may mimic the appearance of chondroblastoma.

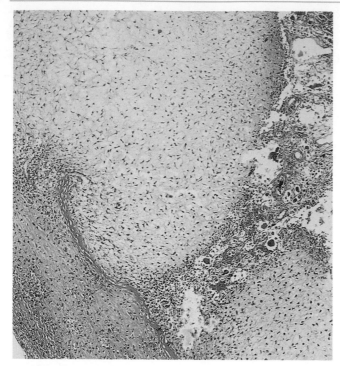

Figure 41–5 At higher magnification, chondromyxoid fibroma has a chondroid appearance in the central portion of the tumor lobules. A small sampling of this portion of the lesional tissue may mimic the appearance of a chondroma or chondrosarcoma.

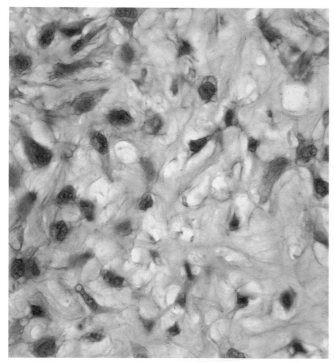

Figure 41–6 At high magnification, the central portion of the tumor is chondromyxoid (well-developed hyaline cartilage is unusual in chondromyxoid fibroma). Cytologically, the cells are stellate in these regions. However, the nuclei are uniform and do not show significant atypia. Longitudinal grooves and a bean shape to the nucleus may simulate the cytologic features seen in chondroblastoma or Langerhans' cell histiocytosis.

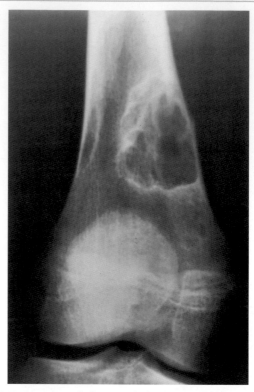

Figure 41–7 This radiograph illustrates the features of a chondromyxoid fibroma in the distal femur. The metaphyseal location is typical, and the lesion is eccentric. The sclerotic and scalloped rim is clearly visible in this case.

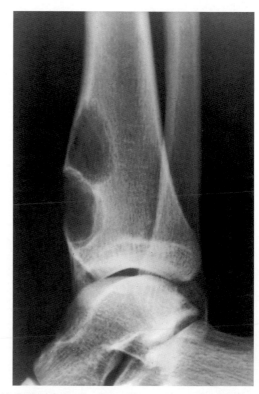

Figure 41–8 The lobulated radiographic appearance of a chondromyxoid fibroma is demonstrated here. The differential diagnosis in such a case includes a metaphyseal fibrous defect (fibroma).

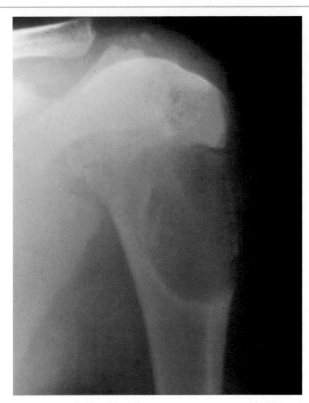

Figure 41–9 This chondromyxoid fibroma of the upper humerus has a lytic and well-marginated radiographic appearance. The lesion abuts but does not cross the physis.

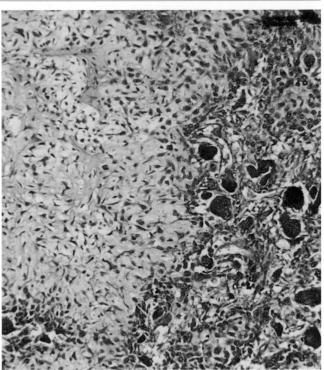

Figure 41–11 Regions of chondromyxoid fibroma may simulate chondroblastoma, as in this photomicrograph. The cytologic features also overlap, suggesting that the two lesions are closely related.

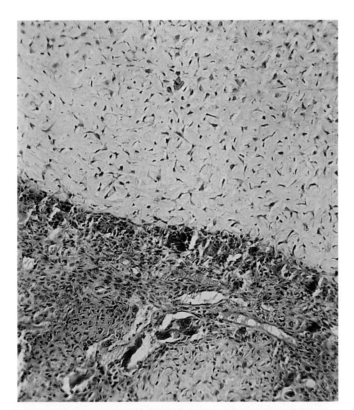

Figure 41–10 The transition from the hyaline cartilage regions of the tumor to the more cellular areas may be abrupt, as shown in this photomicrograph. The tumor may thus exhibit a "bimorphic" histologic pattern.

Figure 41–12 Foci within a chondromyxoid fibroma may be markedly chondroid and thus simulate a chondroma or chondrosarcoma. Chondromyxoid fibromas were commonly mistaken for chondrosarcomas in the past, but the publication of this fact has resulted in more mistaken identification of chondrosarcomas as chondromyxoid fibromas in recent years.

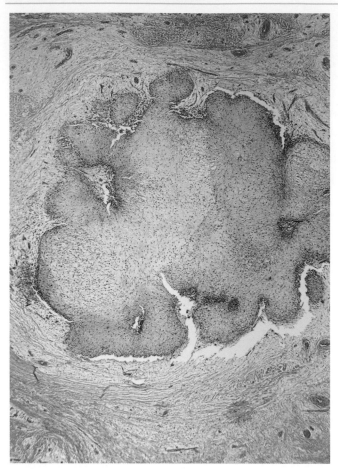

Figure 41–13 As with chondroblastoma, chondromyxoid fibroma may recur if inadequately treated. The recurrence may be within the bone or soft tissues, as shown in this photomicrograph. Such soft tissue recurrences frequently exhibit a rim of calcification radiographically.

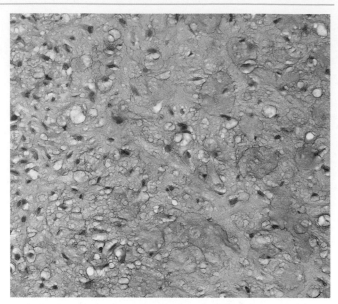

Figure 41–15 At higher magnification, the center of the chondroid lobules in chondromyxoid fibroma may be relatively cellular. This tumor is the same as that illustrated in Figure 41–14. Taken out of context, such regions may lead the pathologist to consider a diagnosis of low-grade chondrosarcoma.

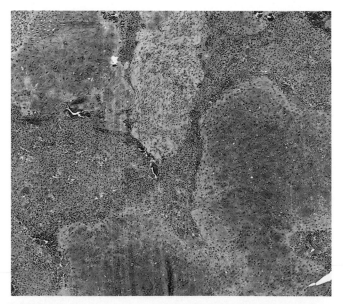

Figure 41–14 The lobulated nature of chondromyxoid fibroma is nicely illustrated in this low-power photomicrograph of a proximal tibial tumor.

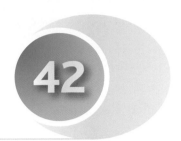

Multiple Chondromas

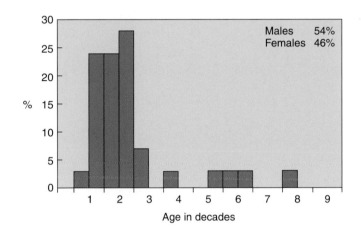

Clinical Signs

1. Multiple mass lesions are palpable.
2. Deformity and shortness of stature are often present because of epiphyseal involvement.
3. There is a tendency to unilaterality in Ollier's disease.
4. Hemangiomas are associated with Maffucci's syndrome.

Clinical Symptoms

1. Symptoms are similar to those of the solitary lesion, with pain and associated pathologic fracture.

Major Radiographic Features

1. Most cases are bilateral, but involvement usually predominates on one side.
2. Affected bones are shortened and deformed.
3. Cartilage masses extend linearly from the physis into the metaphysis.
4. Cartilage masses often have no overlying cortex and may contain stippled calcification.
5. There is a tendency to spare the epiphysis and diaphysis except in severe cases.
6. Affected bones cannot tubulate, and the ends may have a clubbed appearance.
7. The disease tends to regress after puberty.

Radiographic Differential Diagnosis

1. Fibrous dysplasia.
2. Multiple hereditary exostoses.

Major Pathologic Features

Gross

1. The lesional tissue is blue–gray and translucent.
2. No myxoid or cystic change is evident grossly.

Microscopic

1. At low magnification, these lesions are composed predominantly of blue–gray hyaline cartilage matrix.
2. The lesions are generally more cellular than is seen in solitary chondromas. No myxoid stromal change is evident.
3. At higher magnification, the nuclei may be hyperchromic, and binucleated cells may be identified.

Pathologic Differential Diagnosis

Benign lesions

1. Solitary chondroma.
2. Synovial chondromatosis.

Malignant lesions

1. Chondrosarcoma, ordinary type.

Treatment

1. **Primary modality:** Treatment is similar to that for solitary enchondromas, with observation of the lesions if they are asymptomatic.
2. **Other possible approaches:** If the lesion is symptomatic, curettage and bone grafting are performed.

References

Ben-Itzhak I, Denolf FA, Versfeld G, et al: The Maffucci syndrome. *J Pediatr Orthop* 8(3):345–348, 1988.

Gruning T, Franke WG: Bone scan appearances in a case of Ollier's disease. *Clin Nucl Med* 24(11):886–887, 1999.

Liu J, Hudkins PG, Swee RG, et al: Bone sarcomas associated with Ollier's disease. *Cancer* 59(7):1376–1385, 1987.

Loewinger RJ, Lichtenstein JR, Dodson WE, et al: Maffucci's syndrome: a mesenchymal dysplasia and multiple tumour syndrome. *Br J Dermatol* 96(3):317–322, 1977.

Nardell SG: Ollier's disease: dyschondroplasia. *Br Med J* 2(4675):555–557, 1950.

Phelan EM, Carty HM, Kalos S: Generalised enchondromatosis associated with haemangiomas, soft-tissue calcifications and hemihypertrophy. *Br J Radiol* 59(697):69–74, 1986.

Sun TC, Swee RG, Shives TC, et al: Chondrosarcoma in Maffucci's syndrome. *J Bone Joint Surg Am* 67(8):1214–1219, 1985.

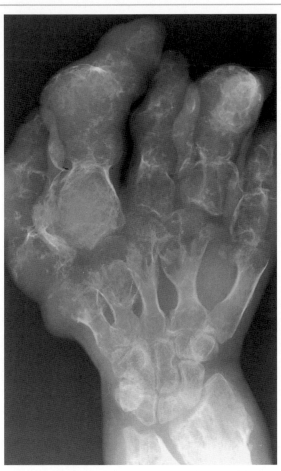

Figure 42–1 This radiograph illustrates extreme deformity of the bones of the hand and wrist by numerous masses of cartilage.

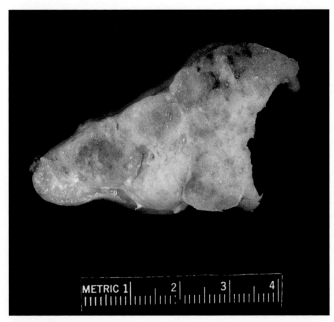

Figure 42–2 This photograph shows the gross features of multiple chondromas in Ollier's disease involving the fifth finger. The disease had resulted in such bony deformity that amputation was done.

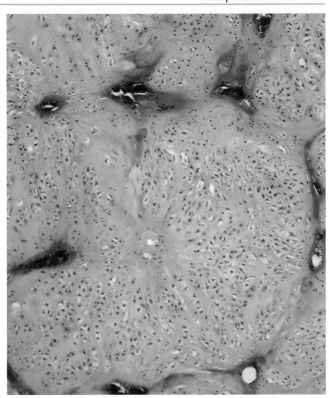

Figure 42–3 This low-power photomicrograph illustrates the lobulated appearance of a chondroma in Ollier's disease. This lesion of the humerus shows somewhat greater cellularity than is seen in many solitary chondromas of the long bones.

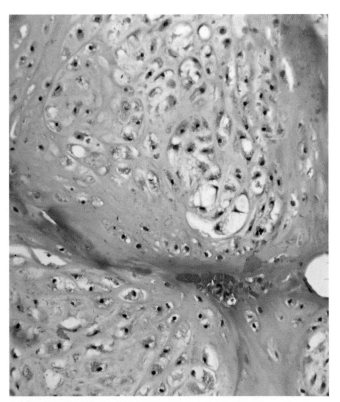

Figure 42–4 The lobulated nature of the chondromas in Ollier's disease is shown at higher magnification in this photomicrograph. Some mild cytologic atypia is also evident in this humeral lesion.

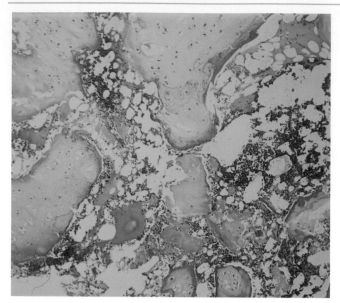

Figure 42–5 The multifocal nature of the chondroma in Ollier's disease is sometimes appreciable histologically, as in this photomicrograph.

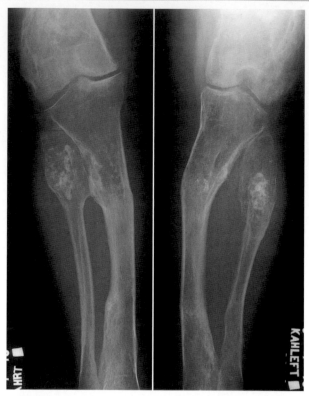

Figure 42–7 Ollier's disease of the lower legs, with bowing, expansion, and deformity of the tibia and fibula, is illustrated in this radiograph. Multiple cartilage masses containing stippled calcification are evident.

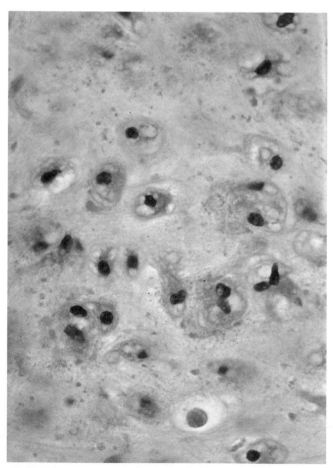

Figure 42–6 The cytologic atypia commonly seen in chondromas of the small bones of the hands and feet can also be seen in Ollier's disease, as demonstrated in this lesion of the thumb.

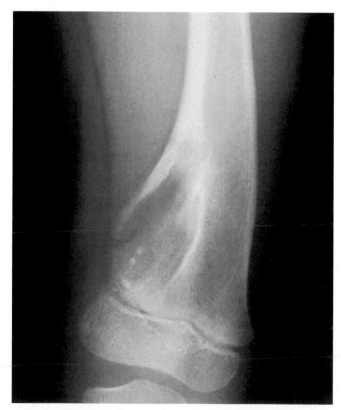

Figure 42–8 Cartilage mass extending linearly from the physis into the metaphysis is noted in this example of Ollier's disease in a 4-year-old male patient. There is absence of overlying cortex, and stippled calcification is present.

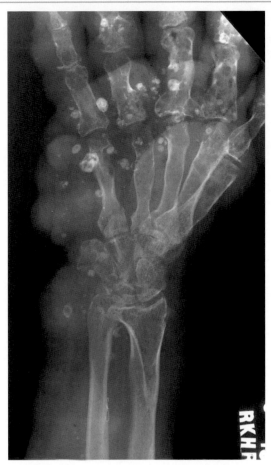

Figure 42–9 Typical changes of Ollier's disease in the bones, associated with soft tissue hemangiomas containing phleboliths, are shown in this example of Maffucci's syndrome.

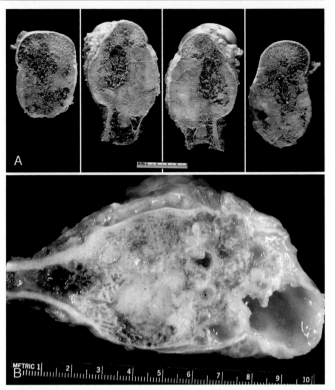

Figure 42–10 Chondrosarcomas can be seen in association with the multiple chondroma syndromes of Ollier's disease (distal femoral tumor shown in *A*) and Maffucci's syndrome (proximal fibular chondrosarcoma shown in *B*).

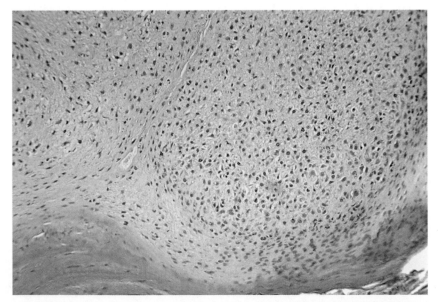

Figure 42–11 Chondrosarcomas in Ollier's disease and Maffucci's syndrome show the cellularity typical of low-grade chondrosarcomas not associated with multiple chondroma syndromes. This Grade 1 chondrosarcoma is from the proximal ulna in a patient with Ollier's disease.

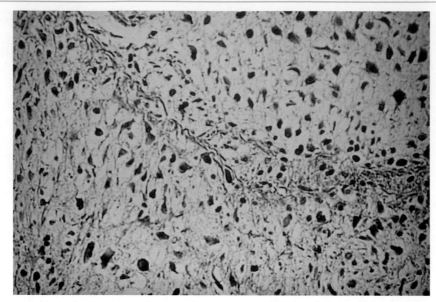

Figure 42–12 The cytologic atypia seen in ordinary chondrosarcomas is also evident in chondrosarcomas complicating Ollier's disease, as illustrated in this case involving the tibia.

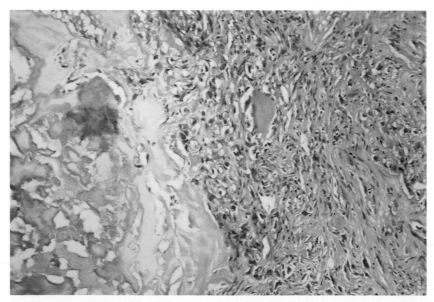

Figure 42–13 Rarely, chondrosarcomas with a dedifferentiated histologic appearance have been identified arising in the background of Ollier's disease, as shown in this case involving the femur.

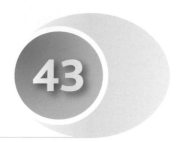

Periosteal Chondroma

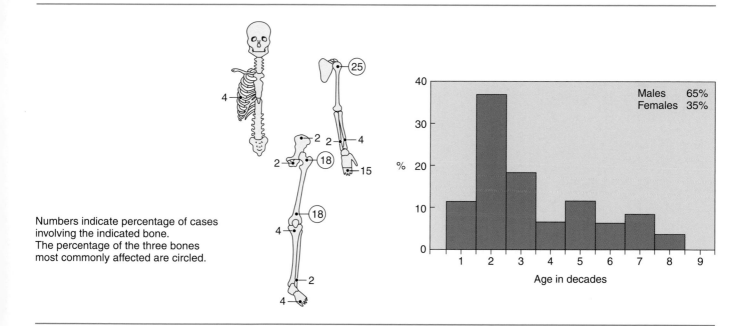

Numbers indicate percentage of cases involving the indicated bone.
The percentage of the three bones most commonly affected are circled.

Males 65%
Females 35%

% / Age in decades

Clinical Signs

1. The lesion may be palpable on physical examination.
2. The lesion is usually not painful to palpation.

Clinical Symptoms

1. Patients usually are asymptomatic.
2. The lesion is most commonly an incidental finding on radiographic examination.

Major Imaging Features

1. The lesion consists of a small surface mass (less than 3 cm) with saucerization of the underlying bone.
2. The location of the lesion is metaphyseal or diaphyseal.
3. Marginal spicules or "buttresses" are present.
4. Approximately 33% are calcified.
5. On magnetic resonance imaging, abnormal signal may be seen within cancellous bone.
6. Larger lesions (greater than 3.5 cm) are more likely to be malignant.

Radiographic Differential Diagnosis

1. Periosteal chondrosarcoma.
2. Periosteal osteosarcoma.
3. Soft tissue neoplasm secondarily involving the cortical bone.

Major Pathologic Features

Gross

1. The tumor is gray–blue and translucent, like all tumors with a prominent hyaline cartilage component.
2. If the margin is present in the specimen, it shows sharp circumscription.
3. The medullary portion of the bone is not involved.
4. The tumor is firm and lacks liquefaction or cystic change.

Microscopic

1. The low-power histologic appearance is that of a lobulated hyaline cartilage tumor that is well circumscribed.
2. The lesion is usually hypercellular.
3. The lesion usually contains binucleated chondrocytes.
4. Nuclear atypia may be prominent.

Pathologic Differential Diagnosis

Benign lesions

1. Synovial chondromatosis.
2. Chondroma.

Malignant lesions

1. Periosteal chondrosarcoma.
2. Periosteal osteosarcoma.

Treatment

1. **Primary modality:** These lesions should be excised en bloc with a marginal or wide margin. Depending on the size of the defect, bone grafting may be necessary.
2. **Other possible approaches:** Observation may be sufficient if a diagnosis is secure and the patient is asymptomatic.

References

Bauer TW, Dorfman HD, Latham JT Jr: Periosteal chondroma: a clinico-pathologic study of 23 cases. *Am J Surg Pathol* 6(7):631–637, 1982.

Boriani S, Bacchini P, Bertoni F, et al: Periosteal chondroma: a review of twenty cases. *J Bone Joint Surg Am* 65(2):205–212, 1983.

Desantos LA, Spjut JH: Periosteal chondroma: a radiographic spectrum. *Skeletal Radiol* 6(1):15–20, 1981.

Lewis MM, Kenan S, Yabut SM, et al: Periosteal chondroma: A report of ten cases and review of the literature. *Clin Orthop Relat Res* 256:185–192, 1990.

Nojima T, Unni KK, McLeod RA, et al: Periosteal chondroma and periosteal chondrosarcoma. *Am J Surg Pathol* 9(9):666–677, 1985.

Robinson P, White LM, Sundaram M, et al: Periosteal chondroid tumors: radiologic evaluation with pathologic correlation. *Am J Roentgenol* 177(5):1183–1188, 2001.

Varma DG, Kumar R, Carrasco CH, et al: MR imaging of periosteal chondroma. *J Comput Assist Tomogr* 15(6):1008–1010, 1991.

Woertler K, Blasius S, Brinkschmidt C, et al: Periosteal chondroma: MR characteristics. *J Comput Assist Tomogr* 25(3):425–430, 2001.

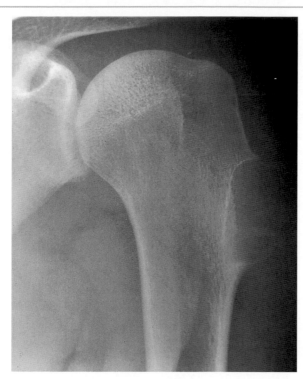

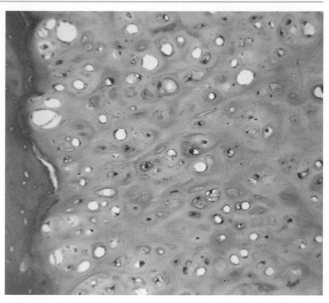

Figure 43–3 At low magnification, a periosteal chondroma is hypocellular and well circumscribed. This photomicrograph shows that the tumor has not penetrated the underlying cortical bone.

Figure 43–1 This radiograph shows a small periosteal chondroma arising on the lateral surface of the upper humeral metaphysis. The sharp margination and thin sclerotic rim, as well as the marginal spicules of calcification, are typical of periosteal chondroma. An incomplete rim of calcification surrounds the soft tissue component of this lesion.

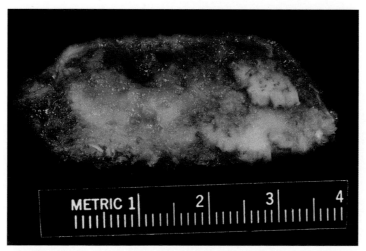

Figure 43–2 The gross pathologic features of this tumor correlate well with its radiographic appearance in Figure 43–1. The small size of the lesion supports a benign diagnosis. As with other hyaline cartilage lesions, the tumor is blue–gray and glistening.

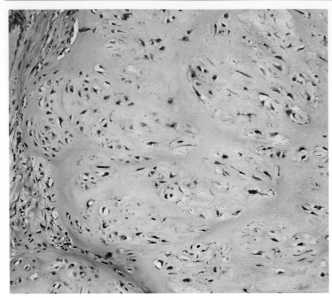

Figure 43–4 The lobulated pattern of a hyaline cartilage tumor is revealed in this photomicrograph. Although periosteal chondromas are benign, they may show greater cellularity at low magnification than their intramedullary counterparts.

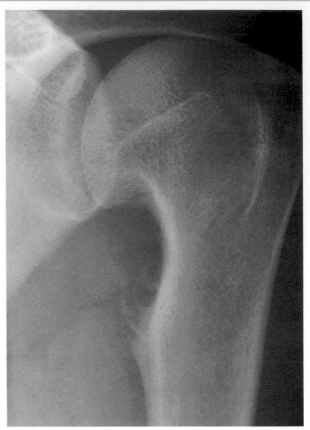

Figure 43–6 This radiograph illustrates a periosteal chondroma of the proximal humerus. The lesion shows a sharp sclerotic margin indicative of slow growth. The marginal spicules and buttresses are typical of periosteal chondroma.

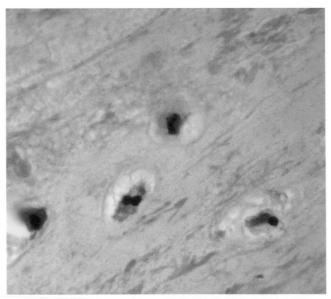

Figure 43–5 At high magnification, the cytologic features of the chondrocytes are uniform. Binucleation, as seen in this photomicrograph, should not dissuade the pathologist from making a diagnosis of periosteal chondroma if the gross and radiographic features are typical.

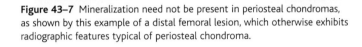

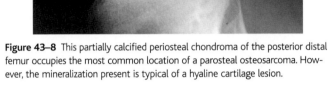

Figure 43–7 Mineralization need not be present in periosteal chondromas, as shown by this example of a distal femoral lesion, which otherwise exhibits radiographic features typical of periosteal chondroma.

Figure 43–8 This partially calcified periosteal chondroma of the posterior distal femur occupies the most common location of a parosteal osteosarcoma. However, the mineralization present is typical of a hyaline cartilage lesion.

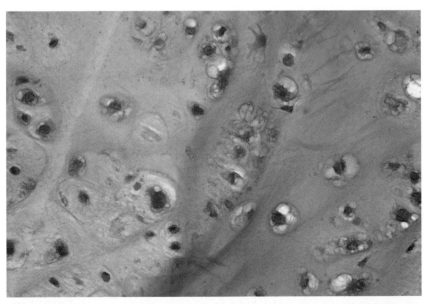

Figure 43–9 At high magnification, periosteal chondromas frequently show greater nuclear pleomorphism and more numerous occurrences of binucleation than intramedullary chondromas. Thus, the histologic features of periosteal chondroma are closer to those of chondromas of the small bones and synovial chondromatosis.

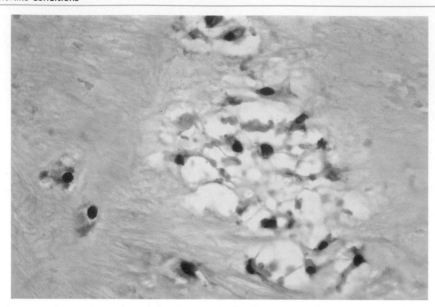

Figure 43–10 Focal myxoid change may be seen in a periosteal chondroma, as in this photomicrograph. Such a feature, however, should alert the pathologist to evaluate the lesion carefully.

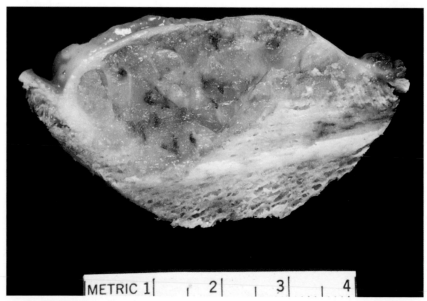

Figure 43–11 This gross specimen shows a periosteal chondrosarcoma. In contrast to periosteal chondromas, which are 3 cm or less, periosteal chondrosarcomas are 5 cm or larger, as is this femoral lesion.

Chondrosarcoma

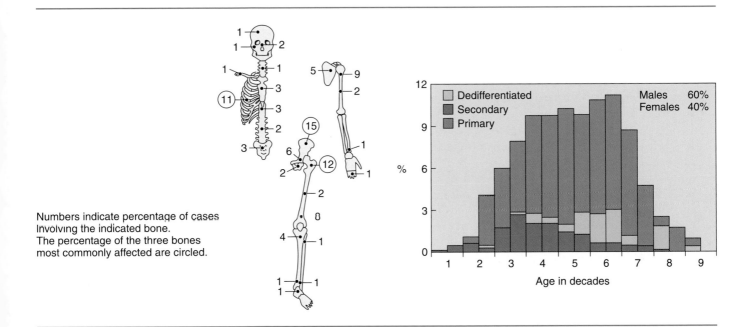

Numbers indicate percentage of cases
Involving the indicated bone.
The percentage of the three bones
most commonly affected are circled.

Clinical Signs

1. Local tenderness is present.
2. A mass may be found on physical examination. The mass is generally hard.

Clinical Symptoms

1. Pain is the usual presenting complaint. The pain is usually local; however, when tumors involve the pelvic girdle or vertebra, referred pain may be the initial manifestation.
2. A mass lesion may be noted but is more commonly present in patients who have tumors involving the appendicular skeleton.

3. A long duration of clinical symptoms—even of one or two decades—is frequently seen because these tumors almost invariably are slow-growing.

Major Radiographic Features

1. There is a predilection for the central skeleton and for the metaphysis or diaphysis of the affected bone.
2. Of lesions, 66% are partially calcified.
3. Cortical erosion or destruction is usually present.
4. The cortex is often thickened, but periosteal reaction is scant or absent.
5. Soft tissue extension is commonly seen in large lesions.

Radiographic Differential Diagnosis

1. Osteosarcoma.
2. Fibrosarcoma.
3. Metastatic carcinoma.
4. Multiple myeloma.

Major Pathologic Features

Gross

1. Chondrosarcomas tend to be homogeneous and blue–gray.
2. Scattered regions of whitish-yellow calcification may be evident.
3. Myxoid foci or frank liquefaction of the tumor help to grossly distinguish chondrosarcoma from chondroma.

Microscopic

1. At low magnification, these tumors show abundant blue–gray chondroid matrix production.
2. The tumors vary in cellularity but generally are more cellular than chondromas. The grade of the tumor correlates in general with its cellularity; higher-grade tumors are more cellular.
3. At higher magnification, the nuclei of the cells are somewhat variable and are more pleomorphic than those in the cells of a chondroma.
4. Binucleation of the cells is frequently evident but does not suffice for a diagnosis of malignancy because some chondromas also show this feature.
5. Myxoid change within the chondroid matrix may be evidenced by an inhomogeneous and "stringy" appearance. This is a particularly important histologic feature to help differentiate chondroma from low-grade chondrosarcoma in long bones.
6. The cytologic atypia evident on high-power examination is generally mild to moderate. If a tumor with marked cytologic atypia is encountered, a careful search should be made for osteoid production to exclude the diagnosis of chondroblastic osteosarcoma.
7. The guidelines for a diagnosis of chondrosarcoma in a small bone of the hand or foot are different. Increased cellularity, binucleated cells, hyperchromasia, and myxoid change may all be seen in a chondroma in this location. To diagnose chondrosarcoma in this location, radiologic evidence of permeation of the tumor through the cortex should be present.

Pathologic Differential Diagnosis

Benign lesions

1. Chondroma.
2. Chondromyxoid fibroma.

Malignant lesions

1. Chondroblastic osteosarcoma.
2. Chondroid chordoma.

Treatment

1. **Primary modality:** Surgical resection with a wide surgical margin is performed. Reconstruction is individualized depending on the location of the lesion. Amputation may be necessary to achieve a wide surgical margin.
2. **Other possible approaches:** Although these tumors are considered resistant to routine chemotherapy and radiation therapy, radiation is used for palliation in surgically inaccessible sites such as the spine or sacrum.

References

Bjornsson J, McLeod RA, Unni KK, et al: Primary chondrosarcoma of long bones and limb girdles. *Cancer* 83(10):2105–2119, 1998.

Cawte TG, Steiner GC, Beltran J, et al: Chondrosarcoma of the short tubular bones of the hands and feet. *Skeletal Radiol* 27(11):625–632, 1998.

Garrison RC, Unni KK, McLeod RA, et al: Chondrosarcoma arising in osteochondroma. *Cancer* 49(9):1890–1897, 1982.

Geirnaerdt MJ, Hermans J, Bloem JL, et al: Usefulness of radiography in differentiating enchondroma from central grade 1 chondrosarcoma. *Am J Roentgenol* 169(4):1097–1104, 1997.

Gitelis S, Bertoni F, Picci P, et al: Chondrosarcoma of bone: the experience at the Istituto Ortopedico Rizzoli. *J Bone Joint Surg Am* 63(8): 1248–1257, 1981.

Mankin JH, Cantley KP, Lippiello L, et al: The biology of human chondrosarcoma. I. Description of the cases, grading, and biochemical analyses. *J Bone Joint Surg Am* 62(2):160–176, 1980.

Masciocchi C, Sparvoli L, Barile A: Diagnostic imaging of malignant cartilage tumors. *Eur J Radiol* 27 (Suppl 1):S86–S90, 1998.

McCarthy EF, Dorfman HD: Chondrosarcoma of bone with dedifferentiation: a study of eighteen cases. *Hum Pathol* 13(1):36–40, 1982.

Murphey MD, Flemming DJ, Boyea SR, et al: Enchondroma versus chondrosarcoma in the appendicular skeleton: differentiating features. *Radiographics* 18(5):1213–1237, 1998.

Murphey MD, Walker EA, Wilson AJ, et al: From the archives of the AFIP: imaging of primary chondrosarcoma: radiologic-pathologic correlation. *Radiographics* 23(5):1245–1278, 2003.

Ogose A, Unni KK, Swee RG, et al: Chondrosarcoma of small bones of the hands and feet. *Cancer* 80(1):50–59, 1997.

Pring ME, Weber KL, Unni KK, et al: Chondrosarcoma of the pelvis. A review of sixty-four cases. *J Bone Joint Surg Am* 83-A(11):1630–1642, 2001.

Pritchard DJ, Lunke RJ, Taylor WF, et al: Chondrosarcoma: a clinicopathologic and statistical analysis. *Cancer* 45(1):149–157, 1980.

Rosenthal DI, Schiller AL, Mankin JH: Chondrosarcoma: correlation of radiological and histological grade. *Radiology* 150(1):21–26, 1984.

Swarts SJ, Neff JR, Nelson M, et al: Chromosomal abnormalities in low grade chondrosarcoma and a review of the literature. *Cancer Genet Cytogenet* 98(2):126–130, 1997.

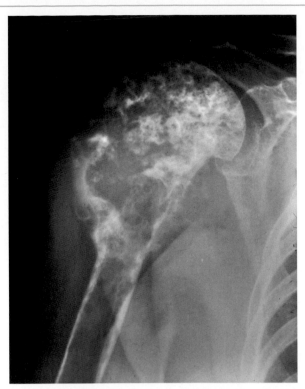

Figure 44–1 This radiograph shows a destructive lesion in the proximal humerus in an adult patient. The lesion is partially calcified, with multiple areas of ringlike calcification. These features are indicative of a hyaline cartilage tumor. The extensive cortical destruction and associated soft tissue extension of the tumor support a malignant diagnosis.

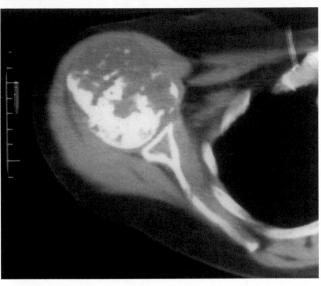

Figure 44–3 A computed tomographic (CT) scan of this lesion shows extensive calcification. CT and magnetic resonance imaging (MRI) are particularly helpful in defining the extent of soft tissue involvement and the relationship of any soft tissue extension to regional neurovascular structures.

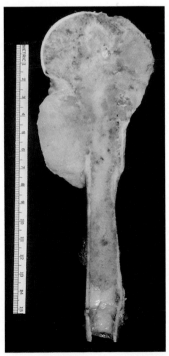

Figure 44–2 The bisected gross specimen of the tumor correlates well with its radiographic appearance shown in Figure 44–1. The tumor has the characteristic blue–gray aura of a hyaline cartilage tumor on cross-section. The cortex has been destroyed, and an associated soft tissue mass is present.

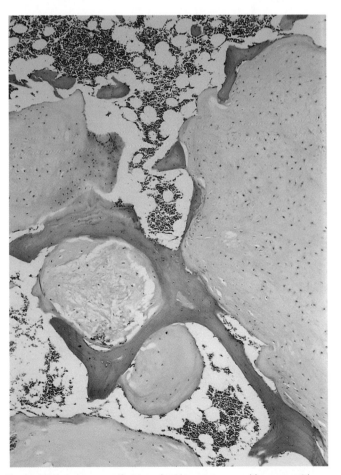

Figure 44–4 At low magnification, chondrosarcomas are blue–gray with hematoxylin-eosin–stained sections. The tumors are generally not highly cellular but are often arranged in a lobulated manner. Adjacent lobules at the periphery of the lesion show an invasive quality of growth, as in this photomicrograph.

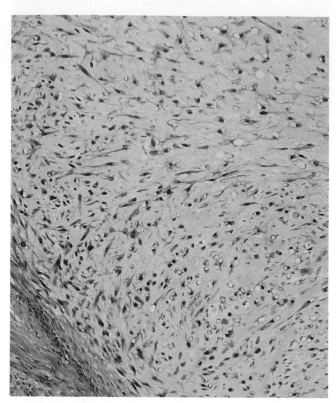

Figure 44–5 Chondrosarcomas are hypercellular when compared with chondromas, as in this example of a chondrosarcoma of the distal femur. The nuclei show greater pleomorphism and hyperchromasia as well.

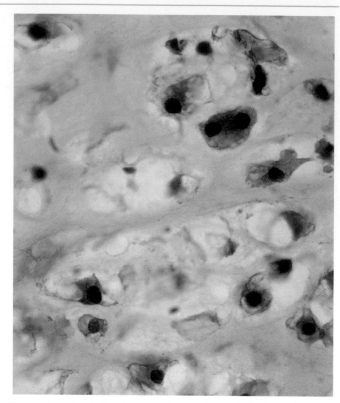

Figure 44–7 Binucleation is commonly stated to be an important feature in the differentiation of chondrosarcoma from chondroma. Binucleated chondrocytes are identifiable in this example of a chondrosarcoma involving the sacroiliac region.

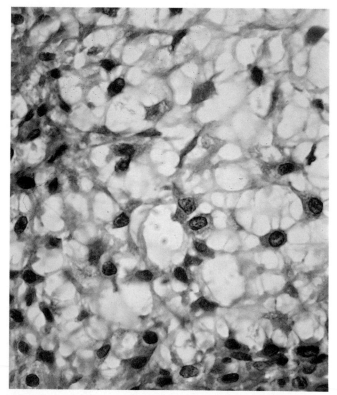

Figure 44–6 At higher magnification, the nuclear pleomorphism is more evident. This tumor also shows a myxoid stromal quality, a feature frequently seen in chondrosarcomas.

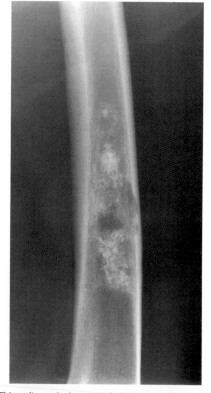

Figure 44–8 This radiograph shows a calcified intramedullary chondrosarcoma of the femoral diaphysis. Central lysis and cortical erosion are present and constitute the major radiographic evidence that the lesion is malignant.

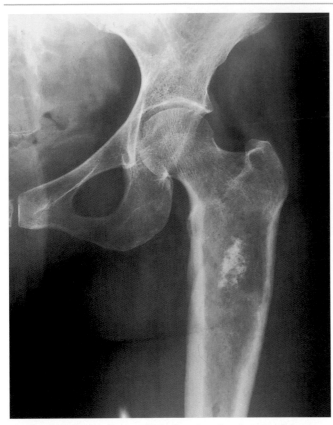

Figure 44–9 This chondrosarcoma is large, partially calcified, and poorly marginated. Expansion of the bone in combination with cortical thickening, as in this example, is unusual in any tumor other than chondrosarcoma.

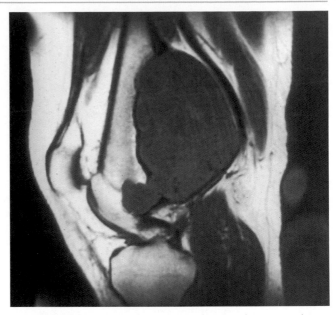

Figure 44–11 MRI provides superior contrast between the tumor and normal marrow and between the tumor and adjacent soft tissues, as demonstrated in this image of the same tumor seen in the CT scan in Figure 44–10. Sagittal images are useful in showing the longitudinal extent of the tumor in a single slice. Calcification is not demonstrated.

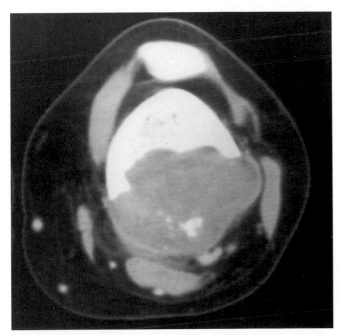

Figure 44–10 Destruction of the cortex is associated with a bulky soft tissue mass in this case. An area of central calcification is also present. CT and MRI are essential for preoperative staging. This CT scan demonstrates the extent of this chondrosarcoma and the presence of subtle calcification, which help identify the tumor as most likely a chondrosarcoma.

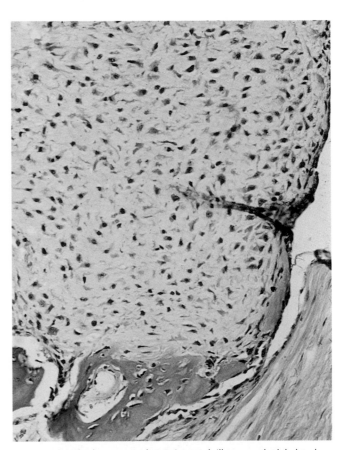

Figure 44–12 This low-power photomicrograph illustrates the lobulated pattern of growth in a chondrosarcoma.

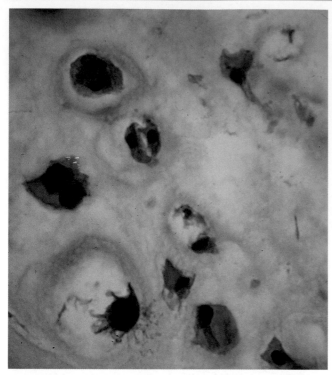

Figure 44–13 Multiple binucleated chondrocytes are identifiable in this high-power photomicrograph of a chondrosarcoma. Nuclear pleomorphism is also evident. Although chondromas of the small bones, periosteal chondromas, and synovial chondromatosis may also share these features, they are not present to the extent illustrated here.

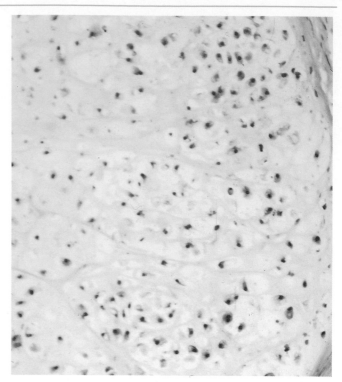

Figure 44–15 Because the majority of chondrosarcomas are low-grade, the histologic features alone may not be sufficient to support a malignant diagnosis. Although the tumor is slightly hypercellular, its location (not small bone and not periosteal) and the radiographic features showing endosteal erosion would be particularly helpful in classifying this tumor as malignant.

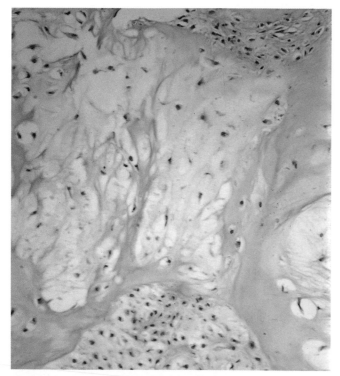

Figure 44–14 At low power, the myxoid quality of the lesion may be the first clue that the hyaline cartilage tumor is not a chondroma. This photomicrograph shows such a stromal myxoid change.

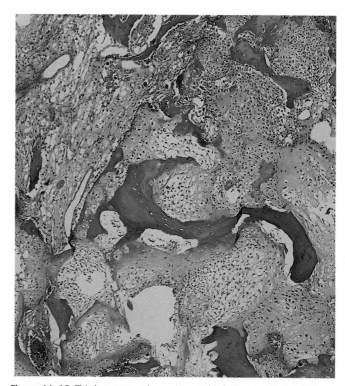

Figure 44–16 This low-power photomicrograph of a low-grade chondrosarcoma from the acetabular region shows the characteristic permeative pattern of medullary bone involvement.

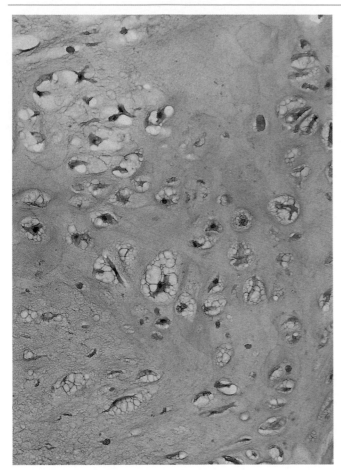

Figure 44–17 Low-grade chondrosarcomas, like this tumor that involved the acetabular region, can be difficult to distinguish from enchondroma. Careful correlation with the radiographic appearance of the tumor is generally helpful in such cases.

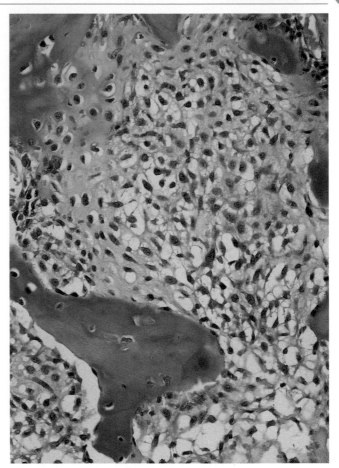

Figure 44–18 Higher-grade chondrosarcomas, like this example from the region of the acetabulum, may be difficult to distinguish from chondroblastic osteosarcomas.

Chondrosarcoma Arising in Osteochondroma

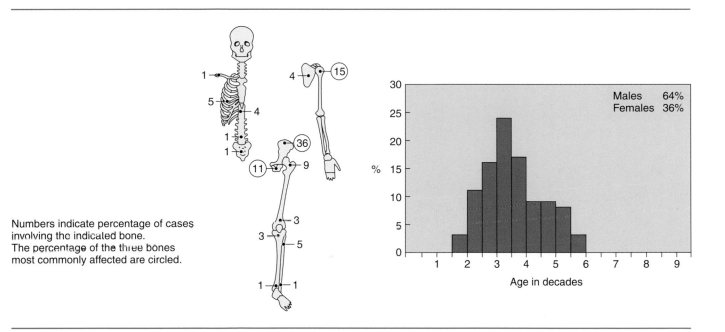

Numbers indicate percentage of cases involving the indicated bone.
The percentage of the three bones most commonly affected are circled.

Males 64%
Females 36%

%

Age in decades

Clinical Signs

1. A tender mass lesion is present.

Clinical Symptoms

1. A mass lesion that may have recently increased in size is found.
2. Pain is present in the region of the lesion.

Major Radiographic Features

1. A thick and indistinct cartilage cap may be seen on a lesion that otherwise has the features of an osteochondroma.

2. When present, radiolucent regions in the lesion are a useful indicator of secondary chondrosarcoma.
3. Destruction of the underlying osteochondroma or adjacent bone is evident in advanced cases.
4. Magnetic resonance imaging (MRI) and computed tomography (CT) are the most sensitive diagnostic techniques for assessing these radiographic features.

Radiographic Differential Diagnosis

1. Osteochondroma with secondary bursa formation.
2. Atypical benign osteochondroma.

Major Pathologic Features

Gross

1. Masses of cartilaginous tissue greater than 1 cm in thickness are present.
2. The cartilaginous tissue may show liquefaction or frank cystification.
3. There is extension into the surrounding soft tissues.

Microscopic

1. On low-power examination, the tumor is composed predominantly of hyaline cartilage.
2. Most tumors are hypocellular but show greater cytologic atypia than is seen in an osteochondroma.
3. The cartilage cap is not arranged in the orderly columnar manner of an osteochondroma; rather, it is disorganized, with clusters of cells scattered in the cartilage matrix.
4. Myxoid change characterized by a loose, watery appearance of the cartilage matrix or by a stringing of the matrix is evident.

Pathologic Differential Diagnosis

Benign lesions

1. Osteochondroma.
2. Periosteal chondroma.

Malignant lesions

1. Periosteal chondrosarcoma.
2. Periosteal osteosarcoma.

Treatment

1. **Primary modality:** surgical resection with a wide margin. Bone grafting of the cortical defect is usually necessary. Other bone and joint reconstructive procedures may be indicated, depending on the size of the defect.
2. **Other possible approaches:** amputation, if a wide margin cannot be achieved by resection owing to soft tissue or neurovascular involvement.

References

Ahmed AR, Tan TS, Unni KK, et al: Secondary chondrosarcoma in osteochondroma: report of 107 patients. *Clin Orthop Relat Res* 411:193–206, 2003.

Garrison RC, Unni KK, McLeod RA, et al: Chondrosarcoma arising in osteochondroma. *Cancer* 49(9):1890–1897, 1982.

Kilpatrick SE, Pike EJ, Ward WG, et al: Dedifferentiated chondrosarcoma in patients with multiple osteochondromatosis: report of a case and review of the literature. *Skeletal Radiol* 26(6):370–374, 1997.

Wuisman PI, Jutte PC, Ozaki T: Secondary chondrosarcoma in osteochondromas. Medullary extension in 15 of 45 cases. *Acta Orthop Scand* 68(4):396–400, 1997.

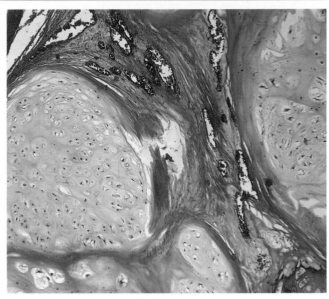

Figure 45–3 At low magnification, the periphery of a chondrosarcoma arising in an osteochondroma may show invasion, as in this photomicrograph. The lobulated nature of the lesion is also evident at low power, and the tumor is more cellular than the cartilage cap of an osteochondroma.

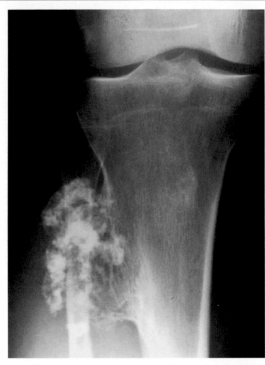

Figure 45–1 The radiograph illustrates a typical osteochondroma arising from the diametaphyseal region of the proximal tibia. The surface is indistinct and irregular, with some areas lacking calcification. These features suggest the possibility of a chondrosarcoma arising in the osteochondroma.

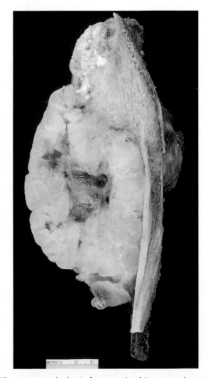

Figure 45–2 The gross pathologic features in this case mirror the radiographic appearance of the lesion (Fig. 45–1). The thickness of the cartilage (more than 2 cm) indicates that the tumor may be malignant. In addition, the central portion of the hyaline cartilage tumor has undergone myxoid degeneration, a gross pathologic feature commonly associated with malignancy.

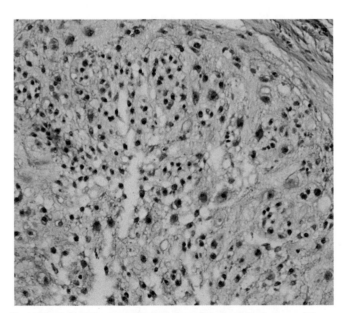

Figure 45–4 At higher magnification, the cellularity of the lesion and the cytologic atypia are evident. The nuclear pleomorphism and cellularity are equivalent to that seen in intramedullary chondrosarcoma.

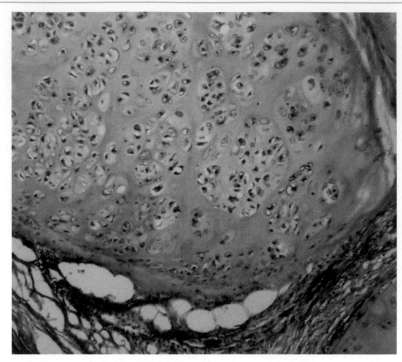

Figure 45–5 Invasion of the soft tissues adjacent to the lesion is helpful in identifying the tumor as malignant. However, bursa formation can occur in the region of an osteochondroma and radiographically mimic the appearance of soft tissue invasion.

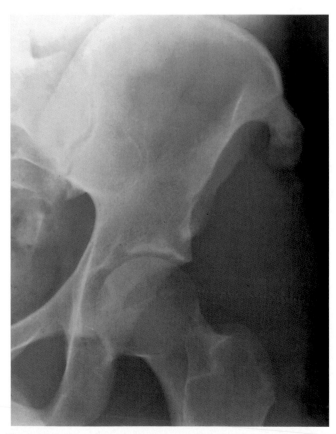

Figure 45–6 This radiograph demonstrates the typical features of an osteo-chondroma involving the iliac bone.

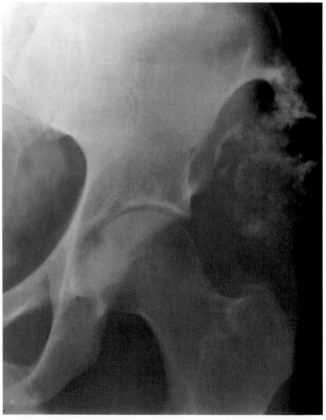

Figure 45–7 Eight years after the initial radiographic evaluation (see Fig. 45–6) the lesion is markedly enlarged, and the periphery is indistinct. A secondary chondrosarcoma has developed in the lesion.

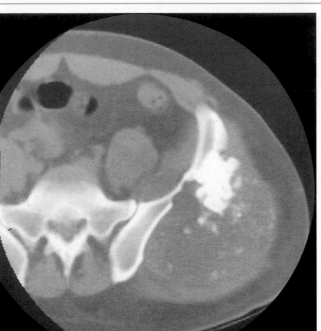

Figure 45–8 This computed tomographic (CT) scan shows a chondrosarcoma arising in an osteochondroma of the iliac bone. Soft tissue masses may be more easily evaluated with this imaging modality. Note that the soft tissue component of this lesion shows scanty calcification.

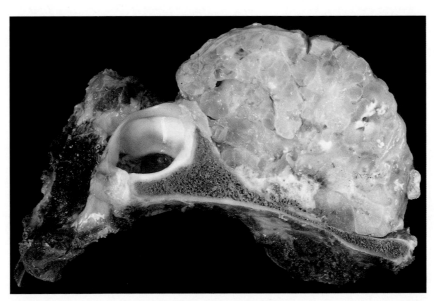

Figure 45–9 This gross specimen shows a secondary chondrosarcoma arising in an osteochondroma of the pelvis. The chondrosarcoma has become so large as to obscure the original osteochondroma.

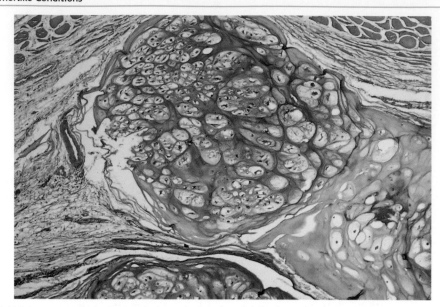

Figure 45–10 This low-power photomicrograph shows the invasion of skeletal muscle adjacent to the secondary chondrosarcoma.

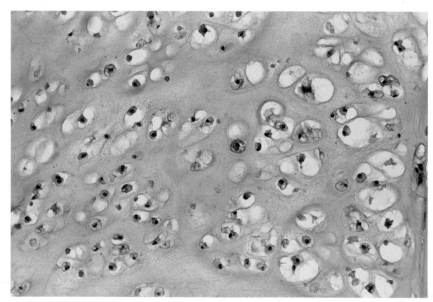

Figure 45–11 Higher magnification of this secondary chondrosarcoma shows the characteristic features of a low-grade hyaline cartilage malignancy: (1) hyper-cellularity, (2) pleomorphism, and (3) binucleation of the chondrocytes.

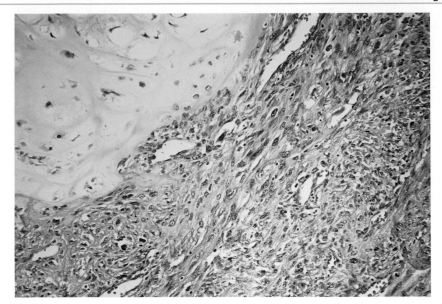

Figure 45–12 Rarely, chondrosarcomas that arise in an osteochondroma may show foci of "dedifferentiation," so-called secondary dedifferentiated chondrosarcoma. In this example, the characteristic pattern of hypercellular spindle cell tumor is superimposed on the low-grade hyaline cartilage malignancy that developed in an osteochondroma.

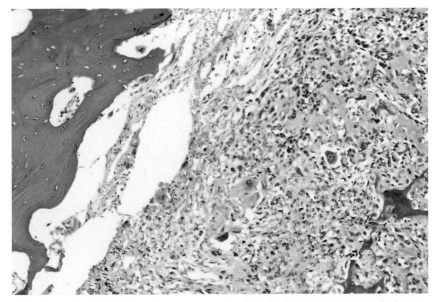

Figure 45–13 Rarely, malignancies other than chondrosarcoma may arise in an osteochondroma. The photomicrograph shows an osteosarcoma that developed in an osteochondroma.

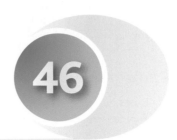

Dedifferentiated Chondrosarcoma

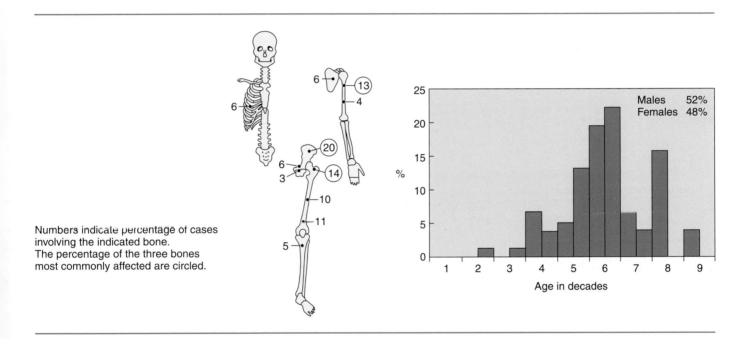

Numbers indicate percentage of cases
involving the indicated bone.
The percentage of the three bones
most commonly affected are circled.

Males 52%
Females 48%

Age in decades

Clinical Signs

1. A soft tissue mass may be the only finding on physical examination.

Clinical Symptoms

1. Pain is a universal symptom, and a mass lesion is frequently present.
2. Some longstanding indolent tumors may show an abrupt change in the pain pattern or accelerated growth of a mass lesion.

Major Radiographic Features

1. An "aggressive" area is superimposed on what is otherwise typical of chondrosarcoma. This usually takes the form of a radiolucent region but may also be a permeative destructive region within the tumor.
2. The lesion is often large and poorly marginated.
3. Intramedullary calcification of a cartilage tumor is usually present.
4. Cortical destruction and an associated soft tissue mass are evident.

5. Many cases are indistinguishable from ordinary intra-medullary chondrosarcomas.

Radiographic Differential Diagnosis

1. Ordinary chondrosarcoma.
2. Sarcoma arising in an old infarct.
3. Mesenchymal chondrosarcoma.
4. Osteosarcoma.

Major Pathologic Features

Gross

1. This tumor shows a bimorphic gross appearance; areas of lobulated gray–white hyaline cartilage coexist with regions of more fleshy yellow–brown soft tumor.
2. There is an abrupt transition from the hyaline cartilage component of the tumor, which is usually centrally located, to the spindle cell component.
3. The anaplastic component of the tumor nearly always dominates the gross lesion and usually has caused cortical destruction of the affected bone with associated production of a soft tissue mass.

Microscopic

1. The grossly evident bimorphic pattern is also appreciable histologically.
2. The low-grade hyaline cartilage component shows the typical features of ordinary chondrosarcoma.
3. Immediately adjacent to the lobules of well-differentiated chondrosarcoma are sheetlike regions of high-grade spindle cell malignancy.
4. Osteoid matrix may be identified in the spindle cell component of the lesion.
5. The spindle cell component of the lesion may show the histologic features of fibrosarcoma or malignant fibrous histiocytoma.

Pathologic Differential Diagnosis

Benign lesions

1. Chondroma, if incompletely sampled.

Malignant lesions

1. Chondrosarcoma, ordinary type.
2. Osteosarcoma.
3. Fibrosarcoma.
4. Malignant fibrous histiocytoma.

Treatment

1. **Primary modality:** Surgical ablation by amputation is usually necessary because of aggressive soft tissue invasion by the tumor.
2. **Other possible approaches:** Limb-saving resection and oncologic reconstruction can be done if an adequately wide margin can be achieved. Adjuvant chemotherapy may be used.

References

Dahlin DC, Beabout JW: Dedifferentiation of low-grade chondrosarcomas. *Cancer* 28(2):461–466, 1971.

Dickey ID, Rose PS, Fuchs B, et al: Dedifferentiated chondrosarcoma: the role of chemotherapy with updated outcomes. *J Bone Joint Surg Am* 86-A(11):2412–2418, 2004.

Kalil RK, Inwards CY, Unni KK, et al: Dedifferentiated clear cell chondrosarcoma. *Am J Surg Pathol* 24(8):1079–1086, 2000.

Littrell LA, Wenger DE, Wold LE, et al: Radiographic, CT, and MR imaging features of dedifferentiated chondrosarcomas: a retrospective review of 174 de novo cases. *Radiographics* 24(5):1397–1409, 2004.

McCarthy EF, Dorfman HD: Chondrosarcoma of bone with dedifferentiation: a study of eighteen cases. *Hum Pathol* 13(1):36–40, 1982.

Mirra JM, Marcove RC: Fibrosarcomatous dedifferentiation of primary and secondary chondrosarcoma: review of five cases. *J Bone Joint Surg Am* 56(2):285–296, 1974.

Mitchell AD, Ayoub K, Mangham DC, et al: Experience in the treatment of dedifferentiated chondrosarcoma. *J Bone Joint Surg Br* 82(1):55–61, 2000.

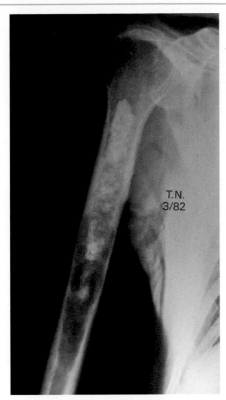

Figure 46–1 This radiograph illustrates a large diaphyseal dedifferentiated chondrosarcoma of the humerus. The aggressive destruction of the area, inferiorly superimposed on an otherwise typical appearance of chondrosarcoma, suggests the correct diagnosis.

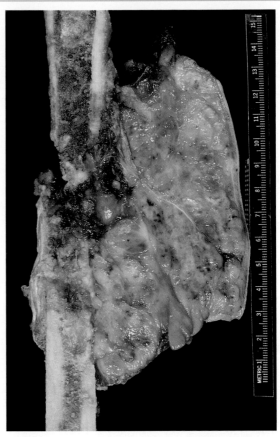

Figure 46–3 Although the majority of the lesion is fleshy and distinctly different grossly from the usual hyaline cartilage tumor, the medullary portion of the tumor shows the characteristic glistening blue–gray aura of the underlying low-grade chondrosarcoma.

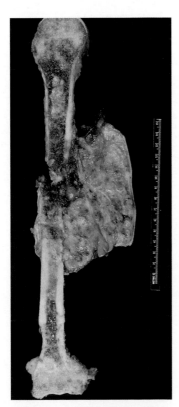

Figure 46–2 The gross appearance of the lesion correlates well with the radiographic evidence of cortical destruction and associated soft tissue extension.

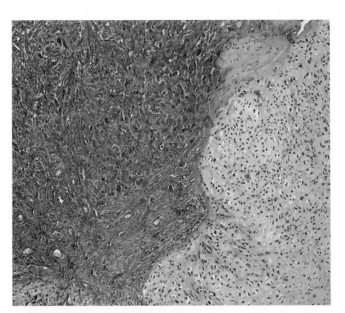

Figure 46–4 At low magnification, dedifferentiated chondrosarcoma shows a bimorphic pattern consisting of a hypocellular cartilage tumor juxtaposed with a high-grade spindle cell sarcoma.

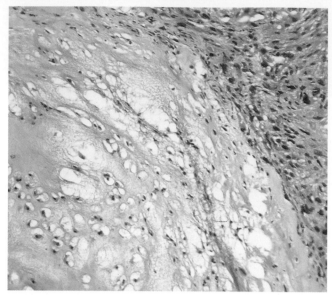

Figure 46–5 At higher magnification, the hyaline cartilage portion of the tumor is indistinguishable from a low-grade chondrosarcoma. In contrast, the hypercellular spindle cell portion of the tumor may be identical with a fibrosarcoma, malignant fibrous histiocytoma, or fibroblastic osteosarcoma.

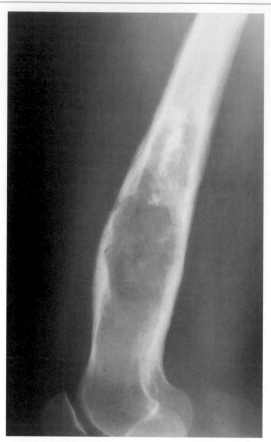

Figure 46–7 This radiograph illustrates the typical features of chondrosarcoma superiorly but shows a very aggressive appearance inferiorly, which is worrisome for a dedifferentiated chondrosarcoma.

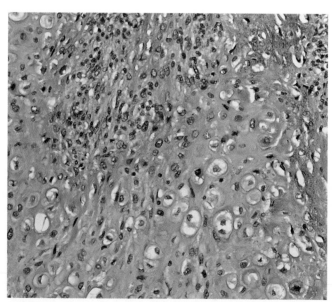

Figure 46–6 At higher magnification, the cytologic atypia associated with the high-grade portion of the tumor is evident. Osteoid may be identified, as in this photomicrograph.

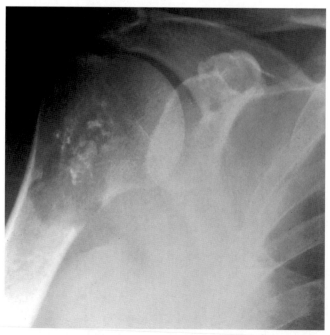

Figure 46–8 This dedifferentiated chondrosarcoma of the proximal humerus shows an aggressive lytic region inferiorly superimposed on an otherwise typical radiographic appearance for chondrosarcoma. The medial cortical destruction is particularly worrisome for dedifferentiation.

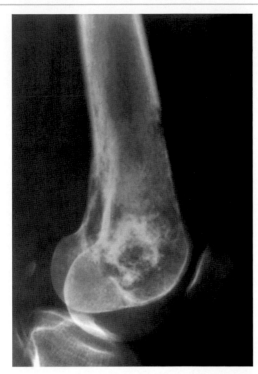

Figure 46–9 This tumor involving the distal femur shows radiographic features typical of chondrosarcoma distally. Again, however, a permeative destructive pattern of growth, seen proximally in the lesion, suggests that the tumor is a dedifferentiated chondrosarcoma.

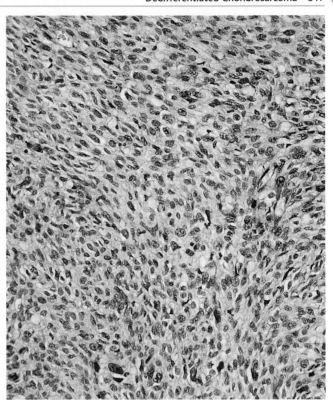

Figure 46–11 At higher magnification, the spindle cell portion of the tumor shows a "herringbone" pattern of growth, as seen in fibrosarcoma.

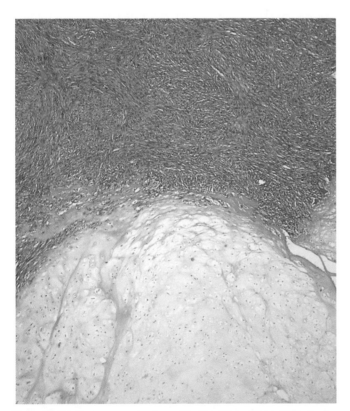

Figure 46–10 The low-power pattern of juxtaposition of hypocellular hyaline cartilage tumor and hypercellular spindle cell sarcoma is characteristic of dedifferentiated chondrosarcoma.

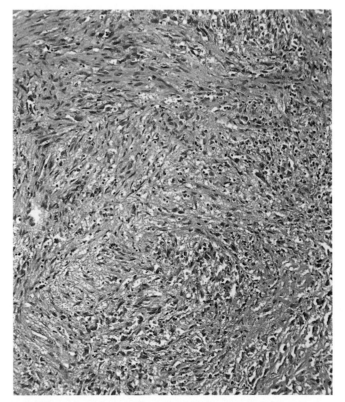

Figure 46–12 A storiform pattern of growth, characteristically associated with malignant fibrous histiocytoma, may also be seen in the dedifferentiated portion of the tumor.

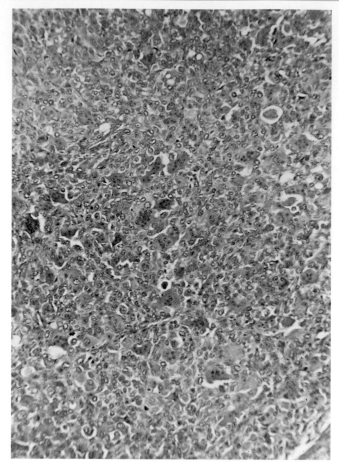

Figure 46–13 Numerous benign multinucleated giant cells may also be seen in the hypercellular portion of the tumor. Such a pattern may histologically mimic the appearance of malignant fibrous histiocytoma or malignant giant cell tumor.

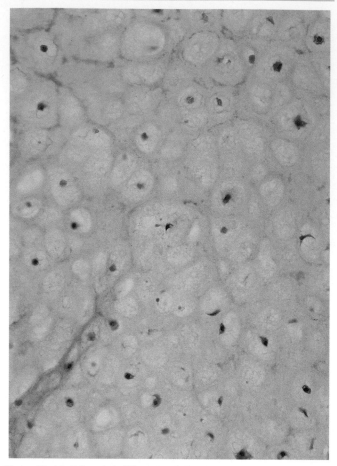

Figure 46–14 Although dedifferentiated chondrosarcoma is a high-grade malignancy, the chondroid portion of the tumor histologically may mimic a benign enchondroma, as in this photomicrograph.

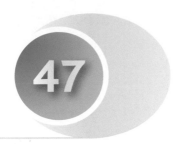

Mesenchymal Chondrosarcoma

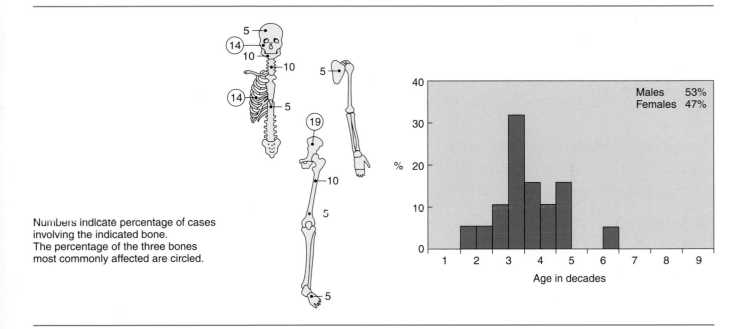

Numbers indicate percentage of cases involving the indicated bone.
The percentage of the three bones most commonly affected are circled.

Clinical Signs

1. A mass lesion is usually the only clinical sign.

Clinical Symptoms

1. Pain and swelling are usually the only symptoms.
2. Approximately one third of patients have had symptoms for longer than 1 year at the time of diagnosis.

Major Radiographic Features

1. Most mesenchymal chondrosarcomas have a malignant radiographic appearance but no specific diagnostic features, or the radiographic features are suggestive of ordinary chondrosarcoma.
2. The tumor usually shows calcification.
3. Poor margination and cortical destruction are present.
4. Frequently there is an associated soft tissue mass.

Radiographic Differential Diagnosis

1. Chondrosarcoma.
2. Osteosarcoma.
3. Fibrosarcoma.

Major Pathologic Features

Gross

1. These tumors are typically gray to pink and vary in consistency from firm to soft.
2. The border of the tumor is usually well defined.
3. Hard calcific foci are usually scattered throughout the tumor.
4. Necrosis and hemorrhage may be evident.

Microscopic

1. The low-power pattern shows a bimorphic appearance with islands of hyaline cartilage embedded within highly cellular zones of small, round to slightly spindled cells.
2. Chondroid zones vary in size and may be more calcified or even ossified.
3. The pattern at low-power magnification in the cellular regions is usually hemangiopericytomatous, with numerous thin-walled branching vessels coursing through the tumor.
4. At higher magnification, the cells within the cellular regions have uniform cytologic characteristics, being round to oval with uniform round to oval nuclei.

Pathologic Differential Diagnosis

Benign lesions

1. Benign hemangiopericytoma.

Malignant lesions

1. Ewing's sarcoma.
2. Dedifferentiated chondrosarcoma.
3. Osteosarcoma.
4. Malignant hemangiopericytoma.

Treatment

1. **Primary modality:** Surgical resection with a wide margin is performed, and reconstruction is individualized according to the location and the patient. This tumor's aggressive behavior with extensive involvement often mandates amputation to achieve an adequate margin.
2. **Other possible approaches:** Adjuvant chemotherapy may be useful. Therapeutic radiation is indicated for surgically inaccessible lesions.

References

Bertoni F, Picci P, Bacchini P, et al: Mesenchymal chondrosarcoma of bone and soft tissues. *Cancer* 52(3):533–541, 1983.

Dabska M, Huvos A: Mesenchymal chondrosarcoma in the young: a clinicopathologic study of 19 patients with explanation of histogenesis. *Virchows Arch (Pathol Anat) Histopathol* 399(1):89–104, 1983.

Huvos AG, Rosen G, Dabska M, et al: Mesenchymal chondrosarcoma: a clinicopathologic analysis of 35 patients with emphasis on treatment. *Cancer* 51(7):1230–1237, 1983.

Nakashima Y, Unni KK, Shives TC, et al: Mesenchymal chondrosarcoma of bone and soft tissue. A review of 111 cases. *Cancer* 57(12):2444–2453, 1986.

Salvador AH, Beabout JW, Dahlin DC: Mesenchymal chondrosarcoma—observations on 30 new cases. *Cancer* 28(3):605–615, 1971.

Steiner GC, Mirra JM, Bullough PG: Mesenchymal chondrosarcoma: a study of the ultrastructure. *Cancer* 32(4):926–939, 1973.

Swanson PE, Lillemoe TJ, Manivel JC, et al: Mesenchymal chondrosarcoma. An immunohistochemical study. *Arch Pathol Lab Med* 114(9):943–948, 1990.

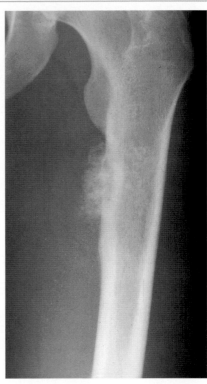

Figure 47–1 This radiograph illustrates the poorly marginated appearance of a mesenchymal chondrosarcoma. The lesion exhibits calcification, a feature suggesting that this is a cartilage tumor. The cortical destruction and associated soft tissue mass are radiographic indications of the malignancy of the process.

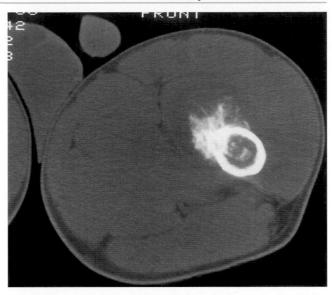

Figure 47–3 A computed tomographic (CT) scan of the tumor shows the soft tissue extent of the lesion and the medullary involvement.

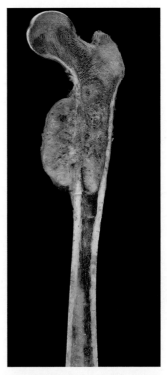

Figure 47–2 The gross pathologic features of the tumor correlate well with the radiographic appearance shown in Figure 47–1. The tumor is fleshy, in contrast with a hyaline cartilage tumor. However, the lesional tissue may be gritty owing to foci of calcification within the tumor.

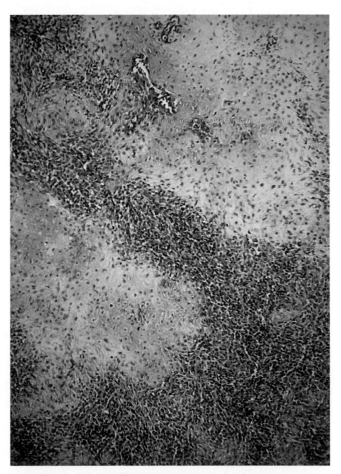

Figure 47–4 At low magnification, mesenchymal chondrosarcomas are bimorphic tumors, composed of relatively hypocellular chondroid zones and hypercellular regions. The hypercellular regions consist of small cells.

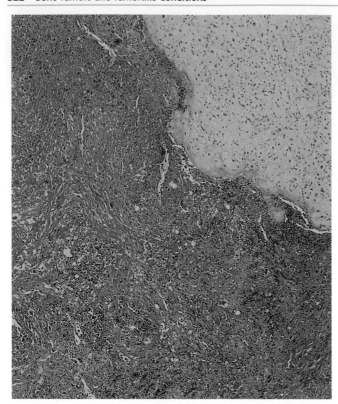

Figure 47–5 Chondroid zones within the tumor are variable in size, some being quite small, as in this photomicrograph.

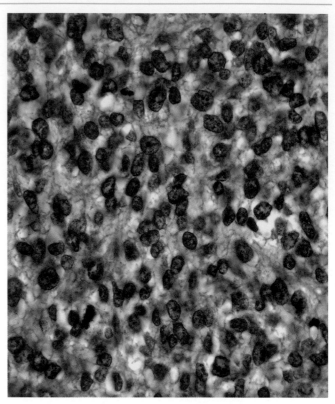

Figure 47–7 At high magnification, the hypercellular portion of the tumor is composed of small cells, which are round to oval. The cytologic features are similar to those of small cell osteosarcoma and hemangiopericytoma.

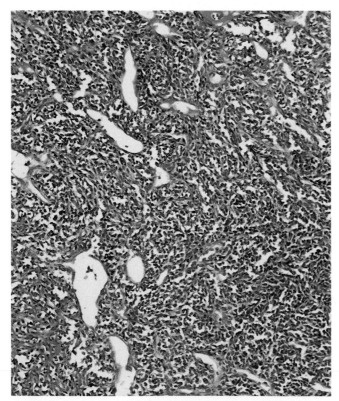

Figure 47–6 The hypercellular zones of the tumor characteristically have a hemangiopericytomatous pattern of growth, as illustrated in this photomicrograph. "Stag horn"–like vascular spaces are evident at low magnification.

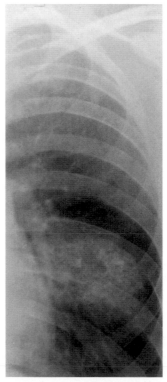

Figure 47–8 Mesenchymal chondrosarcomas are common in flat bone locations, as in this case involving the rib. There is an associated large, partially calcified soft tissue mass with apparent underlying cortical destruction of the affected rib.

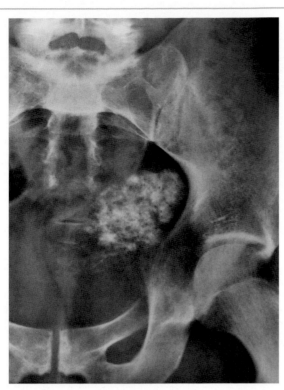

Figure 47–9 This mesenchymal chondrosarcoma involves the acetabular region, a location often involved in ordinary chondrosarcoma. The bone shows lytic destruction, and there is associated calcification in the soft tissue portion of the tumor.

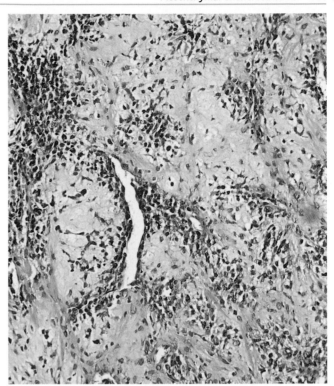

Figure 47–11 This photomicrograph, at low magnification, shows a mesenchymal chondrosarcoma in which the hyaline cartilage portion of the lesion predominates. The small cell portion of the tumor persists in a perivascular pattern.

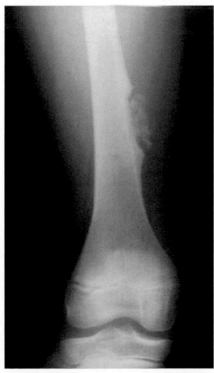

Figure 47–10 This periosteal tumor of the femoral diaphysis proved to be a mesenchymal chondrosarcoma. The buttresses and periosteal location are atypical of mesenchymal chondrosarcoma because the majority of these lesions are centrally located.

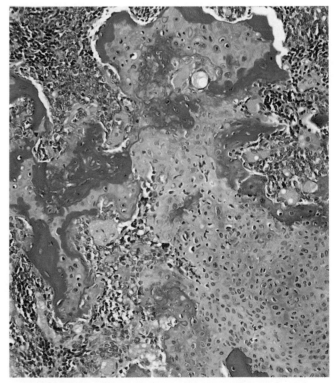

Figure 47–12 Osteoid-like regions may be identified in mesenchymal chondrosarcoma. The differential diagnosis in such cases includes small cell osteosarcoma, a lesion that probably is closely related to mesenchymal chondrosarcoma.

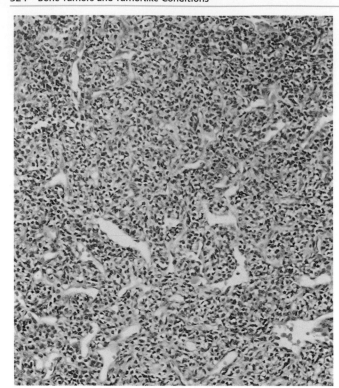

Figure 47–13 The hemangiopericytomatous pattern of growth is particularly prominent in this mesenchymal chondrosarcoma that involves the mandible, a common primary location for the tumor.

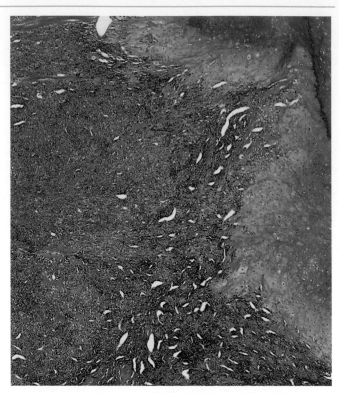

Figure 47–15 This photomicrograph illustrates a mesenchymal chondrosarcoma of the soft tissue of the thigh. Approximately one third of mesenchymal chondrosarcomas are of soft tissue origin.

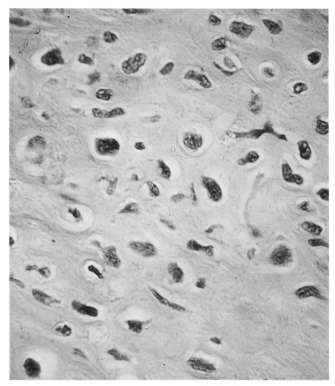

Figure 47–14 The chondroid portions of a mesenchymal chondrosarcoma are indistinguishable from ordinary chondrosarcoma. A small sample from such a region would be identified as an ordinary chondrosarcoma.

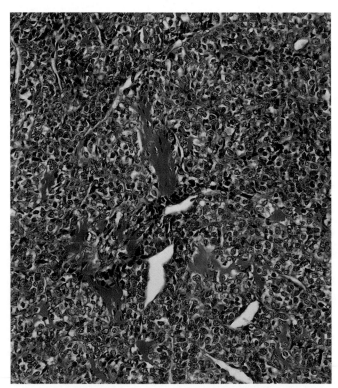

Figure 47–16 This photomicrograph demonstrates the morphology of the tumor shown in Figure 47–15. This tumor has the small cell hemangiopericytomatous pattern commonly present in mesenchymal chondrosarcoma. Rarely, foci of pink osteoid formation also may be seen in this tumor.

Clear Cell Chondrosarcoma

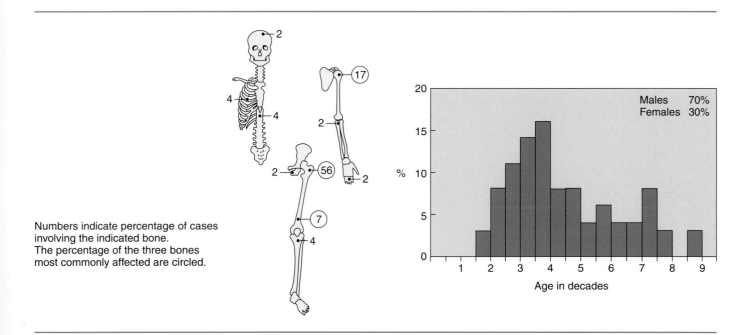

Numbers indicate percentage of cases
involving the indicated bone.
The percentage of the three bones
most commonly affected are circled.

Males 70%
Females 30%

%

Age in decades

Clinical Signs

1. Regional tenderness is present.
2. A mass lesion may be found on physical examination.

Clinical Symptoms

1. Pain is the most common symptom at the time of presentation.
2. These tumors are slow-growing; as such, the symptoms may be of long duration. Of patients in the Mayo Clinic series, 18% had symptoms for longer than 5 years.

Major Radiographic Features

1. The lesion has an epiphyseal location in the proximal femur or humerus.
2. Early lesions look benign, with sharp margination, sclerosis at the periphery, and expansion of the affected bone.
3. Twenty-five percent are calcified on plain radiograph.
4. Larger lesions look malignant, with poor margination and cortical destruction.

Radiographic Differential Diagnosis

1. Chondroblastoma.
2. Chondrosarcoma, ordinary type.
3. Giant cell tumor.

Major Pathologic Features

Gross

1. The curetted fragments are frequently found to contain a cartilaginous bluish-gray translucent matrix.
2. Cystic spaces may be identified; these may represent secondary aneurysmal bone cyst formation.

Microscopic

1. At low magnification, these tumors are faintly lobulated and variable from region to region. Foci of obvious cartilage matrix production may lie adjacent to zones containing numerous mononuclear and multinucleated giant cells.
2. Bony trabeculae are usually identified in this tumor at low power. These are either at the center of lobules of tumor or scattered within the zones of mononuclear cells.
3. At higher magnification, the tumor cells have vesicular nuclei and characteristically show abundant clear cytoplasm. The cell boundaries between such cells are usually distinct.
4. About 50% of the tumors show regions of ordinary chondrosarcoma; in these regions, the multinucleated giant cells are not identified.

Pathologic Differential Diagnosis

Benign lesions

1. Chondroblastoma.
2. Osteoblastoma.
3. Aneurysmal bone cyst.

Malignant lesions

1. Chondrosarcoma, ordinary type.
2. Chondroblastic osteosarcoma.

Treatment

1. **Primary modality:** En bloc resection with a wide surgical margin is performed, with reconstruction of the joint by custom prosthesis, osteochondral allograft, or resection arthrodesis, depending on the location and the needs of the patient.
2. **Other possible approaches:** Amputation may be necessary with large lesions, recurrent lesions, or lesions associated with local contamination resulting from a pathologic fracture or where a wide margin cannot be achieved with resection.

References

Bjornsson J, Unni KK, Dahlin DC, et al: Clear cell chondrosarcoma of bone: observations in 47 cases. *Am J Surg Pathol* 8(3):223–230, 1984.

Cohen EK, Kresell HY, Frank TS, et al: Hyaline-cartilage origin bone and soft tissue neoplasms: MR appearance and histologic correlation. *Radiology* 167(2):477–481, 1988.

Collins MS, Koyama T, Swee RG, et al: Clear cell chondrosarcoma: radiographic, computed tomographic, and magnetic resonance findings in 34 patients with pathologic correlation. *Skeletal Radiol* 32(12):687–694, 2003.

Faraggiana T, Sender B, Glicksman P: Light- and electron-microscopic study of clear cell chondrosarcoma. *Am J Clin Pathol* 75(1):117–121, 1981.

Itala A, Leerapun T, Inwards C, et al: An institutional review of clear cell chondrosarcoma. *Clin Orthop Relat Res* 440:209–212, 2005.

Kaim AH, Hugli R, Bonel HM, et al: Chondroblastoma and clear cell chondrosarcoma: radiological and MRI characteristics with histopathological correlation. *Skeletal Radiol* 31(2):88–95, 2002.

Leggon RE, Unni KK, Beabout JW, et al: Clear cell chondrosarcoma. *Orthopedics* 13(5):593–596, 1990.

Masui F, Ushigome S, Fujii K: Clear cell chondrosarcoma: a pathological and immunohistochemical study. *Histopathology* 34(5):447–452, 1999.

Weiss AP, Dorfman HD: Clear-cell chondrosarcoma: a report of ten cases and review of the literature. *Surg Pathol* 1:123–129, 1988.

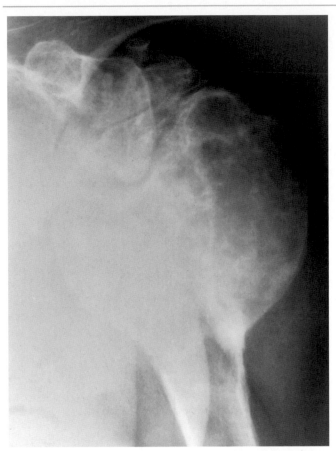

Figure 48–1 This radiograph shows a clear cell chondrosarcoma of the proximal humerus causing marked expansion of the bone and cortical thinning. Mottled calcification is present. At this point in the evolution of the tumor, a radiographic diagnosis of chondrosarcoma, ordinary type, would be most likely. The radiographic features of the lesion 10 years earlier (see Fig. 48–3) are more characteristic of clear cell chondrosarcoma.

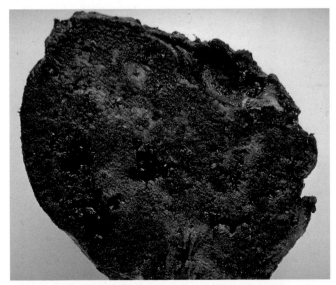

Figure 48–2 The gross features of the tumor shown in Figure 48–1 correlate well with its radiographic appearance. Hemorrhagic cystic spaces are evident in this tumor. Such regions of secondary aneurysmal bone cyst are frequently seen in cases of clear cell chondrosarcoma.

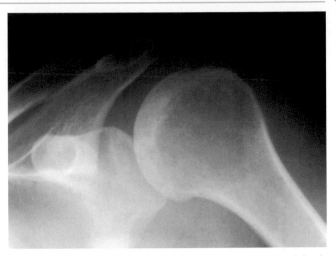

Figure 48–3 The margins of the clear cell chondrosarcoma are better defined in this radiograph of the proximal humerus 10 years prior to definitive surgery. There is only mild expansion of the bone, and no calcification is present. These radiographic features are nonspecific but suggestive of a benign lesion. Early in their evolution, clear cell chondrosarcomas frequently mimic benign conditions.

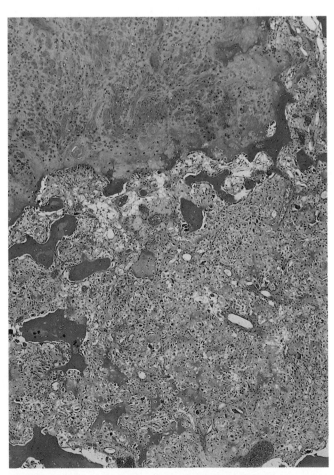

Figure 48–4 At low magnification, clear cell chondrosarcomas show a variable histologic pattern of growth. Hyaline cartilage regions interdigitate with more cellular regions, as shown in this case involving the proximal femur.

Figure 48–5 Calcification similar to that seen in chondroblastoma may be found in clear cell chondrosarcoma. This feature, in combination with the histologic variability and the presence of benign multinucleated giant cells, may result in a mistaken diagnosis of chondroblastoma.

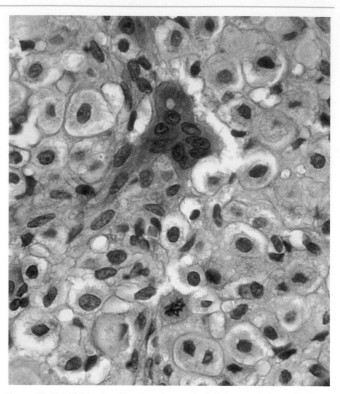

Figure 48–7 At high magnification, the cytologic features of clear cell chondrosarcoma may be deceptively bland. Tumor cells show abundant cytoplasm, as in this photomicrograph. The occurrence of such polygonal cytoplasm, the bland nuclear features, and the presence of multinucleated giant cells mimic the features of chondroblastoma.

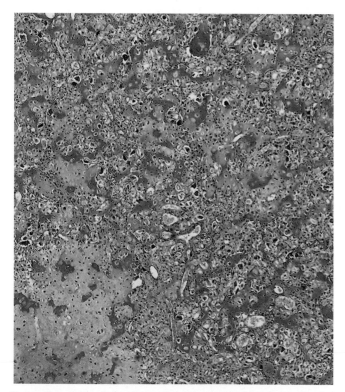

Figure 48–6 Clear cell chondrosarcoma shows an invasive pattern of growth at the periphery of the lesion. In this photomicrograph, permeation through the adjacent medullary bone is evident.

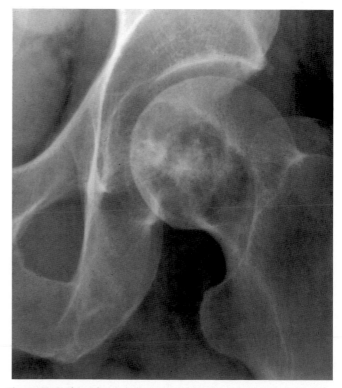

Figure 48–8 This radiograph illustrates the benign features commonly seen in clear cell chondrosarcoma. The sharp sclerotic margin of this tumor is compatible with the appearance of chondroblastoma.

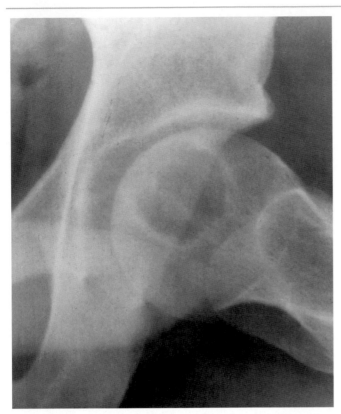

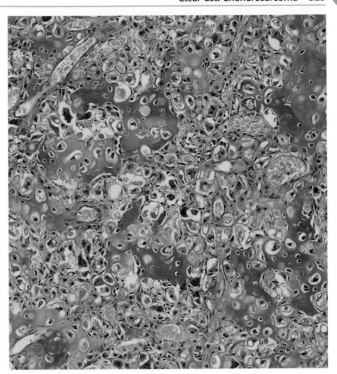

Figure 48–9 Like chondroblastoma, clear cell chondrosarcoma frequently involves the epiphysis of the affected bone. Such is the case with this tumor, which is partially calcified, has sclerotic margins, and involves the epiphysis of the proximal femur.

Figure 48–11 Clear cell chondrosarcoma is histologically variable from region to region, as seen in this low-power photomicrograph. Foci may show pure hyaline cartilage differentiation, whereas other regions may show bone production. Thus, the differential diagnosis may include ordinary chondrosarcoma and chondroblastic osteosarcoma.

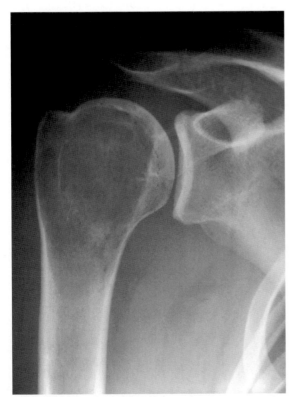

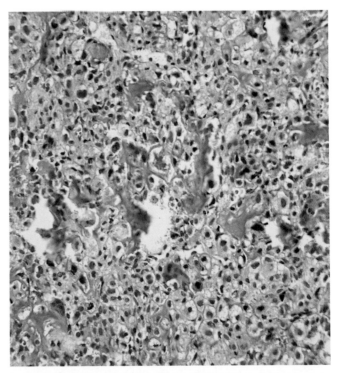

Figure 48–10 This radiograph shows a more advanced lesion in the proximal humerus, presenting as a purely lytic and poorly marginated tumor.

Figure 48–12 Bone production is evident in this low-power photomicrograph. Such foci may mimic the appearance of a chondroblastic osteosarcoma. However, the cytologic atypia is much less pronounced in clear cell chondrosarcoma than in chondroblastic osteosarcoma.

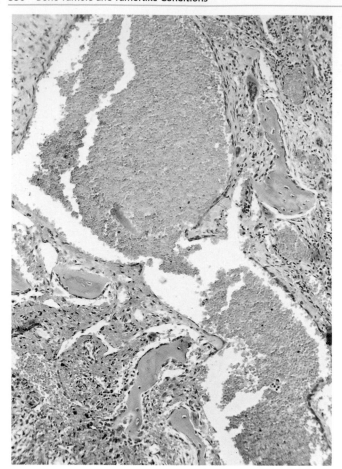

Figure 48–13 This photomicrograph shows a region of secondary aneurysmal bone cyst complicating clear cell chondrosarcoma. Although such secondary aneurysmal bone cysts are more commonly encountered in benign tumors, they frequently occur as a component in clear cell chondrosarcoma.

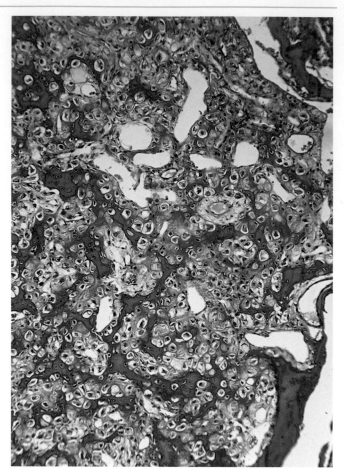

Figure 48–14 Although clear cell chondrosarcoma is a well-differentiated or low-grade tumor, it can recur locally or in other osseous locations or metastasize to the lung. The histologic features of the pulmonary metastases are identical with those of the primary tumor, as illustrated in this photomicrograph.

Section 2C: Fibrous and Fibrohistiocytic Tumors

Fibrosarcoma

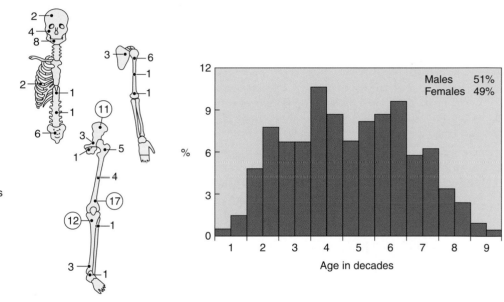

Numbers indicate percentage of cases involving the indicated bone.
The percentage of the three bones most commonly affected are circled.

Males 51%
Females 49%

%

Age in decades

Clinical Signs

1. A mass lesion is generally present in the area of the affected bone.
2. The mass is generally painful to palpation.

Clinical Symptoms

1. Pain and swelling are common, as with all malignant bone tumors.
2. The duration of symptoms is generally short.
3. Fibrosarcoma may arise "secondarily" in a precursor lesion such as a bone infarct or in Paget's disease, but the most common precursor condition is radiation therapy.

Major Radiographic Features

1. The lesion is large and eccentrically located.
2. The lesion may be metaphyseal or diaphyseal within the affected bone.
3. The lesion is purely lytic, with absent or scant sclerosis.
4. The lesion is poorly marginated.
5. Cortical destruction and extension into the adjacent soft tissues are common.
6. A periosteal reaction is uncommonly seen.

7. Approximately 30% of lesions arise secondarily in a preexisting lesion.

Radiographic Differential Diagnosis

1. Osteosarcoma.
2. Myeloma.
3. Metastatic carcinoma.
4. Giant cell tumor.
5. Malignant fibrous histiocytoma.

Major Pathologic Features

Gross

1. The lesional tissue is firm and fleshy.
2. Myxoid qualities may be present, and high-grade tumors may be grossly hemorrhagic, friable, and necrotic.
3. Most tumors will have broken through the cortex.

Microscopic

1. At low magnification, the histologic view is classically that of a spindle cell tumor arranged in a "herringbone" pattern of growth.
2. At its periphery, the lesion grows in a permeative manner, invading between preexisting bony trabeculae.
3. Low-grade tumors may produce abundant collagen and may be relatively hypocellular.
4. High-grade tumors are more cellular, showing less collagen production.
5. At high magnification, the cytologic features vary with the grade of the tumor. Low-grade tumors show homogeneous cytologic features, with dark, spindle-shaped nuclei; high-grade tumors show marked nuclear pleomorphism and abundant mitotic activity.
6. Rarely, the tumor may be markedly myxoid.

Pathologic Differential Diagnosis

Benign lesions

1. Desmoplastic fibroma.

Malignant lesions

1. Malignant fibrous histiocytoma.
2. Fibroblastic osteosarcoma.
3. Metastatic spindling carcinoma.

Treatment

1. **Primary modality:** preoperative chemotherapy and limb-sparing resection with a wide surgical margin and reconstruction as indicated, where feasible. However, amputation may be required to achieve an adequate margin. Adjuvant multidrug chemotherapy programs, similar to those used for osteosarcoma, may be used for patients with high-grade tumors.
2. **Other possible approaches:** radiation therapy for surgically inaccessible lesions and aggressive thoracotomy for pulmonary metastases.

References

Bertoni F, Capanna R, Calderoni P, et al: Primary central (medullary) fibrosarcoma of bone. *Semin Diagn Pathol* 1(3):185–198, 1984.

Campanacci M, Olmi R: Fibrosarcoma of bone. A study of 114 cases. *Ital J Orthop Traumatol* 3(2):199–206, 1977.

Dahlin DC, Ivins JC: Fibrosarcoma of bone. A study of 114 cases. *Cancer* 23(1):35–41, 1969.

Inwards CY, Unni KK, Beabout JW, et al: Desmoplastic fibroma of bone. *Cancer* 68(9):1978–1983, 1991.

Larsson SE, Lorentzon R, Boquist L: Fibrosarcoma of bone: a demographic, clinical and histopathological study of all cases recorded in the Swedish Cancer Registry from 1958 to 1968. *J Bone Joint Surg Br* 58-B:412–417, 1976.

Papagelopoulos PJ, Galanis E, Frassica FJ, et al: Primary fibrosarcoma of bone. Outcome after primary surgical treatment. *Clin Orthop Relat Res* 373:88–103, 2000.

Ruggieri P, Sim FH, Bond JR, et al: Malignancies in fibrous dysplasia. *Cancer* 73(5):1411–1424, 1994.

Sugiura I: Desmoplastic fibroma: case report and review of the literature. *J Bone Joint Surg Am* 58(1):126–130, 1976.

Taconis WK, Van Rijssel TG: Fibrosarcoma of long bones. A study of the significance of areas of malignant fibrous histiocytoma. *J Bone Joint Surg Br* 67(1):111–116, 1985.

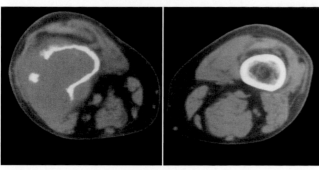

Figure 50–1 This computed tomographic (CT) scan shows a large lytic and eccentric defect in the distal femur. Cortical destruction and soft tissue extension of the lesion attest to its malignant nature; however, the tumor is otherwise nondescript.

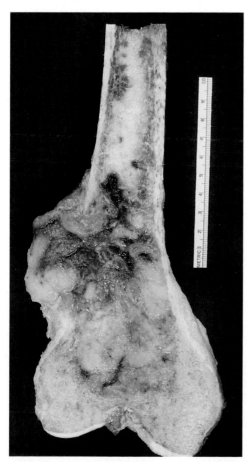

Figure 50–2 The gross pathologic features of the fibrosarcoma in Figure 50–1 are shown in this photograph. The lesional tissue is soft and gray–white to tan. The cortical destruction and soft tissue extension evident radiographically are illustrated grossly in this cross-section of the tumor.

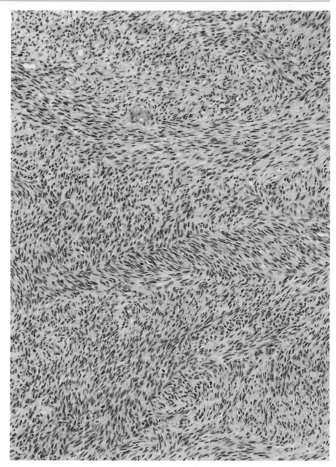

Figure 50–3 At low magnification, fibrosarcomas are composed of spindle cells in a "herringbone" pattern of growth. The high-grade tumors show greater cellularity, mitotic activity, and cytologic pleomorphism.

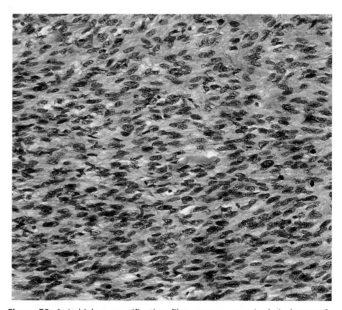

Figure 50–4 At higher magnification, fibrosarcomas vary in their degree of cytologic atypia and mitotic activity. This tumor that involved the maxilla resulted in pulmonary metastasis 34 months after diagnosis, attesting to its high-grade nature.

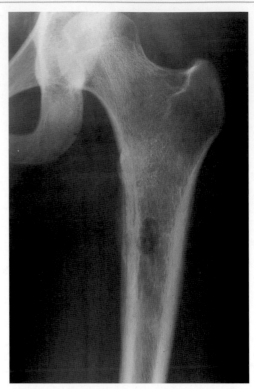

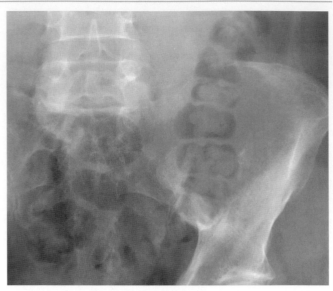

Figure 50–7 This radiograph of the pelvis illustrates a large, purely lytic fibrosarcoma of the left iliac bone and sacrum. There is extensive destruction of the bone.

Figure 50–5 This radiograph shows a poorly marginated lytic fibrosarcoma in the subtrochanteric diaphyseal region of the femur. Scanty periosteal reaction is present in this case.

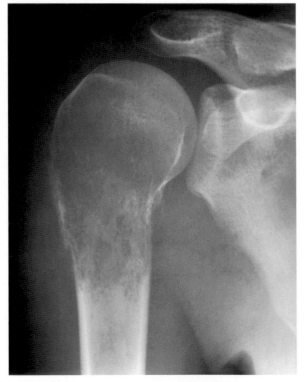

Figure 50–6 This large fibrosarcoma of the proximal humerus presented as a purely lytic metaphyseal lesion. The cortical destruction attests to the aggressiveness of the lesion, and the bone has been sufficiently weakened to have sustained a pathologic fracture.

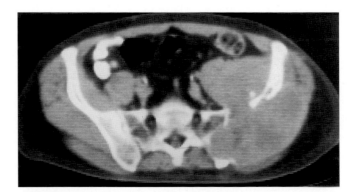

Figure 50–8 A CT scan of the tumor shown in Figure 50–7 demonstrates a large soft tissue component containing low-density areas of necrotic tumor or hemorrhage.

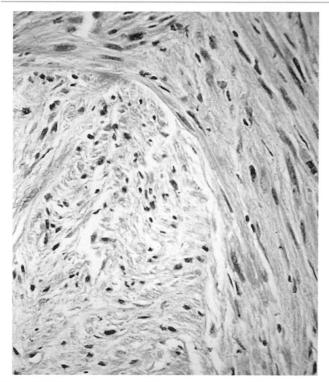

Figure 50–9 This photomicrograph illustrates the hypocellular nature of well-differentiated or low-grade fibrosarcomas. Although nuclear pleomorphism may be present, such tumors lack significant mitotic activity and generally show abundant collagenous stroma.

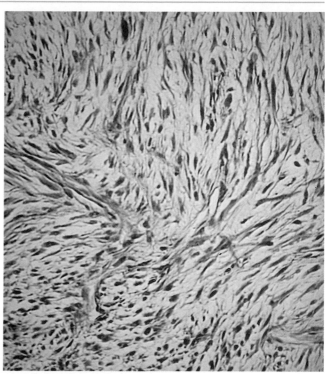

Figure 50–11 Myxoid stromal change may be present and generally accompanies low-grade fibrosarcomas.

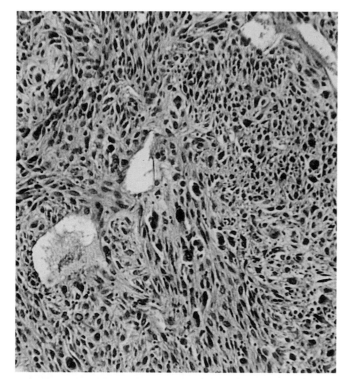

Figure 50–10 In contrast with low-grade tumors (as shown in Fig. 50–9), high-grade tumors are hypercellular and show less collagenous matrix production. Greater nuclear pleomorphism is also evident even at low magnification, as in this example of a high-grade fibrosarcoma.

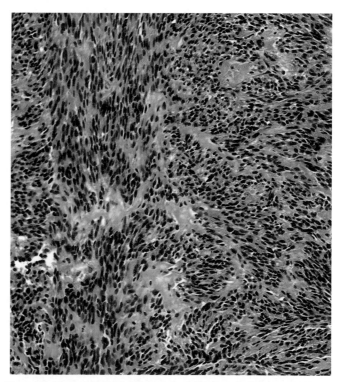

Figure 50–12 The histologic differentiation of high-grade fibrosarcoma from fibroblastic osteosarcoma is made on the basis of identifying osteoid; however, dense collagen can mimic the appearance of osteoid, as in this photomicrograph; thus, the distinction is, at times, subjective.

Figure 50–13 This photomicrograph shows a desmoplastic fibroma. These tumors are histologically identical with soft tissue aggressive fibromatosis of desmoid type.

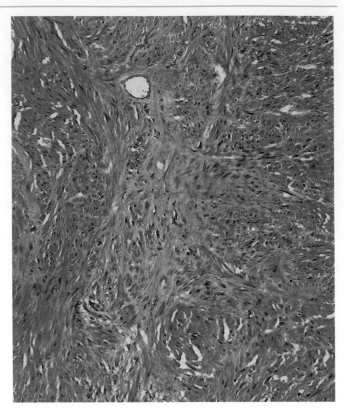

Figure 50–15 Leiomyosarcomas may arise as primary bone tumors. These tumors are commonly in the pathologic differential diagnosis with fibrosarcoma of bone.

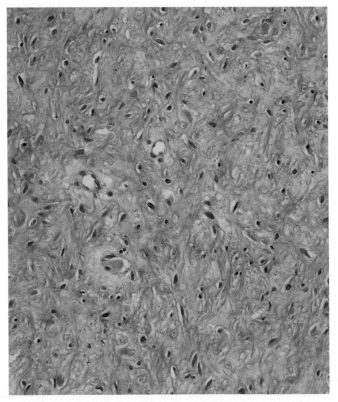

Figure 50–14 This photomicrograph illustrates the densely collagenized stroma seen in desmoplastic fibroma of bone. Such lesions are in the differential diagnosis of low-grade fibrosarcoma.

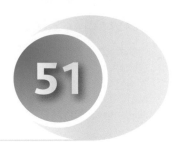

Malignant Fibrous Histiocytoma

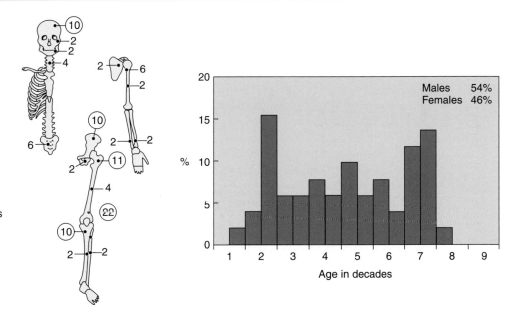

Numbers indicate percentage of cases
involving the indicated bone.
The percentage of the three bones
most commonly affected are circled.

Males 54%
Females 46%

%

Age in decades

Clinical Signs

1. A painful or tender mass lesion is the most common finding on physical examination.

Clinical Symptoms

1. Pain and swelling are the most common symptoms.
2. Symptoms may be of short duration but are generally present for 6 months or longer.
3. This tumor may arise after radiation therapy for an unrelated malignancy or as a malignancy complicating Paget's disease.

Major Radiographic Features

1. The lesion most often arises in a metaphyseal or diaphyseal location in the affected bone.
2. The lesion most often is purely lytic, although a few have mixed sclerosis and lysis.
3. Cortical destruction and associated soft tissue mass are common.
4. Periosteal reaction is absent or scant.
5. The tumor may be identified arising from a preexisting lesion (e.g., a bone infarct).

Radiographic Differential Diagnosis

1. Osteosarcoma.
2. Fibrosarcoma.
3. Malignant lymphoma.
4. Metastatic carcinoma.
5. Myeloma.

Major Pathologic Features

Gross

1. The gross tumor varies in consistency from firm to soft, depending on the cellularity and the amount of collagen being produced.
2. The color varies from tumor to tumor and within a given tumor; it may be yellow, brown, or tan.
3. Necrotic regions are frequently present in high-grade tumors.

Microscopic

1. At low magnification, the appearance is generally that of a spindle cell tumor arranged in a matted or storiform pattern.
2. The cytologic features tend to be variable, with some cells being more rounded and "histiocytic" and others spindled and "fibroblastic."
3. Multinucleated giant cells, lipid-laden histiocytes, and malignant giant cells are scattered throughout the lesion.
4. At higher magnification, the cytologic atypia can be variable from low-grade to high-grade tumors, as can the variability in the mitotic activity present.

Pathologic Differential Diagnosis

Benign lesions

1. Fibroma (metaphyseal fibrous defect).
2. Benign fibrous histiocytoma.
3. Giant cell tumor.
4. Giant cell reparative granuloma (giant cell reaction).

Malignant lesions

1. Metastatic sarcomatoid carcinoma (particularly hypernephroma).
2. Fibrosarcoma.
3. Fibroblastic osteosarcoma.

Treatment

1. **Primary modality:** Preoperative chemotherapy and wide surgical resection are used when possible. Oncologic reconstruction varies with the location. Amputation may be necessary to achieve a margin in large lesions with neurovascular involvement.
2. **Other possible approaches:** Adjuvant chemotherapy may be used. Thoracotomy is useful for patients with pulmonary metastases. Radiation therapy has been effective in some surgically inaccessible lesions.

References

Capanna R, Bertoni F, Bacchini P, et al: Malignant fibrous histiocytoma of bone. The experience at the Rizzoli Institute: report of 90 cases. *Cancer* 54(1):177–187, 1984.

Ghandur-Mnaymneh L, Zych G, Mnaymneh W: Primary malignant fibrous histiocytoma of bone: report of six cases with ultrastructural study and analysis of the literature. *Cancer* 49(4):698–707, 1982.

Huvos AG, Heilweil M, Bretsky SS: The pathology of malignant fibrous histiocytoma of bone. A study of 130 patients. *Am J Surg Pathol* 9(12):853–871, 1985.

McCarthy EF, Matsuno T, Dorfman HD: Malignant fibrous histiocytoma of bone: a study of 35 cases. *Hum Pathol* 10(1):57–70, 1979.

Mirra JM, Gold RH, Marafiote R: Malignant (fibrous) histiocytoma arising in association with a bone infarct in sickle-cell disease: coincidence or cause and effect? *Cancer* 39(1):186–194, 1977.

Nishida J, Sim FH, Wenger DE, et al: Malignant fibrous histiocytoma of bone. A clinicopathologic study of 81 patients [see comments]. *Cancer* 79(3):482–493, 1997.

Ruggieri P, Sim FH, Bond JR, et al: Malignancies in fibrous dysplasia. *Cancer* 73(5):1411–1424, 1994.

Taconis WK, Mulder JD: Fibrosarcoma and malignant fibrous histiocytoma of long bones: radiographic features and grading. *Skeletal Radiol* 11(4):237–245, 1984.

Taconis WK, Van Rijssel TG: Fibrosarcoma of long bones. A study of the significance of areas of malignant fibrous histiocytoma. *J Bone Joint Surg Br* 67(1):111–116, 1985.

Yokoyama R, Tsuneyoshi M, Enjoji M, et al: Prognostic factors of malignant fibrous histiocytoma of bone. A clinical and histopathologic analysis of 34 cases. *Cancer* 72(6):1902–1908, 1993.

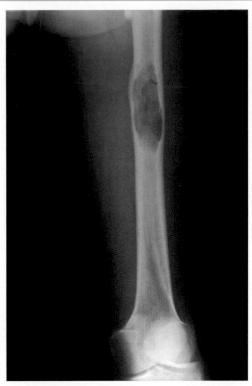

Figure 51–1 This radiograph illustrates an intramedullary malignant fibrous histiocytoma that shows a purely lytic pattern of growth. Mild expansion of the femoral diaphysis and cortical destruction are evident.

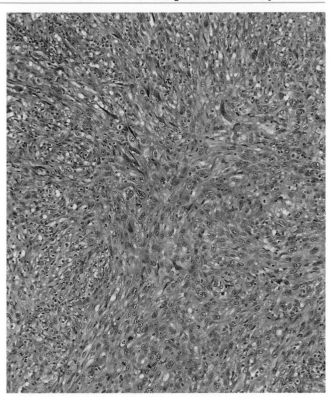

Figure 51–3 At low magnification, the histologic pattern of malignant fibrous histiocytoma may vary from region to region. Classically, the tumor grows in a storiform pattern, as shown in this photomicrograph.

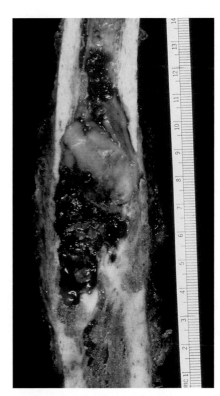

Figure 51–2 The gross pathologic features of this lesion correlate well with its radiographic appearance in Figure 51–1. Grossly, the tumor is soft, fleshy, and variable in color from gray–white to yellow. Foci of hemorrhage, as are visible in this case, may be present.

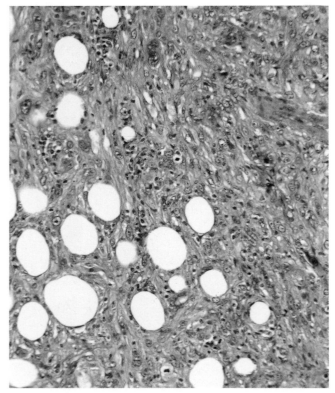

Figure 51–4 At higher magnification, the tumor is seen to be composed of a variety of cell types. Some tumors have a pronounced inflammatory component; others show lesser degrees of inflammatory reaction.

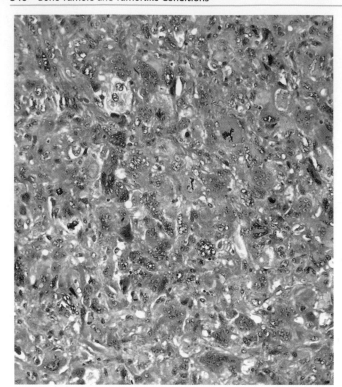

Figure 51–5 At higher magnification, the degree of cytologic atypia present in malignant fibrous histiocytomas is variable. Most commonly, significant cytologic atypia and brisk mitotic activity are present, as shown in this photomicrograph.

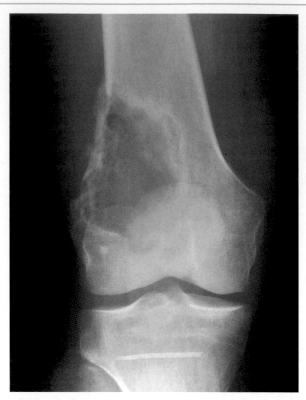

Figure 51–7 This radiograph illustrates a malignant fibrous histiocytoma of the distal femoral metaphysis. The tumor is eccentric and shows a permeative pattern of growth with cortical destruction.

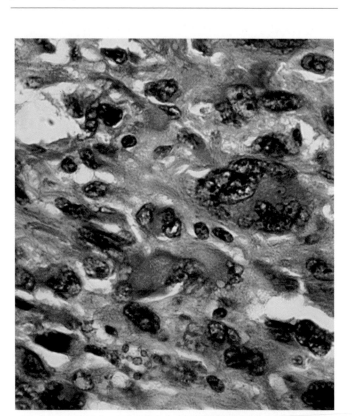

Figure 51–6 At high magnification, marked cytologic atypia characterized by nuclear pleomorphism, hyperchromasia, and an irregular chromatin pattern are common in malignant fibrous histiocytoma. Multinucleation is also common. Such tumors may simulate a giant cell tumor.

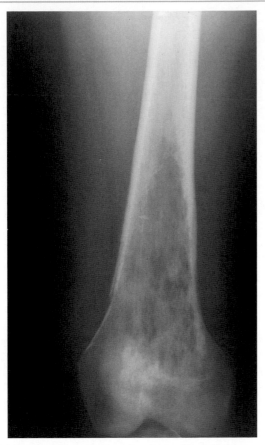

Figure 51–8 A large, poorly marginated, malignant fibrous histiocytoma of the lower femoral diametaphysis is shown in this radiograph. The lesion is irregular in contour and demonstrates a mixed lytic and sclerotic pattern of growth.

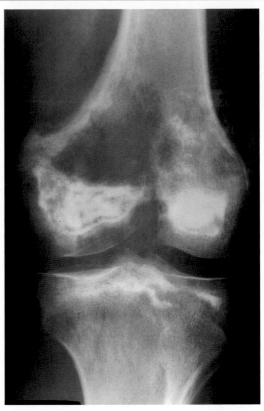

Figure 51–9 Malignant fibrous histiocytoma may arise secondary to a bone infarct, as shown in this radiograph of the distal femur. Infarct is also present in the upper tibia.

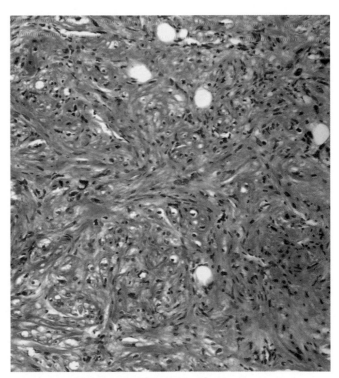

Figure 51–10 At low magnification, an ill-defined storiform pattern of growth is evident in this malignant fibrous histiocytoma of the proximal tibia. The tumor is growing in a permeative manner.

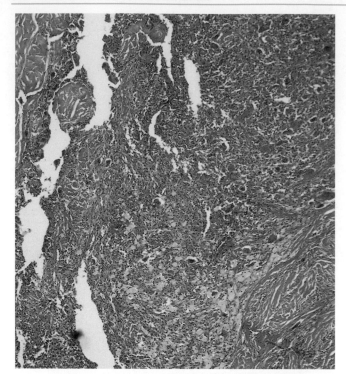

Figure 51–11 Numerous multinucleated giant cells may be present in malignant fibrous histiocytomas, resulting in a histologic appearance simulating that of giant cell tumor. This photomicrograph illustrates such a histologic pattern in a tumor that involved the distal femur.

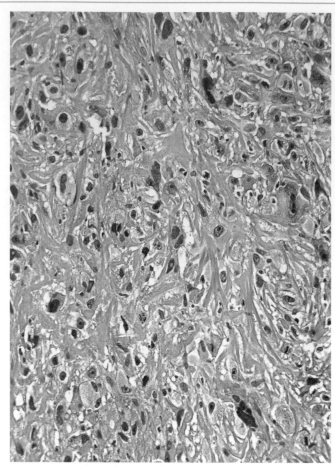

Figure 51–13 Differentiation of fibroblastic osteosarcoma (shown in this photomicrograph) from malignant fibrous histiocytoma can be extremely difficult. Demonstration of "malignant" osteoid in the lesion identifies it as an osteosarcoma; however, fracture callus and reactive new bone formation associated with malignant fibrous histiocytoma may simulate such osteoid. Such a distinction is probably only of academic importance.

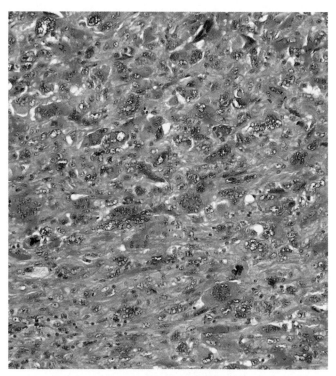

Figure 51–12 When numerous multinucleated giant cells are found in a tumor, careful assessment of the cytologic features of the mononuclear cells is necessary. At high magnification, the nuclei of the mononuclear cells of malignant fibrous histiocytoma are cytologically different from those of the multinucleated giant cells, as this photomicrograph shows.

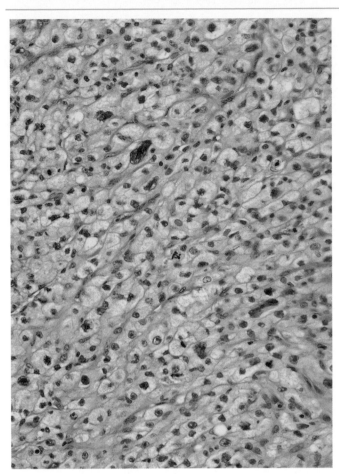

Figure 51–14 Metastatic sarcomatoid renal cell carcinoma can histologically mimic the appearance of malignant fibrous histiocytoma. This photomicrograph illustrates that malignant fibrous histiocytoma may contain clear cells that are somewhat packeted and thus mimic the appearance of renal cell carcinoma.

Section 2D: Hematopoietic Tumors

Malignant Lymphoma

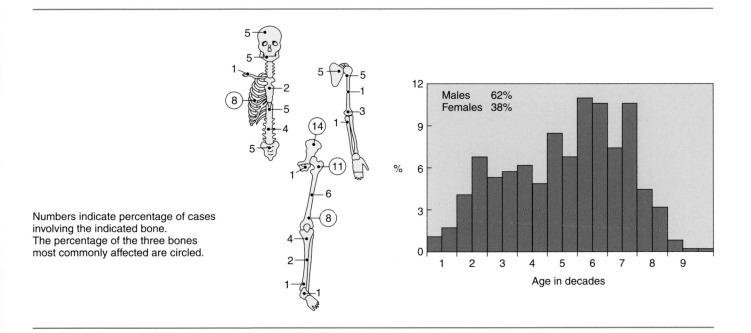

Numbers indicate percentage of cases involving the indicated bone.
The percentage of the three bones most commonly affected are circled.

Males 62%
Females 38%

%

Age in decades

Clinical Signs

1. A tender mass lesion is commonly found on physical examination if the affected bone is superficial.
2. Lymphadenopathy and splenomegaly may be present in disseminated disease.
3. Extension into the soft tissues may result in an associated soft tissue mass.

Clinical Symptoms

1. Malignant lymphoma most commonly is associated with pain and swelling.
2. Pain is variable in intensity but may have been present for years.

3. Neurologic symptoms may be present in those patients who have vertebral involvement related to cord or nerve root compression.
4. The patient may have few complaints, however, and generally feels quite well despite extensive disease.

Major Radiographic Features

1. The lesion is generally characterized by extensive diaphyseal permeative destruction of the affected bone.
2. The pattern may be one of pure lysis or sclerosis, or it may be a mixture of lysis and sclerosis.
3. Periosteal reaction is unusual.
4. The cortex may be thickened, and the lesion shows poor margination at the periphery.

5. An associated soft tissue mass is commonly present.
6. Isotope bone scan, computed tomography, and magnetic resonance imaging are frequently helpful in defining the extent of the lesion and its location.

Radiographic Differential Diagnosis

1. Ewing's sarcoma.
2. Osteosarcoma.
3. Osteomyelitis.
4. Metastatic carcinoma.

Major Pathologic Features

Gross

1. Viable tumor extending into the soft tissues generally shows a whitish, fish flesh–like appearance.
2. Lymphomas generally permeate the bone extensively, leaving residual bony trabeculae that may impart a gritty consistency to the medullary portion of the specimen.

Microscopic

1. At low magnification, lymphomas show a diffuse sheetlike proliferation of cells without matrix production.
2. At higher magnification, osseous lymphomas generally show a mixture of cells, with both small and large cells scattered throughout the lesional tissue.
3. The nuclear characteristics are generally variable, with both cleaved and noncleaved nuclei identifiable.
4. Reticulin stains generally show a fine meshwork of reticulin fibers surrounding individual cells.
5. Immunohistochemical stains for lymphoid markers are positive if optimally fixed tissue is available for analysis. (*Note:* Touch preparations may be used for immunohistochemical analysis, thereby avoiding the use of tissue that has been subjected to decalcification procedures.)

Pathologic Differential Diagnosis

Benign lesions

1. Chronic osteomyelitis.

Malignant lesions

1. Metastatic undifferentiated carcinoma.
2. Malignant fibrous histiocytoma (histiocytic variant).

Treatment

1. **Primary modality:** Radiation therapy is the mainstay of treatment of the local bony lesion. Chemotherapy is used when systemic disease is identifiable.
2. **Other possible approaches:** Surgical intervention with internal fixation or joint replacement for pathologic fractures may be used. Resection or amputation may be required for distal-extremity lesions that have failed to respond to radiation therapy.

References

Clayton F, Butler JJ, Ayala AG, et al: Non-Hodgkin's lymphoma in bone. Pathologic and radiologic features with clinical correlates. *Cancer* 60(10):2494–2501, 1987.

Dosoretz DE, Murphy GF, Raymond AK, et al: Radiation therapy for primary lymphoma of bone. *Cancer* 51(1):44–46, 1983.

Dosoretz DE, Raymond AK, Murphy GF, et al. Primary lymphoma of bone: the relationship of morphologic diversity to clinical behavior. *Cancer* 50(1):1009–1014, 1982.

Kirsch J, Ilaslan H, Bauer T, et al: The incidence of imaging findings and the distribution of skeletal lymphoma in a consecutive patient population seen over 5 years. *Skeletal Radiol* 35(8):590–594, 2006.

Neiman RS, Barcos M, Berard C, et al: Granulocytic sarcoma: a clinicopathologic study of 61 biopsied cases. *Cancer* 48(6):1426–1437, 1981.

Ostrowski ML, Unni KK, Banks PM, et al: Malignant lymphoma of bone. *Cancer* 58(12):2646–2655, 1986.

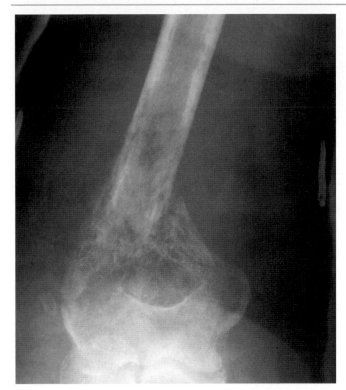

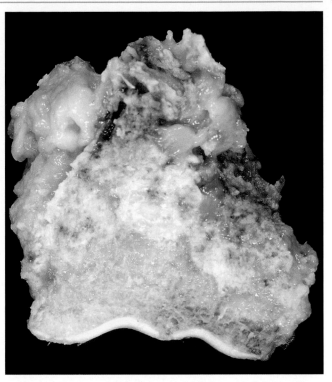

Figure 52–1 This radiograph demonstrates the permeative destructive appearance of a malignant lymphoma involving the distal humerus. An associated soft tissue mass is present, and a pathologic fracture has occurred.

Figure 52–2 The gross pathologic features of malignant lymphoma of bone are demonstrated in this tumor, which was resected owing to the pathologic fracture and loss of bone. Classically, lymphomas are soft, "fish flesh" tumors that are gray–white.

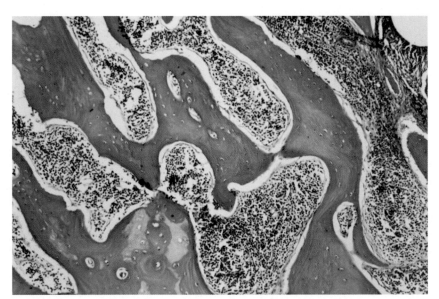

Figure 52–3 At low magnification, malignant lymphoma grows in a permeative pattern, whether it involves bone (as in this photomicrograph) or soft tissue. Residual bony trabeculae are present within the medullary portion of this non-Hodgkin's lymphoma.

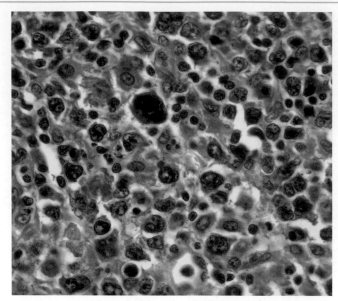

Figure 52–4 At high magnification, the cytologic variability generally present in osseous lymphomas is seen in this photomicrograph. Large and small cells are mixed and generally grow in a sheetlike, diffuse manner. "Multilobulated" cells may be seen, as in this example, and some cases represent neoplasms of T-cell origin; however, most osseous lymphomas are of B-cell lineage.

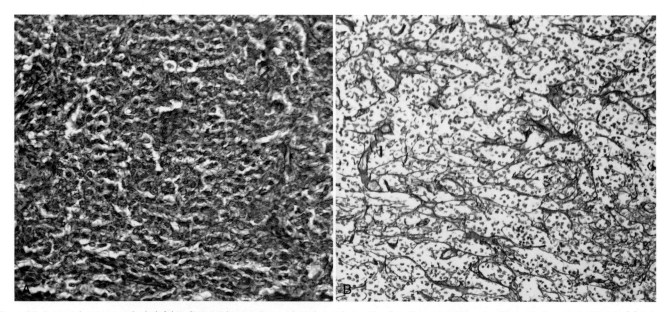

Figure 52–5 Special stains may be helpful in distinguishing malignant lymphoma from other "small round cell" tumors. The periodic acid–Schiff stain (*A*) helps to distinguish lymphoma from Ewing's sarcoma because lymphomas are negative and most Ewing's sarcomas are positive. Lymphomas may show more reticulin fibers (*B*, reticulin stain) than do Ewing's sarcomas.

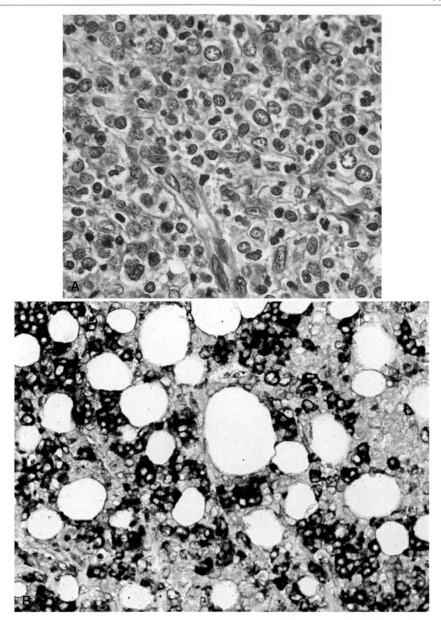

Figure 52–6 Other hematopoietic neoplasms may mimic the appearance of lymphoma. Granulocytic sarcoma is particularly notorious for resembling a lymphoma, as shown in *A*. Special stain may be helpful in differentiating such cases from lymphoma. Myeloperoxidase immunostain (*B*) is positive in granulocytic sarcomas and negative in lymphomas.

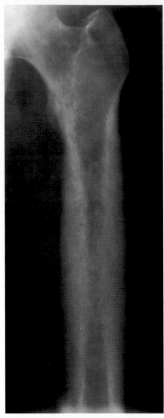

Figure 52–7 This radiograph shows an extensive diaphyseal lymphoma of the femur with poor margination and cortical thickening.

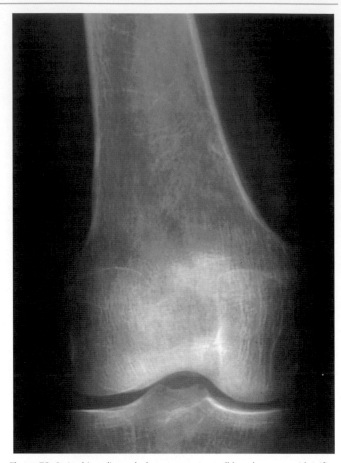

Figure 52–9 As this radiograph demonstrates, not all lymphomas are identifiable with plain radiography. This patient had a tumor involving the distal femur.

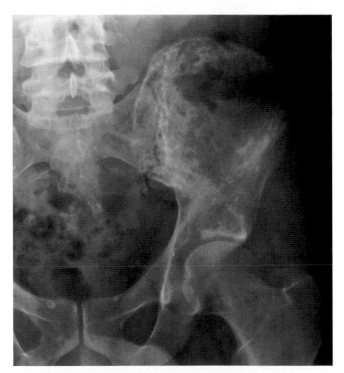

Figure 52–8 Although many lymphomas of bone show a lytic pattern radiographically, mixed lytic and sclerotic lesions, as in this tumor of the ilium, are common. The irregular, permeative pattern of growth of the tumor also favors the radiographic appearance of a malignant process.

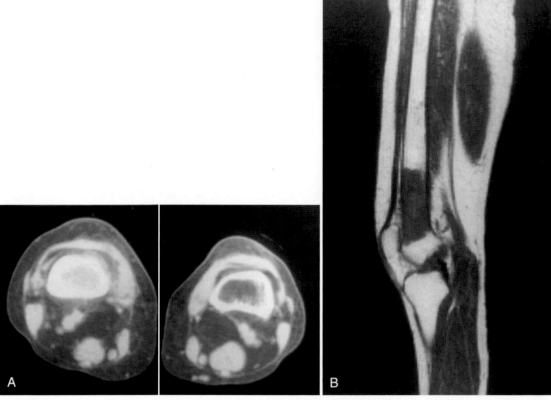

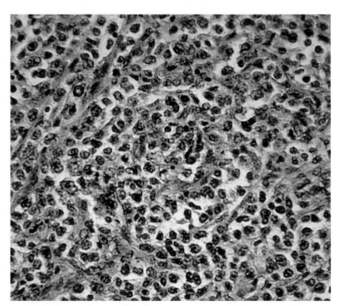

Figure 52–10 *A* and *B:* A computed tomographic (CT) scan of the distal femur seen in Figure 52–9 shows an intramedullary lymphoma. The radiographic density of the marrow in the right femur is greater than in the uninvolved left femur. Magnetic resonance imaging (MRI) may also be helpful in such cases. *B:* The longitudinal extent of the lymphoma appears as a low-signal (black) area as compared with the normal marrow (white) in this sagittal reconstruction.

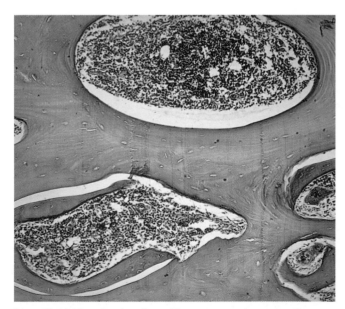

Figure 52–11 The sclerotic radiographic appearance of some lymphomas results from the sclerotic reaction induced by the tumor. Such bony sclerosis is illustrated in this low-power photomicrograph of a calvarial lymphoma showing a permeative pattern of growth.

Figure 52–12 At higher magnification, lymphomas generally are seen to be composed of a pleomorphic discohesive infiltrate, as is the case with this femoral tumor.

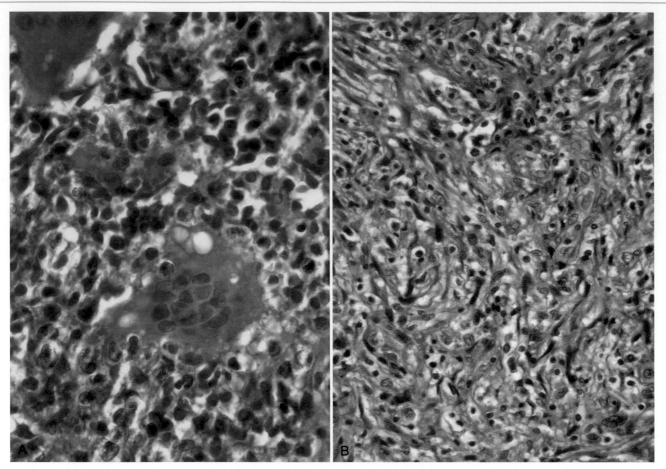

Figure 52–13 Malignant lymphoma can mimic other primary sarcomas of bone. The presence of multinucleated giant cells in a lymphoma is shown (*A*). The "histiocytic" appearance of the large cells in lymphoma and the presence of multinucleated giant cells may suggest the diagnosis of malignant fibrous histiocytoma. Although spindling of the cells is rare in lymphoma, such change may rarely be seen in osseous lymphomas (*B*) and may mimic histologically the appearance of a primary sarcoma.

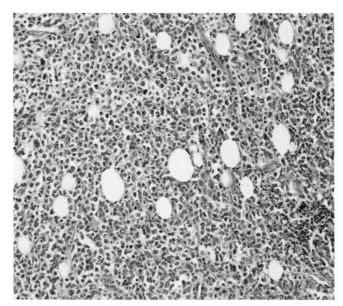

Figure 52–14 At low magnification, malignant lymphoma tends to grow in a permeative pattern that leaves behind parts of the normal architecture. The normal elements left may be bony trabeculae or fatty marrow elements, as this photomicrograph shows.

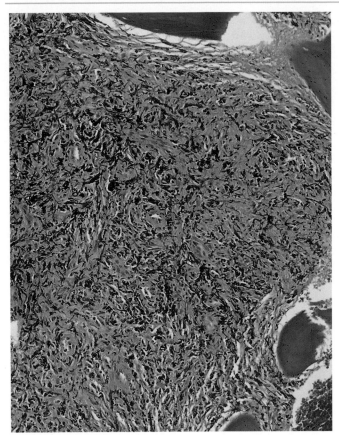

Figure 52–15 Primary lymphomas of bone may show marked crush artifact, as illustrated in this photomicrograph. Such crush artifact may be the first histologic clue that the tumor is a primary osseous lymphoma.

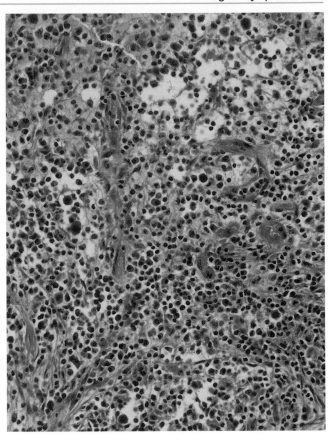

Figure 52–16 A mixed population of lymphocytes, plasma cells, and eosinophils may be appreciated at low magnification in cases of primary Hodgkin's lymphoma of bone. Careful search for Reed-Sternberg cells is essential in such cases. This photomicrograph illustrates an example of Hodgkin's lymphoma of the ilium.

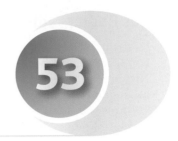

Myeloma

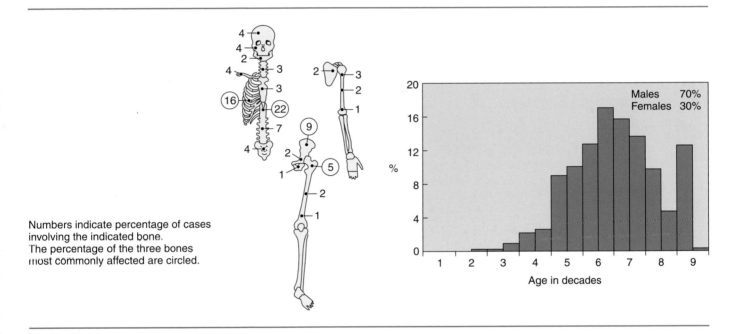

Numbers indicate percentage of cases
involving the indicated bone.
The percentage of the three bones
most commonly affected are circled.

Clinical Signs

1. Local pain and tenderness are common on physical examination.
2. A palpable mass may be found that is the result of extraosseous extension of the tumor or hemorrhage related to it.
3. Peripheral neuropathy may be detected in some patients.
4. Hypercalcemia occurs in fewer than 50% of patients.
5. Hypergammaglobulinemia may manifest itself as rouleaux formation appreciable on peripheral blood smear.
6. Serum electrophoresis and immunoelectrophoresis generally reveal a monoclonal gammopathy, but nonsecretory myelomas rarely occur.

Clinical Symptoms

1. Pain is the most frequent complaint at the time of diagnosis.
2. The duration of the pain is usually less than 6 months.
3. Constitutional symptoms of weakness and weight loss are almost uniformly present.
4. Pathologic fracture results in a sudden onset of pain in many patients.
5. Peripheral neuropathy may be present, particularly in osteosclerotic myeloma.
6. A tendency toward bleeding and fever may also be experienced.

Major Radiographic Features

1. Multiple small, discrete lesions involving one or several bones are identifiable.
2. The tumor occasionally may present as a solitary osseous lesion.
3. The lesion is purely lytic.
4. The surrounding bone does not show a sclerotic reaction, nor is there periosteal reaction.
5. Endosteal scalloping may be identified.
6. Expansion of the affected bone and an associated soft tissue mass are common.
7. Whole-body magnetic resonance imaging and positron emission tomography scanning permit evaluation of the entire skeleton and afford more accurate depiction of lesions than radiographic skeletal surveys.

Radiographic Differential Diagnosis

1. Metastatic carcinoma.
2. Malignant lymphoma.
3. Fibrosarcoma.

Major Pathologic Features

Gross

1. The tumor tissue is generally soft and friable.
2. The color of the tissue varies from reddish to gray–white and grossly may appear similar to that of malignant lymphoma.
3. Extension into soft tissue may be discovered at the time of biopsy.

Microscopic

1. At low magnification, the pattern is that of a cellular tumor lacking production of matrix.
2. The amount of cytoplasm on the cells varies but generally is abundant.
3. At higher magnification, the nuclei generally are eccentrically placed in the cytoplasm and show a clumped chromatin pattern.
4. A cytoplasmic clearing adjacent to the nucleus (perinuclear hof) is frequently discernible.
5. Amyloid may be present as large masses of amorphous eosinophilic material. In such cases, a foreign body giant cell reaction may be elicited by the amyloid.
6. Mitotic activity is generally not brisk.

Pathologic Differential Diagnosis

Benign lesions

1. Chronic osteomyelitis.

Malignant lesions

1. Malignant lymphoma.

Treatment

1. **Primary modality:** The mainstay of treatment is chemotherapy. Radiation therapy is effective in controlling localized lesions that are causing disabling pain or limitation of activity. The patient with solitary myeloma requires high-dose radiation for control of the disease.
2. **Other possible approaches:** Surgical intervention with internal fixation of impending or actual pathologic fractures may be needed. Decompressive laminectomy may be indicated in patients with compressive myelopathy, and spinal stabilization is occasionally warranted.

References

Bataille R, Sany J: Solitary myeloma: clinical and prognostic features of a review of 114 cases. *Cancer* 48(3):845–851, 1981.

Chong ST, Beasley HS, Daffner RH: POEMS syndrome: radiographic appearance with MRI correlation. *Skeletal Radiol* 35(9):690–695, 2006.

Dimopoulos MA, Moulopoulos LA, Maniatis A, et al: Solitary plasmacytoma of bone and asymptomatic multiple myeloma. *Blood* 96(6):2037–2044, 2000.

Frassica FJ, Beabout JW, Unni KK, et al: Myeloma of bone. *Orthopedics* 8(9):1184–1186, 1985.

Haferlach T, Loffler H: Prognostic factors in multiple myeloma: practicability for clinical practice and future perspectives. *Leukemia* 11 (Suppl 5):S5–S9, 1997.

Kelly JJ Jr, Kyle RA, Miles JM, et al: Osteosclerotic myeloma and peripheral neuropathy. *Neurology* 33(2):202–210, 1983.

Kyle RA: Multiple myeloma: review of 869 cases. *Mayo Clin Proc* 50(1):29–40, 1975.

Kyle RA: Long-term survival in multiple myeloma. *N Engl J Med* 308(6):314–316, 1983.

Kyle RA, Elveback LR: Management and prognosis of multiple myeloma. *Mayo Clin Proc* 51(12):751–760, 1976.

Ludwig H, Meran J, Zojer N: Multiple myeloma: an update on biology and treatment. *Ann Oncol* 10 (Suppl 6):31–43, 1999.

Mulligan ME, Badros AZ: PET/CT and MR imaging in myeloma. *Skeletal Radiol* 36(1):5–16, 2007.

Rajkumar SV, Greipp PR: Prognostic factors in multiple myeloma. *Hematol Oncol Clin North Am* 13(6):1295–1314, xi, 1999.

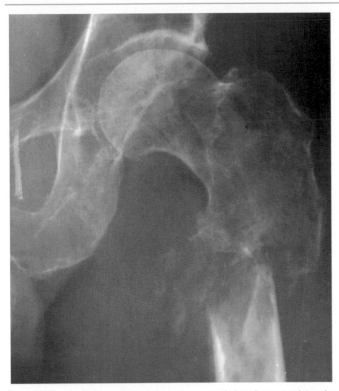

Figure 53–1 This radiograph illustrates a large, purely lytic lesion involving the proximal femur. The tumor has expanded the femur, resulting in pathologic fracture. The underlying process is myeloma.

Figure 53–3 At low magnification, myeloma is a tumor that is uniform in appearance. The tumor is composed of round cells without any evidence of stromal proliferation.

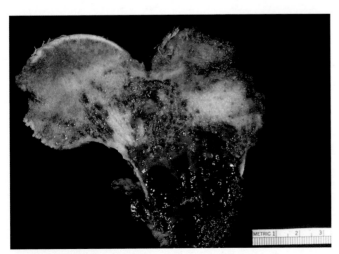

Figure 53–2 The gross pathologic features in this case correlate well with its radiographic features in Figure 53–1. Grossly, myeloma is a soft, fish flesh–like lesion, as shown here. Hemorrhage is commonly seen; in this case it is the result of the pathologic fracture that necessitated resection of the proximal femur.

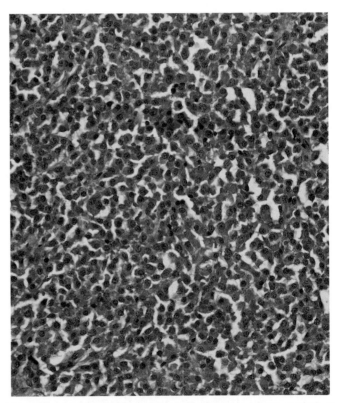

Figure 53–4 In contrast with most cases of malignant lymphoma, myeloma is generally composed of a homogeneous population of cells. This case illustrates such a proliferation of uniform cells.

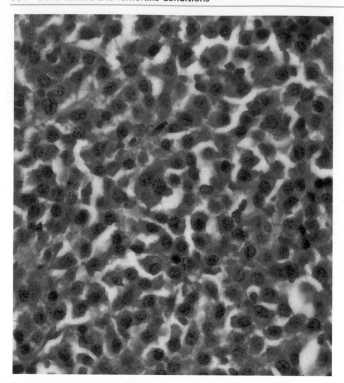

Figure 53–5 At high magnification, the proliferating plasma cells show abundant cytoplasm and an eccentrically located nucleus. Well-differentiated myelomas have cytologic features that deviate minimally from benign plasma cells; in such cases, chronic osteomyelitis may be included in the histologic differential diagnosis.

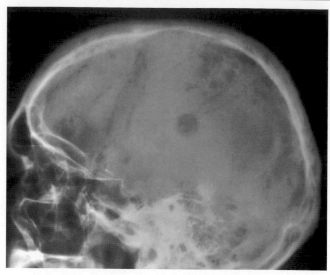

Figure 53–7 Multiple discrete lytic calvarial lesions, seen in this radiograph, are the hallmark of multiple myeloma.

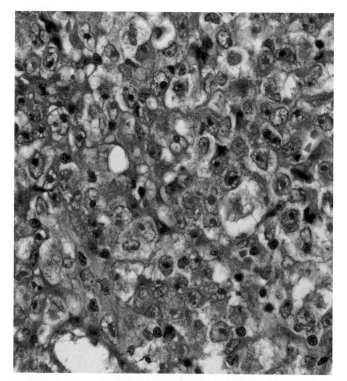

Figure 53–6 Some myelomas show significantly greater nuclear pleomorphism. In such cases, the differential diagnosis includes immunoblastic lymphoma. However, some evidence of plasmacytic differentiation, as illustrated in this case, usually is seen.

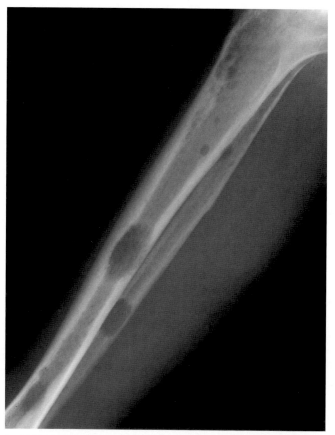

Figure 53–8 The long bone lesions of multiple myeloma show the same general radiographic features as lesions of flat bones, as in this radiograph illustrating tibial and fibular involvement.

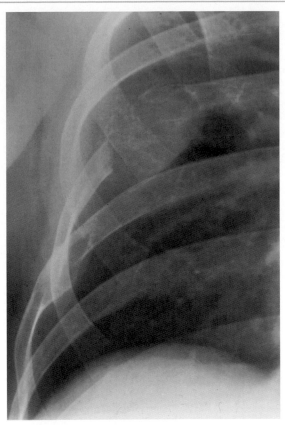

Figure 53–9 When myeloma involves the flat bone, a soft tissue mass may be evident, as in this example of myeloma involving two ribs.

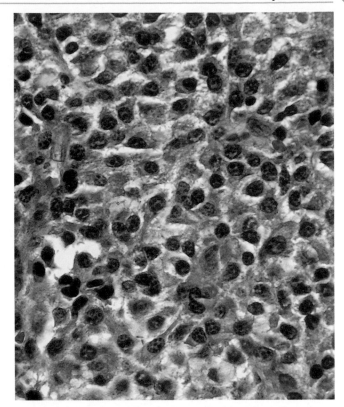

Figure 53–11 At high magnification, the nuclei of myeloma cells are eccentrically placed and lie within abundant cytoplasm. A perinuclear clearing is frequently evident in the cytoplasm, as this photomicrograph illustrates.

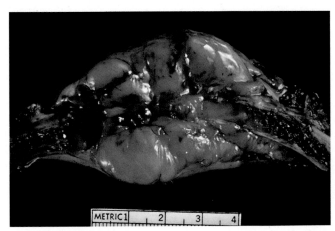

Figure 53–10 The gross appearance of myeloma is similar to that of malignant lymphoma, as in this case involving the rib. Extension of the tumor into the soft tissues, as seen in Figure 53–9, is present.

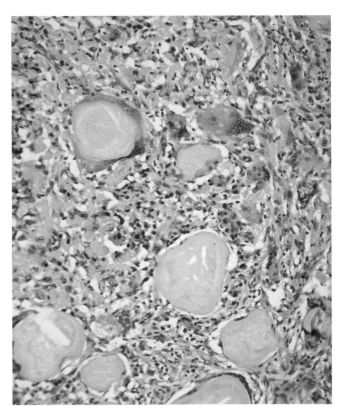

Figure 53–12 Amyloid may be formed in cases of myeloma. Such deposits of amyloid may result in a foreign body type of giant cell reaction, as shown in this photomicrograph.

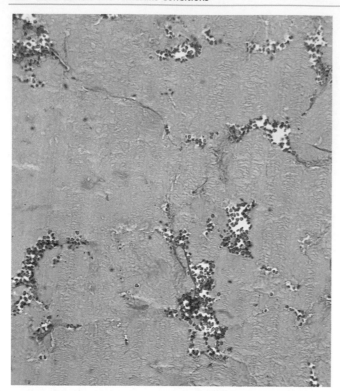

Figure 53–13 In some cases of myeloma, amyloid formation may be so prominent as to overwhelm the plasmacytic proliferation. Such is the case in this tumor involving the fourth thoracic vertebra.

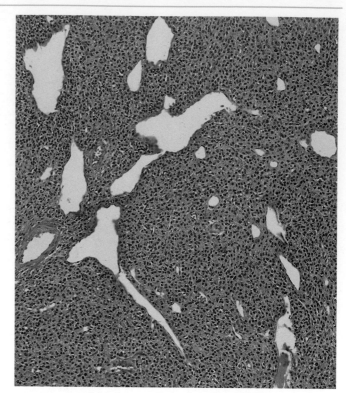

Figure 53–15 Some myelomas may show a prominent vascular pattern, as in this example from a rib lesion. Such tumors may be confused with hemangiopericytomas on initial low-power histologic evaluation.

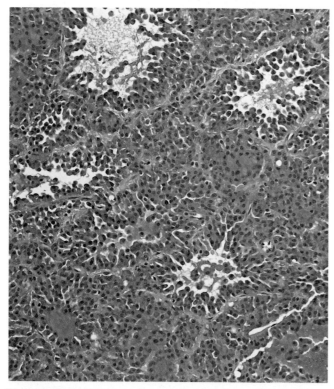

Figure 53–14 Myeloma grows in a noncohesive manner, and, in some cases, the resulting pattern may even resemble gland formation, as in metastatic adenocarcinoma. This case of myeloma shows such a pseudogland histologic pattern of growth.

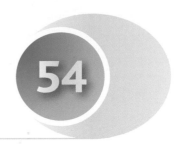

Mastocytosis (Mast Cell Disease)

Clinical Signs

1. The pigmented rash urticates when rubbed (urticaria pigmentosa).
2. Hepatosplenomegaly may be found on physical examination.

Clinical Symptoms

1. Pigmented skin rash may be the patient's presenting complaint (urticaria pigmentosa).
2. Abdominal fullness may be experienced (hepatosplenomegaly).
3. Abdominal cramping and diarrhea may occur.
4. The lesion may be an incidental finding on radiography and is usually mistaken for metastatic carcinoma.

Major Radiographic Features

1. Skeletal involvement is most commonly diffuse; focal lesions are occasionally superimposed on diffuse disease, whereas focal lesions alone are unusual.
2. Diffuse osteopenia is the most common presentation, but diffuse sclerosis or mixed lysis and sclerosis are also seen.
3. Focal lesions are usually sclerotic or mixed.

Radiographic Differential Diagnosis

1. Osteoporosis.
2. Diffuse myeloma.
3. Lymphoma.

Major Pathologic Features

Gross

1. Lesional tissue may be too ossified to cut with frozen section.

Microscopic

1. At low magnification, the bone shows diffuse permeation of the medullary space by a uniform population of small, regular cells. The cells are usually concentrated around bony trabeculae and are associated with fibrosis.
2. The trabeculae may show sclerosis, with increased thickness and greater irregularity than normal.
3. At higher magnification, the cells are uniform, with a faintly granular cytoplasm.
4. The nuclei are regular, are round to oval, and have a finely stippled chromatin pattern.
5. The cells may show a tendency to spindle, and in some areas the proliferation exhibits a granuloma-like quality.
6. Eosinophils may form a prominent part of the infiltrate.
7. Special stains may be used to demonstrate the metachromatic granules within the cytoplasm of the mast cells

Pathologic Differential Diagnosis

Benign lesions

1. Histiocytosis X.
2. Granulomatous osteomyelitis.
3. Nonspecific reactive changes.

Malignant lesions

1. Hairy cell leukemia.
2. Malignant lymphoma.
3. Metastatic breast carcinoma.

Treatment

1. **Primary modality:** depends on the extent of disease. In children with limited disease, the prognosis is good. In patients with skeletal involvement, the prognosis is guarded but good. Rarely is there associated mast cell leukemia. Resection with a marginal or wide surgical margin is applicable in cases with limited disease.
2. **Other possible approaches:** chemotherapy.

References

Bain BJ: Systemic mastocytosis and other mast cell neoplasms. *Br J Haematol* 106(1):9–17, 1999.

Barer M, Peterson LFA, Dahlin DC, et al: Mastocytosis with osseous lesions resembling metastatic malignant lesions in bone. *J Bone Joint Surg Am* 50(1):142–152, 1968.

Havard CWH, Scott RB: Urticaria pigmentosa with visceral and skeletal lesions. *Q J Med* 28:459–470, 1959.

Horny HP, Ruck P, Krober S, et al: Systemic mast cell disease (mastocytosis). General aspects and histopathological diagnosis. *Histol Histopathol* 12(4):1081–1089, 1997.

Webb TA, Li CY, Yam LT: Systemic mast cell disease: a clinical and hematopathologic study of 26 cases. *Cancer* 49(5):927–938, 1982.

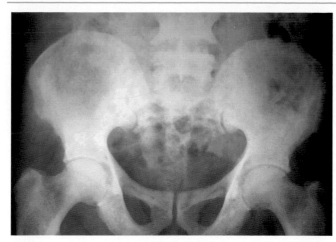

Figure 54–1 Mastocytosis may produce multifocal sclerosing lesions, as in this case involving the pelvic bones. Such lesions are commonly mistaken for metastatic osteoblastic carcinoma.

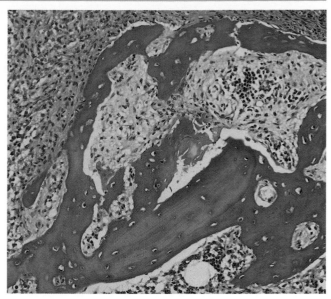

Figure 54–3 At low magnification, the marrow space may show diffuse replacement in cases of mastocytosis. Even at this level of magnification, the uniform cytologic features of the infiltrate are evident.

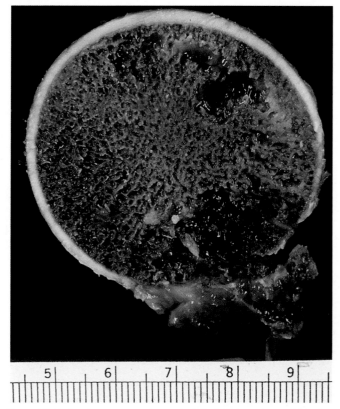

Figure 54–2 Grossly, mastocytosis may be relatively inapparent. Although this femoral head showed diffuse involvement microscopically, only some thickening of the bony trabeculae was grossly evident.

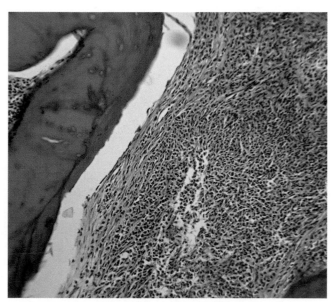

Figure 54–4 Fibrosis of the marrow space and bony sclerosis, evident in this case of mastocytosis involving the ilium, may also be seen.

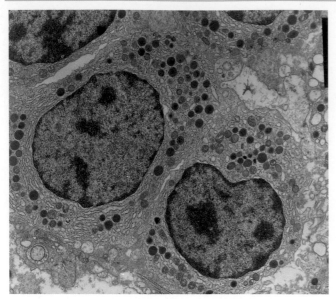

Figure 54–5 Ultrastructurally, mastocytosis is characterized by large cytoplasmic granules, as illustrated in this sample of a lesion involving the femoral head.

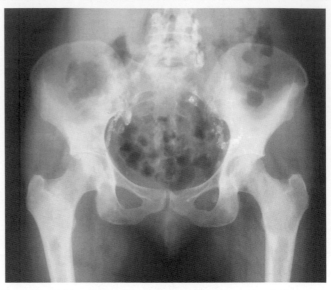

Figure 54–7 This radiograph illustrates the diffuse bony sclerosis that may be seen in mastocytosis.

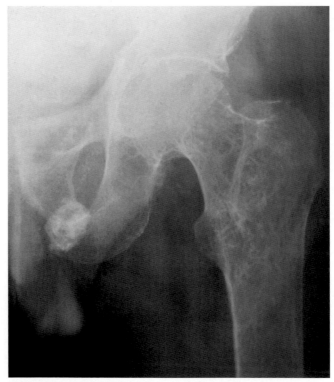

Figure 54–6 This radiograph shows a case of mastocytosis with diffuse skeletal demineralization and fracture of the pubic ramus.

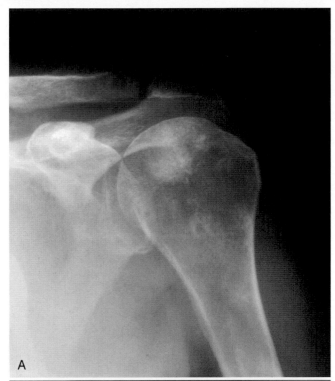

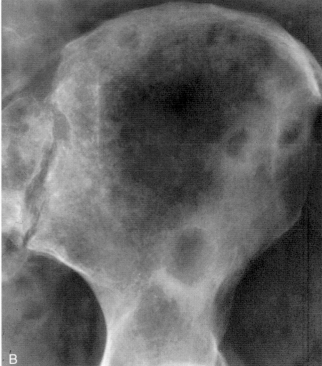

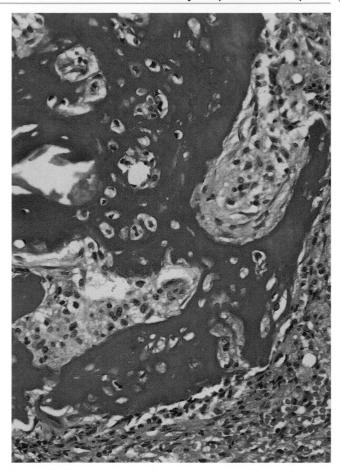

Figure 54–9 Bony sclerosis is commonly seen in mast cell disease, both radiographically and histologically, as shown in this photomicrograph.

Figure 54–8 These radiographs show the shoulder (*A*) and pelvis (*B*) of a patient with mastocytosis. Some of the focal lesions are sclerotic; others are lytic, with surrounding sclerosis.

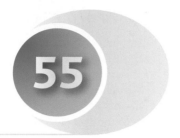

Langerhans' Cell Histiocytosis (Histiocytosis X)

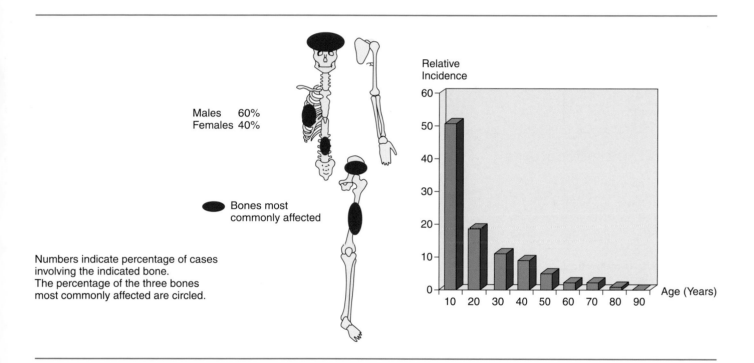

Males 60%
Females 40%

● Bones most
commonly affected

Numbers indicate percentage of cases
involving the indicated bone.
The percentage of the three bones
most commonly affected are circled.

Relative
Incidence

Age (Years)

Clinical Signs

1. A mass may be palpable on physical examination.
2. Cutaneous seborrhea-like lesions may be identified, indicating skin involvement.
3. Hearing loss or decreased balance may indicate involvement of the mastoid region.
4. Marked tenderness in the region of the affected bone may be found on physical examination.

Clinical Symptoms

1. Pain is the most frequent presenting complaint.

2. A swelling may also be noted in the region of the bone involved.
3. Only rarely will the lesion be discovered incidentally on radiographic examination.
4. Protean clinical symptoms are seen in multisystem disease (e.g., Hand-Schüller-Christian or Letterer-Siwe variants).
5. The patient may present with otorrhea.
6. Loose teeth may be the presenting complaint in patients with maxillary or mandibular involvement.
7. Excessive thirst may be a manifestation of associated central nervous system disease.

373

Major Imaging Features

1. The radiographic appearance is highly variable; lesions tend to occur in flat bones, especially the calvarium.
2. Lesions range from solitary to innumerable.
3. Most lesions are lytic, with well-defined margins.
4. Expansion, solid periosteal new bone formation, and surrounding sclerosis may occur.
5. Lesions are often medullary and have an irregular or scalloped margin.
6. Many lesions have a double contour.
7. Spine involvement usually affects the vertebral body and results in uniform compression.
8. Other favored sites include the ribs, the clavicle, the neck of the scapula, and the supra-acetabular iliac bone.
9. Extensive marrow and soft tissue edema with periostitis may be encountered, producing a misleading appearance.

Radiographic Differential Diagnosis

1. Osteomyelitis.
2. Primary osseous malignancies.
3. Metastases.

Major Pathologic Features

Gross

1. Lesional tissue is usually soft and may be "runny."
2. The tissue color varies from gray–tan to pale red or yellow. The eosinophils may impart a greenish hue to the lesional tissue.
3. Pathologic fracture may be identified in resected specimens.

Microscopic

1. At low magnification, the lesional tissue is arranged in a loose fashion. Necrosis is common.
2. The lesion is polymorphous, being composed of a variety of inflammatory cells including polymorphonuclear leukocytes, lymphocytes, plasma cells, multinucleated giant cells, and the characteristic Langerhans' cell histiocytes.
3. The Langerhans' cells are arranged in relatively solid sheets or clusters.
4. At higher magnification, the characteristic cytologic features of the Langerhans' cell include the following:
   a. An indented or folded nucleus.
   b. A crisp nuclear membrane.
   c. A finely stippled chromatin pattern.
   d. Small, inconspicuous nucleoli.
   e. Abundant pale eosinophilic cytoplasm.
5. Eosinophils may be abundant; they may be clustered into small eosinophilic "abscesses."
6. Mitotic activity may be focally brisk.

Pathologic Differential Diagnosis

Benign lesions

1. Osteomyelitis.
2. Erdheim-Chester disease.

Malignant lesions

1. Malignant lymphoma.
2. Malignant fibrous histiocytoma, inflammatory variant.

Treatment

1. **Primary modality:** When surgically accessible, a simple solitary lesion compromising the structural integrity of the bone is managed by curettage and bone grafting. Solitary lesions may be observed and treated with steroid injection or low-dose radiation, depending on the clinical setting.
2. **Other possible approaches:** With multiple lesions, a period of observation for patients with asymptomatic lesions may permit spontaneous healing. Direct injection of methylprednisolone acetate into the lesion has produced encouraging results. For Hand-Schüller-Christian disease and Letterer-Siwe disease, corticosteroids and chemotherapy may be used.

References

Arico M, Egeler RM: Clinical aspects of Langerhans cell histiocytosis. *Hematol Oncol Clin North Am* 12(2):247–258, 1998.

Beltran J, Aparisi F, Bonmati LM, et al: Eosinophilic granuloma: MRI manifestations. *Skeletal Radiol* 22(3):157–161, 1993.

Broadbent V, Gadner H: Current therapy for Langerhans' cell histiocytosis. *Hematol Oncol Clin North Am* 12(2):327–338, 1998.

Enriquez P, Dahlin DC, Hayles AB, et al: Histiocytosis X: a clinical study. *Mayo Clin Proc* 42(2):88–99, 1967.

Garg S, Mehta S, Dormans JP: Langerhans cell histiocytosis of the spine in children. Long-term follow-up. *J Bone Joint Surg Am* 86-A(8):1740–1750, 2004.

Herzog KM, Tubbs RR: Langerhans cell histiocytosis. *Adv Anat Pathol* 5(6):347–358, 1998.

Kilpatrick SE, Wenger DE, Gilchrist GS, et al: Langerhans' cell histiocytosis (histiocytosis X) of bone. A clinicopathologic analysis of 263 pediatric and adult cases. *Cancer* 76(12):2471–2484, 1995.

Stull MA, Kransdorf MJ, Devaney KO: Langerhans cell histiocytosis of bone. *Radiographics* 12(4):801–823, 1992.

Vassallo R, Ryu JH, Colby TV, et al: Pulmonary Langerhans' cell histiocytosis. *N Engl J Med* 342(26):1969–1978, 2000.

Wester SM, Beabout JW, Unni KK, et al: Langerhans' cell granulomatosis (histiocytosis X) of bone in adults. *Am J Surg Pathol* 6(5):413–426, 1982.

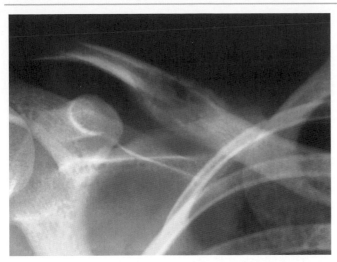

Figure 55–1 This radiograph shows an example of Langerhans' cell histiocytosis of the clavicle. The lesion is poorly marginated, and associated new bone formation is present. A similar appearance could be caused by Ewing's sarcoma or osteomyelitis.

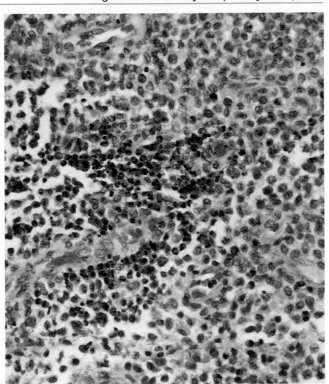

Figure 55–3 At low magnification, Langerhans' cell histiocytosis is a lesion composed of multiple cell types. Eosinophils may be prominent, as in this case, or sparse. In this lesion, the loose nature of the process is evident and an eosinophilic "abscess" is present.

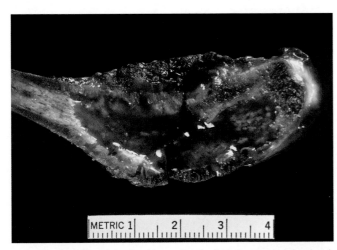

Figure 55–2 Another example of Langerhans' cell histiocytosis of the clavicle demonstrates the gross pathologic features of the condition. The lesional tissue may be loose and runny. Lesions that extend beyond the cortex, as shown here, may simulate the appearance of a malignant neoplasm radiographically.

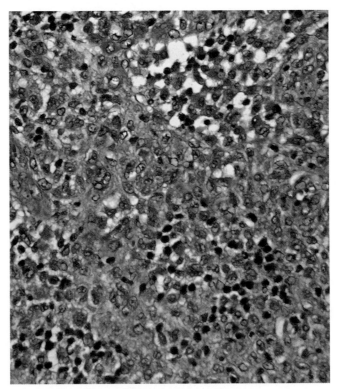

Figure 55–4 At higher magnification, the polymorphous nature of the process is evident. The Langerhans' cell–type histiocytes have abundant cytoplasm and a coffee bean–shaped nucleus. Lymphocytes, plasma cells, and polymorphonuclear leukocytes are scattered throughout the lesional tissue.

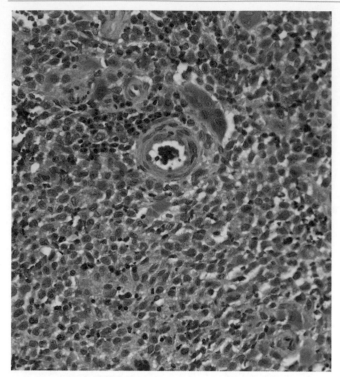

Figure 55–5 Multinucleated giant cells, as shown in this photomicrograph, may be seen in Langerhans' cell histiocytosis. Mitotic activity may be fairly brisk, but this feature does not appear to correlate with the clinical course of the disease.

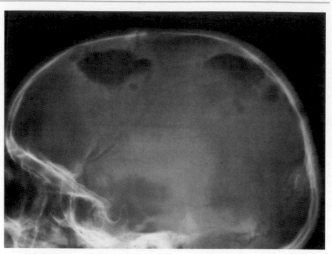

Figure 55–7 This radiograph shows multiple calvarial lesions, most of which are serpiginous with sharp margination. This is one of the radiographic appearances of Langerhans' cell histiocytosis.

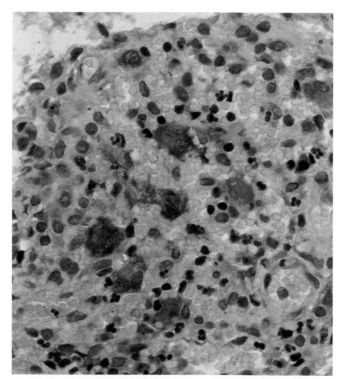

Figure 55–6 Immunohistochemical techniques may be helpful in substantiating the diagnosis of Langerhans' cell histiocytosis. The polymorphous nature of the infiltrate frequently raises consideration of the differential diagnosis of chronic osteomyelitis. In such cases, immunostains for S-100 protein and CDIa may be helpful in identifying the characteristic Langerhans' cells of Langerhans' cell histiocytosis.

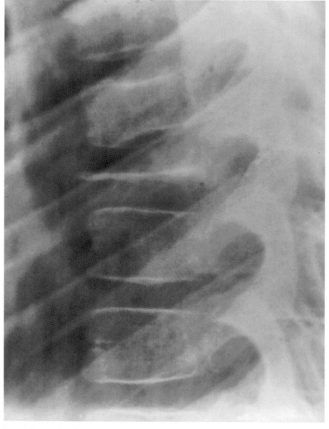

Figure 55–8 Uniform compression of a thoracic vertebra is shown in this radiograph. This condition, termed "vertebra plana," is another presentation of Langerhans' cell histiocytosis.

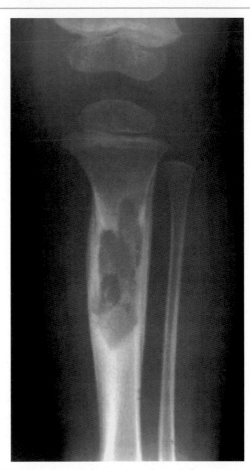

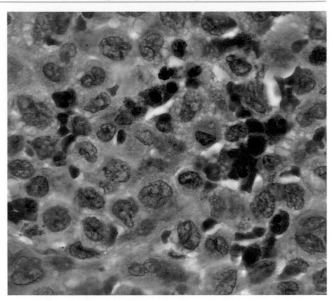

Figure 55–11 At high magnification, the cytologic features of the nuclei of the Langerhans' cells are identifiable. The nucleus is oval or bean-shaped and has a characteristic longitudinal groove if viewed en face.

Figure 55–9 This radiograph demonstrates the typical appearance of Langerhans' cell histiocytosis involving the tibial diaphysis. The medullary lesion has a serpiginous margin that is well defined. The "hole within a hole" appearance and the thick, solid periosteal new bone formation are also characteristic.

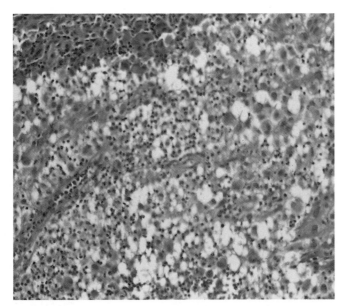

Figure 55–10 At low magnification, lesional tissue in Langerhans' cell histiocytosis often has a loose, edematous appearance, as in this case of an L4 vertebral lesion.

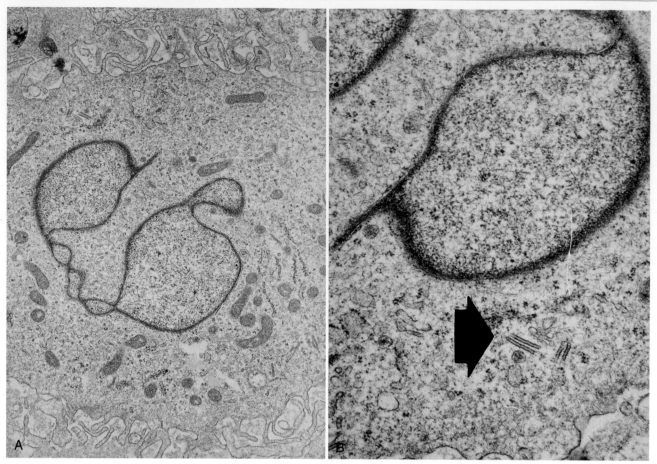

Figure 55–12 Ultrastructural investigation can help in identifying the characteristic features of Langerhans' cell histiocytosis. The lobulated nucleus is identifiable (A), but the feature that is diagnostic of the condition is the presence of the characteristic granules (arrow; B).

Section 2E: Vascular Tumors

Hemangioma

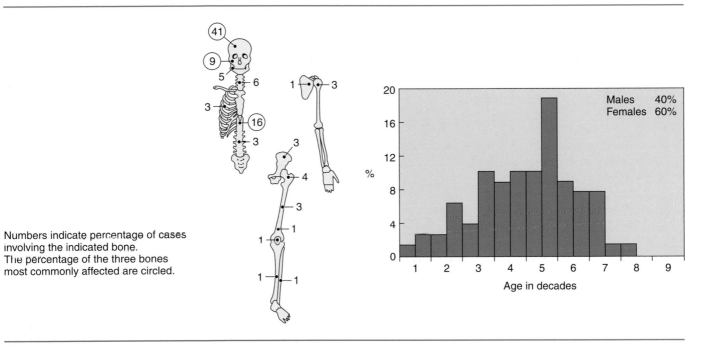

Numbers indicate percentage of cases involving the indicated bone.
The percentage of the three bones most commonly affected are circled.

Males 40%
Females 60%

% — Age in decades

Clinical Signs

1. Local pain and swelling are frequently seen in cases involving the skull and ribs.
2. Vertebral lesions may result in a compression fracture and resultant neurologic signs.
3. Severe hemorrhage may be encountered at the time of surgery.

Clinical Symptoms

1. The majority of hemangiomas are incidental findings on radiography.

2. Swelling is frequently noted and is related to expansion of the affected bone. This is particularly true of lesions involving the skull.
3. Local pain is a less common complaint.
4. Spinal lesions may produce spinal cord compression.

Major Imaging Features

1. In the calvarium the features are as follows:
   a. The lesion is small and oval with sharp margins.
   b. The lesion has a sunburst or granular appearance.
   c. Fifteen percent are multicentric.

2. In the spine the features are as follows:
   a. The lesion has a "corduroy" or honeycomb appearance.
   b. The lesion has a polka-dot appearance on computed tomography scan.
   c. The lesion may have a soft tissue mass or an associated pathologic fracture.
3. In the long bones there is no specific appearance.
4. Magnetic resonance imaging of the spine shows the lesion to have foci of high signal on T1 that gets brighter on T2 fat-saturated sequences.

Radiographic Differential Diagnosis

1. For calvarial lesions:
   a. Langerhans' cell histiocytosis.
   b. Epidermoid cyst.
2. For vertebral lesions:
   a. Paget's disease.
   b. Metastatic carcinoma.
3. For long bone lesions:
   a. Angiosarcoma.
   b. Other sarcomas.

Major Pathologic Features

Gross

1. Grossly, these lesions are soft, friable, red, and bloody.
2. Tumors may be more firm and fleshy if they are capillary in type.
3. Bony trabeculae coursing through the tumor may be grossly evident and are the counterpart of the "sunburst" seen radiographically in some cases.

Microscopic

1. At low magnification, these lesions may show large, cavernous vascular spaces or small capillary-type vascular spaces.
2. The vascular nature is evident at low magnification, with the vascular spaces being lined by a thin, attenuated endothelial lining.
3. At higher magnification, the endothelial cells are inconspicuous, as are their nuclei, which are small and dark.

Pathologic Differential Diagnosis

Benign lesions

1. Disappearing bone disease.
2. Lymphangioma.

Malignant lesions

1. Angiosarcoma.
2. Adamantinoma.

Treatment

1. **Primary modality:** Observation is recommended for the usual lesion with an asymptomatic presentation. Curettage and grafting are used for the symptomatic lesion.
2. **Other possible approaches:** The symptomatic spinal lesion is treated with radiation therapy, with a dose of 3000 to 4000 rads. Surgical treatment with laminectomy is reserved for patients with spinal cord compression. Spinal angiography is helpful in these instances.

References

Asch MJ, Cohen AH, Moore TC: Hepatic and splenic lymphangiomatosis with skeletal involvement: report of a case and review of the literature. *Surgery* 76(2):334–339, 1974.

Dorfman HD, Steiner GC, Jaffe JL: Vascular tumors of bone. *Hum Pathol* 2(3):349–376, 1971.

Karlin CA, Brower AC: Multiple primary hemangiomas of bone. *Am J Roentgenol* 129(1):162–164, 1977.

Keel SB, Rosenberg AE: Hemorrhagic epithelioid and spindle cell hemangioma: a newly recognized, unique vascular tumor of bone. *Cancer* 85(9):1966–1972, 1999.

Kleer CG, Unni KK, McLeod RA: Epithelioid hemangioendothelioma of bone. *Am J Surg Pathol* 20(11):1301–1311, 1996.

Tillman RM, Choong PF, Beabout JW, et al: Epithelioid hemangioendothelioma of bone. *Orthopedics* 20(2):177–180, 1997.

Unni KK, Ivins JC, Beabout JW, et al: Hemangioma, hemangiopericytoma, and hemangioendothelioma (angiosarcoma) of bone. *Cancer* 27(6):1403–1414, 1971.

Wenger DE, Wold LE: Benign vascular lesions of bone: radiologic and pathologic features. *Skeletal Radiol* 29(2):63–74, 2000.

Wold LE, Swee RG, Sim FH: Vascular lesions of bone. *Pathol Annu* 20 Pt 2:101–137, 1985.

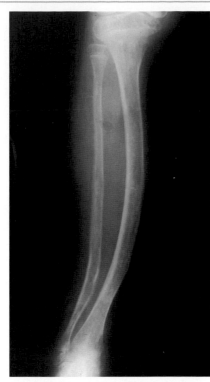

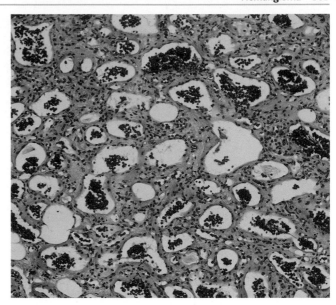

Figure 56–3 At low magnification, hemangiomas may show large, dilated vascular spaces, as seen in this case. Such lesions are termed "cavernous hemangiomas." In other cases, small, capillary-like spaces may predominate; these lesions are termed "capillary hemangiomas."

Figure 56–1 This radiograph shows an extensive hemangioma of the lower leg involving the soft tissues and the tibia and fibula. The bones contain lytic areas and are attenuated and bowed.

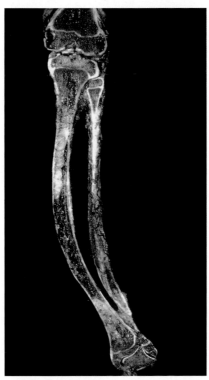

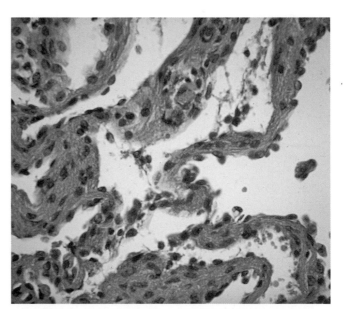

Figure 56–2 A gross specimen from the case shown in Figure 56–1 demonstrates the marked bowing of the tibia and fibula that was evident radiographically. Grossly, hemangiomas are red, hemorrhagic lesions that may bleed extensively at the time of biopsy.

Figure 56–4 At high magnification, the endothelial cells lining the vascular spaces are inconspicuous. This feature helps to distinguish hemangiomas from low-grade angiosarcoma. The nuclei of the endothelial cells in a hemangioma are dark-staining and are flattened adjacent to the vascular lumina.

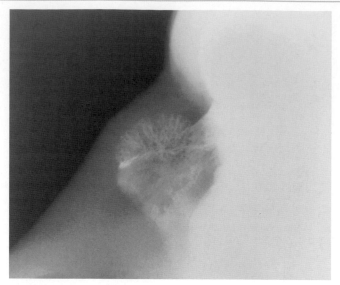

Figure 56–5 This radiograph illustrates the "sunburst" appearance of a hemangioma involving the nasal bones. This appearance is a result of the presence of radiating spicules of bone in the lesion.

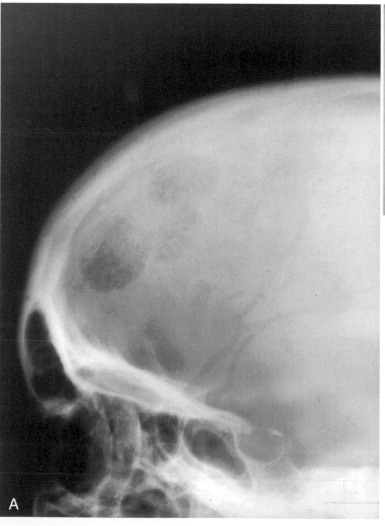

A

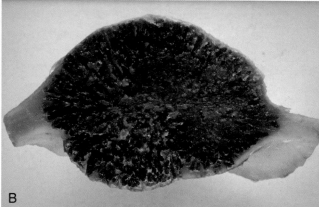

B

Figure 56–6 The calvarium is a common location for hemangiomas. *A*: This radiograph illustrates multicentric involvement showing three frontal bone lesions with sharp margination and a granular appearance. *B*: The gross appearance of such calvarial hemangiomas is shown. The radiating spicules of bone are visible traversing the lesion.

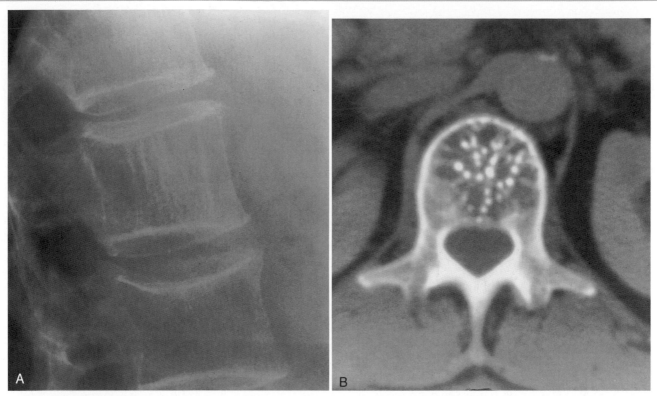

Figure 56–7 *A*: The coarse vertical trabecular appearance of a vertebral hemangioma results in the so-called corduroy vertebra. *B*: The computed tomographic (CT) cross-sectional appearance of a similar vertebral hemangioma is shown. In cross-section, the coarse trabeculae result in a polka-dot pattern.

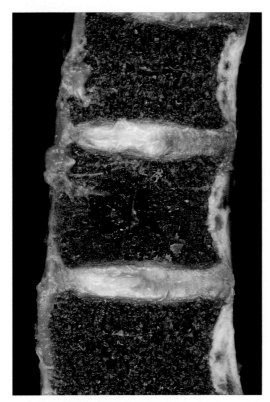

Figure 56–8 Grossly, hemangiomas of the vertebrae, shown in this photograph, are common findings during postmortem examination. Such lesions are small and generally clinically silent.

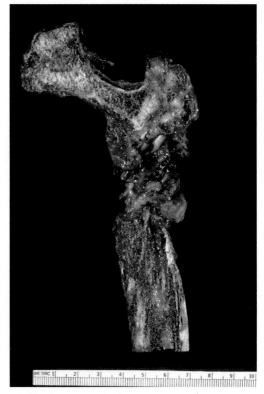

Figure 56–9 This gross specimen of the proximal femur exhibits the bony dissolution associated with phantom bone disease (massive osteolysis, Gorham's disease).

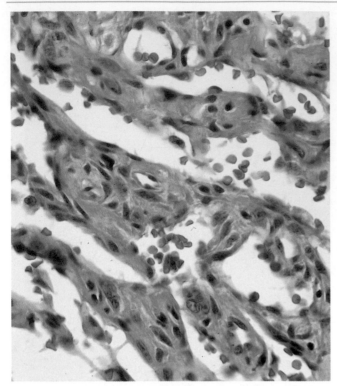

Figure 56–10 The histologic features of phantom bone disease are often indistinguishable from those of a hemangioma, as this femoral lesion demonstrates. The clinical history is often helpful in differentiating these two conditions.

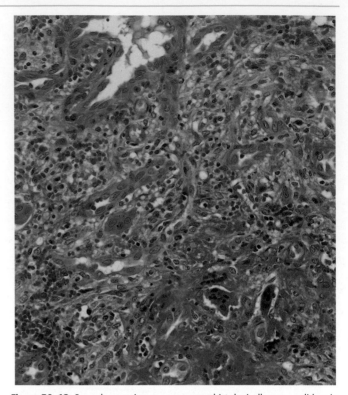

Figure 56–12 Some hemangiomas may appear histologically more solid, as in this example from the fibula. In addition, the endothelial cells of such tumors may become more plump, showing epithelioid cytologic features. Such tumors have been designated "epithelioid hemangiomas."

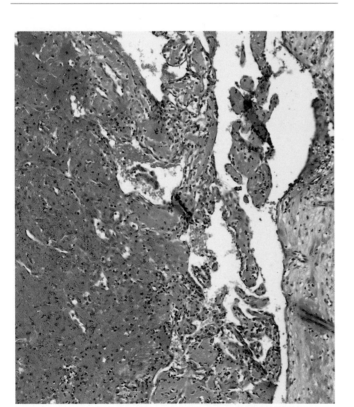

Figure 56–11 Other benign vascular processes may involve the bone and show a histologic pattern similar to that of a hemangioma. This photomicrograph shows an arteriovenous fistula with associated thrombus formation that resulted in a distal fibular defect.

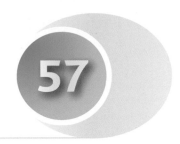

Hemangioendothelioma, Epithelioid Hemangioendothelioma, and Angiosarcoma

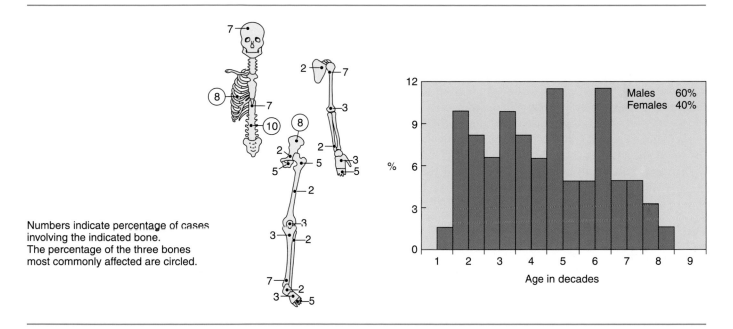

Numbers indicate percentage of cases involving the indicated bone.
The percentage of the three bones most commonly affected are circled.

Clinical Signs

1. Local tenderness may be the only finding on physical examination.

Clinical Symptoms

1. Pain is the usual clinical symptom.
2. Rarely, a mass may be noted if the lesion involves a superficial bone.

Major Radiographic Features

1. There is no specific radiographic appearance.
2. The most common pattern is that of a purely lytic lesion without periosteal reaction.

3. The radiographic appearance correlates with the histologic grade. High-grade lesions appear more permeative and destructive than do low-grade lesions.
4. Multifocal disease may be seen and, when present, frequently tends to cluster in one anatomic region.

Radiographic Differential Diagnosis

1. Osteosarcoma.
2. Fibrosarcoma.
3. Malignant fibrous histiocytoma.
4. Malignant lymphoma.
5. Metastatic carcinoma.
6. Hemangioma.

Major Pathologic Features

Gross

1. The lesional tissue is usually grossly red and bloody.
2. Tumors vary in consistency but are generally soft. Residual bony trabeculae may be present, particularly in low-grade lesions, giving the tumor a firmer consistency.
3. Necrotic tumor may be present but is most often seen in high-grade lesions.

Microscopic

1. The histologic features vary considerably in this group from low-grade tumors, which are obviously vasoformative, to high-grade, which may show areas of spindle cell proliferation without obvious vessel formation.
2. Low-grade tumors show plump endothelial cells lining vascular spaces. At higher magnification, the nuclei may appear histiocytoid or epithelioid. High-grade tumors show greater cytologic variation and mitotic activity and less histologic differentiation than their low-grade counterparts.
3. The radiographic appearance correlates with the histologic grade. High-grade lesions appear more permeative and destructive than do low-grade lesions.
4. Reticulin stains may be helpful in defining the vascular nature of the tumor by showing that the proliferating cells are clustered within a meshwork of reticulin fibers.
5. Immunohistochemical stains for endothelial and mesenchymal markers (e.g., Factor VIII–related antigen and vimentin) are variably positive.

Pathologic Differential Diagnosis

Benign lesions

1. Hemangioma.
2. Disappearing bone disease.

Malignant lesions

1. Metastatic carcinoma.
2. Fibrosarcoma.
3. Telangiectatic osteosarcoma.
4. Adamantinoma.

Treatment

1. **Primary modality:** Treatment is dependent on the grade of the lesion. Low-grade lesions that are unifocal may be treated with en bloc resection with a wide surgical margin. Low-grade multifocal lesions may be effectively treated with radiation therapy or amputation. High-grade lesions may be treated with either radiation therapy or ablative surgery, although some lesions are amenable to limb-saving resection.
2. **Other possible approaches:** Chemotherapy has been used with limited success in some cases of high-grade tumors.

References

Campanacci M, Boriani S, Giunti A: Hemangioendothelioma of bone: a study of 29 cases. *Cancer* 46(4):804–814, 1980.

Dorfman HD, Steiner GC, Jaffe HL: Vascular tumors of bone. *Hum Pathol* 2(3):349–376, 1971.

Evans HL, Raymond AK, Ayala AG: Vascular tumors of bone: A study of 17 cases other than ordinary hemangioma, with an evaluation of the relationship of hemangioendothelioma of bone to epithelioid hemangioma, epithelioid hemangioendothelioma, and high-grade angiosarcoma. *Hum Pathol* 34(7):680–689, 2003.

Garcia-Moral CA: Malignant hemangioendothelioma of bone: review of world literature and report of two cases. *Clin Orthop Relat Res* 82:70–79, 1972.

Kleer CG, Unni KK, McLeod RA: Epithelioid hemangioendothelioma of bone. *Am J Surg Pathol* 20(11):1301–1311, 1996.

Rosai J, Gold J, Landy R: The histiocytoid hemangiomas: a unifying concept embracing several previously described entities of skin, soft tissue, large vessels, bone, and heart. *Hum Pathol* 10(6):707–730, 1979.

Tillman RM, Choong PF, Beabout JW, et al: Epithelioid hemangioendothelioma of bone. *Orthopedics* 20(2):177–180, 1997.

Unni KK, Ivins JC, Beabout JW, et al: Hemangioma, hemangiopericytoma, and hemangioendothelioma (angiosarcoma) of bone. *Cancer* 27(6):1403–1414, 1971.

Volpe R, Mazabraud A: Hemangioendothelioma (angiosarcoma) of bone: a distinct pathologic entity with an unpredictable course. *Cancer* 49(4):727–736, 1981.

Weiss SW, Enzinger FM: Epithelioid hemangioendothelioma: a vascular tumor often mistaken for a carcinoma. *Cancer* 50(5):970–981, 1982.

Wold LE, Unni KK, Beabout JW, et al: Hemangioendothelial sarcoma of bone. *Am J Surg Pathol* 6(1):59–70, 1982.

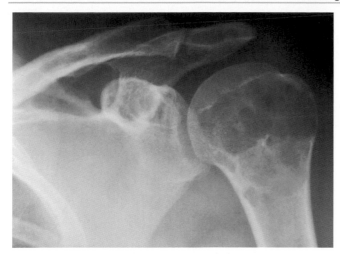

Figure 57–1 This radiograph of the shoulder shows a multicentric, purely lytic process involving the clavicle, scapula, and humerus. The presence of multiple lesions, generally purely lytic in character, in the same anatomic region suggests a diagnosis of angiosarcoma.

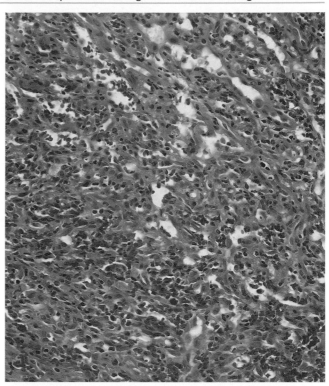

Figure 57–3 At low magnification, these tumors are variable in appearance. In general, however, their vasoformative nature is evident. Most commonly, the vascular spaces are small, as demonstrated in this lesion from the humerus.

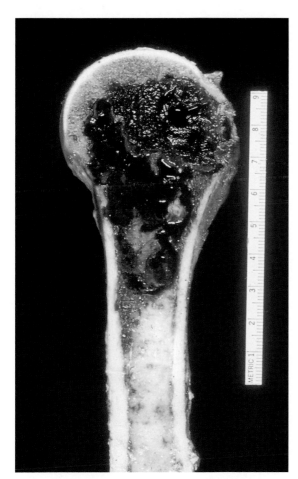

Figure 57–2 The gross specimen in this case of multicentric angiosarcoma correlates well with its radiographic appearance. These tumors generally are red and hemorrhagic. Although the tumor has not extended into the adjacent soft tissue, cortical erosion is evident.

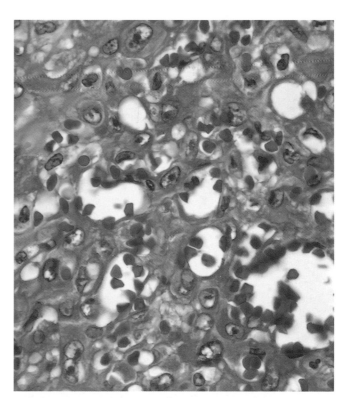

Figure 57–4 At high magnification, the cytologic atypia of these lesions varies from case to case. As this photomicrograph shows, the nuclei are plump, hyperchromatic, and variable in shape. They bulge into the vascular lumina, and tufting may occasionally be seen.

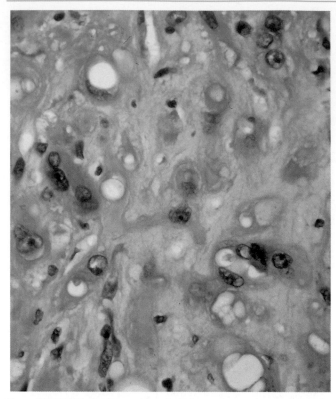

Figure 57–5 Epithelioid hemangioendotheliomas frequently contain a collagenized, chondroid-appearing stroma, as shown in this photomicrograph. Also visible are cells with intracytoplasmic lumina.

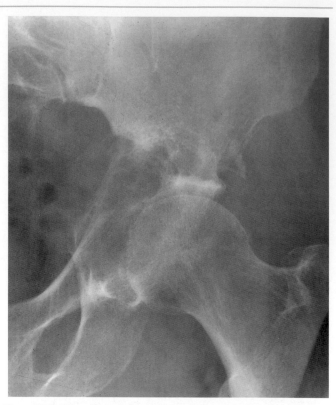

Figure 57–7 This radiograph illustrates the poorly marginated, lytic appearance of a hemangioendothelial sarcoma involving the acetabulum. The radiographic appearance suggests malignancy but is otherwise nonspecific.

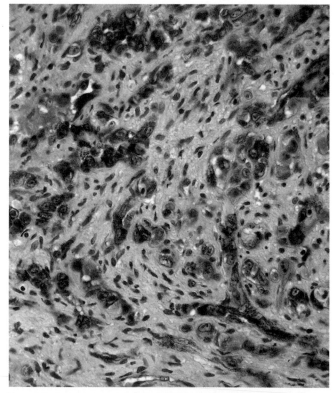

Figure 57–6 Markers of endothelial differentiation may be identified using immunohistochemical analysis. This photomicrograph illustrates positive staining for Factor VIII–related antigen in a low-grade angiosarcoma.

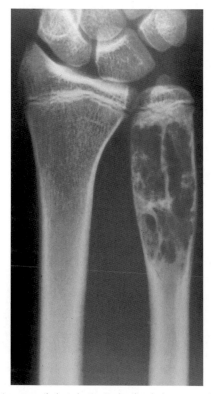

Figure 57–8 An expansile lytic lesion in the distal ulnar metaphysis is shown in this radiograph. Low-grade angiosarcomas often have a benign radiographic appearance.

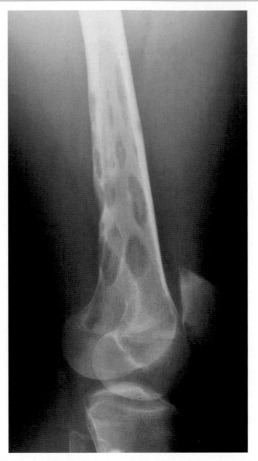

Figure 57–9 This radiograph shows an aggressive, lytic, multicentric process in the distal femur. High-grade angiosarcomas generally demonstrate this aggressive pattern of growth.

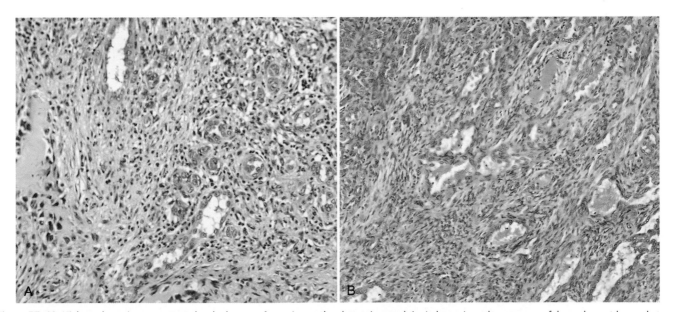

Figure 57–10 High-grade angiosarcomas tend to be less vasoformative, as the photomicrograph in *A* shows. In such cases, a careful search must be made to identify the endothelial nature of the tumor. Although another lesion may be quite vasoformative (*B*), the glandlike appearance of such a lesion may suggest the diagnosis of metastatic adenocarcinoma.

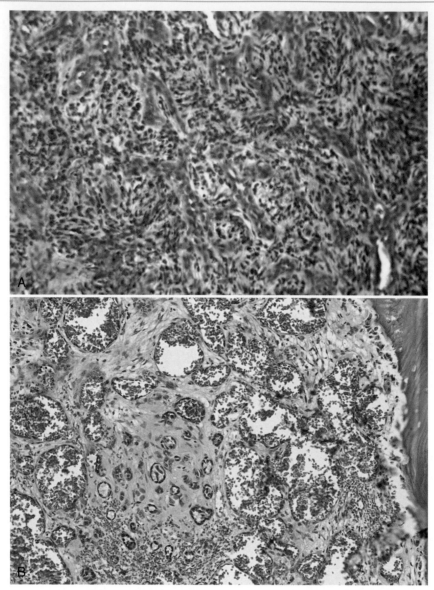

Figure 57–11 *A*: Numerous eosinophils may accompany angiosarcoma, whether they are low- or high-grade. This feature, when taken out of context, may suggest a diagnosis of eosinophilic granuloma. *B*: Other lesions may simulate the appearance of adamantinoma. The location of the lesion is helpful in distinguishing between these two conditions.

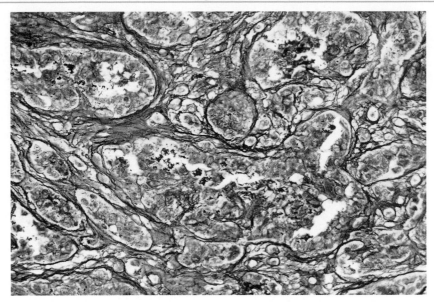

Figure 57–12 Special stains may help to show the clustered pattern of growth that is present in hemangioendothelial sarcomas. This reticulin stain highlights this histologic feature, which may not be obvious in high-grade tumors with hematoxylin and eosin–stained sections.

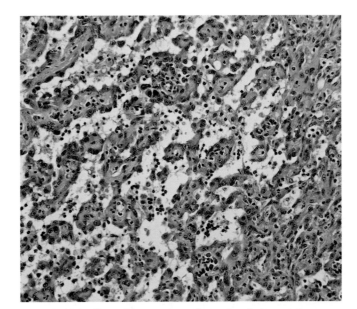

Figure 57–13 Papillary tufting, a common feature in soft tissue angiosarcomas, is uncommon in bony lesions. This femoral lesion in a patient with multicentric disease demonstrates this histologic feature.

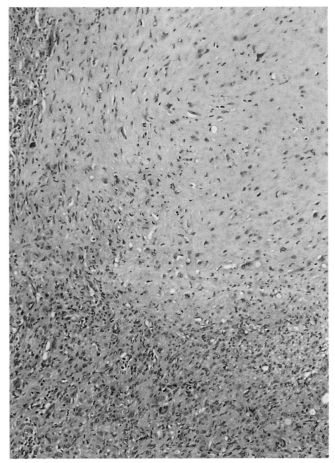

Figure 57–14 This photomicrograph shows the dense eosinophilic hyalin-like matrix that is commonly present in epithelioid hemangioendotheliomas. This tumor involved the ilium. Such regions of dense hyalinized stroma may mimic the appearance of a hyaline cartilage tumor.

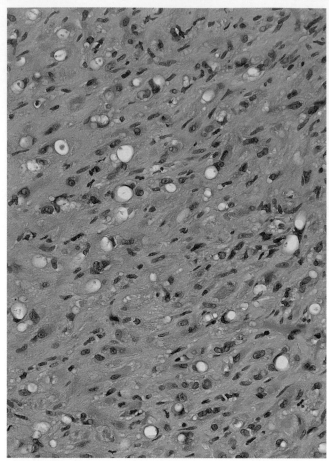

Figure 57–15 This photomicrograph illustrates the cytoplasmic lumina commonly seen in the tumor cells of epithelioid hemangioendothelioma. These tumor cells have a signet ring–like morphology and may therefore be confused with metastatic carcinoma.

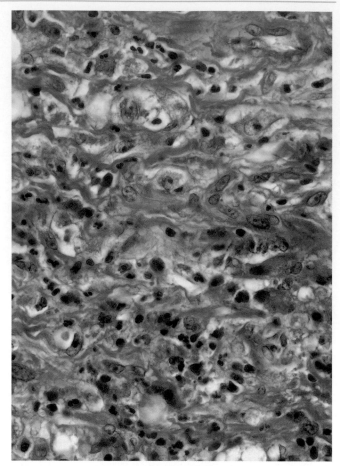

Figure 57–16 Eosinophils are commonly found in benign and malignant vascular tumors. This example of a high-grade angiosarcoma has numerous eosinophils in a region of the tumor that shows little vasoformative morphology.

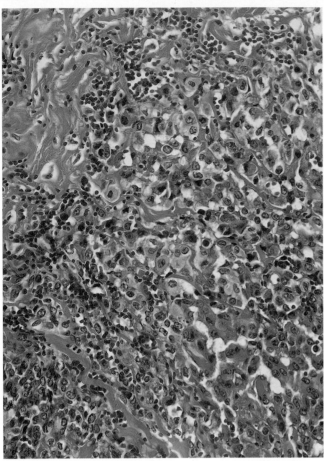

Figure 57–17 High-grade angiosarcomas may show little vasoformation and may even have "epithelioid" cytologic features, as in this tumor of the ilium.

Section 2F: Tumors of Unknown Origin

Hemangiopericytoma

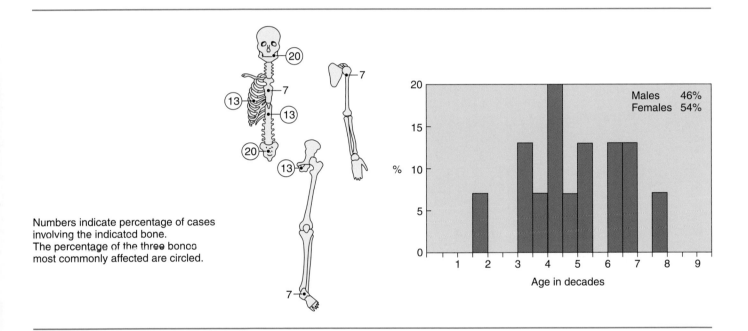

Numbers indicate percentage of cases
involving the indicated bone.
The percentage of the three bones
most commonly affected are circled.

Males 46%
Females 54%

% (y-axis)

Age in decades (x-axis)

Clinical Signs

1. A mass lesion is palpable on physical examination.
2. The mass most commonly is tender to palpation.

Clinical Symptoms

1. Local pain is present.
2. Swelling is noted in the region of the tumor.

Major Radiographic Features

1. This rare primary tumor of bone generally has a non-specific radiographic appearance.
2. More than two thirds are purely lytic.

3. Most have a malignant appearance, and their radiographic appearance roughly correlates with the histologic grade of the tumor.
4. A honeycomb appearance occasionally is seen.

Radiographic Differential Diagnosis

1. Any lytic primary bone tumor.
2. Lytic metastatic tumors of bone.

Major Pathologic Features

Gross

1. The tumor is usually firm.
2. The lesional tissue is most often red and bloody.

Microscopic

1. At low magnification, this tumor is composed of round to oval cells.
2. The tumor is hypercellular.
3. Numerous thin-walled blood vessels course through the tumor.
4. The blood vessels are branched and "staghorn" in shape.
5. At higher magnification, the degree of cytologic atypia is variable.
6. Mitotic activity in the tumor is also variable.
7. No matrix is produced by the tumor cells.

Pathologic Differential Diagnosis

Benign lesions

1. Glomus tumor.
2. Capillary hemangioma.

Malignant lesions

1. Mesenchymal chondrosarcoma.
2. Small cell osteosarcoma.
3. Metastatic hemangiopericytoma (particularly common with hemangiopericytomas of the meninges).

Treatment

1. **Primary modality:** En bloc resection with a wide margin and skeletal reconstruction if feasible. Amputation may be necessary to achieve an adequately wide margin.
2. **Other possible approaches:** Radiotherapy for surgically inaccessible lesions. Multiple drug chemotherapy protocols used in an adjuvant setting may be employed.

References

Dunlop J: Primary haemangiopericytoma of bone: report of two cases. *J Bone Joint Surg Br* 55(4):854–857, 1973.

Tang JS, Gold RH, Mirra JM, et al: Hemangiopericytoma of bone. *Cancer* 62(4):848–859, 1988.

Vang PS, Falk E: Haemangiopericytoma of bone. Review of the literature and report of a case. *Acta Orthop Scand* 51(6):903–907, 1980.

Wold LW, Unni KK, Cooper KL, et al: Hemangiopericytoma of bone. *Am J Surg Pathol* 6(1):53–58, 1982.

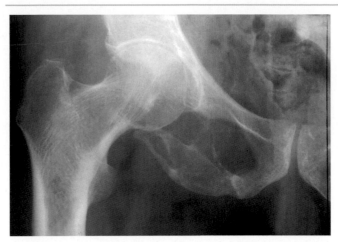

Figure 58–1 This radiograph shows a purely lytic hemangiopericytoma of the ischium. The lesion exhibits features of a malignant lesion but is otherwise nonspecific.

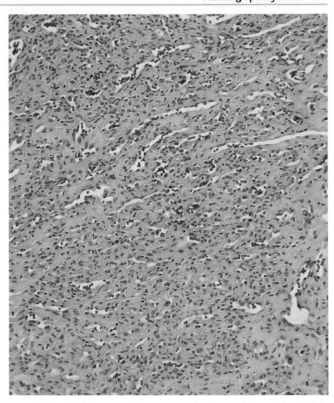

Figure 58–3 This low-power photomicrograph shows a relatively hypocellular tumor composed of void cells arranged around vascular spaces. This tumor of the thoracic vertebra in a 38-year-old man exhibits histologic features of a "benign" hemangiopericytoma.

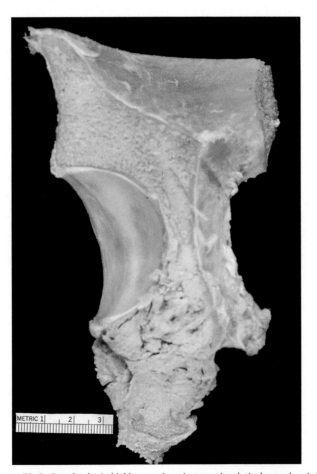

Figure 58–2 Grossly, the ischial hemangiopericytoma is relatively nondescript. The lesional tissue is firm and fibrous. Such tissue may be reddish and bloody.

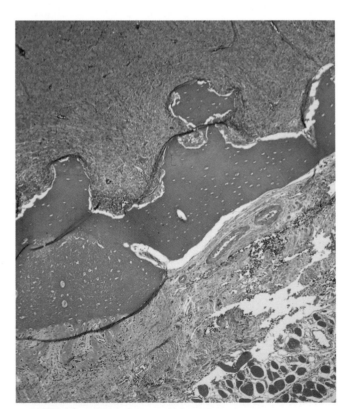

Figure 58–4 At low magnification, more aggressive hemangiopericytomas may show cortical erosion, as is evident in this lesion involving a rib.

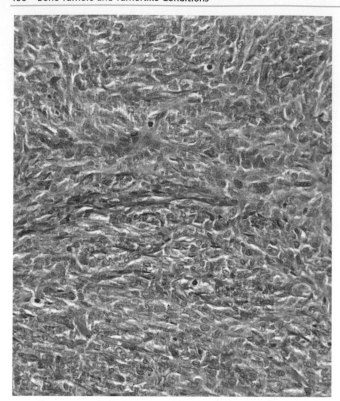

Figure 58–5 Frankly malignant hemangiopericytomas show greater cellular pleomorphism and atypia, as can be seen in this photomicrograph of a primary osseous tumor that also shows moderate mitotic activity.

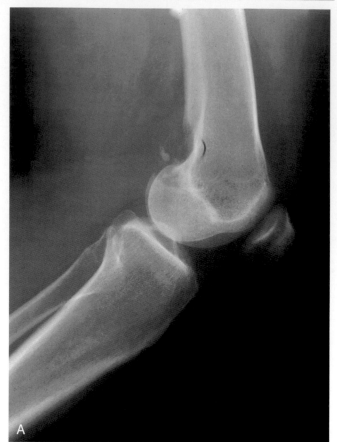

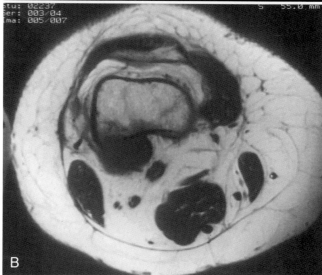

Figure 58–7 A radiograph (*A*) and an axial magnetic resonance imaging (MRI) scan (*B*) of a hemangiopericytoma of the posterior lower femur show destruction of the cortex and extension into the soft tissues. The appearance favors malignancy. The lesion is seen best on MRI.

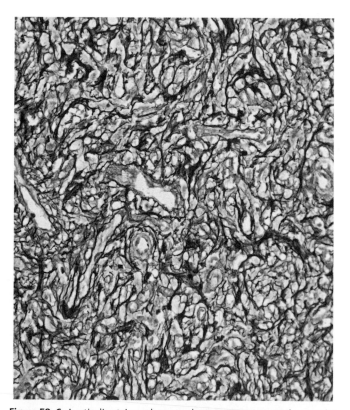

Figure 58–6 A reticulin stain, such as seen here, may accentuate the vascular nature of these tumors. The fine reticulin meshwork that surrounds each cell is helpful in identifying the lesion as a hemangiopericytoma.

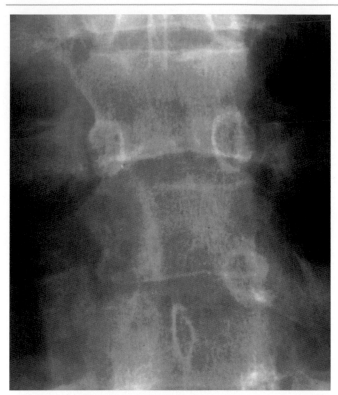

Figure 58–8 Hemangiopericytomas of the meninges show a propensity to osseous metastases, as can be seen in this radiograph of the thoracic spine. Note the lytic destruction of the left pedicle and adjacent vertebral body.

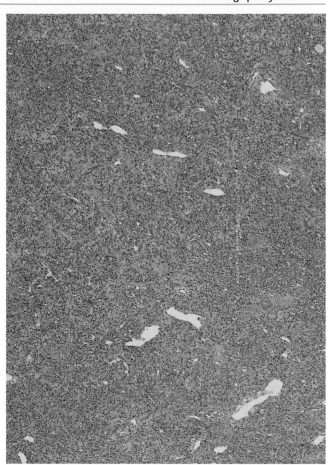

Figure 58–10 The low-power hemangiopericytomatous pattern illustrated in this case of an ischial tumor can also be seen in mesenchymal chondrosarcoma, small cell osteosarcoma, and Ewing's sarcoma. Careful search for matrix in the tumor and immunohistochemical evaluation of the tumor will by exclusion lead to a diagnosis of hemangiopericytoma.

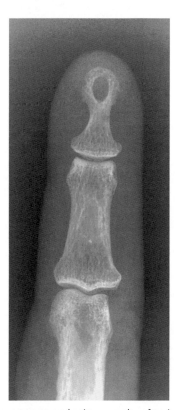

Figure 58–9 Glomus tumors are benign examples of pericytic tumors. These lesions are most commonly identified in the distal phalanx radiographically. Note the well-circumscribed lytic defect of the distal phalangeal tuft in this case.

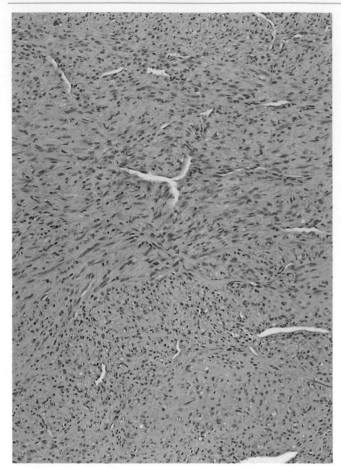

Figure 58–11 A hemangiopericytomatous pattern is commonly seen in cases of congenital fibromatosis, as in this photomicrograph of a skull lesion from a young patient.

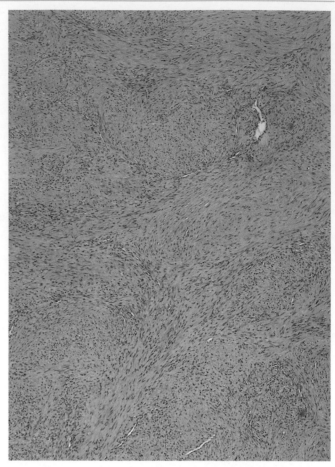

Figure 58–12 A vaguely lobulated pattern is often present in congenital fibromatosis, as in this photomicrograph. Hemangiopericytomas are more uniform in their histologic appearance.

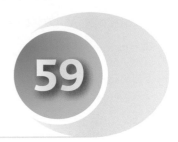

Giant Cell Tumor

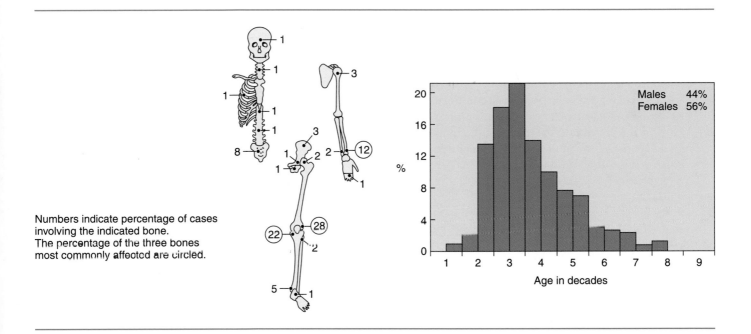

Numbers indicate percentage of cases involving the indicated bone.
The percentage of the three bones most commonly affected are circled.

Males 44%
Females 56%

%

Age in decades

Clinical Signs

1. Of patients, 80% present with a tender, palpable mass.
2. Regional musculature may show atrophic changes secondary to disuse.

Clinical Symptoms

1. Pain of variable severity is almost uniformly present.
2. Approximately 75% of patients discover a swelling in the region of the affected bone.
3. Pathologic fracture may occur.
4. Limited range of motion of the joint adjacent to the affected bone may be noticed.

5. Weakness of the extremity containing the affected bone may be present.

Major Radiographic Features

1. The lesion is purely lytic and epiphyseal in location, extending to the end of the bone.
2. There is neither sclerosis at the periphery of the lesion nor periosteal reaction.
3. Although the tumor is classically epiphyseal in location, it may also arise in an apophysis.
4. The radiographic appearance may mimic that of a malignant tumor.

Radiographic Differential Diagnosis

1. Chondroblastoma.
2. Osteosarcoma.
3. Fibrosarcoma.
4. Malignant fibrous histiocytoma.

Major Pathologic Features

Gross

1. The curetted fragments of tissue are soft and friable.
2. The color of the lesion varies from gray–brown to reddish; there may also be yellow regions containing numerous lipid-laden macrophages.
3. Necrosis with resultant cyst formation may be seen.
4. Tumors may be confined to the bone or may have extended through the cortex into the surrounding soft tissues.

Microscopic

1. Although these tumors may show regions of necrosis and cyst formation, in general they have a uniform pattern of growth at low magnification.
2. Multinucleated giant cells lie scattered uniformly in a "sea" of mononuclear cells, which are round to oval.
3. At higher magnification, the nuclei of the mononuclear cells and those of the multinucleated giant cells are similar in appearance and uniform in their cytologic characteristics.
4. Mitotic figures may be abundant.
5. The tumor lacks matrix production; when pathologic fracture has occurred, however, the reactive new bone formation may alter the histology of the tumor.

Pathologic Differential Diagnosis

Benign lesions

1. Giant cell reparative granuloma (giant cell reaction).
2. Aneurysmal bone cyst.
3. Chondroblastoma.

Malignant lesions

1. Malignant fibrous histiocytoma.
2. Malignancy in giant cell tumor (malignant giant cell tumor).
3. Osteosarcoma containing numerous giant cells.

Treatment

1. **Primary modality:** surgical excision, with the extent of surgery depending on the size and local extent of the tumor. The three primary therapeutic options are (1) curettage and bone grafting for less extensive lesions; (2) resection with bone and joint reconstruction for the very aggressive lesions with associated soft tissue extension, loss of articular cartilage, or pathologic fracture; and (3) curettage and cementation for lesions between these two ends of the spectrum.
2. **Other possible approaches:** cryosurgery or chemical cautery as an adjuvant to curettage and grafting. Radiation therapy should be reserved for surgically inaccessible lesions (e.g., extensive sacral involvement) because of the subsequent risk of malignant "transformation."

References

Cooper KL, Beabout JW, Dahlin DC: Giant-cell tumor: ossification in soft tissue implants. *Radiology* 153(3):597–602, 1984.

Frassica FJ, Sanjay BK, Unni KK, et al: Benign giant cell tumor. *Orthopedics* 16(10):1179–1183, 1993.

Kransdorf MJ, Sweet DE, Buetow PC, et al: Giant cell tumor in skeletally immature patients. *Radiology* 184(1):233–237, 1992.

Larsson SE, Lorentzon R, Boquist L: Giant-cell tumor of bone: a demographic, clinical and histopathological study of all cases recorded in the Swedish Cancer Registry for years 1958 through 1968. *J Bone Joint Surg Am* 57(2):167–173, 1975.

Marcove RC, Weis LD, Vaghaiwalla MR, et al: Cryosurgery in the treatment of giant cell tumors of bone: a report of 52 consecutive cases. *Cancer* 41(3):957–969, 1978.

Peimer CA, Schiller AL, Mankin JH, et al: Multicentric giant-cell tumor of bone. *J Bone Joint Surg Am* 62(4):652–656, 1980.

Picci P, Manfrini M, Zucchi V, et al: Giant-cell tumor of bone in skeletally immature patients. *J Bone Joint Surg Am* 65(4):486–490, 1983.

Rock MG, Pritchard DJ, Unni KK: Metastases from histologically-benign, giant-cell tumor of bone. *J Bone Joint Surg Am* 66(2):269–274, 1984.

Sanerkin NG: Malignancy, aggressiveness, and recurrence in giant cell tumor of bone. *Cancer* 46(7):1641–1649, 1980.

Schajowicz F, Granato DB, McDonald DJ, et al: Clinical and radiological features of atypical giant cell tumours of bone. *Br J Radiol* 64(766):877–889, 1991.

Shih HN, Hsu RW, Sim FH: Excision curettage and allografting of giant cell tumor. *World J Surg* 22(5):432–437, 1998.

Tubbs WS, Brown LR, Beabout JW, et al: Benign giant-cell tumor of bone with pulmonary metastases: clinical findings and radiologic appearance of metastases in 13 cases. *Am J Roentgen* 158(2):331–334, 1992.

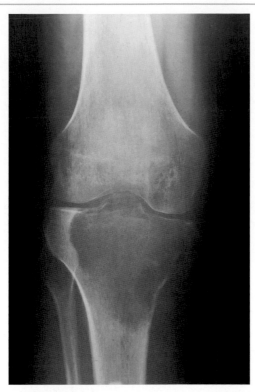

Figure 59–1 This anteroposterior radiograph of the knee shows a large, purely lytic, eccentric lesion involving the proximal tibia. The lesion extends to the end of the bone, and there is expansion of the bone and associated cortical destruction. The features are typical of giant cell tumor.

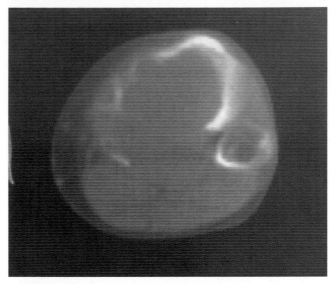

Figure 59–3 The computed tomographic (CT) scan in this case also shows the lesion to be purely lytic, a feature that helps support a diagnosis of giant cell tumor. Cortical destruction and soft tissue extension, evidence of aggressive behavior, are commonly seen in giant cell tumor.

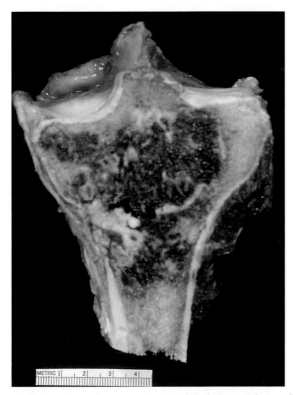

Figure 59–2 The gross pathologic appearance of the lesion correlates well with its radiographic appearance in Figure 59–1. The tumor varies in color from brown to yellow and extends to the articular surface.

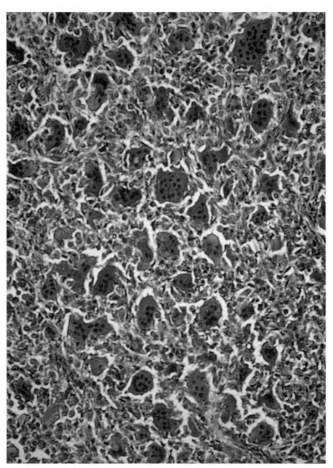

Figure 59–4 At low magnification, giant cell tumor consists of a "sea" of mononuclear cells within which multinucleated giant cells are scattered in a uniform manner.

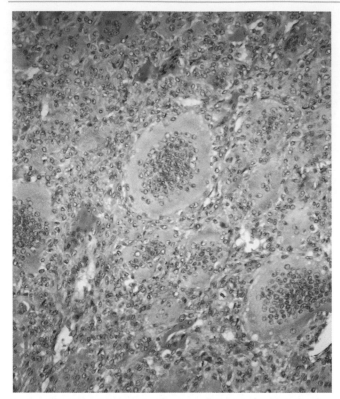

Figure 59–5 Although the histologic appearance of this tumor from the proximal humerus is typical of giant cell tumor, the aggressive radiographic features exhibited by the lesion suggested the possibility of telangiectatic osteosarcoma.

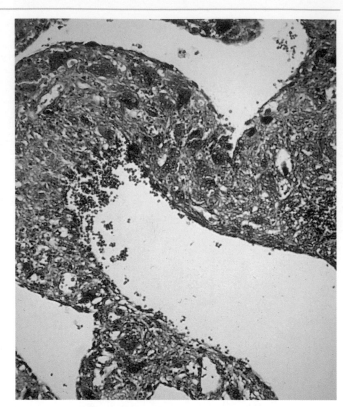

Figure 59–7 Secondary aneurysmal bone cyst may complicate giant cell tumor. In cases such as this, identification of the underlying giant cell tumor may be difficult.

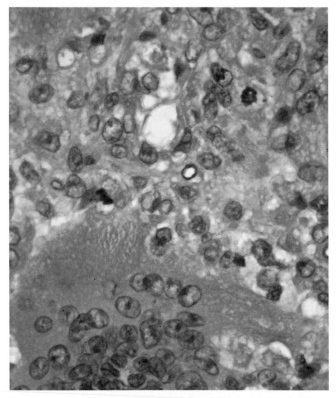

Figure 59–6 At high magnification, the nuclei of the mononuclear stromal cells are similar to those of the multinucleated giant cells. This feature is evident in this tumor from the proximal humerus. Mitotic activity may be brisk in giant cell tumors.

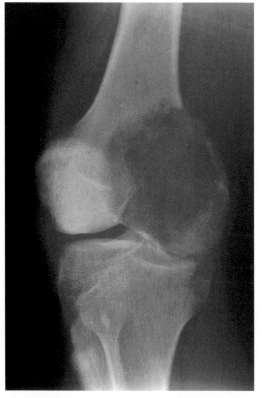

Figure 59–8 This radiograph shows a large, eccentric, aggressive-appearing giant cell tumor of the distal femur. The purely lytic nature of the lesion, its extension to the articular surface, and its eccentric location favor a diagnosis of giant cell tumor.

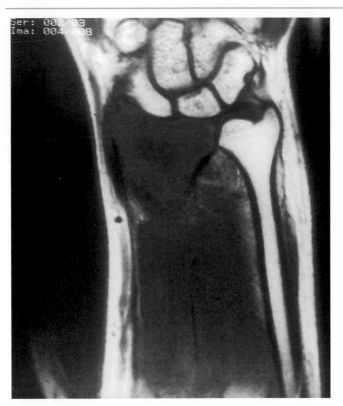

Figure 59–9 This magnetic resonance image of a giant cell tumor of the distal radius demonstrates the utility of this imaging modality, particularly for tumors in peripheral locations. The distal radius is a common site for giant cell tumor.

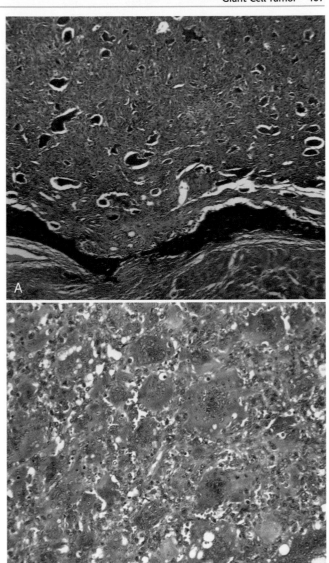

Figure 59–11 A rim of reactive tumor (*A*) frequently surrounds soft tissue recurrences of giant cell tumor. The recurrences—whether osseous, soft tissue, or pulmonary metastases—show the same histologic features as the primary tumor (*B*).

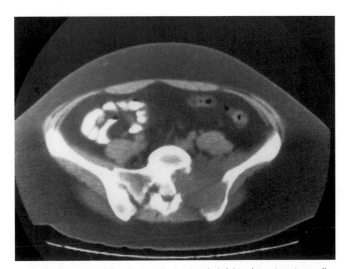

Figure 59–10 As with chordoma, CT scans are helpful in detecting giant cell tumors of the sacrum. These tumors (such as the one shown in this radiograph) may cause extensive destruction of the bone, and the soft tissue involvement generally is better appreciated with CT.

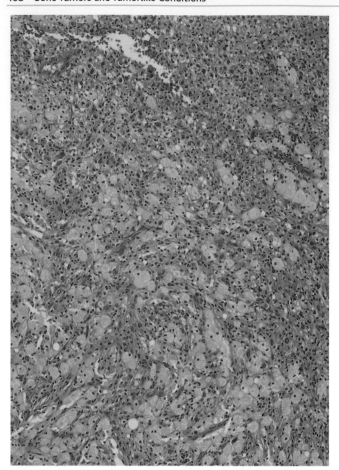

Figure 59–12 Degeneration is common within giant cell tumor. Xanthomatous change is illustrated in this photomicrograph of a distal femoral tumor.

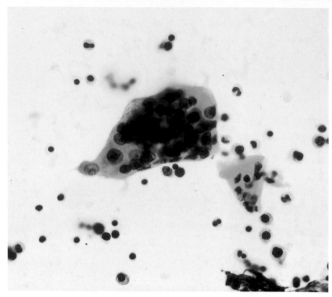

Figure 59–14 Aspiration biopsy of giant cell tumors generally shows numerous multinucleated giant cells, as seen in this aspirate of a sacral lesion.

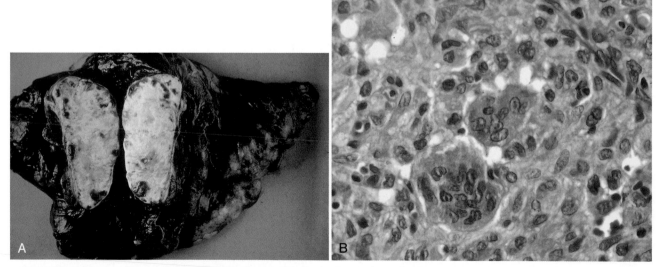

Figure 59–13 The pulmonary metastases, gross pathologic features (*A*), that rarely complicate the clinical course of treated giant cell tumor exhibit the same cytologic similarity between mononuclear and multinucleated cells, as shown in this photomicrograph (*B*).

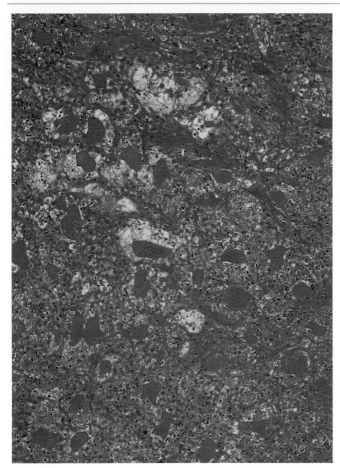

Figure 59–15 Giant cell tumors may become infarcted, as in this tumor from the proximal humerus. "Ghost" tumor cells and giant cells may be seen in such cases.

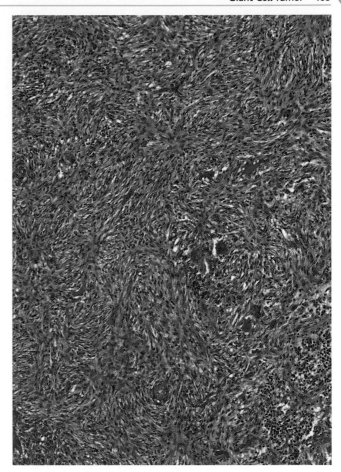

Figure 59–16 Although giant cell tumor typically does not contain spindle cells, some tumors show a fibrous histiocytoma-like pattern, as in this case of a giant cell tumor of the proximal fibula.

Malignancy in Giant Cell Tumor (Malignant Giant Cell Tumor)

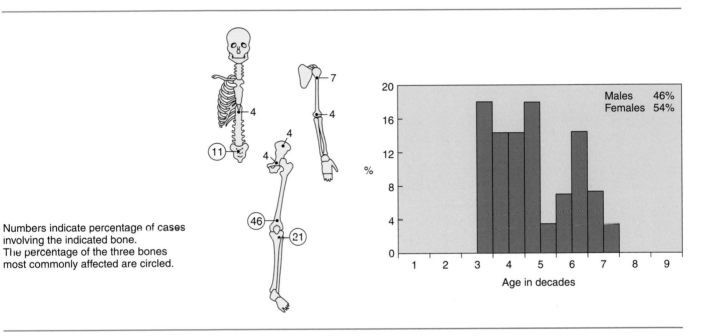

Numbers indicate percentage of cases involving the indicated bone.
The percentage of the three bones most commonly affected are circled.

Males 46%
Females 54%

%

Age in decades

Clinical Signs

1. A tender mass lesion in the region of a previously treated giant cell tumor is commonly present on physical examination.
2. Cutaneous changes from prior radiation therapy are commonly found.

Clinical Symptoms

1. Pain is the most common symptom.
2. Nearly all patients give a history of a previous giant cell tumor having been treated more than 10 years (on average) before the recent onset of pain.

3. Of patients, 75% have received prior radiation therapy as part of treatment for the giant cell tumor.
4. Only rarely is an abrupt change in the symptoms related to the development of a "malignant giant cell tumor" in a patient who has not received prior radiation therapy.

Major Radiographic Features

1. A de novo malignant giant cell tumor has the same radiographic appearance as a benign giant cell tumor, and the two cannot be distinguished.
2. A secondary malignant giant cell tumor is usually seen many years (average of 10 to 13 years) after treatment that included radiation therapy.

411

3. Serial changes that occur more than 3 years after the original treatment are highly suspect for secondary malignant giant cell tumor.

Radiographic Differential Diagnosis

1. Benign giant cell tumor.
2. Recurrent giant cell tumor.
3. Osteomyelitis.

Major Pathologic Features

Gross

1. The tumor expands the end of the bone and generally has broken through the cortex.
2. Zones of necrosis are identifiable; however, necrosis can be seen in benign giant cell tumors as well.
3. Extension into the surrounding soft tissue is generally present.
4. Hemorrhagic foci may also be identified.

Microscopic

1. At low magnification, the tumor is hypercellular and generally is composed of spindle cells.
2. Matrix production may be, but generally is not, present.
3. The arrangement of the spindle cells may be in a "herringbone," storiform, or haphazard pattern.
4. At higher magnification, the spindle cells show marked pleomorphism and nuclear atypia characterized by variation in size, shape, and staining qualities.
5. In general, mitotic activity is brisk.
6. Most commonly, no residual benign giant cell tumor is identifiable in the lesion. On rare occasions, however, zones of otherwise typical giant cell tumor may be identified adjacent to the high-grade sarcoma.

Pathologic Differential Diagnosis

Benign lesions

1. Giant cell tumor.
2. Metaphyseal fibrous defect (fibroma).

Malignant lesions

1. Osteosarcoma.
2. Fibrosarcoma.
3. Malignant fibrous histiocytoma.

Treatment

1. **Primary modality:** preoperative chemotherapy and wide surgical resection. Aggressive behavior and extensive involvement often mandate amputation to achieve an adequate margin.
2. **Other possible approaches:** chemotherapy, radiation therapy for surgically inaccessible lesions, and thoracotomy for metastatic pulmonary disease.

References

Hutter RVP, Worcester JN Jr, Francis KC, et al: Benign and malignant giant cell tumors of bone: a clinicopathological analysis of the natural history of the disease. *Cancer* 15:653–690, 1962.

Meis JM, Dorfman HD, Nathanson SD, et al: Primary malignant giant cell tumor of bone: "dedifferentiated" giant cell tumor. *Mod Pathol* 2(5):541–546, 1995.

Nascimento AG, Huvos AG, Marcove RC: Primary malignant giant cell tumor of bone: a study of eight cases and review of the literature. *Cancer* 44(4):1393–1402, 1979.

Ortiz-Cruz EJ, Quinn RH, Fanburg JC, et al: Late development of a malignant fibrous histiocytoma at the site of a giant cell tumor. *Clin Orthop Relat Res* 318:199–204, 1995.

Rock MG, Sim FH, Unni KK, et al: Secondary malignant giant-cell tumor of bone. Clinicopathological assessment of nineteen patients. *J Bone Joint Surg Am* 68(7):1073–1079, 1986.

Sanerkin NG: Malignancy, aggressiveness, and recurrence in giant cell tumor of bone. *Cancer* 46(7):1641–1649, 1980.

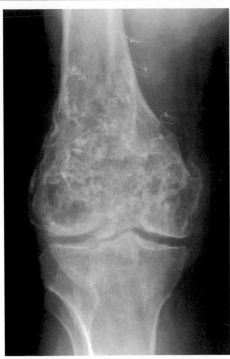

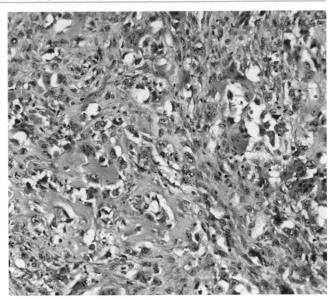

Figure 60–1 This radiograph shows a sarcoma arising from the site of a prior benign giant cell tumor. The development of the sarcoma is often obscured by the distortion caused by the previous tumor. In many cases, serial studies are essential to make the diagnosis with confidence.

Figure 60–3 In contrast with benign giant cell tumors, in which the mononuclear cells contain nuclei similar to those in the multinucleated giant cells, malignancies arising in giant cell tumors show marked nuclear pleomorphism, as this photomicrograph illustrates.

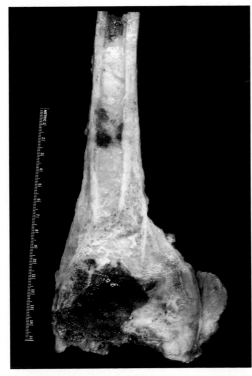

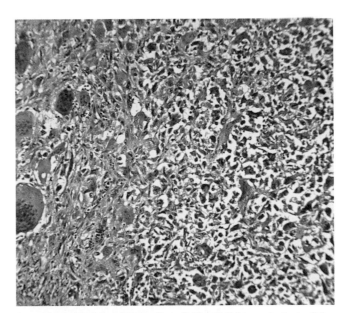

Figure 60–2 In this gross specimen of the tumor seen in Figure 60–1, the distal femur has been replaced by a firm fibrous tumor, which has destroyed the medial cortex of the femur. This sarcoma, which showed the histologic pattern of growth of a fibrosarcoma, occurred in a patient who had received radiation therapy for a giant cell tumor 12 years previously.

Figure 60–4 Although malignancy is rarely identified de novo in giant cell tumors, when such cases are encountered, both a benign giant cell tumor component and a sarcoma should be histologically identifiable. This photomicrograph shows a distal femoral tumor from a 28-year-old man that radiographically was classic for a benign giant cell tumor. Histologically, the lesion shows a pattern typical of benign giant cell tumor and a sarcomatous component.

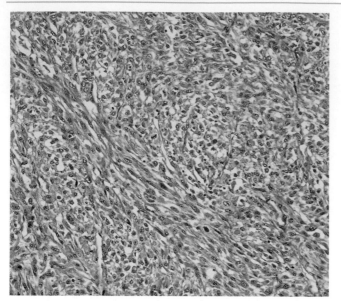

Figure 60–5 Malignancies that arise in the region of a prior giant cell tumor almost uniformly consist of spindle-shaped cells. This tumor shows some features of a malignant fibrous histiocytoma. Osseous and chondroid matrix production may also be evident in these tumors.

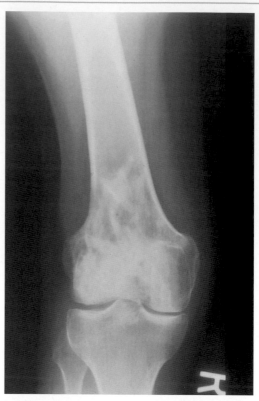

Figure 60–7 This radiograph demonstrates the appearance of a distal femur 16 years after curettage, grafting, and radiation therapy for a benign giant cell tumor.

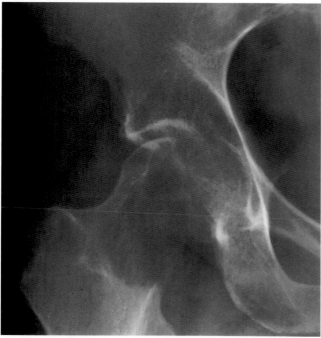

Figure 60–6 This radiograph shows a de novo malignant giant cell tumor of the proximal femur, characterized by an aggressive appearance and lytic destruction extending to the bone end. Benign giant cell tumors may also cause this type of change.

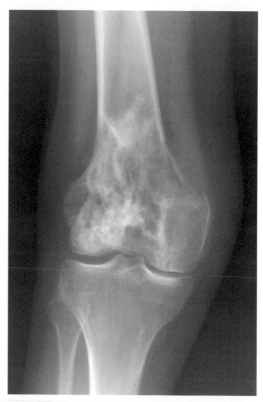

Figure 60–8 In this view, taken 5 months after the radiograph shown in Figure 60–7, the appearance of the lesion has changed. Lytic destruction resulting from secondary fibrosarcoma has developed.

Adamantinoma

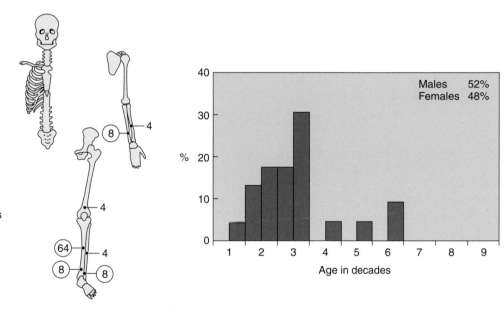

Numbers indicate percentage of cases involving the indicated bone.
The percentage of the three bones most commonly affected are circled.

Males 52%
Females 48%

% — Age in decades

Clinical Signs

1. A mass lesion is the only usual finding on physical examination.

Clinical Symptoms

1. Pain is the most common initial symptom.
2. A mass lesion is rarely the initial symptom.
3. The duration of symptoms may be several months to many years.

Major Radiographic Features

1. The lesion occurs in the diaphysis of the tibia.
2. Eccentric lucencies are connected by sclerosis.

3. A dominant central lesion is present.
4. Expansion of the affected bone is common.
5. Multicentricity of the lesion may be present.
6. The fibula may be affected as well.

Radiographic Differential Diagnosis

1. Osteofibrous dysplasia.
2. Fibrous dysplasia.
3. Fibroma.

Major Pathologic Features

Gross

1. These tumors tend to be well circumscribed at their periphery and arranged in a lobulated fashion.

2. The tumor is generally gray or white.
3. The consistency varies from firm and fibrous to soft.
4. Cystic spaces containing blood or straw-colored fluid may be encountered.

Microscopic

1. The tumors may show a myriad of histologic patterns; however, they share an epithelioid low-power pattern.
2. The most common pattern is that of epithelioid islands of cells with peripheral columnar cells showing nuclear palisading.
3. Toward the center of the epithelioid islands, the cells are arranged in a looser pattern with spindling (stellate reticulum–like appearance).
4. Hypocellular fibrous connective tissue occupies the space between the epithelioid islands, and disorganized bone may be seen in these regions, resulting in a pattern that mimics osteofibrous dysplasia.
5. The epithelioid islands may show squamous cytologic features and even keratin production.
6. A vascular pattern with the spaces merging into the epithelial islands is common.
7. The tumor may be purely spindle celled, mimicking fibrosarcoma; however, a cortical location and a lack of cytologic atypia should suggest a diagnosis of adamantinoma.

Pathologic Differential Diagnosis

Benign lesions

1. Osteofibrous dysplasia.
2. Fibrous dysplasia.

Malignant lesions

1. Metastatic carcinoma.
2. Angiosarcoma.

Treatment

1. **Primary modality:** En bloc removal with a wide surgical margin is done. Reconstruction of the bone can be achieved with an intercalary allograft or vascularized fibular graft. Amputation may be necessary for large or recurrent lesions.
2. **Other possible approaches:** Simple excision with a marginal margin is discouraged because of a high recurrence rate. Therapeutic lymph node dissection has occasionally been necessary for metastatic disease.

References

Campanacci M, Giunti A, Bertoni F, et al: Adamantinoma of the long bones: the experience at the Istituto Ortopedico Rizzoli. *Am J Surg Pathol* 5(6):533–542, 1981.

Desai SS, Jambhekar N, Agarwal M, et al: Adamantinoma of tibia: a study of 12 cases. *J Surg Oncol* 93(5):429–433, 2006.

Hazelbag HM, Taminiau AH, Fleuren GJ, et al: Adamantinoma of the long bones. A clinicopathological study of thirty-two patients with emphasis on histological subtype, precursor lesion, and biological behavior. *J Bone Joint Surg Am* 76(10):1482–1499, 1994.

Keeney GL, Unni KK, Beabout JW, et al: Adamantinoma of long bones. A clinicopathologic study of 85 cases. *Cancer* 64(3):730–737, 1989.

Knapp RH, Wick MR, Scheithauer BW, et al: Adamantinoma of bone: an electron microscopic and immunohistochemical study. *Virchows Arch A Pathol Anat Histopathol* 398(1):75–86, 1982.

Rock MG, Beabout JW, Unni KK, et al: Adamantinoma. *Orthopedics* 6:472–477, 1983.

Rosai J, Pinkus GS: Immunohistochemical demonstration of epithelial differentiation in adamantinoma of the tibia. *Am J Surg Pathol* 6(5):427–434, 1982.

Sweet DE, Vinh TN, Devaney K: Cortical osteofibrous dysplasia of long bone and its relationship to adamantinoma. A clinicopathologic study of 30 cases. *Am J Surg Pathol* 16(3):282–290, 1992.

Van der Woude HJ, Hazelbag HM, Bloem JL, et al: MRI of adamantinoma of long bones in correlation with histopathology. *Am J Roentgenol* 183(6):1737–1744, 2004.

Weiss SW, Dorfman HD: Adamantinoma of long bones: an analysis of nine new cases with emphasis on metastasizing lesions and fibrous dysplasia–like changes. *Hum Pathol* 8(2):141–153, 1977.

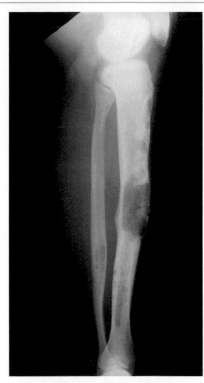

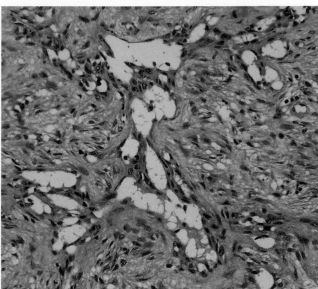

Figure 61–3 The low-power pattern of adamantinoma is that of a lesion composed of islands of epithelioid cells lying within a hypocellular fibrous connective tissue. At the periphery of these islands is a palisading of the nuclei. Toward the center of the islands, the cells have a looser arrangement and a more stellate appearance (so-called stellate reticulum).

Figure 61–1 Multicentric adamantinoma involving the tibia and fibula is shown in this radiograph of the lower extremity. Multiple lytic areas with surrounding sclerosis are present. Note the dominant central expansile lesion.

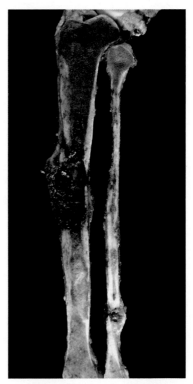

Figure 61–2 The bisected gross specimen in this case reveals the involvement of both the tibia and the fibula, as shown in Figure 61–1. Such multicentric disease is not uncommon; indeed, this gross appearance is virtually diagnostic. The multicentric nature of the disease may explain recurrences in cases treated with marginal excision.

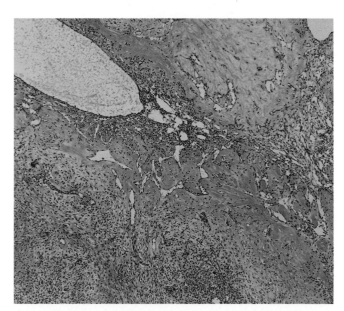

Figure 61–4 Some adamantinomas contain more open spaces; when these are blood-filled, the appearance may mimic that of a vascular neoplasm.

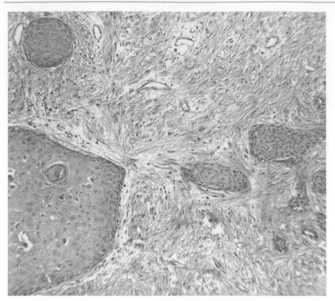

Figure 61–5 Squamous differentiation, as shown in this case, may be so prominent as to mimic the appearance of a squamous cell carcinoma. Other tumors may appear glandular and therefore look like metastatic adenocarcinoma.

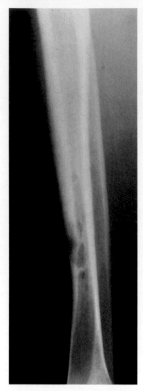

Figure 61–7 Multiple small cortical lucencies are apparent in this example of an adamantinoma involving the tibia. The lucencies are connected by sclerotic regions.

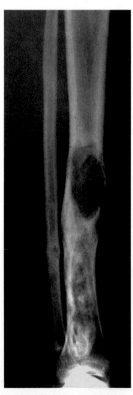

Figure 61–6 The typical appearance of a multicentric adamantinoma involving the tibia and fibula is shown in this radiograph. The dominant lesion involves the diaphysis of the tibia and is centrally located.

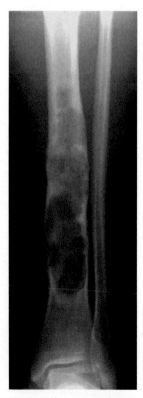

Figure 61–8 Adamantinomas are slow-growing lesions and, as such, may result in significant expansion of the affected bone prior to diagnosis of the lesion. This example shows diaphyseal expansion of the tibia with a sclerotic margin, another feature indicating slow growth.

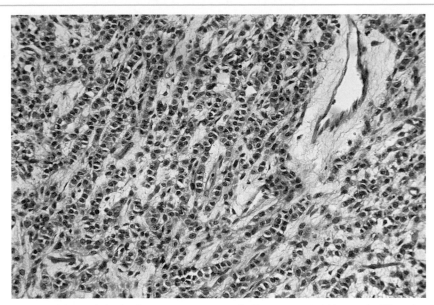

Figure 61–9 At times, the arrangement of the epithelioid cells may give rise to a single-file pattern, mimicking poorly differentiated adenocarcinoma. This tumor had been present in the tibia for 50 years.

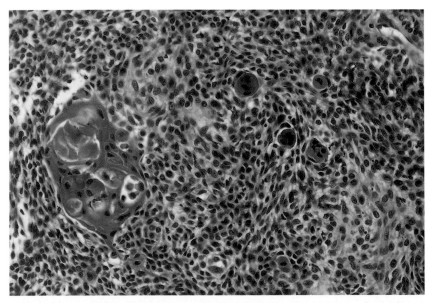

Figure 61–10 Squamous differentiation may be so prominent that squamous pearl formation occurs. Such cases may have a deceptively bland cytologic appearance and suggest the diagnosis of squamous cell carcinoma arising in chronic osteomyelitis.

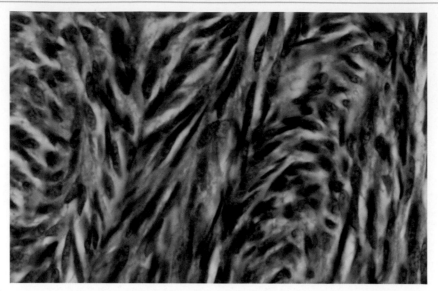

Figure 61–11 Regions of adamantinoma may show a predominantly spindle cell morphology as illustrated in this photomicrograph. Cases with a predominant spindle cell morphology may be mistaken for a spindle cell sarcoma.

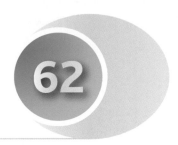

Chordoma

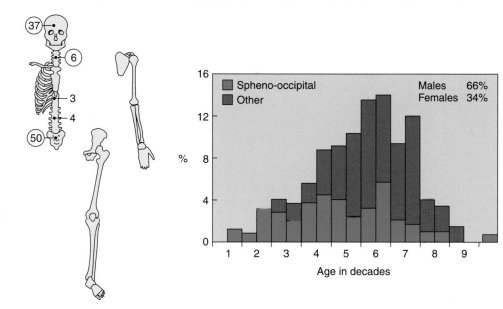

Numbers indicate percentage of cases involving the indicated bone.
The percentage of the three bones most commonly affected are circled.

Clinical Signs

1. Sacral tumors generally extend anteriorly and thus produce a presacral mass appreciable on rectal examination.
2. Spheno-occipital tumors cause cranial nerve VI palsy but may also result in cranial nerve VII and VIII abnormalities. Downward growth may produce a nasopharyngeal mass lesion.
3. Vertebral chordomas give rise to nerve root compression or spinal cord compression signs, but those in the cervical region may also result in symptoms suggestive of a chronic retropharyngeal abscess.

Clinical Symptoms

1. Symptoms and duration are variable and depend on tumor location (sacral, spheno-occipital, or vertebral); however, they are usually of long duration.
2. Sacral tumors nearly always are associated with pain in the sacral or coccygeal region. Constipation may be experienced.
3. Spheno-occipital tumors generally cause symptoms related to involvement of cranial nerves. Of these, cranial nerves VI, VII, and VIII are the most frequently involved.
4. Vertebral chordomas may cause symptoms owing to nerve root or spinal cord compression.

Major Radiographic Features

1. The lesion is in the sacrum or clivus.
2. Midline destruction is seen. (Regardless of location—sacral, clival, or vertebral—all chordomas are midline lesions.)
3. Poor margination and an associated soft tissue mass are commonly present.
4. Of all chordomas, 50% are seen to be calcified on radiography.
5. Computed tomography and magnetic resonance imaging are the best modalities to delineate the extent of the lesion.

Radiographic Differential Diagnosis

1. Metastatic carcinoma.
2. Myeloma.
3. Giant cell tumor.
4. Neurogenic tumor.

Major Pathologic Features

Gross

1. Chordomas generally are soft, grayish tumors that have a gelatinous consistency grossly.
2. The tumor tends to be well circumscribed and may even show gross lobulation.
3. In both the sacral and the spheno-occipital regions, the tumor tends to elevate the periosteum of the affected bone, extending into the presacral and cranial cavities, respectively.

Microscopic

1. At low magnification, chordomas characteristically are arranged in a lobulated fashion, with fibrous septa separating the lobules.
2. The tumor generally is arranged in chords or strands of cells.
3. Between the chords of cells is abundant intercellular mucoid matrix.
4. At higher magnification, the cells have abundant eosinophilic vacuolated cytoplasm (physaliferous cells). The boundaries between cells in the strands are indistinct, resulting in a syncytial quality.
5. In the spheno-occipital region, some tumors have a histologic appearance very similar to that of chondrosarcoma (chondroid chordoma).

Pathologic Differential Diagnosis

Benign lesions

1. Chondromyxoid fibroma.

Malignant lesions

1. Metastatic carcinoma.
2. Chordosarcoma.

Treatment

1. **Primary modality:** En bloc resection with a marginal or wide margin is performed; sacrificing involved nerve roots provides the best chance for cure. Sacral lesions below the third sacral vertebra can be removed with a posterior approach; lesions above this level are approached both anteriorly and posteriorly.
2. **Other possible approaches:** Adjuvant radiation therapy is used for narrow or contaminated margins and surgically inaccessible lesions. Radiation therapy is particularly helpful for tumors in the spheno-occipital region.

References

Bjornsson J, Wold LE, Ebersold MJ, et al: Chordoma of the mobile spine. *Cancer* 71(3):735–740, 1993.

Chambers PW, Schwinn CP: Chordoma: a clinicopathologic study of metastasis. *Am J Clin Pathol* 72(5):765–776, 1979.

Erdem E, Angtuaco EC, Van Hemert R, et al: Comprehensive review of intracranial chordoma. *Radiographics* 23(4):995–1009, 2003.

Eriksson B, Gunterberg B, Kindblom LG: Chordoma: a clinicopathologic and prognostic study of a Swedish national series. *Acta Orthop Scand* 52(1):49–58, 1981.

Kaiser TE, Pritchard DJ, Unni KK: Clinicopathologic study of sacrococcygeal chordoma. *Cancer* 53(11):2574–2578, 1984.

Meis JM, Raymond AK, Evans JL, et al: "Dedifferentiated" chordoma. *Am J Surg Pathol* 11(7):516–525, 1987.

Mindell ER: Current concepts review: chordoma. *J Bone Joint Surg Am* 63(3):501–505, 1981.

Mitchell A, Scheithauer BW, Unni KK, et al: Chordoma and chondroid neoplasms of the spheno-occiput. An immunohistochemical study of 41 cases with prognostic and nosologic implications. *Cancer* 72(10):2943–2949, 1993.

Rosenthal DI, Scott JA, Mankin JH, et al: Sacro-coccygeal chordoma: magnetic resonance imaging and computed tomography. *Am J Roentgenol* 145(1):143–147, 1983.

Volpe R, Mazabraud A: A clinicopathologic review of 25 cases of chordoma (a pleomorphic and metastasizing neoplasm). *Am J Surg Pathol* 7(2):161–170, 1983.

Wold LE, Laws ER Jr: Cranial chordomas in children and young adults. *J Neurosurg* 59(6):1043–1047, 1983.

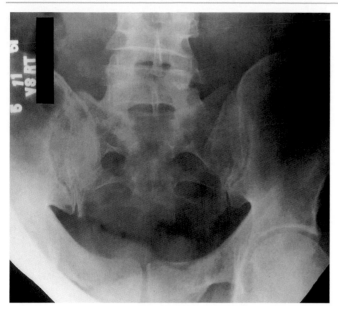

Figure 62–1 This radiograph illustrates how difficult it may be to demonstrate a chordoma in the sacrum with a routine anteroposterior view.

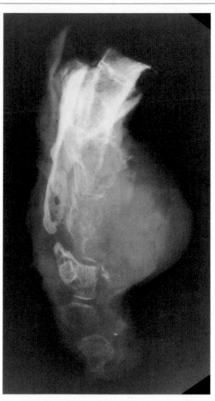

Figure 62–3 The specimen radiogram exhibits the same features seen in the gross specimen. Lateral radiographs of the pelvis may help visualize a sacral chordoma, as do computed tomography (CT) and magnetic resonance imaging (MRI).

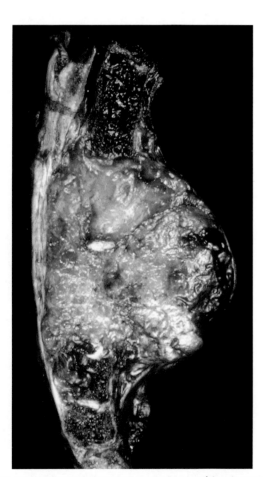

Figure 62–2 The gross pathologic features in this case (also shown in Fig. 62–1) demonstrate destruction of a significant portion of the sacrum and extension of the tumor into the presacral space.

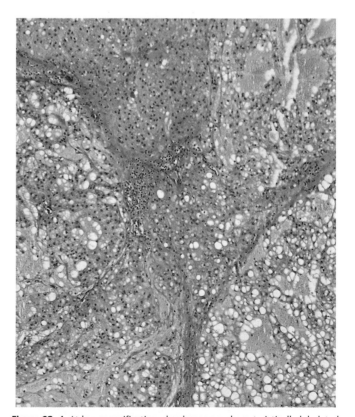

Figure 62–4 At low magnification, chordomas are characteristically lobulated tumors, as this photomicrograph shows.

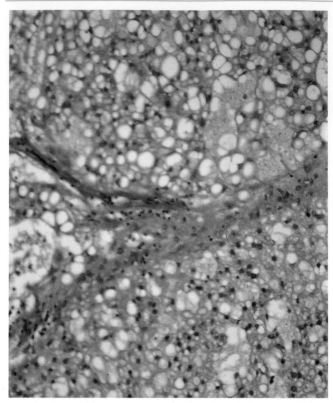

Figure 62–5 Within the lobules, the tumor is mildly cellular, and numerous cytoplasmic vacuoles are identifiable even at medium magnification. Chording of the cells is a feature that varies from tumor to tumor and need not be prominent.

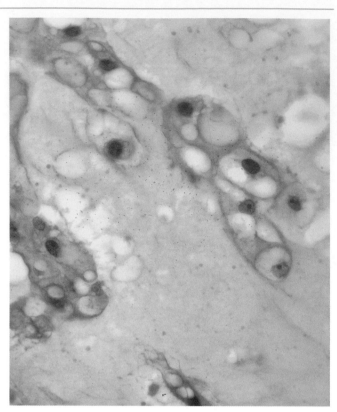

Figure 62–7 Chording of the cells, as seen in this photomicrograph, is a feature that can result in a histologic pattern similar to that of a mucinous adenocarcinoma.

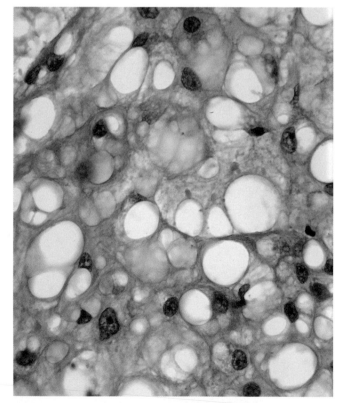

Figure 62–6 At high magnification, the cytologic features show that the cells have abundant vacuolated cytoplasm. Such cells have been termed "physaliferous."

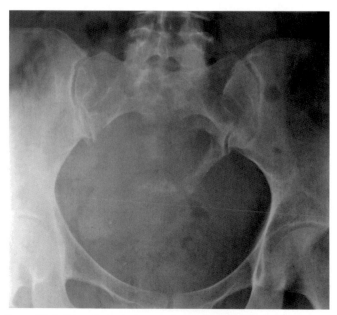

Figure 62–8 This radiograph shows a chordoma presenting as a large, poorly marginated, midline, destructive tumor of the sacrum. An area of central calcification is present.

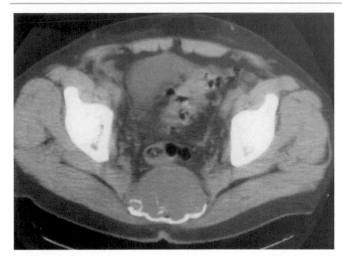

Figure 62–9 This CT scan shows the typical features of a sacral chordoma, with bony destruction and anterior extension of the lesion.

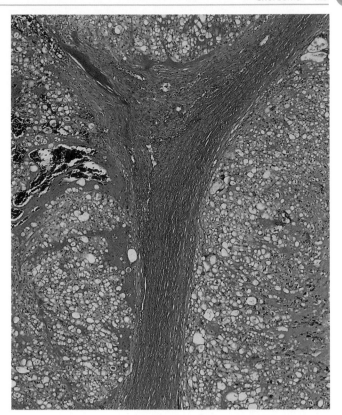

Figure 62–11 The lobulated pattern of growth of a chordoma is evident in this sacral tumor. Soft tissue extensions of the tumor maintain this pattern.

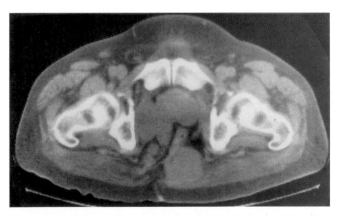

Figure 62–10 Multiple soft tissue nodules of recurrent chordoma are identifiable in this CT scan. These tumors have a propensity for such recurrences, and CT or MRI usually is needed to detect them.

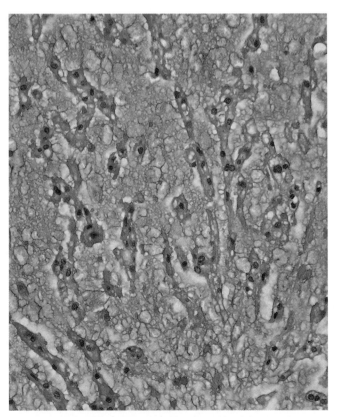

Figure 62–12 Chording and the physaliferous quality of the cytoplasm are evident in this photomicrograph.

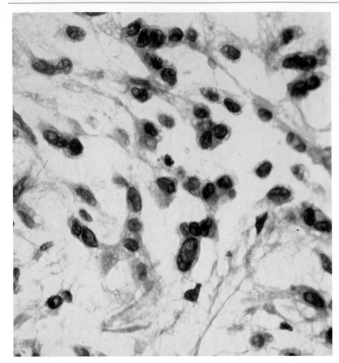

Figure 62–13 Chording is also evident in this tumor involving the seventh thoracic vertebra. Although some mesenchymal and even epithelial tumors may exhibit a similar pattern of chorded growth, the diagnosis of chordoma is valid only for midline tumors.

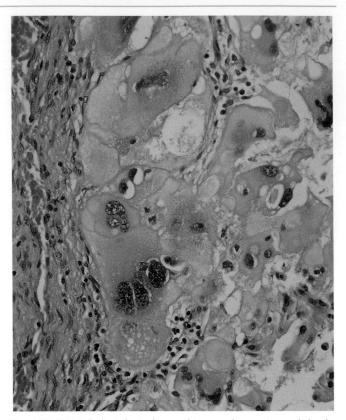

Figure 62–15 Marked cytologic pleomorphism may be seen in sacral chordomas, as illustrated in this photomicrograph. Such atypia is most commonly seen after radiation therapy or with recurrence of a tumor.

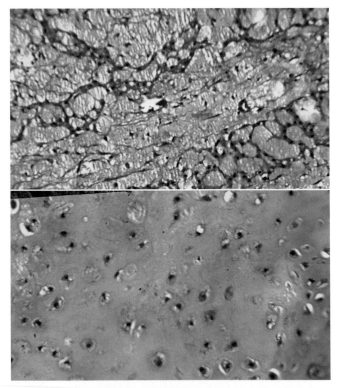

Figure 62–14 In the spheno-occipital region, some tumors show a mixture of chondroid and chordoid features histologically. Such tumors have been termed "chondroid chordomas."

Ewing's Sarcoma

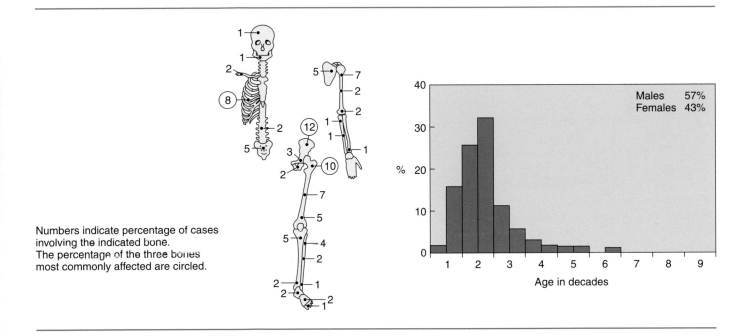

Numbers indicate percentage of cases
involving the indicated bone.
The percentage of the three bones
most commonly affected are circled.

Males 57%
Females 43%

Clinical Signs

1. A palpable, tender mass lesion is found.
2. Fever and an increased erythrocyte sedimentation rate may be seen.
3. Anemia and leukocytosis may also be present.

Clinical Symptoms

1. Local pain is the first symptom in 50% of patients. Although it may be intermittent at first, pain tends to increase in severity over time.
2. Swelling is commonly present at the time of diagnosis but is rarely the first symptom.

3. Fever and other constitutional symptoms suggestive of an infection may be present.

Major Radiographic Features

1. The tumor most commonly presents as an extensive diaphyseal lesion.
2. The lesion has a permeative pattern of growth and is poorly marginated.
3. The lesion may be lytic or sclerotic, or it may have regions of both lysis and sclerosis evident radiographically.
4. Characteristically, there is prominent periosteal new bone formation.

427

5. A soft tissue mass most commonly accompanies the osseous lesion.
6. An isotope bone scan, computed tomography, and magnetic resonance imaging are helpful in defining the lesion.

Radiographic Differential Diagnosis

1. Malignant lymphoma.
2. Osteosarcoma.
3. Osteomyelitis.
4. Langerhans' cell histiocytosis.

Major Pathologic Features

Gross

1. The tumor is characteristically gray–white.
2. The tumor is moist and glistening.
3. The tumor may be almost liquid and can mimic the appearance of pus.

Microscopic

1. The low-power appearance is that of a "small round cell tumor" with little intercellular stroma.
2. Between the areas of highly cellular tumor, fibrous strands that compartmentalize the tumor may be identified.
3. At high magnification, the cells are uniform and round to oval.
4. The nuclei are round to oval and have a delicate, finely dispersed chromatin pattern.
5. Nucleoli, if present, are inconspicuous.
6. Mitotic figures are not abundant.
7. The majority of tumors have glycogen identifiable in the cytoplasm (periodic acid–Schiff–positive and diastase-sensitive).
8. The tumor is reticulin-poor and does not show evidence of matrix production.

Pathologic Differential Diagnosis

Benign lesions

1. Chronic osteomyelitis.

Malignant lesions

1. Malignant lymphoma.
2. Mesenchymal chondrosarcoma.
3. Small cell osteosarcoma.
4. Metastatic neuroblastoma.

Treatment

1. **Primary modality:** radiation therapy to control the primary lesion. An effort is made to avoid irradiating an actively growing physis. Combination chemotherapy to control occult systemic disease is used in conjunction with the radiotherapy.
2. **Other possible approaches:** preoperative chemotherapy followed by resection with or without postoperative radiation therapy. Increased emphasis is being placed on the addition of surgical treatment to the overall management of Ewing's tumor.

References

Bacci G, Picci P, Gitelis S, et al: The treatment of localized Ewing's sarcoma: the experience at the Istituto Ortopedico Rizzoli in 163 cases treated with and without adjuvant chemotherapy. *Cancer* 49(8):1561–1570, 1982.

Bernstein M, Kovar H, Paulussen M, et al: Ewing's sarcoma family of tumors: current management. *Oncologist* 11(5):503–519, 2006.

Burchill SA: Ewing's sarcoma: diagnostic, prognostic, and therapeutic implications of molecular abnormalities. *J Clin Pathol* 56(2):96–102, 2003.

Devoe K, Weidner N: Immunohistochemistry of small round-cell tumors. *Semin Diagn Pathol* 17(3):216–224, 2000.

Eggli KD, Quiogue T, Moser RP Jr: Ewing's sarcoma. *Radiol Clin North Am* 31(2):325–337, 1993.

Kennedy JG, Frelinghuysen P, Hoang BH: Ewing sarcoma: current concepts in diagnosis and treatment. *Curr Opin Pediatr* 15(1):53–57, 2003.

Kissane JM, Askin FB, Foulkes M, et al: Ewing's sarcoma of bone: clinicopathologic aspects of 303 cases from the Intergroup Ewing's Sarcoma Study. *Hum Pathol* 14(9):773–779, 1983.

Mendenhall CM, Marcus RB Jr, Enneking WF, et al: The prognostic significance of soft tissue extension in Ewing's sarcoma. *Cancer* 51(5):913–917, 1983.

Nascimento AG, Unni KK, Pritchard DJ, et al: A clinicopathologic study of 20 cases of large-cell (atypical) Ewing's sarcoma of bone. *Am J Surg Pathol* 4(1):29–36, 1980.

Rosen G, Caparros B, Nirenberg A, et al: Ewing's sarcoma: ten-year experience with adjuvant chemotherapy. *Cancer* 47(9):2204–2213, 1981.

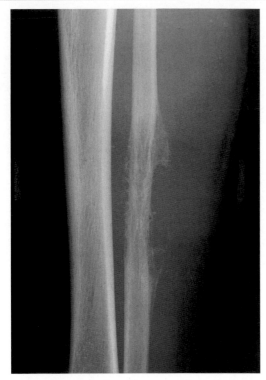

Figure 63–1 This radiograph of Ewing's sarcoma shows the characteristic lytic appearance of such tumors. A diaphyseal location, as in this case involving the fibula, is most common. The periosteum is generally elevated in such cases, resulting in Codman's triangle and an associated soft tissue mass.

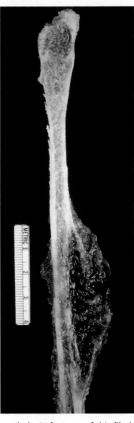

Figure 63–2 The gross pathologic features of this fibular Ewing's sarcoma correlate well with the radiographic features shown in Figure 63–1. The lesional tissue is frequently soft and hemorrhagic, as in this case. A small incisional biopsy may yield a loose gray–white tissue that mimics the gross features of an osteomyelitis.

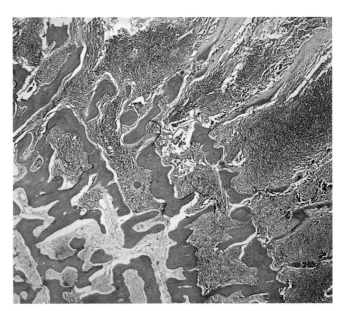

Figure 63–3 At low magnification, Ewing's sarcoma is a highly cellular tumor composed of small round cells. The periosteum is elevated by this cellular proliferation, resulting in a layering of periosteal new bone that may appear as an "onion skin" radiographically. The reactive new bone is shown in this photomicrograph.

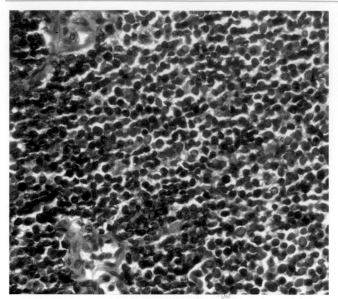

Figure 63–4 At higher magnification, Ewing's sarcoma is composed of small round cells; frequently, however, two cell types are identifiable. The nuclei of the most prominent type are round with a regular chromatin pattern; if nucleoli are present, they are indistinct. The second cell type contains a dark, hyperchromatic nucleus and is thought to represent a degenerative change.

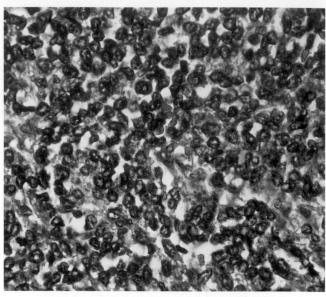

Figure 63–5 Ewing's sarcoma is homogeneous at high magnification, and no matrix is identifiable within the tumor. In contrast, small cell osteosarcoma should have identifiable osteoid within the tumor.

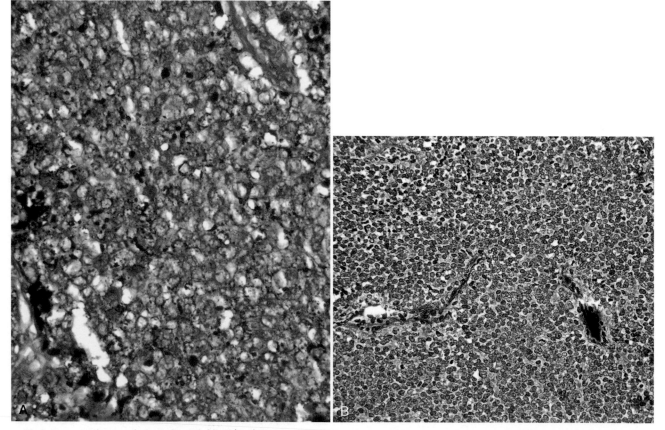

Figure 63–6 Two special stains, the periodic acid–Schiff (PAS) stain and the reticulin stain, are helpful in confirming the diagnosis of Ewing's sarcoma. Ewing's sarcoma is generally, but not uniformly, PAS-positive (*A*) and reticulin-poor (*B*).

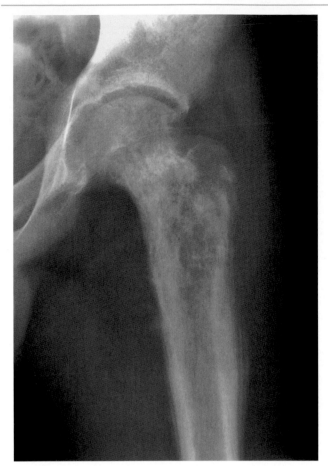

Figure 63–7 This radiograph shows Ewing's sarcoma of the proximal femur. The lesion is long and poorly marginated. The multilaminae, or "onion skin," periosteal reaction is evident.

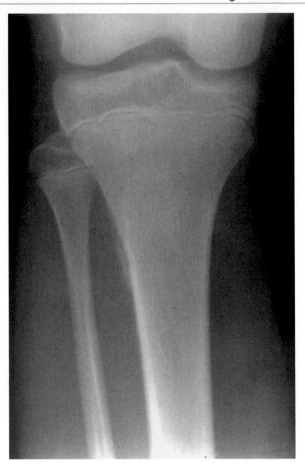

Figure 63–9 This plane radiograph shows only new bone formation associated with Ewing's sarcoma of the proximal tibia.

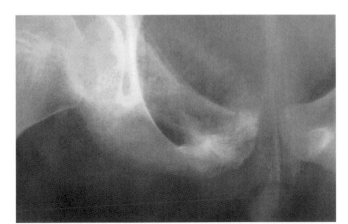

Figure 63–8 This Ewing's sarcoma of the pubic ramus shows irregular lysis, spiculated new bone, and an associated soft tissue mass. These features are frequently seen with this tumor.

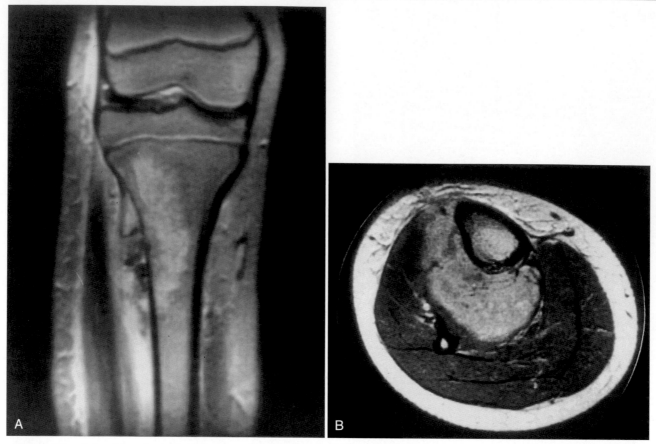

Figure 63–10 Although the plane radiographic features are unimpressive (see Fig. 63–9), coronal magnetic resonance imaging (MRI) shows a fairly large intramedullary tumor with cortical destruction and elevation of the periosteum (*A*). Axial MRI of the same tumor shows a large soft tissue mass typical of this tumor (*B*). This case demonstrates the utility of computed tomography (CT) and MRI in the evaluation of cases that are inconspicuous on plane radiographic evaluation.

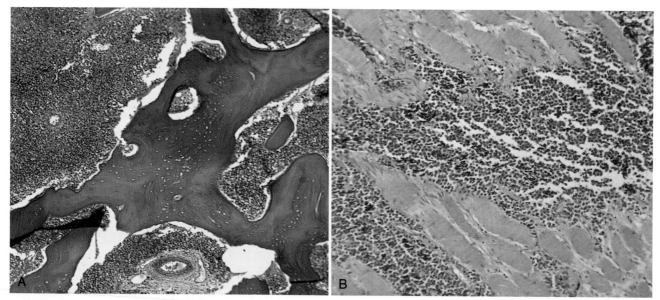

Figure 63–11 These photomicrographs illustrate the permeative nature of the pattern of growth of Ewing's sarcoma, whether it is in bone (*A*) or involves the soft tissues adjacent to the affected bone (*B*).

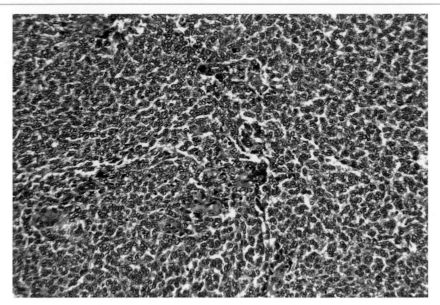

Figure 63–12 The cytologic features of Ewing's sarcoma are homogeneous, as this photomicrograph shows. Foci of necrosis may be present.

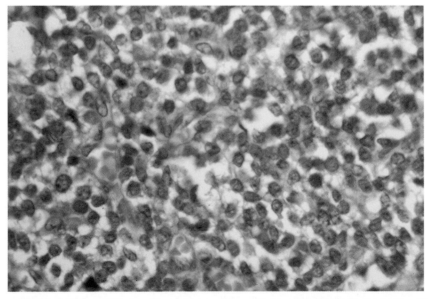

Figure 63–13 At high magnification, the nuclei are uniform and show a finely granular chromatin pattern.

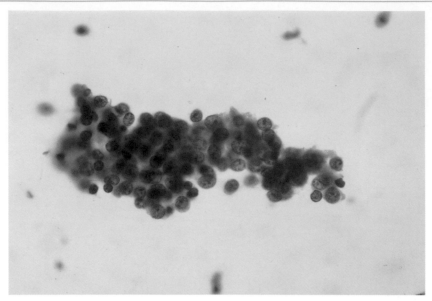

Figure 63–14 Fine-needle aspiration of Ewing's sarcoma yields small, uniform cells, which may be found in clusters but are generally noncohesive in smear preparations. Although diagnosis of the primary tumor with this technique is possible, its main utility is in confirming metastatic disease, as in this case of a transthoracic needle aspirate in a patient with a primary tumor in the ilium.

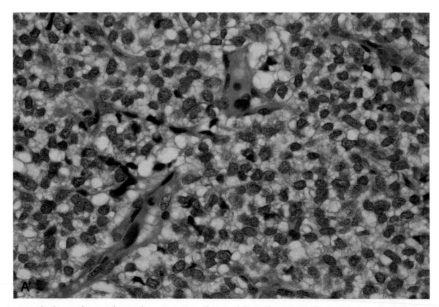

Figure 63–15 *A*: The photomicrograph shows the cytologic characteristics of typical Ewing's sarcoma in contrast to the "atypical" Ewing's sarcoma shown in *B*.

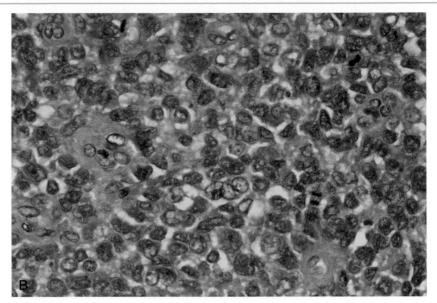

Figure 63–15 Cont'd, *B*: Atypical Ewing's sarcoma demonstrates greater cytologic pleomorphism than the uniform small cell cytology of typical Ewing's sarcoma.

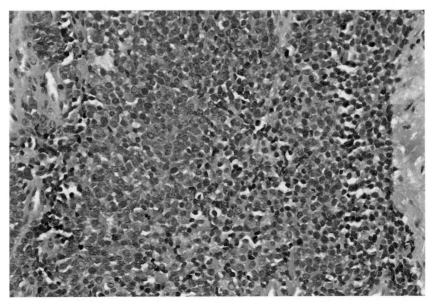

Figure 63–16 Ewing's sarcoma of the small bones is associated with a better prognosis than Ewing's sarcoma in other locations. The tumor shown in this photomicrograph involved a carpal bone.

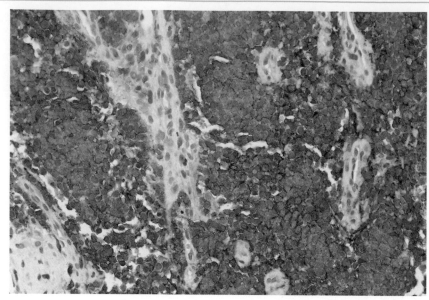

Figure 63–17 Immunohistochemical stains for lymphoid markers and CD99 (MIC2) can be helpful in distinguishing Ewing's sarcoma from lymphoma and other "small round cell tumors." This Ewing's sarcoma of the small bones of the hand shows strong CD99 positivity.

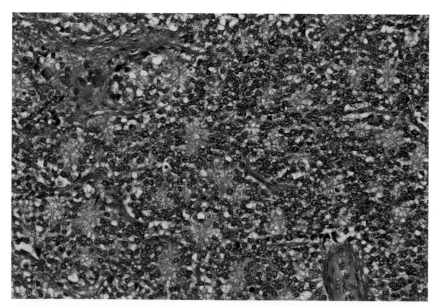

Figure 63–18 Ewing's sarcoma shows a spectrum of histologic patterns ranging from a sheetlike proliferation of small cells to the pattern of primitive neuroectodermal tumor (PNET) illustrated in this photomicrograph. Tumors that show the typical pattern of Ewing's sarcoma may show a PNET histologic pattern with recurrence.

Section 2G: Secondary Sarcomas

Paget's Sarcoma

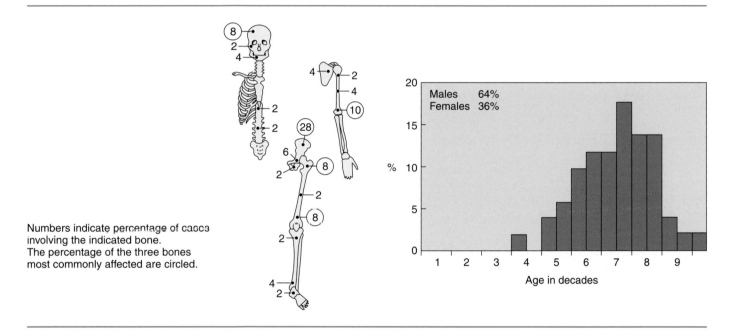

Numbers indicate percentage of cases involving the indicated bone.
The percentage of the three bones most commonly affected are circled.

Males 64%
Females 36%

%

Age in decades

Clinical Signs

1. A painful mass lesion is felt in the region of the affected bone.
2. Symptoms are rapidly progressive.

Clinical Symptoms

1. Pain is felt in the affected region. An increase in pain in one bone in a patient with Paget's disease should arouse suspicion of the development of a sarcoma.
2. Swelling may result from soft tissue extension of the tumor.

Major Radiographic Features

1. Most tumors are purely lytic, although sclerotic and mixed lesions do occur.
2. The bone of origin usually shows changes of Paget's disease.
3. The tumor extends into the surrounding soft tissue.
4. There is a pattern of "geographic" bone destruction.
5. Computed tomography or magnetic resonance imaging may be useful for detection when a soft tissue component is present. Compared with uncomplicated Paget's disease with respect to location, these sarcomas have a predilection for the humerus and only rarely arise in the spine.

Radiographic Differential Diagnosis

1. Paget's disease with marked lysis.
2. Florid Paget's disease extending into soft tissues.
3. Magnetic resonance imaging will show preservation of marrow fat when massive osteolysis is a result of the exacerbation of the lytic phase of Paget's and will show replacement of marrow fat on T1-weighted sequences when it is a result of sarcoma.

Major Pathologic Features

Gross

1. A destructive lesion involves the bone and extends into the soft tissues.
2. The soft, fleshy tumor generally is whitish to brown.

Microscopic

1. At low magnification, the tumor is highly cellular.
2. The tumor generally is composed of spindle cells.
3. At higher magnification, the spindle cells show significant pleomorphism and cytologic atypia.
4. The specific diagnosis may be that of osteosarcoma, fibrosarcoma, or malignant fibrous histiocytoma.

Pathologic Differential Diagnosis

Benign lesions

1. Lytic phase of Paget's disease (radiographic, primarily).
2. Fracture callus.
3. Myositis ossificans (heterotopic ossification).

Malignant lesions

1. Malignant lymphoma.
2. Osteosarcoma.
3. Fibrosarcoma.
4. Malignant fibrous histiocytoma.

Treatment

1. **Primary modality:** Usually, the tumor's aggressive behavior, with extensive local involvement, requires amputation to achieve an adequately wide surgical margin.
2. **Other possible approaches:** Preoperative chemotherapy and limb-saving resection may be chosen if surgical staging suggests that an adequately wide margin can be achieved. Radiation therapy is used for surgically inaccessible lesions, and an aggressive approach with thoracotomy is used for pulmonary metastases.

References

Boutin RD, Spitz DJ, Newman JS, et al: Complications in Paget disease at MR imaging. *Radiology* 209(3):641–651, 1998.

Donath J, Szilagyi M, Fornet B, et al: Pseudosarcoma in Paget's disease. *Eur J Radiol* 10(10):1664–1668, 2000.

Haibach H, Farrell C, Dittrich FJ: Neoplasms arising in Paget's disease of bone: a study of 82 cases. *Am J Clin Pathol* 83(5):594–600, 1985.

Lamovec J, Rener M, Spiler M: Pseudosarcoma in Paget's disease of bone. *Ann Diagn Pathol* 3(2):99–103, 1999.

Mankin HJ, Hornicek FJ: Paget's sarcoma: a historical and outcome review. *Clin Orthop Relat Res* 438:97–102, 2005.

Sundaram M, Khanna G, El-Khoury G: T1 weighted MR imaging for distinguishing large osteolysis of Paget's disease from sarcomatous degeneration. *Skeletal Radiol* 30(7):378–383, 2001.

Wick MR, Siegal GP, McLeod RA, et al: Sarcomas of bone complicating osteitis deformans (Paget's disease): fifty years' experience. *Am J Surg Pathol* 5(1):47–59, 1981.

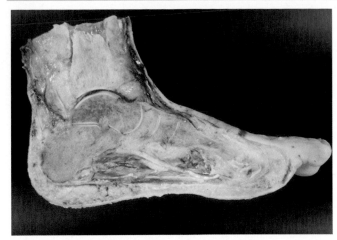

Figure 64–1 This gross specimen shows a case of Paget's sarcoma involving the distal tibia. The patient initially had suffered a pathologic fracture of the distal tibia and had been treated conservatively for the fracture because the underlying malignancy was radiographically subtle. The tumor has broken through the cortex and extended into the soft tissues of the foot.

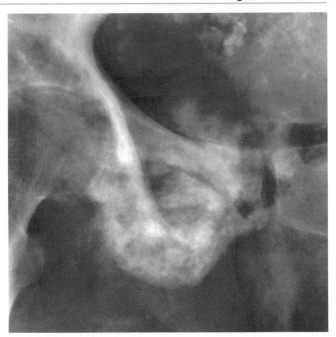

Figure 64–3 A blastic Paget sarcoma, arising in the ischium and pubis in a region of preexisting Paget's disease, is shown in this radiograph. The soft tissue component of the tumor contains bony mineralization indicative of an osteosarcoma.

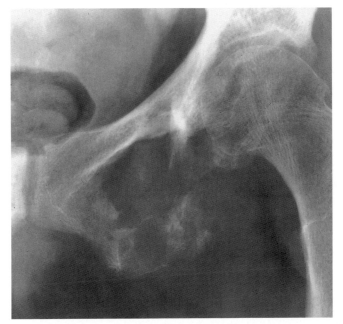

Figure 64–2 This radiograph shows a lytic Paget sarcoma arising in the ischium with preexisting Paget's disease and causing considerable bone destruction.

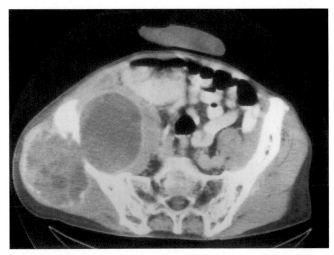

Figure 64–4 This computed tomographic (CT) scan shows Paget's sarcoma of the pelvis with a large soft tissue component surrounding the iliac bone. Both innominate bones show evidence of Paget's disease as well.

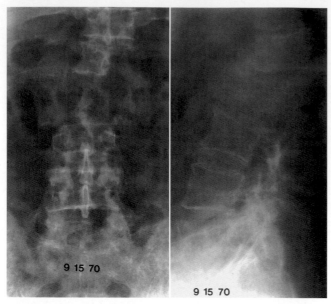

Figure 64–5 This radiograph reveals extensive lysis of a vertebra resulting from uncomplicated Paget's disease. The radiographic appearance is that of a malignancy; however, the spine is a rare site for this complication of Paget's disease.

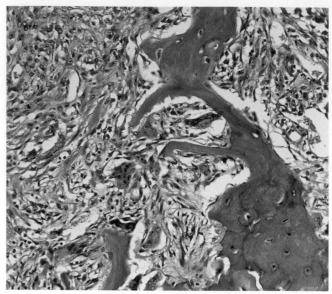

Figure 64–7 Some sarcomas that complicate Paget's disease do not demonstrate matrix production. This photomicrograph shows such a case. These lesions may be classified as fibrosarcomas or as malignant fibrous histiocytomas, depending on other features evident in the tumor.

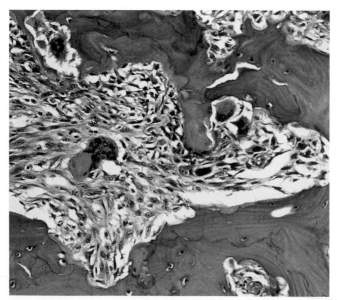

Figure 64–6 Paget's sarcomas may show a variety of histologic patterns. As this photomicrograph illustrates, osteosarcoma is the most common.

Postradiation Sarcoma

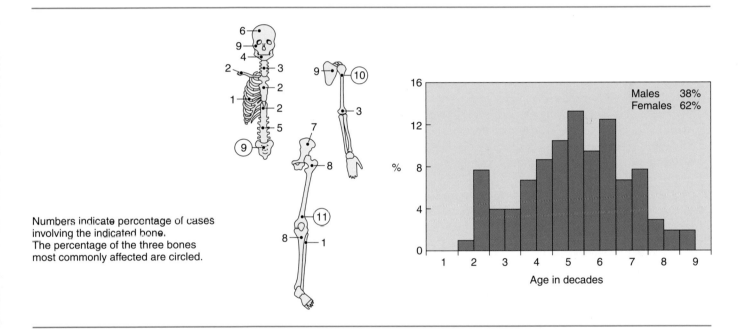

Numbers indicate percentage of cases involving the indicated bone.
The percentage of the three bones most commonly affected are circled.

Males 38%
Females 62%

% / Age in decades

Clinical Signs

1. A tender mass lesion is found on physical examination.
2. Skin changes compatible with prior radiation therapy may be present.

Clinical Symptoms

1. Pain is felt in the region of prior radiation therapy.
2. The interval between radiation therapy and diagnosis of sarcoma has varied from 2.75 to 55 years in cases treated at the Mayo Clinic, with an average interval of 15.1 years.
3. A swelling may be noted by the patient.

Major Radiographic Features

1. The tumor may arise from normal bone or in an area of a preexisting lesion within the radiation portal.
2. The underlying bone often is altered by radiation, surgery, the preexisting abnormality, or some combination of these.
3. The underlying changes in the affected bone may obscure the lesion early in the course of the disease.
4. The latent period ranges from 2.75 to 55 years, with an average of 15.1 years.
5. Postradiation sarcomas are radiographically similar to conventional tumors.
6. A soft tissue mass, cortical destruction, and extraosseous bone production are indicative of sarcoma.

Radiographic Differential Diagnosis

1. Metastatic disease.
2. Radiation-induced change without sarcoma.
3. Osteoporosis.
4. Insufficiency stress fracture.

Major Pathologic Features

Gross

1. These tumors tend to be soft and fleshy.
2. The tumor has most commonly extended beyond the confines of the affected bone and has an associated soft tissue mass.
3. Foci of hemorrhage and necrosis may be identifiable.
4. Matrix production in the form of osteoid or even cartilage may be seen, and calcification may be present on a degenerative basis.

Microscopic

1. At low magnification, the pattern varies from tumor to tumor. Of postradiation sarcomas compiled by the Mayo Clinic, the majority (approximately 50%) showed osteoid production and were classified as osteosarcomas.
2. Spindle cell tumors lacking osteoid matrix production were the second largest group, accounting for 42% of the total, with the majority of these being classified as fibrosarcomas and the remainder as malignant fibrous histiocytomas.
3. At higher magnification, the cytologic characteristics are those of a pleomorphic high-grade sarcoma. The nuclei vary in size, shape, and nuclear-staining characteristics.

Pathologic Differential Diagnosis

Benign lesions

1. Reactive spindle cell proliferation in the region of prior irradiation.
2. Fracture callus at a site of pathologic fracture after radiation therapy.

Malignant lesions

1. Osteosarcoma.
2. Fibrosarcoma.
3. Malignant fibrous histiocytoma.

Treatment

1. **Primary modality:** Preoperative chemotherapy and limb-saving resection if a wide surgical margin can be achieved. Reconstruction is individualized and depends on the location of the tumor. Amputation will be necessary if surgical staging indicates that an adequately wide margin cannot be achieved to preserve the neurovascular structures.
2. **Other possible approaches:** Radiation therapy for lesions in inaccessible sites, thoracotomy for pulmonary metastases, or chemotherapy protocols similar to those used for osteosarcoma may be done.

References

Brady LW: Radiation-induced sarcomas of bone. *Skeletal Radiol* 4(2):72–78, 1979.

Ergun H, Howland WJ: Postradiation atrophy of mature bone. *CRC Crit Rev Diagn Imaging* 12(3):225–243, 1980.

Frassica FJ, Frassica DA, Wold LE, et al: Postradiation sarcoma of bone. *Orthopedics* 16(1):105–106, 109, 1993.

Frassica FJ, Sim FH, Frassica DA, et al: Survival and management considerations in postirradiation osteosarcoma and Paget's osteosarcoma. *Clin Orthop Relat Res* (270):120–127, 1991.

Unni KK, Dahlin DC: Premalignant tumors and conditions of bone. *Am J Surg Pathol* 3(1):47–60, 1979.

Weatherby RP, Dahlin DC, Ivins JC: Postradiation sarcoma of bone: review of 78 Mayo Clinic cases. *Mayo Clin Proc* 56(5):294–306, 1981.

Williams HJ, Davies AM: The effect of X-rays on bone: a pictorial review. *Eur Radiol* 16(3):619–633, 2006.

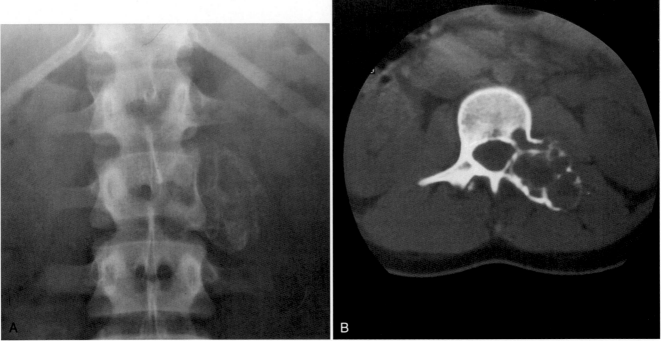

Figure 67–9 This radiograph (*A*) and CT scan (*B*) demonstrate an aneurysmal bone cyst involving the L2 vertebra. When the vertebrae are involved, it is generally the posterior or dorsal elements that are affected; the radiographic appearance is that of an expansile, lytic defect.

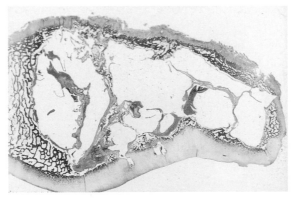

Figure 67–10 Multiple septa are present in an aneurysmal bone cyst, as shown in this low-power photomicrograph in which the fibrous septa are seen traversing the cystic space.

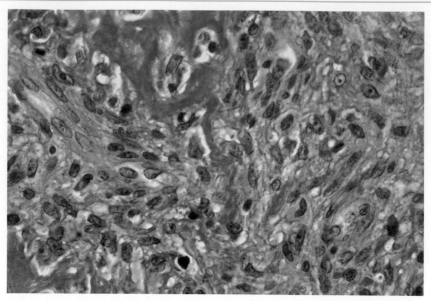

Figure 67–11 The fibrous bone present in the septa of the lesion may suggest the possibility that the lesion is an osteosarcoma. However, the loose arrangement of the lesion, its vascular appearance, and the presence of bone may also mimic the appearance of osteoblastoma.

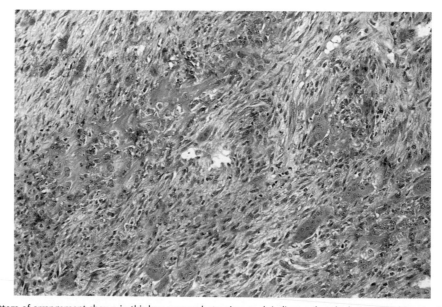

Figure 67–12 The loose pattern of arrangement shown in this low-power photomicrograph indicates that the lesion is proliferative in nature and not neoplastic.

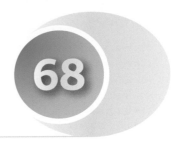

Unicameral Bone Cyst (Simple Cyst)

Clinical Signs

1. The majority of these lesions are incidental radiographic "abnormalities."
2. A painful mass occasionally may be identified on physical examination.

Clinical Symptoms

1. The majority of tumors are asymptomatic.
2. The onset of pain is abrupt (associated with pathologic fracture).
3. Rarely, swelling in the region of the lesion may be noticed.

Major Radiographic Features

1. Cysts usually occur in the upper humerus or upper femur.
2. They frequently abut the epiphyseal plate.
3. They are often large and elongated.
4. Expansion is usually present but does not exceed the width of the epiphyseal plate.
5. There is sharp margination, often with trabeculation.
6. Pathologic fracture occurs and may result in healing or bone fragment settling to the dependent part of the lesion, indicative of fluid.

Radiographic Differential Diagnosis

1. Aneurysmal bone cyst.
2. Fibrous dysplasia.

Major Pathologic Features

Gross

1. The cystic cavity usually contains a straw-colored fluid.
2. If there has been bleeding into the cyst, pathologic fracture, or a previous attempt to insert a needle into the lesion, the fluid may be blood-tinged or frankly bloody.
3. Occasionally, partial or complete septation of the cyst may be seen.

Microscopic

1. At low magnification, the lining of the cyst appears as a thin rim of fibrous connective tissue.
2. Thicker areas of the cyst wall contain multinucleated giant cells.
3. Amorphous eosinophilic debris (probably fibrin) frequently is identified in the hypocellular fibrous connective tissue. This may undergo calcification, resulting in an appearance simulating that of cementum.
4. At higher magnification, no cytologic atypia is appreciated.

Pathologic Differential Diagnosis

Benign lesions

1. Aneurysmal bone cyst.
2. Giant cell tumor.

Malignant lesions

1. Osteosarcoma. Rarely, this has been mistakenly treated as a simple cyst. Radiographic features should aid in avoiding this mistake.

Treatment

1. **Primary modality:** Treatment consists of dual-needle aspiration of the cyst and injection of methylprednisolone. Multiple steroid injections may be necessary to promote healing of the cyst.
2. **Other possible approaches:** In patients with loss of structural integrity in a weightbearing bone associated with a large cyst, curettage and grafting are indicated.

References

Bauer TW, Dorfman HD: Intraosseous ganglion: a clinicopathologic study of 11 cases. *Am J Surg Pathol* 6(3):207–213, 1982.

Boseker EH, Bickel WH, Dahlin DC: A clinicopathologic study of simple unicameral bone cysts. *Surg Gynecol Obstet* 127(3):550–560, 1968.

Capanna R, Campanacci DA, Manfrini M: Unicameral and aneurysmal bone cysts. *Orthop Clin North Am* 27(3):605–614, 1996.

Capanna R, Dal Monte A, Gitelis S, et al: The natural history of unicameral bone cyst after steroid injection. *Clin Orthop Relat Res* 166:204–211, 1982.

Hecht AC, Gebhardt MC: Diagnosis and treatment of unicameral and aneurysmal bone cysts in children. *Curr Opin Pediatr* 10(1):87–94, 1998.

Keenan S, Bui-Mansfield LT: Musculoskeletal lesions with fluid-fluid level: a pictorial essay. *J Comput Assist Tomogr* 30(3):517–524, 2006.

Lokiec F, Wientroub S: Simple bone cyst: etiology, classification, pathology, and treatment modalities. *J Pediatr Orthop B* 7(4):262–273, 1998.

Schajowicz F, Sainz MC, Slullitel JA: Juxta-articular bone cysts (intra-osseous ganglia): a clinicopathological study of eighty-eight cases. *J Bone Joint Surg Br* 61(1):107–116, 1979.

Wilkins RM: Unicameral bone cysts. *J Am Acad Orthop Surg* 8(4):217–224, 2000.

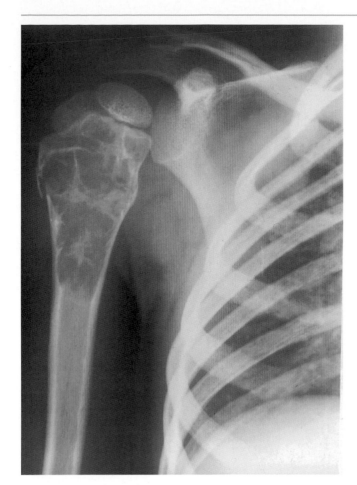

Figure 68–1 This radiograph shows a unicameral bone cyst abutting against the physis of the upper humerus. The lesion has resulted in mild expansion of the bone and shows sharp margination. A pathologic fracture is present, and trabeculation is evident.

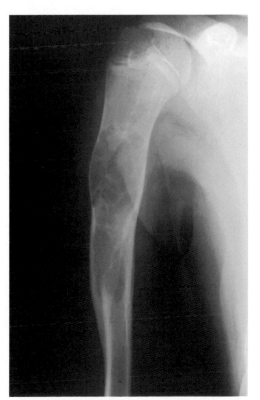

Figure 68–2 Migration of this unicameral bone cyst of the humerus has resulted in a diaphyseal location for the lesion.

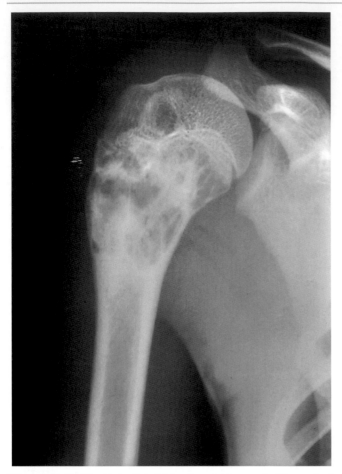

Figure 68–3 Considerable healing of this unicameral bone cyst of the proximal humerus has occurred after a pathologic fracture sustained 8 months earlier.

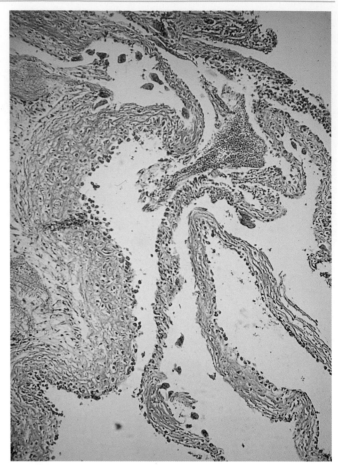

Figure 68–5 At low magnification, curetted fragments of tissue from a simple cyst may demonstrate septa similar to those seen in aneurysmal bone cyst. Usually, they show only a thin lining on the bone.

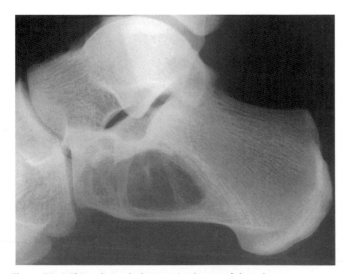

Figure 68–4 This radiograph shows a simple cyst of the calcaneus.

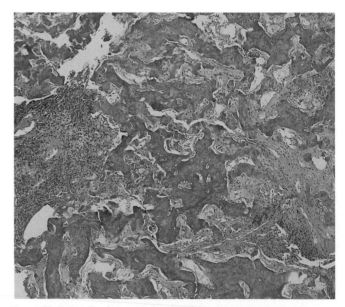

Figure 68–6 Reactive bone may be identified adjacent to simple cysts.

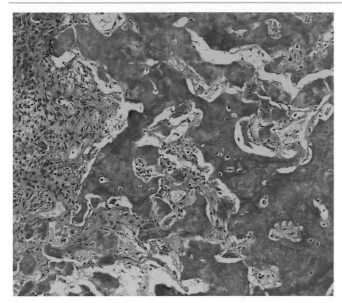

Figure 68–7 Some regions of the wall may contain multinucleated giant cells and have histologic features identical with those of aneurysmal bone cyst.

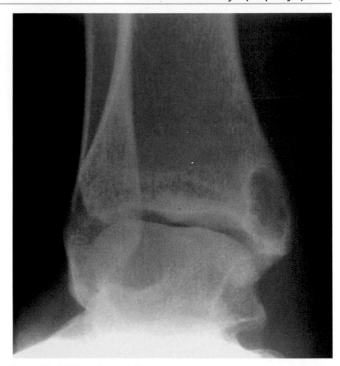

Figure 68–9 This radiograph illustrates an intraosseous ganglion of the distal tibia. Such lesions most commonly involve bones adjacent to the ankle, hip, and knee. Most are eccentric in location as compared with unicameral bone cysts, which are central in location.

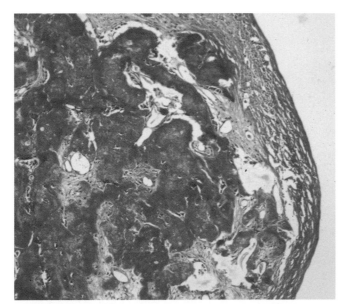

Figure 68–8 Eosinophilic aggregates of calcified fibrinous debris may be identified in the wall of the cyst. The histologic features of such debris may resemble cementum.

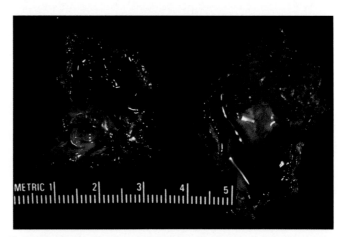

Figure 68–10 This photograph shows the gross pathologic features of an intraosseous ganglion involving the proximal tibia. The thin-walled cyst is filled with mucoid clear fluid similar to that in a ganglion cyst of the soft tissues.

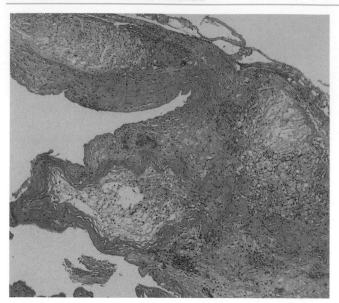

Figure 68—11 The histologic features of an intraosseous ganglion are illustrated in this photomicrograph. The lesion is histologically identical with the soft tissue lesion.

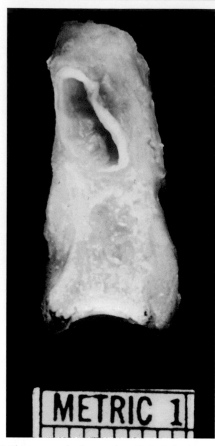

Figure 68–13 The gross and microscopic pathologic features of osseous epidermoid cyst are similar to those of the more common soft tissue lesions, as illustrated in this case involving a distal phalanx of a finger.

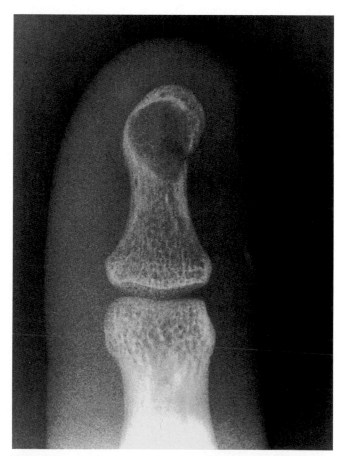

Figure 68–12 Osseous epidermoid cysts most commonly involve the cranial bones and small bones of the hand, as shown in this case involving the distal phalanx of a finger. Such lesions commonly are included in the radiographic differential diagnosis with enchondroma.

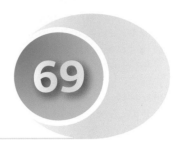

Giant Cell Reaction (Giant Cell Reparative Granuloma)

Clinical Signs

1. A mass lesion may be discovered on physical examination.
2. The mass may be tender to palpation.
3. There are no findings on physical examination in many cases.

Clinical Symptoms

1. Approximately 50% of patients present with local pain as their primary complaint.
2. Approximately 50% of patients present with a localized swelling.
3. Rarely, the lesion is asymptomatic and incidentally discovered on radiographic examination.

Major Imaging Features

1. Most lesions are purely lytic, although occasional sclerosis or calcification is seen.
2. Expansion and cortical thinning, as well as sharp margination, are invariably seen.
3. Cortical breakthrough and new periosteal bone are occasionally seen.
4. Lesions may be intramedullary or rarely surface.
5. On magnetic resonance imaging (MRI), fluid–fluid levels amid solid components may be identified akin to secondary ABCs.
6. On MRI, marrow edema is a frequent finding.

Radiographic Differential Diagnosis

1. Aneurysmal bone cyst.
2. Giant cell tumor.
3. Enchondroma.

Major Pathologic Features

Gross

1. Curetted fragments of bone are reddish-brown.
2. In contrast to aneurysmal bone cyst, the volume of tissue curetted approximates the size of the lesion as identified radiographically.

Microscopic

1. At low magnification, the lesional tissue is composed of spindle cells lying in a fibrous stroma.
2. Numerous multinucleated giant cells are present; these tend to be arranged in a vaguely clustered manner.
3. Reactive new bone with prominent osteoblastic activity resembling osteoblastoma is present.
4. At higher magnification, the mononuclear stromal cells and the giant cells lack cytologic atypia.
5. Mitotic figures may be identified, but in general the mitotic rate is low.

Pathologic Differential Diagnosis

Benign lesions

1. Aneurysmal bone cyst.
2. Brown tumor of hyperparathyroidism.
3. Giant cell tumor.
4. Fracture callus.

Malignant lesions

1. Malignant fibrous histiocytoma.
2. Osteosarcoma.

Treatment

1. **Primary modality:** Excision by curettage and bone grafting as necessary are usually adequate.

2. Other possible approaches: En bloc resection and skeletal reconstruction may be done when they can be performed without significant compromise in function.

References

Averill RM, Smith RJ, Campbell CJ: Giant-cell tumors of the bones of the hand. *J Hand Surg* 5(1):39–50, 1980.

Bertoni F, Bacchini P, Capanna R, et al: Solid variant of aneurysmal bone cyst. *Cancer* 71(3):729–734, 1993.

D'Alonzo RT, Pitcock JA, Milford LW: Giant-cell reaction of bone: report of two cases. *J Bone Joint Surg Am* 54(6):1267–1271, 1972.

Glass TA, Mills SE, Fechner RE, et al: Giant-cell reparative granuloma of the hands and feet. *Radiology* 149(1):65–68, 1983.

Ilaslan H, Sundaram M, Unni KK: The solid variant of aneurysmal bone cyst in long tubular bones: giant cell reparative granuloma. *Am J Roentgenol* 180(6):1681–1687, 2003.

Lorenzo JC, Dorfman HD: Giant-cell reparative granuloma of short tubular bones of the hands and feet. *Am J Surg Pathol* 4(6):551–563, 1980.

Ratner V, Dorfman HD: Giant cell reparative granuloma of the hand and foot bones. *Clin Orthop Relat Res* 260:251–258, 1990.

Wold LE, Dobyns JH, Swee RG, et al: Giant cell reaction (giant cell reparative granuloma) of the small bones of the hands and feet (30 cases). *Am J Surg Pathol* 10(7):491–496, 1986.

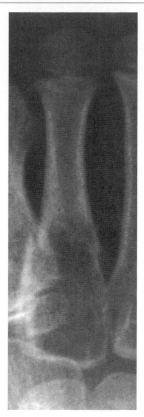

Figure 69–1 This radiograph shows a giant cell reaction of the proximal second metacarpal. There is cortical expansion and thinning by this purely lytic process.

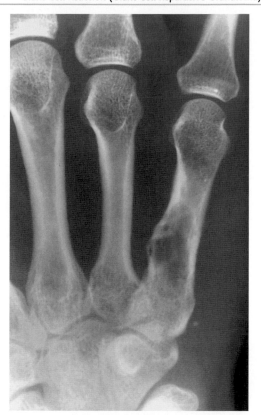

Figure 69–3 In this purely lytic giant cell reaction of the proximal metacarpal, the lesion is well marginated and shows cortical expansion and thinning.

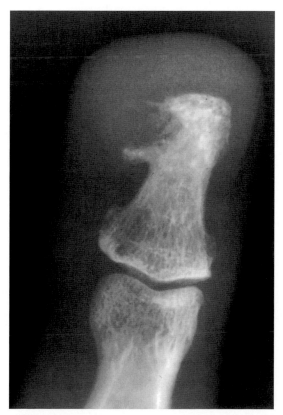

Figure 69–2 A giant cell reaction of the distal phalanx is shown in this radiograph. The lesion arose eccentrically and has extended into the soft tissues.

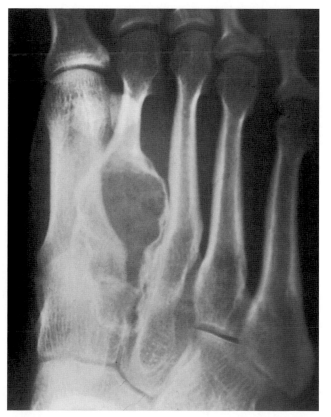

Figure 69–4 Marked bony expansion has resulted from the presence of this large, lytic giant cell reaction of the proximal second metatarsal.

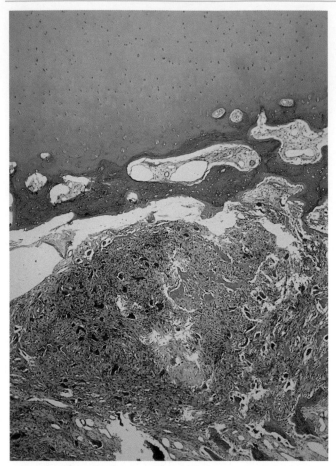

Figure 69–5 This photomicrograph shows a giant cell reaction extending to the end of a small bone in the hand. At low magnification, giant cells may be seen to slightly cluster in these lesions.

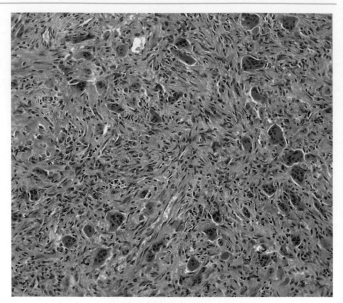

Figure 69–6 Giant cell reactions show a distinctly spindled mononuclear stromal component, as in this photomicrograph. This is in contrast with benign giant cell tumors, in which the mononuclear stromal component is round to oval.

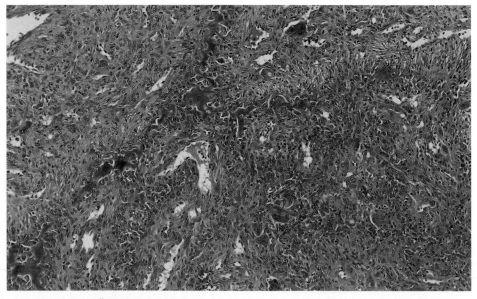

Figure 69–7 The stromal component of giant cell reactions is generally more collagenous than that of giant cell tumors. Osteoid may be seen in the stroma as well.

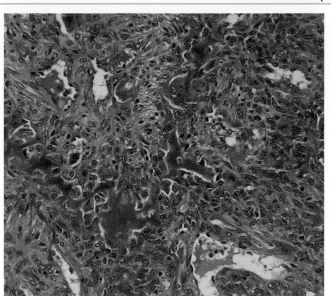

Figure 69–8 Giant cell reactions, like this lesion involving the fifth metacarpal, have histologic features similar to those of the solid variant of aneurysmal bone cyst.

Fibroma (Metaphyseal Fibrous Defect)

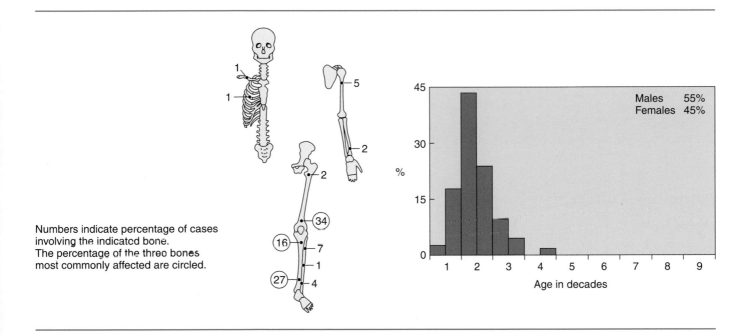

Numbers indicate percentage of cases involving the indicated bone.
The percentage of the three bones most commonly affected are circled.

Males 55%
Females 45%

%

Age in decades

Clinical Signs

1. Physical examination is usually unrevealing in these cases.
2. A slight swelling may be present if the affected bone is near the skin (e.g., the distal tibia).

Clinical Symptoms

1. These lesions are usually asymptomatic and are discovered on radiographic examination for an unrelated condition.
2. Local pain of short duration may be present.
3. Pathologic fracture may be the first clinical symptom.

Major Radiographic Features

1. The location of the lesion is metaphyseal.
2. The lesion is expansile and sharply marginated and is located in the cortex.
3. The lesion appears multilocular and has a scalloped margin.
4. The long axis of the lesion generally parallels that of the affected bone, and a sclerotic rim surrounds it.
5. Multiple lesions may be present.

Radiographic Differential Diagnosis

1. Chondromyxoid fibroma.
2. Fibrous dysplasia.

471

Major Pathologic Features

Gross

1. The cortex may be attenuated in the area of the lesion but remains intact unless pathologic fracture has occurred.
2. The lesion is well demarcated from the surrounding bone.
3. Curetted fragments are fibrous and vary from yellow to brown, depending on the proportion of fibrous tissue to lipid-laden or hemosiderin-laden histiocytes present in the lesion.

Microscopic

1. At low magnification, the pattern is variable from region to region. Zones of spindle cells are arranged in a storiform pattern and interspersed with other foci containing more abundant histiocytic cells.
2. Giant cells are scattered throughout the lesion in irregular clusters. (In general, these cells contain fewer nuclei than the giant cells of giant cell tumor.)
3. Clusters of lipophages are scattered irregularly throughout the lesion.
4. Clusters of hemosiderin-laden macrophages are similarly dispersed.
5. At higher magnification, the nuclei of the spindled cells and histiocytes are regular. Mitotic figures may be present.
6. When pathologic fracture occurs, there may be associated reactive new bone formation.

Pathologic Differential Diagnosis

Benign lesions

1. Giant cell tumor.
2. Benign fibrous histiocytoma.
3. Giant cell tumor of tendon-sheath type.
4. Pigmented villonodular synovitis.

Malignant lesions

1. Malignant fibrous histiocytoma.
2. Osteosarcoma (if pathologic fracture and reactive new bone are misinterpreted).

Treatment

1. **Primary modality:** If the diagnosis is certain and the lesion does not threaten the strength of the bone, observation alone is indicated.
2. **Other possible approaches:** Large lesions occupying more than 50% of the bone diameter pose the risk of fracture. Curettage and bone grafting are curative. Pathologic fractures should be allowed to heal prior to surgical intervention.

References

Arata MA, Peterson HA, Dahlin DC: Pathological fractures through non-ossifying fibromas. Review of the Mayo Clinic experience. *J Bone Joint Surg Am* 63(6):980–988, 1981.

Hod N, Levi Y, Fire G, et al: Scintigraphic characteristics of non-ossifying fibroma in military recruits undergoing bone scintigraphy for suspected stress fractures and lower limb pains. *Nucl Med Commun* 28(1):25–33, 2007.

Ritschl P, Hajek PC, Pechmann U: Fibrous metaphyseal defects. Magnetic resonance imaging appearances. *Skeletal Radiol* 18(4):253–259, 1989.

Steiner GC: Fibrous cortical defect and nonossifying fibroma of bone: a study of the ultrastructure. *Arch Pathol* 97(4):205–210, 1974.

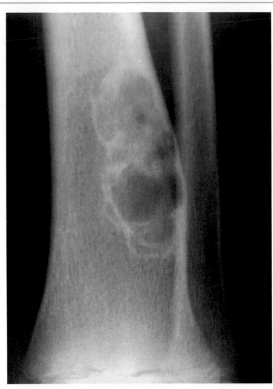

Figure 70–1 Metaphyseal fibrous defects, or fibromas, characteristically have a sharp peripheral margin and a sclerotic rim. These features are well demonstrated in this lesion of the distal diametaphyseal region of the tibia. The affected bone may be expanded, as in this case, and the lesion characteristically has a scalloped margin.

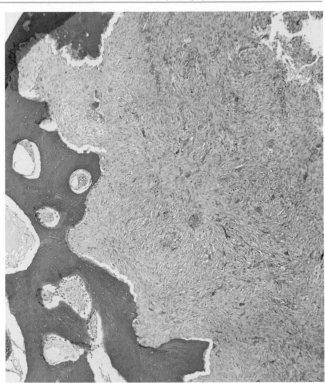

Figure 70–3 At low magnification, the well-circumscribed nature of a metaphyseal fibrous defect is evident at the periphery of the lesion. This photomicrograph shows the edge of a fibular lesion.

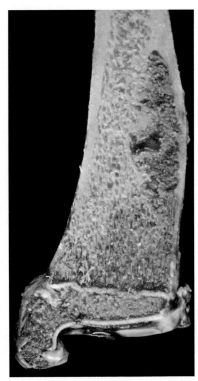

Figure 70–2 The gross pathologic features in this case correlate closely with the radiographic features shown in Figure 70–1. The patient had an incidental fibroma identified at the time of diagnosis of a distal femoral osteosarcoma, for which an above-the-knee amputation was performed.

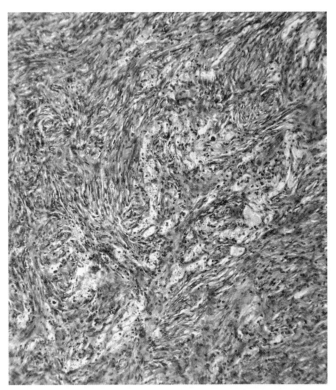

Figure 70–4 The histologic features of a fibroma vary from region to region within the lesion. The cells vary from spindled to round; some show phagocytic activity resulting in hemosiderin-laden or lipid-laden cytoplasm, as illustrated in this photomicrograph.

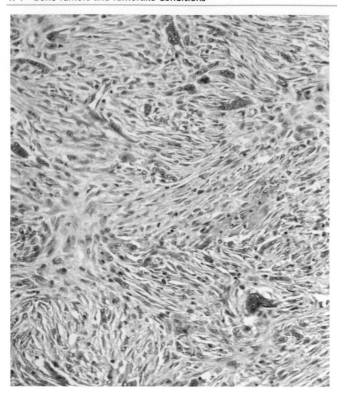

Figure 70–5 The pattern of cell arrangement at low magnification is frequently storiform, as shown in this field from a proximal tibial lesion.

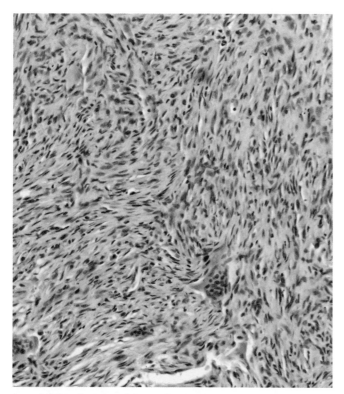

Figure 70–6 Multinucleated giant cells generally are scattered in the lesion; however, they may cluster slightly. This feature may suggest the histologic diagnosis of giant cell tumor; however, the location, radiographic features, ages, and spindled nature of the stromal cells are all characteristics that militate against such a diagnosis.

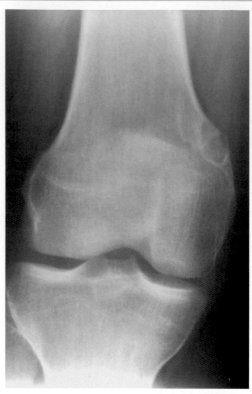

Figure 70–7 This radiograph reveals a small metaphyseal fibroma with a sharp sclerotic margin and slight expansion involving the distal femur. Such a lesion can be confidently identified on the basis of the radiographic features, and surgical intervention is unnecessary.

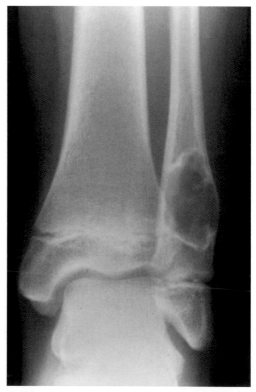

Figure 70–8 This fibroma of the distal fibula also shows the sharp margination and peripheral sclerosis characteristic of this group of lesions.

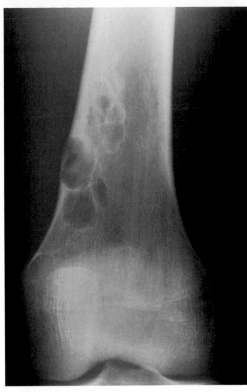

Figure 70–9 This radiograph illustrates the multilocular appearance of a fibroma involving the distal femur.

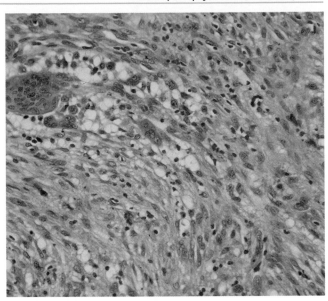

Figure 70–11 Fibroma and benign fibrous histiocytoma share histologic features; both lesions show phagocytic activity and a storiform pattern of growth. The diagnosis of benign fibrous histiocytoma is only viable in a clinical setting in which fibroma is rare. This fibroma shows the characteristic histologic features of these two lesions.

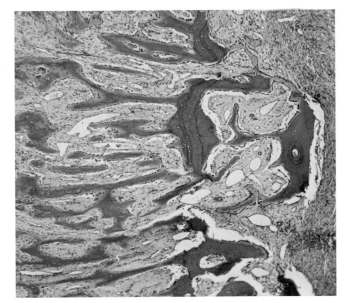

Figure 70–10 If pathologic fracture has occurred through a fibroma, a prominent periosteal reaction may be present. Although the orderly arrangement of the reaction at low magnification is a clue to its benign nature, disregarding this feature may result in a mistaken diagnosis of malignancy based on the mitotic activity and production of osteoid that are evident at high magnification.

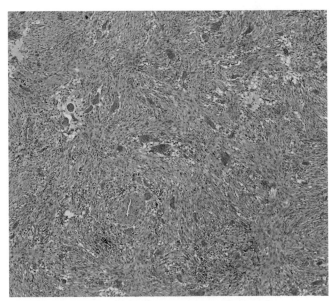

Figure 70–12 Numerous multinucleated giant cells may be present in a fibroma, as in this case involving the proximal tibia.

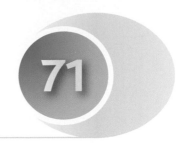

Avulsive Cortical Irregularity (Fibrous Cortical Defect, Periosteal Desmoid)

Clinical Signs

1. There are no findings on physical examination.

Clinical Symptoms

1. These lesions are invariably silent clinically.
2. They are discovered as incidental radiographic findings, often following some trauma.

Major Radiographic Features

1. The lesion is characteristically located along medial posterior supracondylar ridges 1 to 2 cm above the epiphyseal plate, best seen in external rotation.
2. There is cortical fuzziness, irregularity, or spiculation.
3. There may be a small cortical defect.
4. There is no soft tissue mass.
5. The lesion is usually found in boys (3:1), and one third are bilateral.

Radiographic Differential Diagnosis

1. Osteosarcoma.

Major Pathologic Features

Gross

1. In general, these lesions are identified radiographically; biopsy is not necessary.
2. If biopsy is performed, the lesional tissue is found to be nondescript, fibrous, and soft.

Microscopic

1. At low magnification, the lesion is composed of spindle cells.

2. Lesional tissue is hypocellular, and abundant collagen is produced by the spindle cell component of the lesion.
3. At higher magnification, the fibroblasts show no cytologic atypia.
4. Mitotic figures are not identified.

Pathologic Differential Diagnosis

Benign lesions

1. Fibroma.
2. Fibromatosis.

Malignant lesions

1. Fibrosarcoma, well differentiated.

Treatment

1. **Primary modality:** If the radiographic features are classic, no therapy need be initiated.
2. **Other possible approaches:** If the radiographic features are sufficiently atypical to suggest possible tumor, biopsy or curettage is indicated.

References

Pennes DR, Braunstein EM, Glazer GM: Computed tomography of cortical desmoid. *Skeletal Radiol* 12(1):40–42, 1984.

Posch TJ, Puckett ML: Marrow MR signal abnormality associated with bilateral avulsive cortical irregularities in a gymnast. *Skeletal Radiol* 27(9):511–514, 1998.

Resnick D, Greenway G: Distal femoral cortical defects, irregularities, and excavations. *Radiology* 143(2):345–354, 1982.

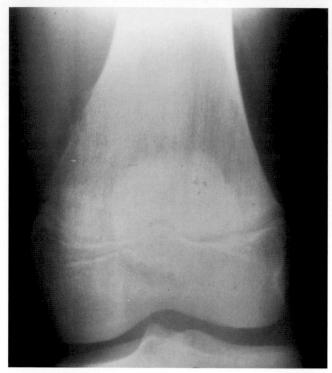

Figure 71–1 This radiograph of the knee shows an elongated area of cortical irregularity along the posterior medial cortex. This region is the most common location for an avulsive cortical irregularity.

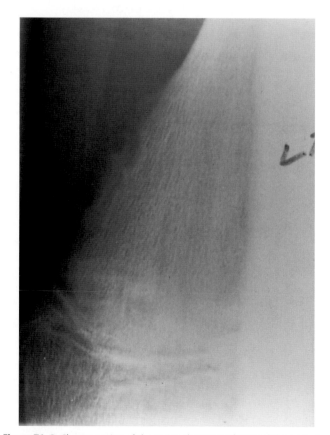

Figure 71–2 Closer scrutiny of the region shows spiculation of the posterior medial cortex in the region of the supracondylar ridge. Such avulsive cortical irregularities are nearly always incidental radiographic findings.

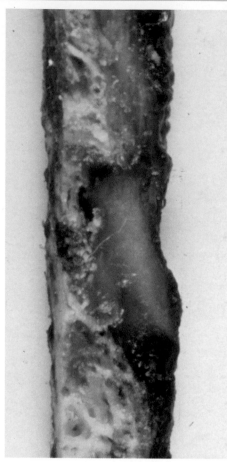

Figure 71–3 Grossly, the lesion presents the pathologic appearance of a small, nondescript region of fibrous tissue associated with the underlying cortical abnormality.

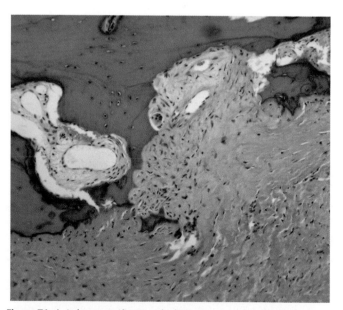

Figure 71–4 At low magnification, the lesion is composed of spindle cells. The lesion is hypocellular, and abundant collagen production may be present.

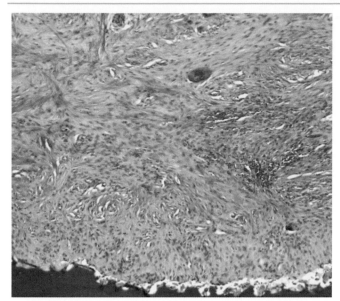

Figure 71–5 At higher magnification, the irregularity of the underlying cortical bone is evident, as this photomicrograph shows. The spindle cells lack cytologic atypia, and the nuclei are uniform, round, and normochromic.

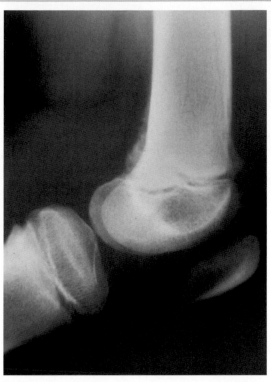

Figure 71–7 This lateral radiograph shows an avulsive cortical irregularity of the distal femur with associated new bone formation. Such reactive new bone may alarm the attending physician and raise suspicion that the lesion represents a malignancy; however, the characteristic location is helpful in correctly identifying the lesion radiographically.

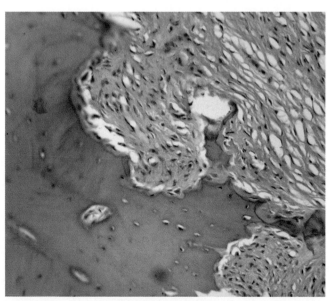

Figure 71–6 At high magnification, no mitotic activity is evident, and the cytologic features are those of mature fibroblasts.

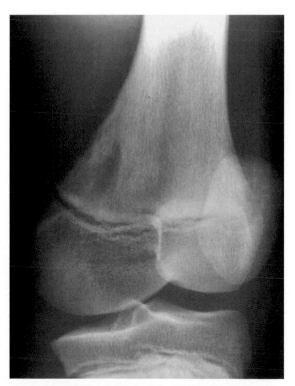

Figure 71–8 This oblique radiograph of the distal femur also demonstrates the cortical irregularity of the femur, as well as the lytic defects and fuzzy, irregular cortical surface commonly associated with this condition.

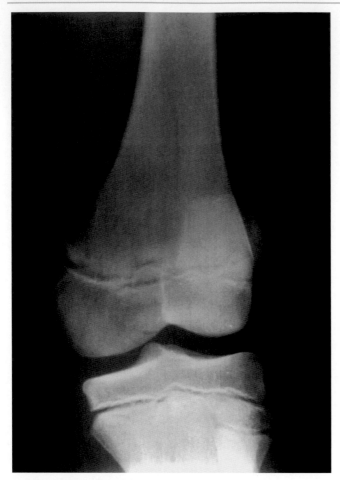

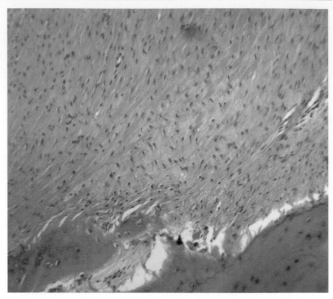

Figure 71–11 Avulsive cortical irregularities histologically are composed of bland spindle cells and abundant collagen. Although these lesions are reactive in origin, they do not show the mitotic activity associated with more common reactive bone and soft tissue lesions, such as aneurysmal bone cyst, proliferative fasciitis, and nodular fasciitis.

Figure 71–9 Some cases may lack periosteal reaction and present as a primarily lytic cortical irregularity, as in this example.

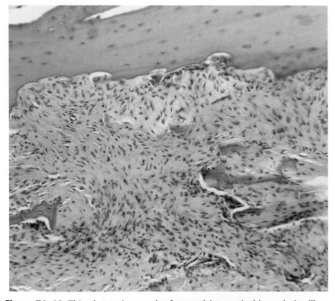

Figure 71–10 This photomicrograph of an avulsive cortical irregularity illustrates the admixture of bone that may be seen in such lesions. A pathologist may mistake this lesion for a bone-forming tumor, particularly when the radiographic features suggest an aggressive neoplastic process.

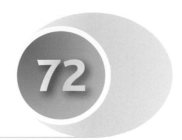

Mesenchymal Hamartoma of the Chest Wall

Clinical Signs

1. A mass lesion is present in the chest wall.
2. Respiratory distress, which varies depending on the size of the lesion, is experienced.

Clinical Symptoms

1. The lesion may be asymptomatic.
2. Difficulty in breathing as a result of mechanical compromise of the underlying lung may occur.
3. The majority of lesions are identified at birth but may not be appreciated until after the child is 6 months of age.
4. A localized swelling of the chest is usually seen.

Major Radiographic Features

1. This is a chest wall lesion of infants.
2. It is often large and usually partially mineralized.
3. One or more ribs are involved, with a combination of erosion and destruction.

Radiographic Differential Diagnosis

1. Aneurysmal bone cyst.
2. Soft tissue tumor.

Major Pathologic Features

Gross

1. The lesional tissue is well circumscribed.
2. Cystic blood-filled spaces may make up a significant proportion of the lesional tissue.
3. The lesional tissue is variable in consistency, but fibrous and chondroid regions may be identified.

4. Calcification may be focally present, particularly at the periphery of the lesion.

Microscopic

1. At low magnification, the lesion varies from region to region.
2. Islands of cartilage resembling epiphyseal plate are identified with regions of spindled cells.
3. Ossifying trabeculae of bone may be identified in the regions of fibroblastic proliferation.
4. The cystic regions are blood-filled and resemble aneurysmal bone cyst.
5. At higher magnification, the proliferating cells lack cytologic atypia.
6. Although mitotic activity may be seen, the lesion is well circumscribed, and atypical mitoses are not present.

Pathologic Differential Diagnosis

Benign lesions

1. Aneurysmal bone cyst.
2. Fibrocartilaginous dysplasia.

Malignant lesions

1. Osteosarcoma.
2. Fibrosarcoma.

Treatment

1. **Primary modality:** resection with a marginal or wide surgical margin.
2. **Other possible approaches:** may regress without treatment.

References

Cohen MC, Drut R, Garcia C, et al: Mesenchymal hamartoma of the chest wall. *Pediatr Pathol* 12(4):525–534, 1992.

Dounies R, Chwals WJ, Lally KP, et al: Hamartomas of the chest wall in infants. *Ann Thorac Surg* 57(4):868–875, 1994.

McCarthy EF, Dorfman HD: Vascular and cartilaginous hamartoma of the ribs in infancy with secondary aneurysmal bone cyst formation. *Am J Surg Pathol* 4(3):247–253, 1980.

McLeod RA, Dahlin DC: Hamartoma (mesenchymoma) of the chest wall in infancy. *Radiology* 131(3):657–661, 1979.

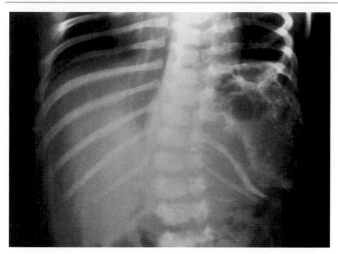

Figure 72–1 This radiograph shows a large mesenchymal hamartoma of the wall of the left lower side of the chest. The lesion is irregularly calcified and shows partial destruction of the seventh through tenth ribs.

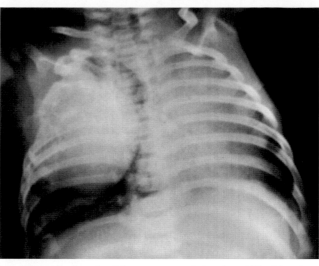

Figure 72–3 The size of such hamartomatous lesions is variable. This radiograph shows a very large lesion involving the right upper part of the chest; it contains a small amount of calcification in the upper portion of the soft tissue mass.

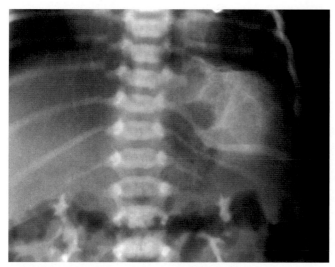

Figure 72–2 This radiograph illustrates the features of a mesenchymal hamartoma of the eighth through tenth ribs on the left side.

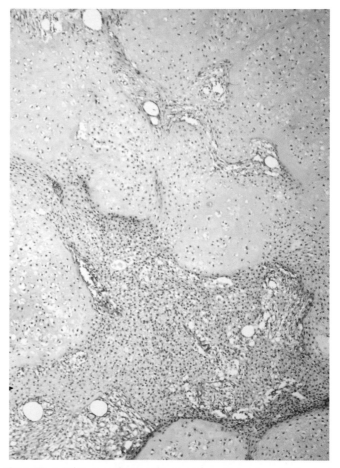

Figure 72–4 At low magnification, the mesenchymal hamartoma of the chest wall shows a variable histology. Chondroid regions are separated by more cellular regions, as in this photomicrograph.

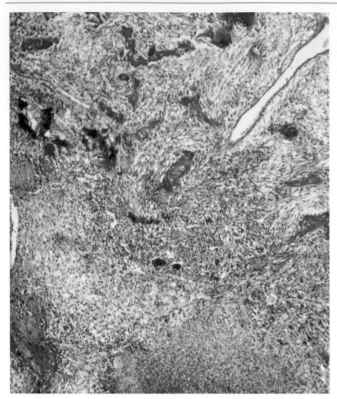

Figure 72–5 Although the solid portions of the lesion may demonstrate a worrisome spindle cell proliferation, mature bony trabeculae appear to arise from the spindle cell portion of the lesion, as this photomicrograph shows.

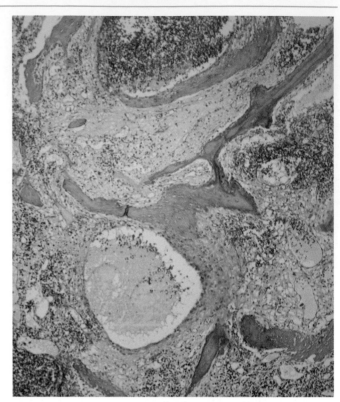

Figure 72–7 Aneurysmal bone cystlike regions are commonly found in mesenchymomas of the chest wall. Such a region is shown in this photomicrograph.

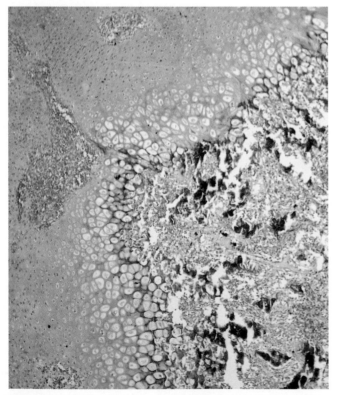

Figure 72–6 This photomicrograph illustrates the juxtaposition of normal cartilage and lesional cartilage in a mesenchymal hamartoma of the chest wall in a male newborn.

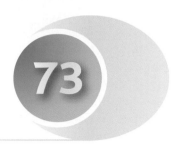

Osteomyelitis

Clinical Signs

1. Children are most commonly affected.
2. Pain is the most common sign; however, this may be minimal in infants.
3. Restricted range of motion and tenderness may be present.
4. In adults, osteomyelitis often complicates other conditions (e.g., chronic debilitating disease, drug addiction, and urinary tract infection).
5. A peripheral blood leukocytosis with a left shift in the differential is usually present; however, this is highly variable.
6. The erythrocyte sedimentation rate (ESR) is elevated.

Clinical Symptoms

1. Fever may occur.
2. Local pain may be present (found most commonly around the knee in children because of involvement of the distal femur or proximal tibia).
3. Swelling in the region of the affected bone may be seen.

Major Radiographic Features

1. A permeative destructive pattern within the medullary cavity may be present.
2. A periosteal reaction may be present.
3. The radiographic identification of bony abnormality usually lags behind the clinical symptoms of the patient by 7 to 10 days.

Radiographic Differential Diagnosis

1. Osteoid osteoma.
2. Osteosarcoma.
3. Ewing's sarcoma.

Major Pathologic Features

Gross

1. Lesional tissue is often loose and "runny" and is surrounded by sclerotic bone.
2. Liquefactive change may be present.

Microscopic

1. An admixture of inflammatory cells may infiltrate the medullary space.
2. There may be loss of normal fatty or hematopoietic marrow.
3. Proliferation of loose edematous connective tissue may be seen within the medullary space.
4. Abscess formation may be present.
5. Necrotic bone (sequestrum) may be seen.
6. Approximately 95% of cases of "uncomplicated" acute osteomyelitis result from staphylococcal infection.

Pathologic Differential Diagnosis

1. Langerhans' cell histiocytosis (histiocytosis X).
2. Malignant lymphoma.
3. Myeloma.

Treatment

Medical

1. An accurate diagnosis is obtained by the following:
   a. Aspiration of organisms for culture.
   b. Positive agglutination titers (e.g., Brucella and Salmonella infections).
2. Key comorbidity and risk factors (i.e., diabetes, intravenous (IV) drug use, human immunodeficiency virus (HIV) infection, and hemoglobinopathies) must be identified.

3. High-dose, organism-specific, parenteral antibiotic therapy is instituted.

Surgical

Treatment varies with the stage of infection (i.e., acute, subacute, or chronic).

1. Open drainage of acute infection is done.
2. Saucerization and excision of infected and dead bone, as well as debridement of tissues, are performed.
3. When necessary, local muscle flaps are used to provide coverage.

References

Chung T: Magnetic resonance imaging in acute osteomyelitis in children. *Pediatr Infect Dis J* 21(9):869–870, 2002.

Connolly LP, Connolly SA: Skeletal scintigraphy in the multimodality assessment of young children with acute skeletal symptoms. *Clin Nucl Med* 28(9):746–754, 2003.

Hanssen AD, Rand JA, Osmon DR: Treatment of the infected total knee arthroplasty with insertion of another prosthesis: the effect of antibiotic-impregnated bone cement. *Clin Orthop Relat Res* 309:44–55, 1994.

Kraemer WJ, Saplys R, Waddell JP, et al: Bone scan, gallium scan and total hip arthroplasty. *J Arthoplasty* 8(6):611–616, 1993.

Langerman RJ, Hawkins BJ, Calhoun JH, et al: Osteomyelitis: diagnosing an often challenging infection. *J Musculoskel Med* 11:56–68, 1994.

Laughlin RT, Wright DG, Mader JT, et al: Osteomyelitis. *Curr Opin Rheumatol* 7(4):315–321, 1995.

Lazzarini L, Mader JT, Calhoun JH: Osteomyelitis in long bones. *J Bone Joint Surg Am* 86-A(10):2305–2318, 2004.

Murray SD, Kehl DK: Chronic recurrent multifocal osteomyelitis. *J Bone Joint Surg Am* 66(7): 1110–1112, 1984.

Patzakis MJ, Calhoun JH, Cierny G 3rd, et al: Symposium on current concepts in the management of osteomyelitis. *Contemp Orthop* 28:157–185, 1994.

Sonnen GM, Henry NK: Pediatric bone and joint infections. *Pediatr Clin North Am* 43(4):933–947, 1996.

Sorsdahl OA, Goodhart GL, Williams HT, et al: Quantitative bone gallium scintigraphy in osteomyelitis. *Skeletal Radiol* 22(4):239–242, 1993.

Termaat MF, Raijmakers PG, Scholten HJ, et al: The accuracy of diagnostic imaging for the assessment of chronic osteomyelitis: a systematic review and meta-analysis. *J Bone Joint Surg Am* 87(11):2464–2471, 2005.

Tuson CE, Hoffman EB, Mann MD: Isotope bone scanning for acute osteomyelitis and septic arthritis in children. *J Bone Joint Surg Br* 76(2): 306–310, 1994.

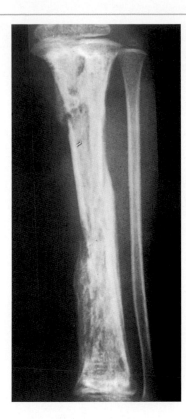

Figure 73–1 This radiograph illustrates bony destruction of a child's tibia caused by acute osteomyelitis. Such destruction may occur relatively rapidly. The tibia and femur are the most common sites of involvement in acute osteomyelitis.

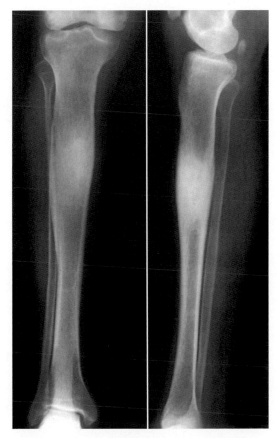

Figure 73–2 This radiograph shows another presentation pattern of acute osteomyelitis. Bony sclerosis, as in this case of osteomyelitis involving the femur, may simulate the radiographic appearance of an osteoid osteoma.

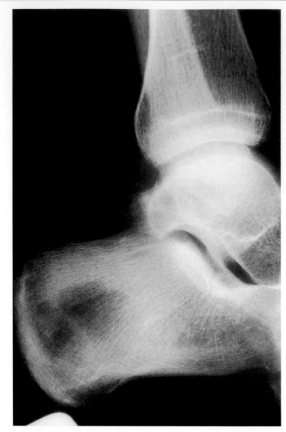

Figure 73–3 This radiograph reveals a relatively ill-defined lesion in the calcaneus that proved to be osteomyelitis on biopsy. Most cases of hematogenous osteomyelitis in the lower extremity involve the femur or tibia, and those in the upper extremity involve the humerus preferentially.

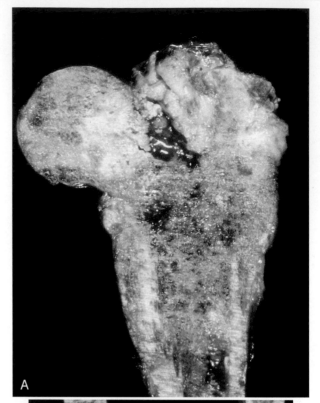

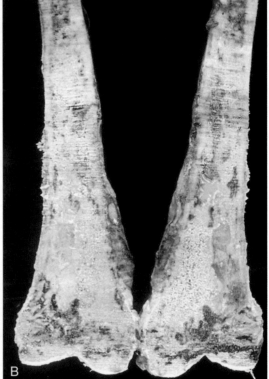

Figure 73–4 *A* and *B*: These two photographs of gross specimens show the marked bony destruction that may result from acute osteomyelitis. At the center of such regions of inflammatory reaction, fragments of dead bone (sequestra) may be present. Removal of the sequestra is necessary if the risk for reactivating osteomyelitis is to be minimized.

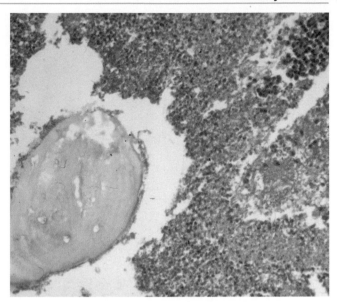

Figure 73–7 This photomicrograph illustrates osteomyelitis with an associated sequestrum. The dead bone is identified by the absence of viable osteocytes.

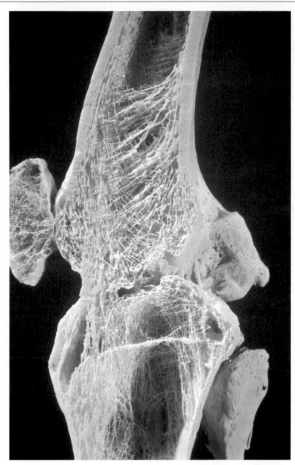

Figure 73–5 This photograph of a gross macerated specimen illustrates bony ankylosis across the knee joint in an adult patient who had longstanding osteomyelitis.

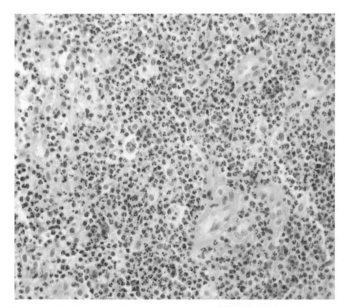

Figure 73–6 This photomicrograph shows one of the microscopic patterns of osteomyelitis. The inflammatory infiltrate in such cases may vary from being predominantly leukocytic to predominantly lymphocytic. Varying numbers of histiocytes are also commonly present.

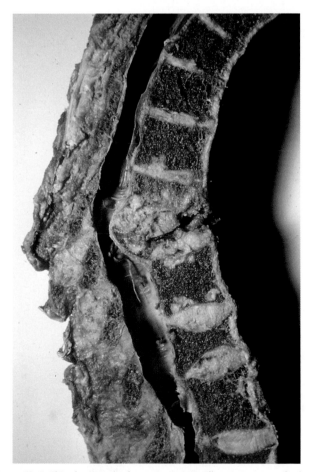

Figure 73–8 This photograph of a gross specimen illustrates a case of tuberculous osteomyelitis of the spine with bony destruction of a vertebral body. Tuberculous osteomyelitis may appear grossly "cheesy" because of granulomatous necrosis.

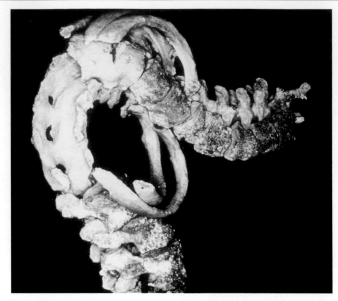

Figure 73–9 This photograph of a gross macerated specimen shows a spinal gibbus secondary to tuberculous osteomyelitis.

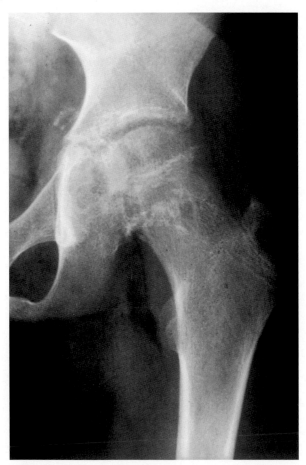

Figure 73–10 This radiograph illustrates bony destruction of the hip secondary to *Mycobacterium tuberculosis* infection.

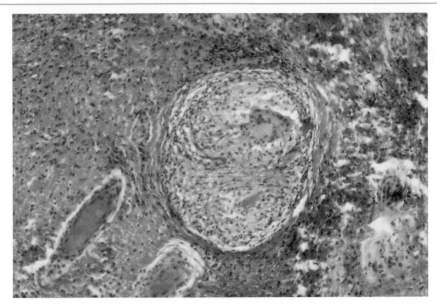

Figure 73–11 This photomicrograph reveals the granulomatous inflammation related to tuberculous osteomyelitis. Similar granulomatous reaction may be present in the synovium adjacent to the involved bone.

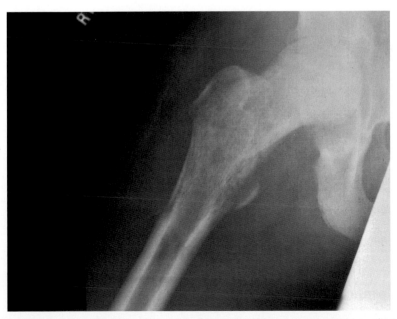

Figure 73–12 This radiograph demonstrates acute osteomyelitis of the proximal femur. The lesion shows a permeative radiographic pattern of destruction that is suggestive of a malignant tumor such as Ewing's sarcoma.

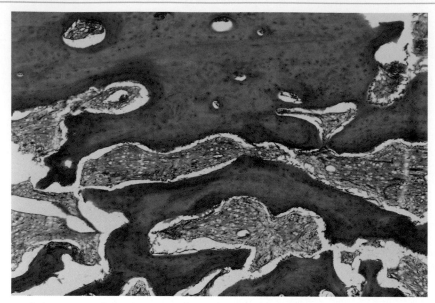

Figure 73–13 This photomicrograph shows a case of chronic osteomyelitis with marked bony sclerosis. The low-power appearance of the condition simulates that of a low-grade parosteal osteosarcoma.

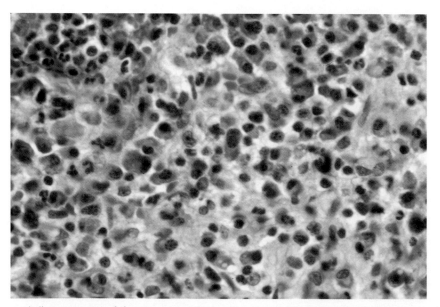

Figure 73–14 This photomicrograph illustrates a case of chronic osteomyelitis in which plasma cells predominate. Such cases can mimic myeloma in appearance.

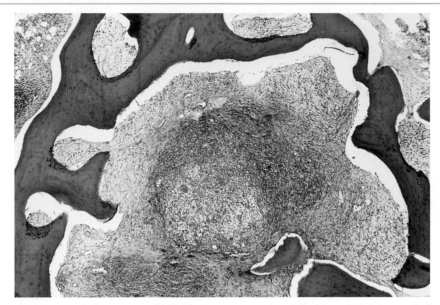

Figure 73–15 This low-power photomicrograph demonstrates the histologic appearance of Brodie's abscess. Such lesions typically simulate osteoid osteoma radiographically.

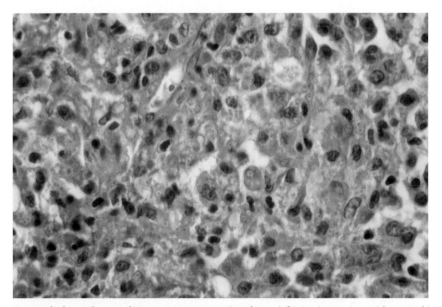

Figure 73–16 This photomicrograph shows the granulomatous response to Histoplasma infection in a patient with a prior history of Hodgkin's disease.

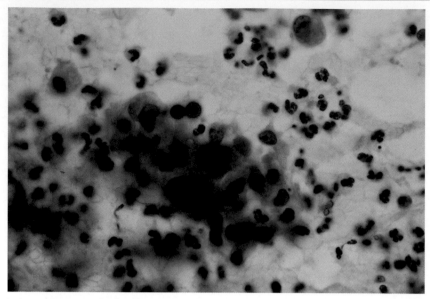

Figure 73–17 Fine-needle aspiration, with associated culture, can frequently help in diagnosing osteomyelitis. This case of blastomycotic osteomyelitis involved the ileum.

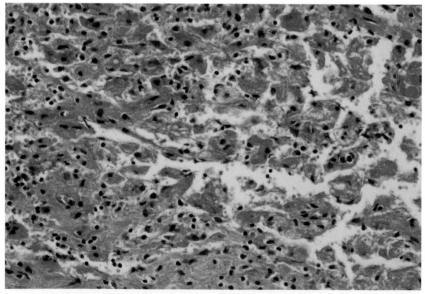

Figure 73–18 Whenever a diagnosis of xanthogranulomatous osteomyelitis is considered, the pathologist should also consider sinus histiocytosis with massive lymphadenopathy (SHML). SHML can present as bony disease, as in this case that involved the sacrum.

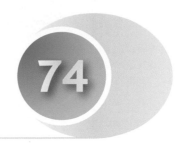

Avascular Necrosis

Risk Factors and Approximate Incidence

1. Corticosteroids are a risk factor in approximately 33% of cases. (In these cases more than 50% of patients have multiple lesions.)
2. Alcohol abuse is a risk factor in approximately 30% of cases.
3. Trauma is a risk factor in approximately 5% of cases.

Clinical Signs

1. Nearly 20% of patients with prior subcapital fracture of the femoral neck will develop avascular necrosis of the femoral head.
2. Avascular necrosis is also associated with steroid therapy, alcoholism, Gaucher's disease, sickle cell disease, and caisson disease.
3. Any condition that interrupts the blood flow to the affected bone can result in avascular necrosis. Conditions such as systemic lupus erythematosus and related collagen vascular diseases may be associated with avascular necrosis.
4. Pathologic fracture may occur through the affected bone.

Clinical Symptoms

1. There may be a sudden onset of pain in the affected joint.
2. The hip is most commonly involved (femoral head).

Major Radiographic Features

1. A change in the contour of the affected bone secondary to collapse of the infarcted area may be seen.
2. Increased density of the affected bone in the subchondral region may be present.

3. Approximately 50% of patients have multiple joints involved.
4. Magnetic resonance imaging is highly sensitive and specific when the clinical setting suggests a diagnosis of avascular necrosis.

Radiographic Differential Diagnosis

1. Osteoarthritis.
2. Chondroblastoma.
3. Malignant lymphoma.

Major Pathologic Features

Gross

1. The necrotic bone separates from the adjacent articular cartilage.
2. Hyperemia results in reddish discoloration of the bone just beyond the region of necrosis.
3. The necrotic bone is yellowish.
4. The necrotic bone may collapse into the remaining bone, flattening the contour of the articular surface.

Microscopic

1. The triangular sequestrum of dead bone retains the trabecular architecture of the native bone, but osteocytes are absent.
2. Fatty and hematopoietic marrow undergoes necrosis with the accumulation of lipid-laden histiocytes.
3. Fibrovascular connective tissue may proliferate in response to the ischemic injury at the periphery of the ischemic region.
4. Liquefactive necrosis may be present early in the course of the process.

Pathologic Differential Diagnosis

1. Storage disease.
2. Metabolic bone disease.
3. Acute osteomyelitis.

Treatment

Medical

1. The underlying disorder must be identified and treated.
2. Symptomatic measures are taken for joint symptoms (e.g., nonsteroidal anti-inflammatory drugs [NSAIDs], physical therapy, ambulatory aids).

Surgical

Surgical treatment is individualized and varies with underlying disease.

1. Core decompression may be performed for early disease (i.e., stages I and II [remains controversial]).
2. Nonvascularized or vascularized fibular bone graft may be undertaken for intermediate disease (i.e., stages II and III [remains controversial]).
3. Total joint replacement may be indicated for advanced disease (i.e., stages IV and V).

References

Aglietti P, Buzzi JN, Buzzi R, et al: Idiopathic osteonecrosis of the knee. Aetiology, prognosis and treatment. *J Bone Joint Surg Br* 65(5): 588–597, 1983.

Bachiller FG, Caballer AP, Portal LF: Avascular necrosis of the femoral head after femoral neck fracture. *Clin Orthop Relat Res* 399:87–109, 2002.

Catto M: A histological study of avascular necrosis of the femoral head after transcervical fracture. *J Bone Joint Surg Br* 47(4):749–776, 1965.

Mont MA, Hungerford DS: Non-traumatic avascular necrosis of the femoral head. *J Bone Joint Surg Am* 77(3):459–474, 1995.

Sissons HA, Nuovo MA, Steiner GC: Pathology of osteonecrosis of the femoral head. A review of experience at the Hospital for Joint Diseases, New York. *Skeletal Radiol* 21(4):229–238, 1992.

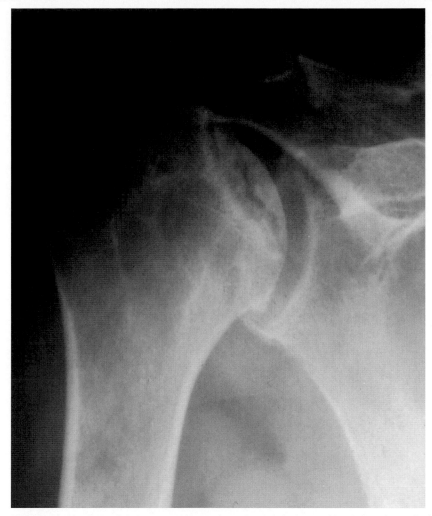

Figure 74–1 This radiograph of the proximal humerus shows a region of avascular necrosis in the humeral head. The subarticular bone shows a wedge-shaped region of radiopacity with the base adjacent to the articular cartilage.

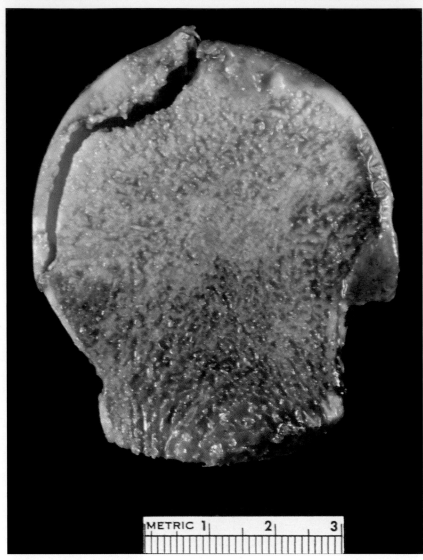

Figure 74–2 This photograph of a gross specimen of the femoral head illustrates an example of avascular necrosis. Note that the wedge-shaped region of yellowish discoloration corresponds to the area of infarction. The articular cartilage has been lifted from the underlying dead bone, resulting in alteration of the mechanical properties of the joint surface, which predisposes to degenerative joint disease.

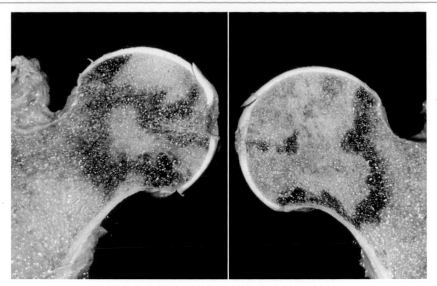

Figure 74–3 This photograph of a gross specimen of the femoral head illustrates a more recent example of avascular necrosis than that seen in Figure 74–2. The entire femoral head is infarcted, and the hyperemic region of bone at the edge of the infarct is easily identified.

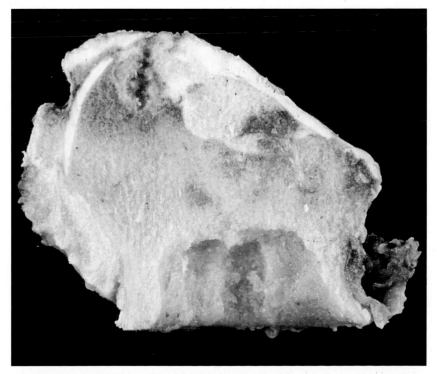

Figure 74–4 Altered mechanical properties of the articular cartilage secondary to avascular necrosis can lead to degenerative joint disease, as illustrated in this example in the femoral head. The underlying cause of the degenerative joint disease may be obscured by the marked degenerative changes.

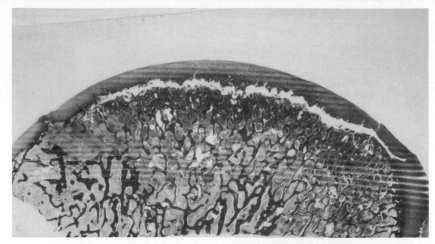

Figure 74–5 This low-power photomicrograph shows avascular necrosis in the femoral head of a patient with systemic lupus erythematosus. The wedge-shaped region identifiable radiographically is also appreciated in this specimen. Note that the region of infarction is also associated with loss of connection to the articular cartilage.

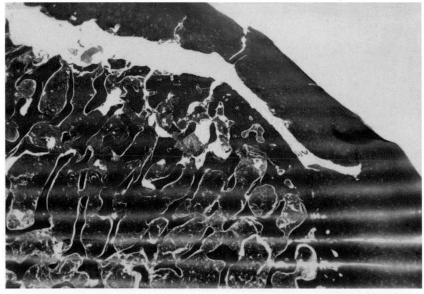

Figure 74–6 The avascular necrosis of Figure 74–5 is illustrated in this photomicrograph at higher magnification. Necrosis is characterized variably by dropout of the cellular elements in the bony trabeculae and marrow and by hemorrhage in the early stages and at the periphery of the lesion.

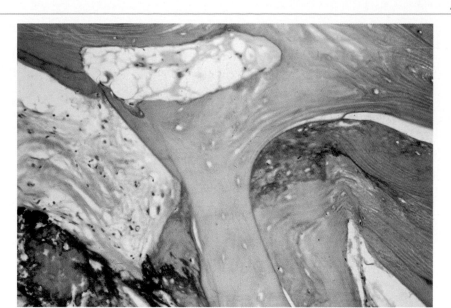

Figure 74–7 This photomicrograph illustrates the healing phase of avascular necrosis. Appositional new bone formation that uses the "scaffolding" of the preexisting necrotic bone is evident.

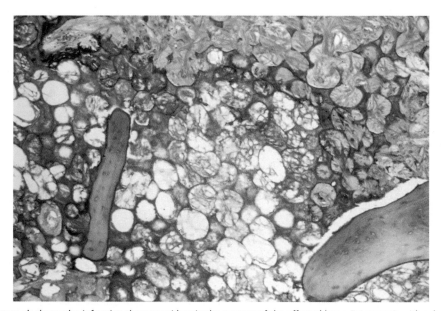

Figure 74–8 This photomicrograph shows the infarctive changes evident in the marrow of the affected bone. Fat necrosis with subsequent calcification is commonly identified as the infarct evolves.

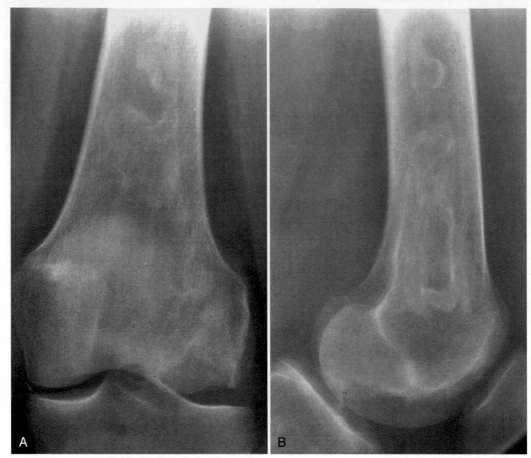

Figure 74–9 Anteroposterior (AP) (*A*) and lateral roentgenograms (*B*) of the distal femur and knee showing bone infarcts. Note the large osteochondral defect in the lateral femoral condyle, consistent with osteonecrosis. There is also patchy sclerosis in the distal femoral metaphysis, consistent with medullary infarcts. These have a linear peripheral margin.

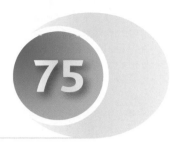

Massive Osteolysis (Gorham's Disease)

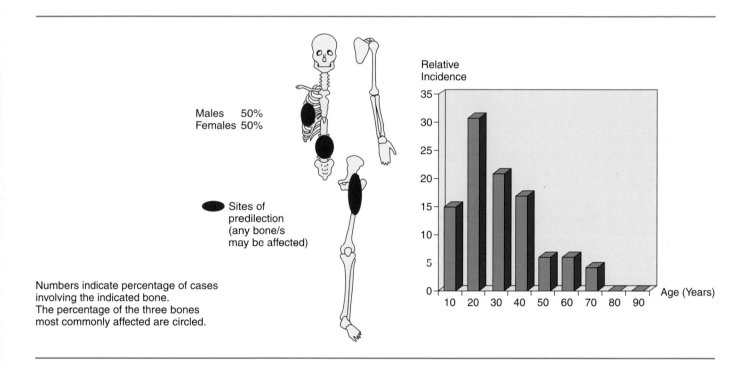

Males 50%
Females 50%

● Sites of
predilection
(any bone/s
may be affected)

Numbers indicate percentage of cases
involving the indicated bone.
The percentage of the three bones
most commonly affected are circled.

Relative
Incidence

Age (Years)

Clinical Signs

1. Most affected individuals experience disease onset before they are 40 years of age.
2. Pelvis, shoulder, and mandible are common sites of involvement.
3. Chylothorax may be associated with disease involving the chest wall or shoulder.
4. A clinical history of trauma is present in two thirds of cases.

Clinical Symptoms

1. Symptoms depend on which bone is affected.

2. Spinal involvement may result in neurologic symptoms.
3. Thoracic involvement may result in pulmonary symptoms.

Major Radiographic Features

1. Initially, the process is characterized by well-circumscribed regions of osteolysis involving the subcortical or intramedullary portion of the bone.
2. Bony sclerosis is absent until healing begins.
3. In the later stages of disease, the affected bone is concentrically tapered.
4. End-stage disease shows complete resorption of the affected bone.

5. The process may extend to involve adjacent bones or soft tissues.

6. Approximately one third of cases appear to arise from bone, one third arise from soft tissue, and one third involve both bone and soft tissue at the time of presentation.

7. When the first radiographic manifestation of the disease is in the soft tissues, then thinning and tapering of the circumference of the adjacent bone may subsequently be seen radiographically.

Radiographic Differential Diagnosis

1. Osseous hemangioma.
2. Idiopathic multicentric osteolysis.
3. Early osseous involvement may mimic a neoplasm of bone or a dysplastic condition such as fibrous dysplasia or neurofibromatosis.

Major Pathologic Features

1. Histologically, this condition is characterized by a proliferation of blood vessels and associated osteolysis. The vessels are usually thin-walled and capillary-like. Occasionally, they may show a more cavernous histologic appearance.

2. Reactive bone is not present in the region of the affected bone.

3. The affected bone is thinned and has been described as having a spongy consistency, evident grossly.

4. In areas where the bone has totally disappeared, there may be residual excess fibrous connective tissue.

Pathologic Differential Diagnosis

1. Hemangioma.
2. Lymphangioma.

Treatment

1. Supportive care is given because most cases resolve spontaneously.

2. Surgical treatment involves wide resection of involved bone and soft tissue in surgically reconstructable areas (i.e., reconstruction of the hip, knee, shoulder with custom prosthetic implants).

3. Radiation therapy can be given for lesions that may be associated with significant morbidity (e.g., vertebral lesions). Moderate doses (e.g., 40 to 45 Gy) may be successful in eradicating the disease.

References

Assoun J, Richardi G, Railhac JJ, et al: CT and MRI of massive osteolysis of Gorham. *J Comput Assist Tomogr* 18(6):981–984, 1994.

Dominguez R, Washowich TL: Gorham's disease or vanishing bone disease: plain film, CT, and MRI findings of two cases. *Pediatr Radiol* 24(5): 316–318, 1994.

Dunbar SF, Rosenberg A, Mankin H, et al: Gorham's massive osteolysis: the role of radiation therapy and a review of the literature [review]. *Int J Radiat Oncol Biol Physics* 26(3):491–497, 1993.

Patel DV: Gorham's disease or massive osteolysis. *Clin Med Res* 3(2): 65–74, 2005.

Shives TC, Beabout JW, Unni KK: Massive osteolysis. *Clin Orthop Relat Res* (294):266–276, 1993.

Vinee P, Tanyu MO, Hauenstein KH, et al: CT and MRI of Gorham syndrome [review]. *J Comput Assist Tomogr* 18(6):985–859, 1994.

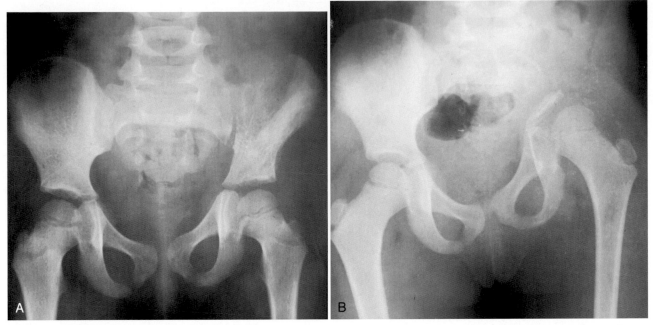

Figure 75–1 *A* and *B*: These two radiographs of the pelvis show the dramatic progression of bony dissolution over a period of 2 months in a patient with massive osteolysis.

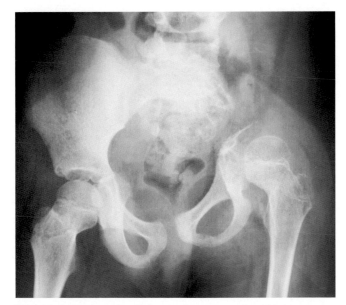

Figure 75–2 One year after the onset of symptoms, the pelvic bony dissolution has ceased and the affected bone begins to show healing with bony sclerosis.

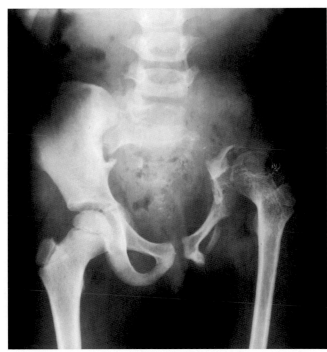

Figure 75–3 Three years after the onset of the disease illustrated in Figures 75–1 through 75–3, the process is stable. Bony deformity remains in the pelvis, but the bone has shown sclerotic changes related to healing.

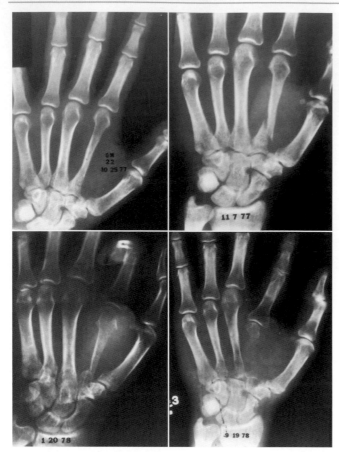

Figure 75–4 This series of radiographs illustrates massive osteolysis involving the metacarpal. Progressive bony dissolution with resultant tapering of the bone is characteristic of this process. Pathologic fracture may occur, as shown in this case.

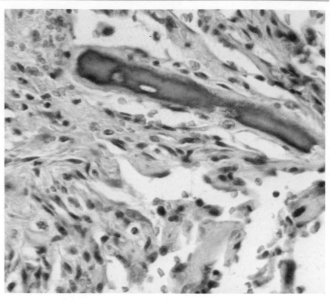

Figure 75–6 This photomicrograph shows the bland cytologic features of the endothelial cells lining the vessels of the bone in massive osteolysis. A thin bony trabecula is present. The vascular changes seen in some cases of massive osteolysis may suggest a diagnosis of hemangioma, or they may be relatively subtle.

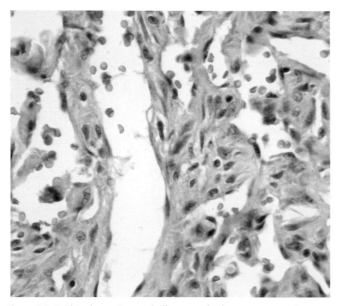

Figure 75–5 This photomicrograph illustrates the features commonly seen histologically in massive osteolysis. Hypervascularity or angiomatous changes may be present in the bone or soft tissues, as in this case.

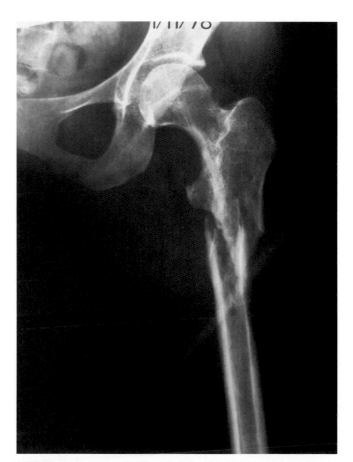

Figure 75–7 This radiograph illustrates massive osteolysis involving the proximal femur. There is an associated pathologic fracture through the diseased bone.

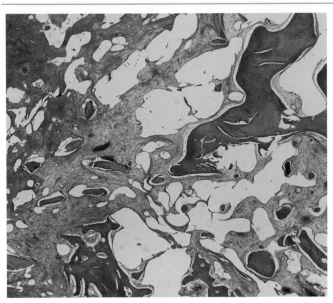

Figure 75–8 This photomicrograph reveals the hypervascular nature of diseased bone in massive osteolysis. Some cases show significantly less vascular transformation of the connective tissue than is evident in this case involving the femur.

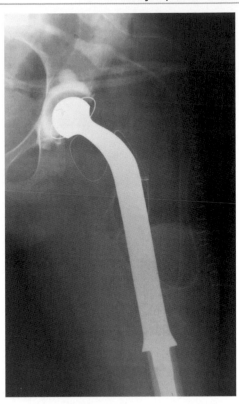

Figure 75–10 This radiograph illustrates the proximal femoral replacement used for reconstruction of the femur seen in Figures 75–7 and 75–9.

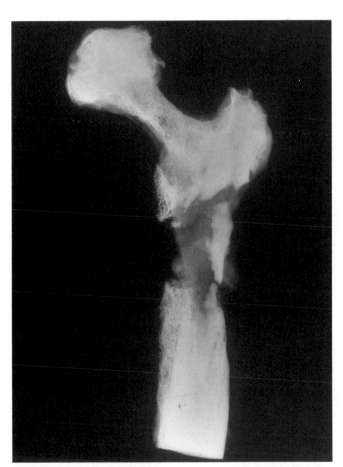

Figure 75–9 This radiograph shows the specimen taken after resection of the proximal femur illustrated in Figure 75–7. The pathologic fracture is also evident in the specimen radiograph.

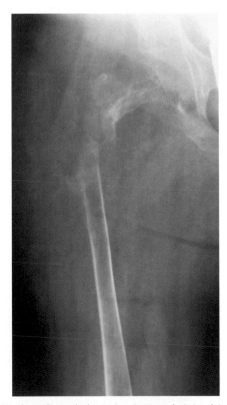

Figure 75–11 This radiograph shows massive osteolysis involving the right proximal femur. Pathologic fracture is present. Concentric narrowing of the femoral neck and the "sucked candy" appearance of the proximal end of the distal fragment are characteristic radiographic features of massive osteolysis.

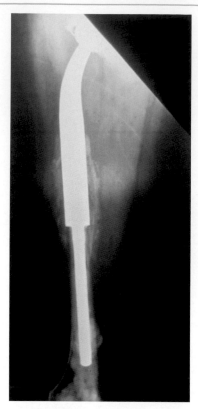

Figure 75–12 A custom prosthesis was used to reconstruct the defect remaining after resection of the proximal femoral lesion illustrated in Figure 75–11.

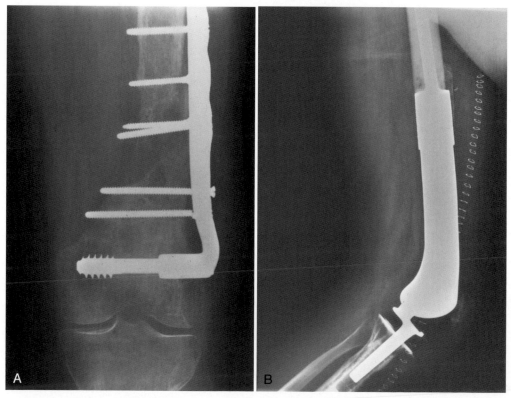

Figure 75–13 *A:* A case of massive osteolysis was treated by internal fixation. Progressive disease resulted in the need for total joint arthroplasty using a custom knee prosthesis (*B*).

Hemophilia

Clinical Signs

1. The gene for factor VIII has a high mutation rate; therefore, patients may present with a wide variation in signs and symptoms dependent on the severity of the factor VIII deficiency.
2. Bloody joint effusion may be seen.
3. Scattered bruises are common.
4. Intramuscular bleeding and hemarthrosis usually do not occur until a child is learning to walk.
5. Young patients may present with limping related to hemarthrosis.
6. Recurrent hemarthroses frequently involve the same joint ("target joint") owing to the synovial proliferation related to prior bleeds and the increased risk of trauma to the hyperplastic synovium.
7. Intramuscular bleeding is particularly common in the thigh, calf, forearm, and iliopsoas.
8. Late arthropathy with joint destruction may occur.

Clinical Symptoms

1. A warm, painful, swollen joint secondary to hemorrhage into the joint space (most common in knees, ankles, and elbows) may be found.
2. Minor trauma results in joint space hemorrhage.
3. A tingling sensation in the region of the affected joint often precedes painful distention of the joint in hemarthrosis.
4. Occasionally, a large intramuscular hemorrhage in the forearm may cause a compartment syndrome.
5. Secondary contractures of the knees and elbows and equinus of the ankles may be seen.

Major Radiographic Features

1. Narrowing of the joint space may be seen.
2. Cartilage destruction may be evident.

3. Bony erosion may be present.
4. Juxta-articular bony cystic changes may be seen.
5. Osteophyte formation may be evident.
6. Juxtaepiphyseal osteoporosis may be found.
7. Subperiosteal hematomas may be seen to result in subperiosteal lytic pseudotumors.
8. Magnetic resonance imaging may define cartilage changes and hypertrophied synovium.

Radiographic Differential Diagnosis

1. Other causes of recurrent hemarthrosis (e.g., pigmented villonodular synovitis).
2. Arthropathy in advanced disease.

Major Pathologic Features

1. Grossly, the synovium is mahogany brown secondary to hemosiderin deposition related to joint space hemorrhage.
2. The synovium is hyperplastic and papillary.
3. Numerous hemosiderin-laden macrophages fill the synovium.
4. Loss of articular cartilage and associated pannus-like proliferation may be evident.
5. Degenerative changes in the articular cartilage may be found, including fissuring of the cartilage. (The pannus contains considerable quantities of iron.)
6. Clustering of the chondrocytes in the articular cartilage may be seen.

Pathologic Differential Diagnosis

1. Pigmented villonodular synovitis.
2. Rheumatoid arthritis.

Treatment

Medical

1. Supportive care (e.g., counseling to avoid activities related to increased risk of trauma and subsequent risk of bleeding) along with physical therapy to maintain joint motion and muscle strength are given.
2. Factor VIII replacement (factor IX for hemophilia B) is instituted.
3. Radionucleotide synovectomy has been successful in some cases.
4. Desmopressin may be used to treat patients with mild hemophilia.

Surgical

1. Pseudotumors should be recognized and excised.
2. Arthroscopic synovectomy may be done.
3. Total joint replacement may be performed for advanced disease.

References

Barber FA, Prudich JF: Acute traumatic knee hemarthrosis. *Arthroscopy* 9(2):174–176, 1993.

Bender JM, Unalan M, Balon HR, et al: Hemophiliac arthropathy. Appearance on bone scintigraphy. *Clin Nucl Med* 19(5):465–466, 1994.

Hoots WK: Pathogenesis of hemophilic arthropathy. *Sem Hematol* 43(1 Suppl 1):S18–22, 2006.

Idy-Peretti I, Le Balc'h T, Yvart J, et al: MR imaging of hemophilic arthropathy of the knee: classification and evolution of the subchondral cysts. *Magn Reson Imaging* 10(1):67–75, 1992.

Lillicrap D: The molecular pathology of hemophilia A [review]. *Transfus Med Rev* 5(3):196–206, 1991.

Ljung R: Genetic diagnosis of hemophilia A. *Pediatr Hematol Oncol* 11(1):9–11, 1994.

Lusher JM, Warrier I: Hemophilia A [review]. *Hematol Oncol Clin North Am* 6(5):1021–1033, 1992.

Magallon M, Monteagudo J, Altisent C, et al: Hemophilic pseudotumor: multicenter experience over a 25-year period. *Am J Hematol* 45(2):103–108, 1994.

Nuss R, Kilcoyne RF, Geraghty S, et al: Utility of magnetic resonance imaging for management of hemophilic arthropathy in children. *J Pediatr* 123(3):388–392, 1993.

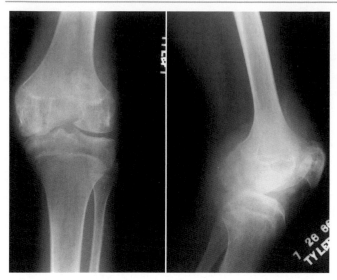

Figure 76–1 This radiograph shows the knee of a patient with hemophilia. The knees, elbows, and ankles are most often affected by hemophilia. Narrowing of the joint space is commonly identified in hemophilic arthropathy.

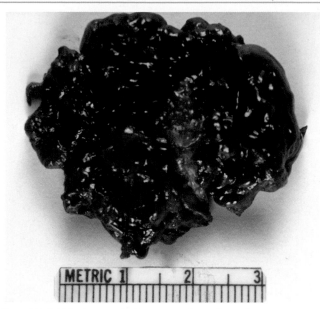

Figure 76–3 This photograph of a gross specimen shows the synovium in a patient with hemophilia who has had multiple intraarticular bleeds. The synovium is dark brown and grossly may mimic the appearance of pigmented villonodular synovitis. Villous hyperplasia of the synovium may be present, but this process is not, in general, tumefacient.

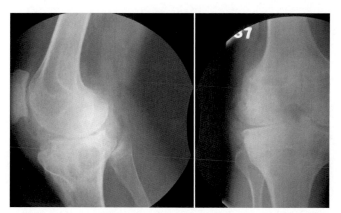

Figure 76–2 This radiograph of the knee of a patient with hemophilia shows joint space narrowing from loss of articular cartilage after repeated intraarticular bleeds. Other features that may be seen radiographically in patients with hemophilia include bony erosion, juxta-articular cysts, and subperiosteal hematomas.

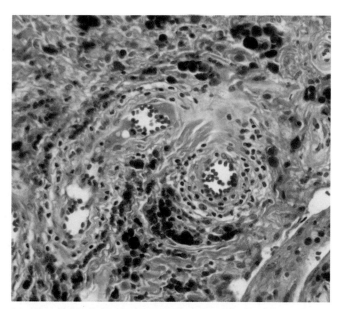

Figure 76–4 This photomicrograph illustrates the numerous hemosiderin-laden macrophages that are seen after an intraarticular bleed. In contrast to pigmented villonodular synovitis, this process lacks multinucleated giant cells and lipid-laden histiocytes.

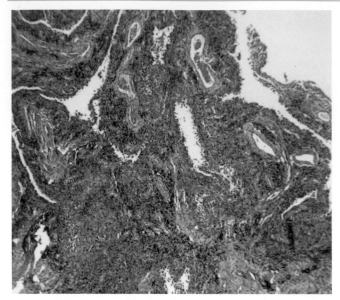

Figure 76–5 Villous hyperplasia of the synovium may accompany the deposition of hemosiderin pigment in hemophilic arthropathy, as shown in this photomicrograph.

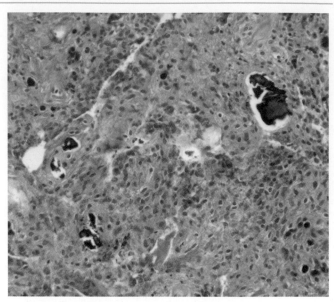

Figure 76–6 As the synovium becomes hyperplastic and the articular cartilage undergoes degenerative changes, bits of cartilage may become embedded in the synovium, as shown in this photomicrograph.

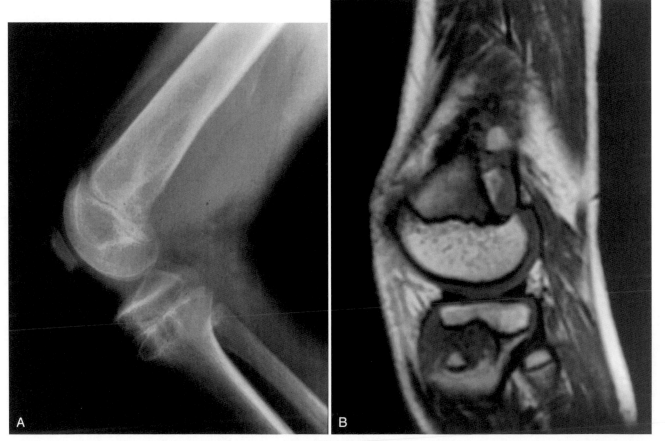

Figure 76–7 This lateral roentgenogram (*A*) and magnetic resonance imaging (MRI) scan (*B*) show the knee of a patient with hemophilia. A pseudotumor is apparent in the proximal tibial metaphysis.

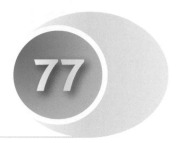

Metastatic Carcinoma

Clinical Signs

1. Tenderness is noted in the region of the affected bone.
2. A mass lesion is found.
3. Pathologic fracture is present.

Clinical Symptoms

1. Pain is the most common symptom; however, metastatic lesions may be asymptomatic and discovered incidentally on radiographic evaluation for an unrelated problem.
2. Swelling may be noticed in the region of the affected bone.

Major Radiographic Features

1. Solitary or, more commonly, multiple lesions arise centrally in a patient with a known primary malignancy.
2. They are usually detected by combined use of radiographic survey and isotope bone scan.
3. Presentations are diverse, with lytic, blastic, or mixed lesions all common.

Radiographic Differential Diagnosis

1. Multiple myeloma.
2. Lymphoma.
3. "Brown tumor" of hyperparathyroidism.
4. Many primary malignancies of bone, if solitary.

Major Pathologic Features

Gross

1. The consistency of metastatic lesions varies from firm in those tumors that elicit a desmoplastic stromal reaction to soft in those that do not.
2. The color of the lesions is variable, depending on the presence or absence of hemorrhage, necrosis, or lipidization of the tumor (as in hypernephroma).
3. The tumors tend to be poorly circumscribed and grow in an invasive, permeative manner.

Microscopic

1. The majority of carcinomas metastatic to bone show obvious glandular or squamous differentiation at low magnification.
2. If obvious glandular or squamous differentiation is lacking, growth in a clustered or organoid pattern is helpful in identifying the lesion as epithelial in origin.
3. Poorly differentiated carcinomas may grow in a sarcomatous pattern and may consist almost entirely of spindled cells. This is particularly common with renal cell carcinomas.
4. Ultrastructural and immunohistochemical investigation of sarcomatous malignancies in patients older than 60 years of age without predisposing factors for developing a primary sarcoma (e.g., Paget's disease and prior radiation) may reveal epithelial characteristics.

Pathologic Differential Diagnosis

Malignant lesions

1. Fibrosarcoma.
2. Malignant fibrous histiocytoma.

Treatment

1. **Primary modality:** requires multidisciplinary team approach that includes (1) careful attention to the patient's general health and correction of nutritional and metabolic problems; (2) aggressive systemic treatment to control the basic neoplastic process; and (3) the use

of radiation therapy as the primary modality to control local symptoms, which provides effective pain relief for up to 1 year in 80% of patients.

2. **Other possible approaches:** internal fixation or prosthetic replacement for actual or imminent pathologic fractures.

References

Fitzgerald RH Jr, Brewer NS, Dahlin DC: Squamous-cell carcinoma complicating chronic osteomyelitis. *J Bone Joint Surg Am* 58(8): 1146–1148,1976.

Sim FH (ed): *Diagnosis and Treatment of Metastatic Bone Disease: A Multidisciplinary Approach to Management.* New York: Raven Press, 1987.

Simon MA, Karluk MB: Skeletal metastases of unknown origin: diagnostic strategy for orthopedic surgeons. *Clin Orthop Relat Res* (166):96–103, 1982.

Tomera KM, Farrow GM, Lieber MM: Sarcomatoid renal carcinoma. *J Urol* 130(4):657–659, 1983.

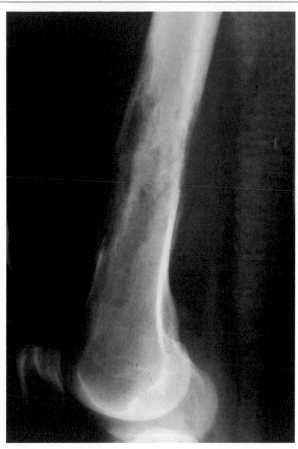

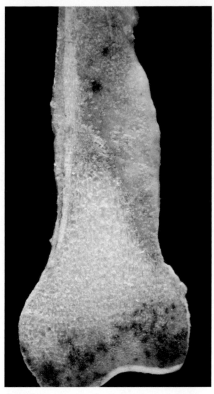

Figure 77–2 The gross specimen corresponding to the radiograph in Figure 77–1 shows a diametaphyseal tumor with diaphyseal cortical destruction. The tumor is firm, white, and fibrous.

Figure 77–1 This radiograph shows a large, poorly marginated lytic lesion of the lower diametaphyseal region of the lower femur. This elderly male patient had a known carcinoma of the lung.

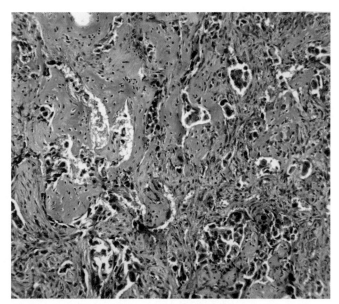

Figure 77–3 At low magnification, metastatic adenocarcinomas generally can be seen to show gland formation, as in this photomicrograph. An osteoblastic response by the bone, if it is pronounced, may obscure the metastatic tumor.

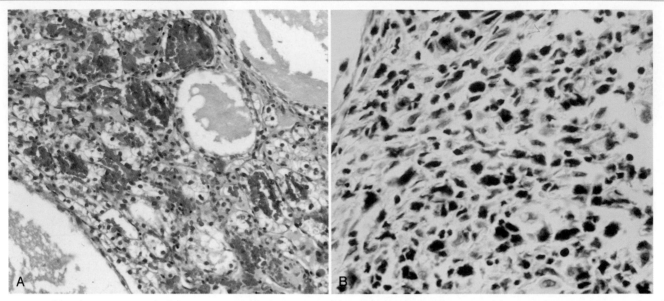

Figure 77–4 Although metastatic renal cell carcinomas generally show a clear cell histologic pattern of differentiation (*A*), metastases from a sarcomatoid renal cell carcinoma may mimic a primary bone tumor (*B*). Fortunately for diagnostic purposes, in general there will be a history of a preceding renal malignancy.

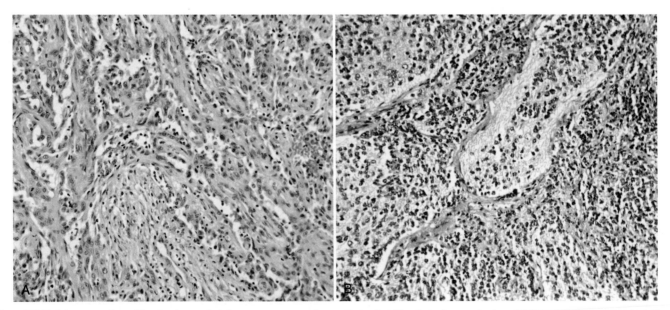

Figure 77–5 *A:* A metastatic papillary carcinoma that, in some areas, grew in a pattern mimicking that of a vascular tumor. Although uncommon, metastatic neuroblastoma (*B*) can mimic a "small blue cell tumor" if rosettes and neutrophil are not recognized.

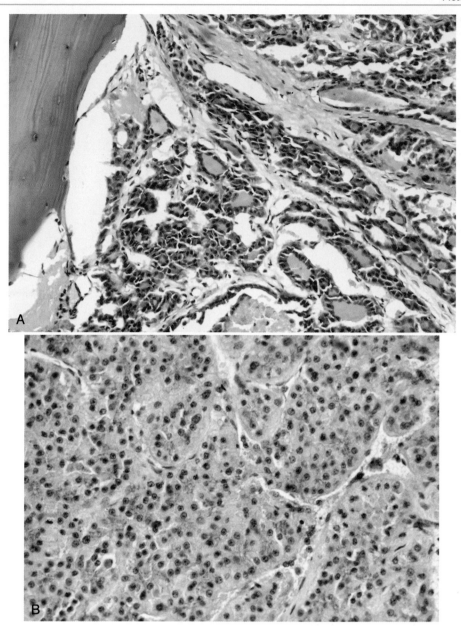

Figure 77–6 At times, it may be possible to suggest a site of origin of an osseous metastasis on the basis of its histologic pattern of growth. *A*: A metastatic follicular carcinoma of the thyroid. *B*: A metastatic hepatocellular carcinoma in which bile could be seen.

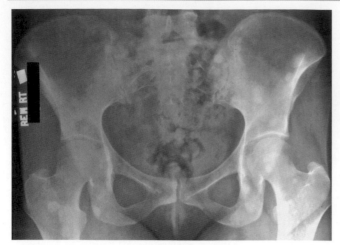

Figure 77–7 Multiple sclerotic metastases are visible in the pelvis of this elderly woman with a prior diagnosis of carcinoma of the breast.

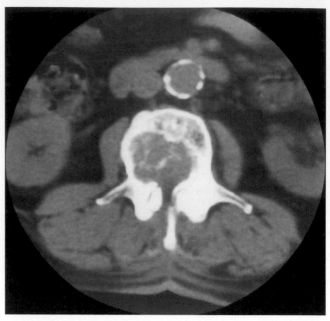

Figure 77–9 A computed tomographic (CT) scan may be helpful in identifying metastasis, as demonstrated by this view showing a mixed lytic and sclerotic metastasis in the lumbar vertebra.

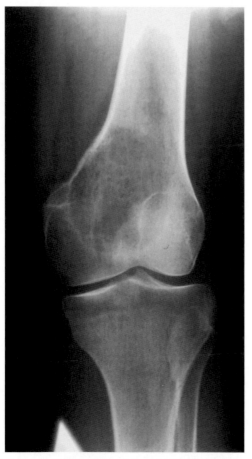

Figure 77–8 This solitary lytic lesion of the distal femur was shown on biopsy to represent metastatic renal cell carcinoma. In this location, a giant cell tumor could also be considered in the differential diagnosis.

Sarcoidosis

Incidence

In the United States, sarcoidosis most often affects African Americans. In the United Kingdom, the disease is rare in blacks and common in whites. It is an uncommon disease of the musculoskeletal system and infrequently considered in contrast to thoracic manifestations of the disease. An accurate incidence of musculoskeletal involvement is difficult to ascertain, but with widespread use of imaging an increasing number of cases are being discovered. Studies have variably reported skeletal involvement in from 3% to 13% of cases of sarcoidosis.

Clinical Signs

1. Acute and chronic polyarthritis.
2. Bone–muscle pain on examination.

Clinical Symptoms

1. Acute and chronic polyarthritis.
2. Bone–muscle pain.
3. Asymptomatic.

Major Radiographic Features

1. Bilateral distribution, commonly involving the small bones of the hands and feet, is seen.
2. Lesions often involve the cortex with preservation of the periosteum and involvement of the ends of the affected bones.
3. Lattice-like or honeycombed phalanges is the most familiar radiographic sign. Although well recognized, it is relatively uncommon.
4. There are foci of sclerosis or osteolysis on radiographs.

5. Magnetic resonance imaging (MRI) features include the following:
   a. Multiple discrete intramedullary lesions in long bones, pelvis, vertebrae.
   b. Cortical destruction with small bone involvement.
   c. Nodular lesions in muscle.
   d. Nonspecific synovitis.

Radiographic Differential Diagnosis

1. Metastatic carcinoma, in the axial skeleton and long tubular bones (particularly on MRI).
2. Multiple myeloma, in the axial skeleton and long tubular bones (particularly on MRI).
3. Lymphoma.

Note: The diagnosis may be considered if the characteristic nodular, low-signal, starlike pattern is identified within muscle.

Major Pathologic Features

Gross

1. The involved bone tends to be soft.
2. True bony cysts and liquefaction are not evident.

Microscopic

1. Characteristically a noncaseating granulomatous inflammation is present.
2. Reactive fibrosis may be seen adjacent to granulomatous foci.
3. Minimal inflammatory infiltrate with lymphocytes may be present, but the lesions do not show significant neutrophilic infiltration.
4. No significant eosinophilic infiltrate is seen.

Pathologic Differential Diagnosis

Benign lesions

1. Granulomatous infection.
2. Sinus histiocytosis massive lymphadenopathy.
3. Erdheim-Chester disease.

Malignant lesions

1. Malignant lymphoma.
2. Malignant fibrous histiocytoma.

Treatment

Medical

1. Careful follow-up and monitoring of disease.
2. Steroids.

Surgical

1. Surgical stabilization of destructive vertebral lesions.

References

Knutsson F: Skeletal changes in sarcoidosis. *Acta Radiologica* 51(6): 429–432, 1959.

Moore SL, Teirstein A, Golimbu C: MRI of sarcoidosis patients with musculoskeletal symptoms. *Am J Roentgenol* 185:154–159, 2005.

Moore SL, Teirstein AE: Musculoskeletal sarcoidosis: spectrum of appearances at MR imaging. *Radiographics* 23(6):1389–1399, 2003.

Otake S, Ishigaki T: Muscular sarcoidosis. *Semin Musculoskeletal Radiol* 5:167–170, 2001.

Sundaram M, Place H, Shaffer WO, et al: Progressive destructive vertebral sarcoid leading to surgical fusion. *Skeletal Radiol* 28(12):717–722, 1999.

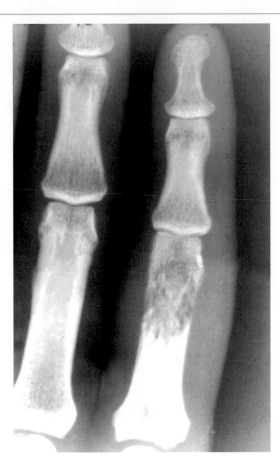

Figure 78–1 Lacelike honeycomb pattern of lysis and sclerosis in the proximal phalanx of the index finger showing an appearance characteristic of phalangeal sarcoidosis. The aggressive radiographic appearance is associated with complete resorption of the adjacent endosteum and significant soft tissue swelling.

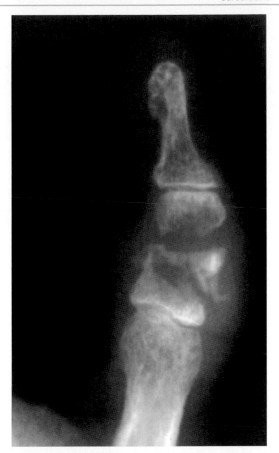

Figure 78–3 Comminuted fracture through an osteolytic phalangeal lesion that does not have features of sarcoid and is relatively nonspecific in appearance. However, the intact proximal and distal phalanges show the honeycomb pattern of sarcoidosis.

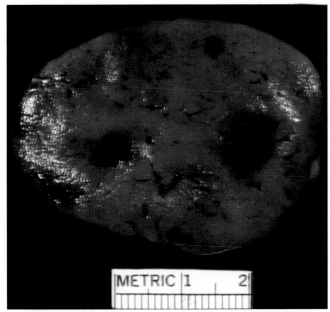

Figure 78–2 Gross photograph of a lymph node involved by sarcoidosis. The nodal architecture is grossly altered as a result of the diffuse involvement by noncasseating granulomatous inflammation.

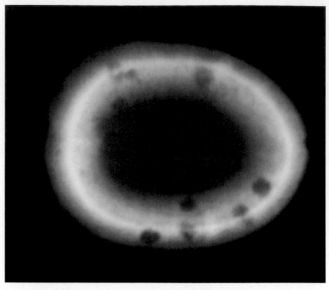

Figure 78–5 Cross-sectional computed tomography (CT) image unequivo-cally showing confined intracortical lesions of sarcoidosis. This is a finding rarely ever observed on radiographs because of the inherent limitations of radiography, but it will be increasingly encountered with widespread use of cross-sectional imaging.

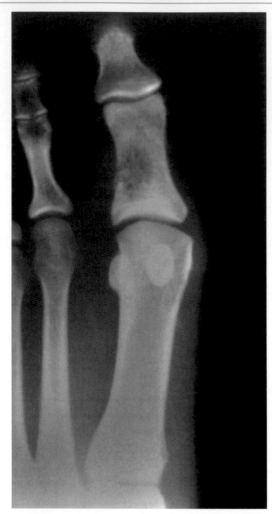

Figure 78–4 Phalangeal sarcoid in the great toe showing a fine lacelike pattern within a predominantly osteolytic lesion.

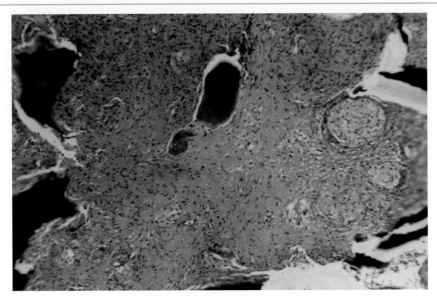

Figure 78–6 This photomicrograph illustrates the fibrosis that is often seen in cases of sarcoidosis and a multinucleated giant cell typical of the disease. A bony trabeculum is being destroyed by the fibroinflammatory process.

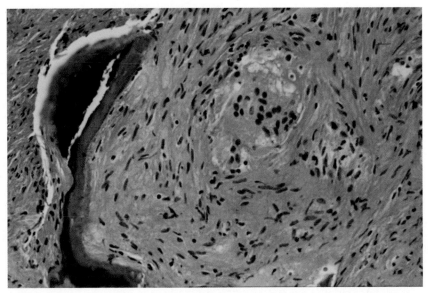

Figure 78–7 This photomicrograph illustrates the infiltrative nature of sarcoidosis involving bone. Little lymphocytic infiltrate is evident, and no necrosis is seen. Careful search for the granulomatous nature of the process may be necessary in cases such as this.

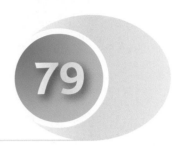

Bizarre Parosteal Osteochondromatous Proliferation (BPOP)

Clinical Signs

1. Radiographically identifiable periosteal mass.
2. Palpable mass adjacent to small bones in the hands or foot.
3. Pain in the region of a periosteal mass.

Clinical Symptoms

1. Mass.
2. Pain, low grade, may be present.

Major Radiographic Features

1. The surface lesion is of variable appearance, depending on the maturity of the lesion.
2. The patient may have fine periostitis with prominent soft tissue swelling (florid reactive periostitis stage).
3. In later stages calcification/ossification of soft tissues and maturing of periosteal reaction, which may develop a solid uninterrupted appearance, may be seen.
4. Magnetic resonance imaging evaluation may show profound marrow edema.

Radiographic Differential Diagnosis

1. Osteomyelitis.
2. Osteosarcoma.

Major Pathologic Features

Gross

1. Grossly, these lesions frequently resemble osteochondromata.
2. The lesional tissue is composed of bone and cartilage, and there may be an overlying fibrovascular pseudocapsule.

3. The lesions are typically small (commonly less than 2 cm in greatest dimension).
4. There is no continuity of the lesion with the underlying medullary bone (as seen in osteochondromata).

Microscopic

1. The lesional tissue is composed of bone, cartilage, and fibrovascular connective tissue.
2. The cartilage tends to be less well organized than is the case in osteochondromata.
3. The endochondral ossification present in the lesional tissue tends to be less well organized than in osteochondromata.
4. The spindle cell component of the lesion may show some mitotic activity, but no atypia is evident.
5. A distinctive feature of BPOP is the presence of irregular calcified matrix, which stains blue (hematoxylin and eosin) and has been referred to as "blue bone."
6. The lesion is very well circumscribed at the periphery.

Pathologic Differential Diagnosis

Malignant lesions

1. Parosteal osteosarcoma.

Benign lesions

1. Osteochondroma.
2. Reactive periostitis.

Treatment

1. **Primary modality:** surgical excision.
2. **Other possible approaches:** careful clinical follow-up ("watchful waiting").

References

Abramovici L, Steiner GC: Bizarre parosteal osteochondromatous proliferation (Nora's lesion): a retrospective study of 12 cases, 2 arising in long bones. *Hum Pathol* 33(12):1205–1210, 2002.

Dhondt E, Oudenhoven L, Khan S, et al: Nora's lesion, a distinct radiological entity? *Skeletal Radiol* 35(7):497–502, 2006.

Ly JQ, Bui-Mansfield LT, Taylor DC: Radiologic demonstration of temporal development of bizarre parosteal osteochondromatous proliferation. *Clin Imaging* 28(3):216–218, 2004.

Meneses MF, Unni KK, Swee RG: Bizarre parosteal osteochondromatous proliferation of bone (Nora's lesion). *Am J Surg Pathol* 17(7):691–697, 1993.

Michelsen H, Abramovici L, Steiner G, et al: Bizarre parosteal osteochondromatous proliferation (Nora's lesion) in the hand. *J Hand Surg Am* 29(3):520–525, 2004.

Murphey MD, Choi JJ, Kransdorf MJ, et al: Imaging of osteochondroma: variants and complications with radiologic-pathologic correlation. *Radiographics* 20(5):1407–1434, 2000.

Nora FE, Dahlin DC, Beabout JW: Bizarre parosteal osteochondromatous proliferation of the hands and feet. *Am J Surg Pathol* 7:245–250, 1983.

Spjut HJ, Dorfman HD: Florid reactive periostitis of the tubular bones of the hands and feet: a benign lesion which may simulate osteosarcoma. *Am J Surg Pathol* 5(5):423–433, 1981.

Sundaram M, Wang L, Kotman M, et al: Florid reactive periostitis and bizarre parosteal osteochondromatons proliferation: pre-biopsy imaging evolution, treatment and outcomes. *Skeletal Radiol* 30(4):192–198, 2001.

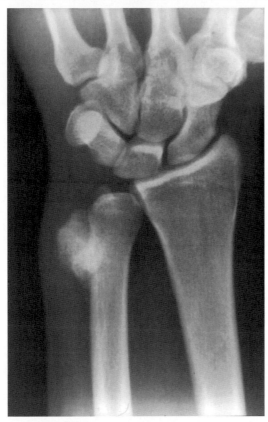

Figure 79–1 This 30-year-old female presented with a bony mass in the region of the distal ulna. No continuity between the cortex of the underlying bone or the medulla—features that help to exclude the diagnosis of osteochondroma—are evident.

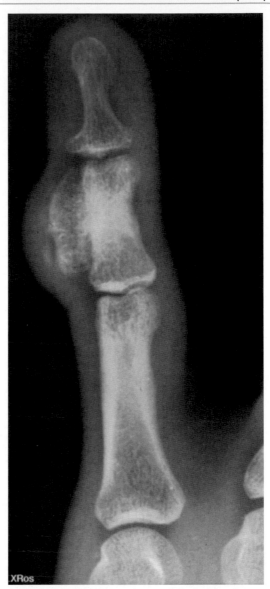

Figure 79–3 This example of a bizarre parosteal osteocartilaginous proliferation involves the middle phalanx of a finger. The lesion is somewhat irregular in contour and is not as heavily mineralized as many examples.

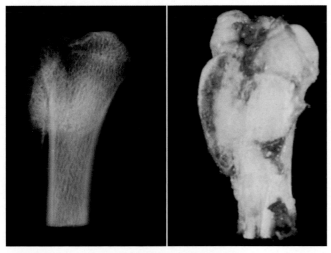

Figure 79–2 This specimen radiograph and gross specimen are from the case shown in Figure 79–1.

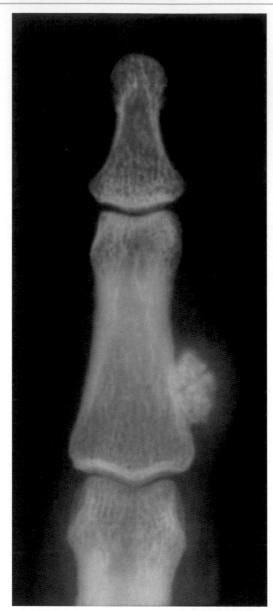

Figure 79–4 This example of a BPOP is heavily mineralized and involves the middle phalanx of a finger, a common location for this condition.

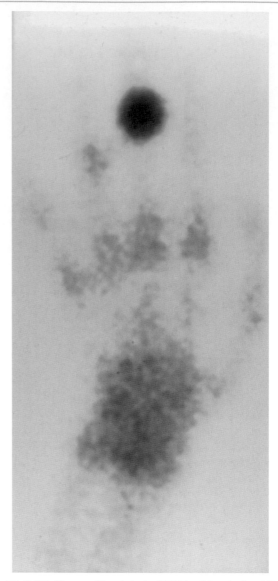

Figure 79–5 This 21-year-old male had a BPOP involving the hand. Bone scan reveals that the lesional tissue shows intense accumulation of radio tracer, correlating with the active osteoblastic activity in the lesional tissue.

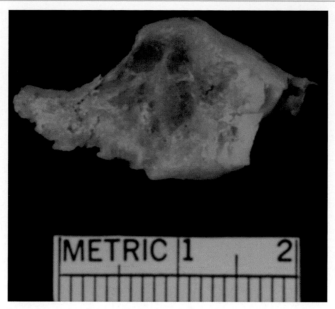

Figure 79–6 This photograph illustrates the gross features of a BPOP that involved the left fifth metacarpal. The cartilage cap and underlying bone in such cases can mimic the gross appearance of an osteochondroma.

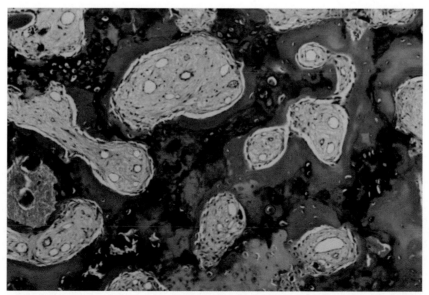

Figure 79–7 The characteristic "blue bone" commonly seen in bizarre parosteal osteochondromatous proliferations is evident in this photomicrograph of a lesion from the hand.

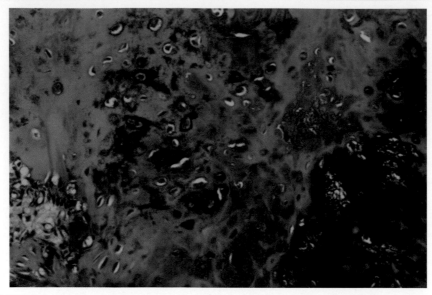

Figure 79–8 The cartilage of BPOP lesions is frequently less well organized than in osteochondromata, as illustrated in this photomicrograph of a lesion that involved the hand.

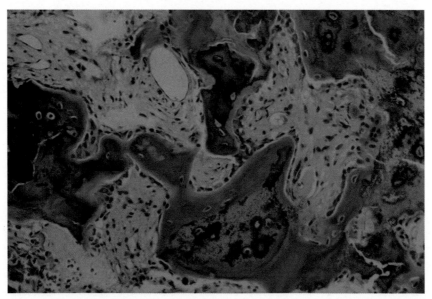

Figure 79–9 In BPOP lesions, a fibroblastic spindle cell component is frequently seen admixed with the bone, as illustrated in this photomicrograph.

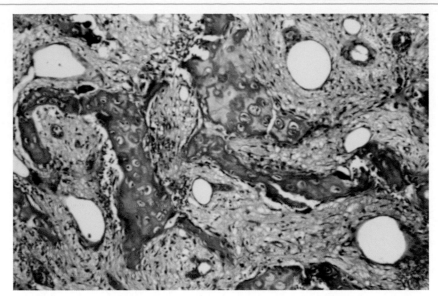

Figure 79–10 Although BPOP most commonly involves the small bones of the hands and feet, rare examples of these lesions have been identified involving long bones. This photomicrograph shows the typical histology of a BPOP lesion, but the lesion was on the surface of the humerus.

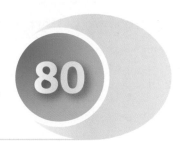

Erdheim-Chester Disease

Incidence

1. Rare non-Langerhans' cell histiocytosis with almost universal bone involvement and 60% extraosseous involvement. Extraosseous involvement is highly variable and may be life threatening.

Clinical Signs

1. The osseous findings may be incidentally discovered following radiography for bone pain.
2. Diabetes insipidus, painless bilateral exophthalmos, and bone pain constitute the classic Erdheim-Chester diagnostic triad.

Clinical Symptoms

1. Bone pain, typically involving the lower extremities and commonly bilateral.
2. Fever.
3. Weight loss.
4. Weakness.
5. Exophthalmos.
6. Abdominal pain.
7. Dysuria.
8. Diabetes insipidus.

Major Radiographic Features

1. Radiographic disease is typically manifested as a bilateral symmetric sclerosis of the diaphyses of long bones. In decreasing order of frequency, they are the femur, humerus, tibia and radius–ulna.
2. Periostitis and endosteal thickening are frequent findings, with resultant reduction of the medullary space.

3. In about 45% of patients, the epiphyseal equivalent may be involved and the axial skeleton and pelvis are spared.
4. Technetium scintigraphy shows increased tracer uptake without exception.
5. Magnetic resonance imaging (MRI) shows markedly low signal on T1-weighted sequences and intermediate to high signal (in relation to muscle) on T2-weighted sequences. When the epiphyseal equivalent is involved, MRI shows sparing of the subchondral bony plate.

Radiographic Differential Diagnosis

1. Camurati-Engelmann disease.

Major Pathologic Features

Gross

1. Tumor masses are commonly soft, particularly when involving nonosseous sites.
2. Fatlike yellow masses may be present.

Microscopic

1. Infiltration of tissue by an admixture of mononuclear cells and foamy histiocytes, lymphocytes, and giant cells is seen.
2. Fibrosis is variable.
3. Nuclei of the mononuclear cells are round and lack the characteristic contour of the Langerhans' histiocytes.
4. The mononuclear cells are immunohistochemically CD68 positive and negative for S-100 protein and CD1a.

Pathologic Differential Diagnosis

Benign lesions

1. Langerhans' cell histiocytosis.
2. Osteomyelitis.

Malignant lesions

1. Malignant fibrous histiocytoma.

Treatment

1. **Primary modality:** No treatment is directed at the bony lesions other than pain reduction, if severe. Treatment is directed at the visceral lesions and is influenced by location and extent of disease.

2. **Other possible approaches:** Corticosteroids, chemotherapy, radiotherapy, and surgical resection have all been tried, particularly for the extraskeletal disease. No consensus exists regarding the best treatment for this unusual condition.

References

Bancroft LW, Berquist TH: Erdheim-Chester disease: radiographic findings in five patients. *Skeletal Radiol* 27(3):127–132, 1998.

Dion E, Graef C, Miquel A, et al: Bone involvement in Erdheim-Chester disease: imaging findings including periostitis and partial epiphyseal involvement. *Radiology* 238(2):632–639, 2006.

Gotthardt M, Welcke U, Brandt D, et al: The role of bone scintigraphy in patients with Erdheim-Chester disease. *Clin Nucl Med* 25(6):414–420, 2000.

Vencio EF, Jenkins RB, Schiller JL, et al: Clonal cytogenetic abnormalities in Erdheim-Chester disease. *Am J Surg Pathol* 31(2):319–321, 2007.

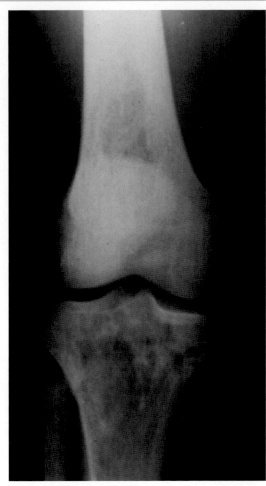

Figure 80–1 This patient was a 39-year-old male who presented with bone pain. The sclerosis in the metaphyses of the femur and tibia extend to the joint line, an increasingly encountered location, whereas in the fibula it is confined to the diaphysis.

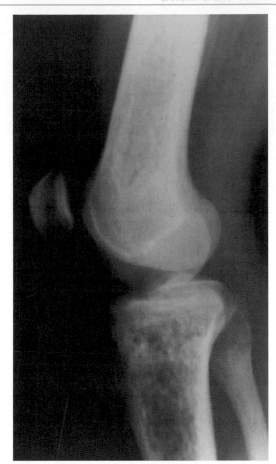

Figure 80–2 This figure illustrates the lateral radiograph corresponding to the anteroposterior view illustrated in Figure 80–1.

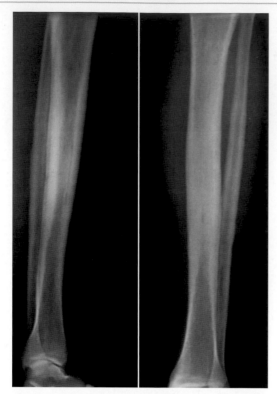

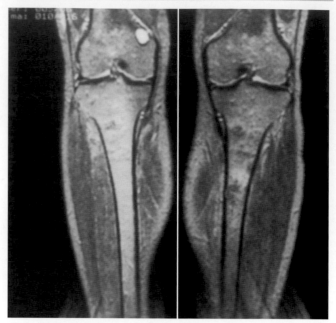

Figure 80–5 This T2-weighted MRI is from the case illustrated in Figure 80–4. Note most of the round lesions are of low signal because the lesions are sclerotic. Lytic metastases and myeloma would have a high signal on T2-weighted sequences.

Figure 80–3 This radiograph illustrates the typical diaphyseal bone sclerosis in the tibia seen in a patient with Erdheim-Chester disease. Such lesions resemble the radiographic appearance of Camurati-Engelmann disease.

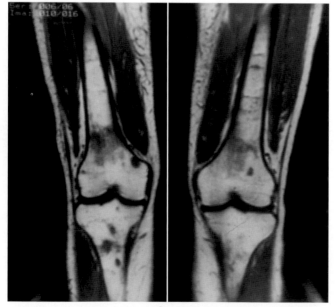

Figure 80–4 This T1-weighted magnetic resonance image (MRI) illustrates an example of Erdheim-Chester disease in a 35-year-old-female. The disease involves the distal femora and proximal tibia bilaterally. Several of the lesions are round and nonconfluent, mimicking metastases and multiple myeloma.

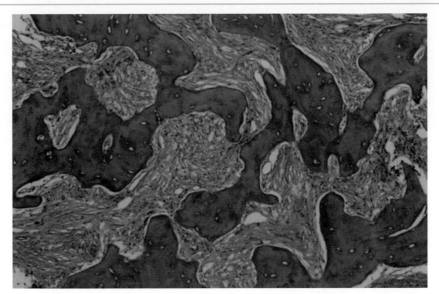

Figure 80–6 The histologic features of Erdheim-Chester disease are relatively nonspecific, consisting of variable fibrosis of the medullary bone with an admixture of mononuclear cells and lipid-laden histiocytes.

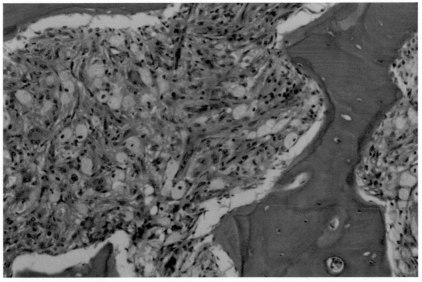

Figure 80–7 Erdheim-Chester disease may diffusely replace the fatty and hematopoietic marrow, as illustrated in this photomicrograph.

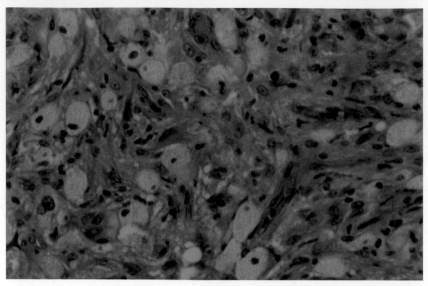

Figure 80–8 Regions within the lesional tissue of Erdheim-Chester disease may show numerous lipid-laden histiocytes, as illustrated in this photomicrograph.

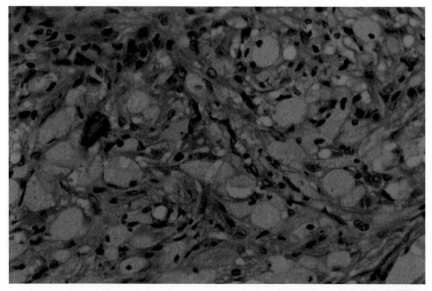

Figure 80–9 No significant cytologic atypia is generally evident in the mononuclear cells of Erdheim-Chester disease.

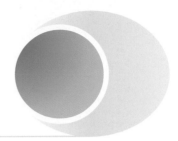

Index

Note: Page numbers followed by "f" refer to illustrations.

A

Acetabulum
    chondrosarcoma in, 302f, 303f
    hemangioendothelial sarcoma in, 390f
    mesenchymal chondrosarcoma in, 323f
    pigmented villonodular synovitis in, 184f
Achilles tendon rupture, and ochronosis, 122
Adamantinoma, 415–420
    angiosarcoma vs., 392f
    differential diagnosis of, 415, 416
    osteofibrous dysplasia vs., 159, 160, 162f, 165f
    pathology of, 415–416
        gross, 415–416, 417f
        histologic, 416, 417f, 418f, 419f, 420f
    radiography of, 415, 417f, 418f
    signs and symptoms of, 415
    treatment of, 416
Adenocarcinoma
    metastatic, 515f
        adamantinoma vs., 418f
        angiosarcoma vs., 391f
        myeloma vs., 366f
    mucinous, chordoma vs., 424f
    poorly differentiated, adamantinoma vs., 419f
Adenoma, parathyroid, 7f
Albers-Schönberg disease, 73. *See also* Osteopetrosis.
Albright's syndrome, 151, 154f, 155f
    fibrocartilaginous dysplasia in, 270f
Alkaptonuria, 121, 122
Amyloid
    in myeloma, 362, 365f, 366f
    in renal osteodystrophy, 17, 18
Amyloidomas, 140
Amyloidosis, 138–143
    differential diagnosis of, 139
    pathology of, 139, 141f, 142f
    radiography of, 139, 141f, 143f
    signs and symptoms of, 139, 143f
    treatment of, 139–140
Aneurysmal bone cyst, 453–458
    avulsive cortical irregularity vs., 480f
    and chest wall hamartoma, 484f
    and chondroblastoma, 274, 275f, 276f
    in clear cell chondrosarcoma, 326, 327f, 330f

Aneurysmal bone cyst *(Continued)*
    differential diagnosis of, 454
    giant cell reaction vs., 465, 469f
    and giant cell tumor, 43f, 406f
    in osteofibrous dysplasia, 162f
    pathology of, 454
        gross, 454, 455f
        histologic, 454, 455f, 456f, 457f, 458f
    radiography of, 453, 455f, 456f, 457f
    signs and symptoms of, 453
    telangiectatic osteosarcoma vs., 241, 242, 243f, 245f, 246f
    treatment of, 454
    unicameral bone cyst vs., 462f, 463f
Angiosarcoma, 387–395
    differential diagnosis of, 387, 388
    hemangiomas vs., 382, 383f
    pathology of, 388
        gross, 388, 389f
        histologic, 388, 389f, 390f, 391f, 392f, 393f, 394f, 395f
    radiography of, 387, 389f, 390f, 391f
    signs and symptoms of, 387
Ankle
    Charcot's joint and, 107f, 108f
    hypertrophic osteoarthropathy in, 63f
    postradiation osteosarcoma of, 447f
Ankylosing spondylitis, 167–171
    differential diagnosis of, 168
    vs. hyperparathyroidism, 4
    incidence and prevalence of, 167
    pathology of, 168
        gross, 169f, 170f
        histologic, 170f
    radiography of, 168, 169f, 171f
    signs and symptoms of, 167–168
    treatment of, 168
Ankylosis, and osteomyelitis, 489f
Arteriovenous fistula, hemangioma vs., 386f
Arthritis. *See also* Osteoarthritis; Rheumatoid arthritis.
    in gout, 125–126
    and ochronosis, 122
Arthroplasty
    hemophilic, 511f, 512f
    knee, 508f
    osteolysis and, 190f

Arthroplasty effect, 189–191
    differential diagnosis of, 189
    pathology of, 189
        gross, 190f
        histologic, 191f
    radiography of, 189, 190f
    signs and symptoms of, 189
    treatment of, 189
Avascular necrosis (AVN), 495–502
    differential diagnosis of, 495, 496
    in Gaucher's disease, 94, 96f, 97f, 98f
    incidence of, 495
    pathology of, 495
        gross, 495, 498f, 499f
        histologic, 495, 500f, 501f
    radiography of, 495, 497f, 502f
    risk factors for, 495
    signs and symptoms of, 495
    treatment of, 496
Avulsive cortical irregularity, 477–480
    differential diagnosis of, 477
    pathology of, 477
        gross, 477, 478f
        histologic, 477, 478f, 479f, 480f
    radiography of, 477, 478f, 479f, 480f
    signs and symptoms of, 477
    treatment of, 477

B

Bamboo spine, 168, 169f
Banana fracture, 46, 48f
Benign bone tumors, xanthomatosis vs., 147f
Bisphosphonates
    for osteoporosis, 12
    for Paget's disease, 47
Bizarre parosteal osteochondromatous proliferation (BPOP), 525–531
    differential diagnosis of, 525
    pathology of, 525
        gross, 525, 527f, 529f
        histologic, 525, 529f, 530f, 531f
    radiography of, 525, 527f, 528f
    signs and symptoms of, 525
    treatment of, 525
Blade of grass sign, 46, 52f
Blue bone, 525, 529f
Blue sclerae, 81, 82

Bone
   cortical
      in Camurati-Engelmann disease,
         55f, 56f, 57f
      in osteofibrous dysplasia, 159, 161f, 162f
      in osteoporosis, 15f
   in melorheostosis, 68, 71f
   in osteomalacia, 32, 35f, 36f
   resorption
      in hyperparathyroidism, 4, 5f, 6f, 7f, 8f
      in renal osteodystrophy, 17, 21f
   in rickets, 26f, 30f
   trabeculae
      in chest wall hamartoma, 481, 484f
      in fibrous dysplasia, 152, 154f
      fluorosis and, 91f, 92f
      in low-grade central osteosarcoma,
         248, 249f, 250f
      in malignant lymphoma, 353f
      in osteoblastoma, 206f, 207f
      in osteochondroma, 261f, 263f
      in osteofibrous dysplasia, 163f, 164f, 165f
      in osteogenesis imperfecta, 86f
      in osteoid osteoma, 196, 198f
      in osteoporosis, 11, 13f, 14f, 15f, 16f
      as osteosarcoma, 216f
      in Paget's disease, 46, 48f, 49f, 50f
      parosteal osteosarcoma in, 223f
      in renal osteodystrophy, 19f, 20f
Bone cyst
   aneurysmal. See Aneurysmal bone cyst.
   simple. See Unicameral bone cyst.
Bone deformities
   in osteogenesis imperfecta, 85f, 87f
   of Paget's disease, 48f, 49f
Bone density
   fluorosis and, 91f, 92f
   in rickets, 24
Bone erosion
   in pigmented villonodular synovitis,
      182f, 184f
   in rheumatoid arthritis, 112, 116f
Bone infarction
   and avascular necrosis, 498f, 499f, 500f,
      501f, 502f
   malignant fibrous histiocytoma and, 347f
Bone sclerosis. See Osteosclerosis.
Bone scan
   in Gaucher's disease, 94
   in Paget's disease, 46
   periosteal new bone formation in, 65f
Bone within a bone appearance, 74
Bowing
   in osteofibrous dysplasia, 159
   in osteogenesis imperfecta, 85f
   with osteomalacia, 34f
   in Paget's disease, 49f
BPOP. See Bizarre parosteal osteochondromatous proliferation.
Breast carcinoma, metastases with, 518f
Brodie's abscess, 493f
Brown tumor
   of hyperparathyroidism, 4, 5f, 6f, 8f, 9f
   and renal osteodystrophy, 17, 18

C
Calcaneous
   osteomyelitis in, 488f
   unicameral bone cyst of, 462f
Calcification
   in chest wall hamartoma, 481, 483f
   chicken wire, 274, 276f
   in chondroblastoma, 274, 276f
   in chondrocalcinosis, 136, 137f

Calcification (Continued)
   in chondrosarcomas, 298, 299f, 301f
      clear cell, 328f
      mesenchymal, 321, 323f
      with osteochondroma, 307f, 309f
   in chordoma, 424f
   in fluorosis, 90, 92f
   in ochronosis, 122
   in periosteal chondroma, 293f
   in phosphaturic mesenchymal tumors, 44f
   in pigmented villonodular synovitis, 182f
   in renal osteodystrophy, 17
   stippled, with multiple chondromas, 288f
Calcific bodies, in synovial chondromatosis,
   173, 174, 175f
Calcinosis, tumoral, 70f
Calcitonin
   for osteoporosis, 12
   for Paget's disease, 47
Calcium, supplemental
   for osteomalacia, 32
   for rickets, 24
Calcium pyrophosphate deposition disease, 135.
   See also Chondrocalcinosis.
Camurati-Engelmann disease, 53–57
   Erdheim-Chester disease vs., 536f
   differential diagnosis of, 54
   pathology of, 54, 56f
   radiography of, 54, 55f, 56f, 57f
   signs and symptoms of, 53–54
   treatment of, 54
Capillary hemangiomas, 383f
Carcinoma, metastatic, 513–518
   Charcot's joint vs., 109f
   differential diagnosis of, 513
   epithelioid hemangioendothelioma vs., 394f
   osteoblastic, mastocytosis vs., P369f
   osteosarcoma vs., 217f
   Paget's disease vs., 48f
   pathology of, 513
      gross, 513, 515f
      histologic, 513, 515f, 516f, 517f
   radiography of, 513, 515f, 518f
   signs and symptoms of, 513
   treatment of, 513–514
Carpal bone, Ewing's sarcoma in, 435f
Carpal tunnel syndrome, amyloidosis and,
   139, 142f
Cartilage, 112, 267f, 268f
   in avascular necrosis, 498f, 499f, 500f
   in Charcot's joint, 106, 108f
   in chondrocalcinosis, 136, 137f
   in chondromas, 266
      chondromyxoid fibroma vs., 280, 282f
   in chondrosarcomas
      clear cell, 327f, 329f
      dedifferentiated, 314, 316f
      mesenchymal, 320, 323f
      with osteochondroma, 306
   clefting in, 102f, 103f
   in hemophilia, 509, 511f, 512f
   in multiple chondromas, 286
   in ochronosis, 122, 123f, 124f
   in osteoarthritis, 100, 101f, 102f, 103f
   in osteogenesis imperfecta, 83, 86f
   osteopetrosis and, 77f, 78f, 79f
   in rickets, 27f, 28f
   in synovial chondromatosis, 174, 176f, 177f
Cartilage tumor, chondroma vs., 268f, 269f, 271f
Cartilaginous cap
   in chondrosarcoma with osteochondroma,
      305, 306, 307f
   in osteochondroma, 260, 261f, 262f, 263f
   in parosteal osteosarcoma, 220, 224f

Caseating granulomatous infectious disease,
   gout vs., 133f
Cavernous hemangiomas, 383f
Cement lines, in Paget's disease, 50f, 51f
Cementoblastomas, 204, 207f
Cementum, and unicameral bone cysts,
   459, 463f
Cervical nerve root, neurilemmoma in, 452f
Charcot's joint, 105–109
   differential diagnosis of, 106
   incidence of, 105
   pathology of, 106
      gross, 106, 107f, 108f
      histologic, 106, 108f, 109f
   radiography of, 106, 107f, 109f
   signs and symptoms of, 105–106
   treatment of, 106
Chest wall hamartoma, 481–484
   differential diagnosis of, 481
   pathology of, 481, 483f, 484f
   radiography of, 481, 483f
   signs and symptoms of, 481
   treatment of, 481
Children, osteopetrosis in, 73
Cholecalciferol
   for osteomalacia, 32
   for rickets, 24
Cholesterol, xanthomatosis and, 146, 147f, 149f
Chondroblastoma, 273–278
   chondromyxoid fibroma vs,
      281f, 282f, 284f
   clear cell chondrosarcoma vs., 328f, 329f
   differential diagnosis of, 274
   pathology of, 274
      gross, 274, 275f
      histologic, 274, 275f, 276f, 277f, 278f
   radiography of, 273–274, 275f, 276f, 277f
   signs and symptoms of, 273
   treatment of, 274
Chondrocalcinosis, 135–137
   differential diagnosis of, 136
   pathology of, 136, 137f
   radiography of, 136, 137f
   signs and symptoms of, 135–136
   treatment of, 136
Chondrocytes
   in chondromas, 268f, 269f
   in chondrosarcoma, 302f
   in osteochondroma, 260, 261f, 262f
   in parosteal osteosarcoma, 220
   in periosteal chondroma, 292
Chondroid chordomas, 422, 426f.
Chondroid differentiation, in high-grade
   surface osteosarcoma, 236
Chondroid matrix
   in chondrosarcomas, 298
   in periosteal osteosarcoma, 228, 229f, 231f
Chondroid zones, in mesenchymal
   chondrosarcoma, 320, 321f, 322f
Chondroma(s), 265–271
   chondrosarcoma vs., 298, 300f, 302f
   differential diagnosis of, 266
   multiple, 285–290
      differential diagnosis of, 286
      gross pathology of, 286, 287f, 289f
      histology of, 286, 287f, 288f, 289f, 290f
      radiography of, 285, 287f, 288f, 289f
      signs and symptoms of, 285
      treatment of, 286
   pathology of, 266
      gross, 266, 267f, 268f
      histologic, 266, 267f, 268f, 269f, 270f,
         271f
   periosteal, 270f, 291–296

Chondroma(s) *(Continued)*
    differential diagnosis of, 291, 292
    gross pathology of, 292, 293f, 296f
    histology of, 292, 293f, 294f, 295f, 296f
    periosteal osteosarcoma vs.,
        227, 228, 230f
    radiography of, 291, 293f, 294f, 295f
    signs and symptoms of, 291
    treatment of, 292
  radiography of, 265, 266, 267f, 268f, 269f
  signs and symptoms of, 265
  treatment of, 266
Chondromyxoid fibroma, 279–284
  differential diagnosis of, 279–280
  oncogenic osteomalacia in, 41f
  pathology of, 280
    gross, 280, 281f
    histologic, 280, 281f, 282f, 283f, 284f
  radiography of, 279–280, 281f, 282f, 283f
  signs and symptoms of, 279
  treatment of, 280
Chondrosarcoma, 297–303, 422
  chondroma vs., 266
  chondromyxoid fibroma vs, 282f, 284f
  clear cell, 325–330
    differential diagnosis of, 326
    gross pathology of, 326, 327f
    histology of, 326, 327f, 328f, 329f, 330f
    radiography of, 325, 327f, 328f, 329f
    signs and symptoms of, 325
    treatment of, 326
  dedifferentiated, 313–318
    differential diagnosis of, 314
    gross pathology of, 314, 315f
    histology of, 314, 315f, 316f, 317f, 318f
    radiography of, 313, 315f, 316f, 317f
    signs and symptoms of, 313
    treatment of, 314
  differential diagnosis of, 298
  intramedullary, 307f
  mesenchymal, 319–324
    differential diagnosis of, 319, 320
    gross pathology of, 320, 321f
    hemangiopericytoma vs., 401f
    histology of, 320, 321f, 322f, 323f, 324f
    radiography of, 319, 321f, 322f, 323f
    signs and symptoms of, 319
    small cell osteosarcoma vs., 255f
    treatment of, 320
  multiple chondromas vs., 289f, 290f
  osteoarthritis vs., 101f
  and osteochondroma, 260, 305–311
    differential diagnosis of, 305, 306
    gross pathology of, 306, 307f, 309f
    histology of, 306, 307f, 308f, 310f, 311f
    radiography of, 305, 307f, 308f, 309f
    signs and symptoms of, 305
    treatment of, 306
  osteosarcoma vs., 214f, 232f
  pathology of, 298
    gross, 298, 299f
    histologic, 298, 299f, 300f, 301f, 302f,
      303f
  periosteal
    chondroma vs., 296f
    gross pathology of, 296f
    osteosarcoma vs., 230f
  radiography of, 297, 299f, 300f, 301f
  signs and symptoms of, 297
  synovial chondromatosis vs., 174, 176f
  treatment of, 298
Chordoma, 421–426
  differential diagnosis of, 422
  pathology of, 422

Chordoma *(Continued)*
    gross, 422, 423f
    histologic, 422, 423f, 424f, 425f, 426f
  radiography of, 422, 423f, 424f, 425f
  signs and symptoms of, 421
  treatment of, 422
Clavicle
  angiosarcoma in, 389f
  Langerhans' cell histiocytosis of, 375f
Clear cell chondrosarcoma, 325–330
  differential diagnosis of, 326
  pathology of, 326
    gross, 326, 327f
    histologic, 326, 327f, 328f, 329f, 330f
  radiography of, 325, 327f, 328f, 329f
  signs and symptoms of, 325
  treatment of, 326
Clear cells, in malignant fibrous
  histiocytoma, 349f
Clubbing, 61f, 62f, 63f
Codfish vertebrae, 32, 83
Codman's triangle
  in Ewing's sarcoma, 429f
  in osteosarcoma, 212, 213f
  in periosteal osteosarcoma, 227
  in telangiectatic osteosarcoma, 244f
Colchicine, 126
Collagen, in fibrosarcoma, 338, 341f, 342f
Collagen vascular disease, and avascular
  necrosis, 495
Compression fractures
  in Gaucher's disease, 94
  in osteomalacia, 34f
  osteoporotic, 13f, 14f
Congenital osteosclerosis, 73. *See also*
  Osteopetrosis.
Corduroy vertebrae, 385f
Cortical hyperostosis, in melorheostosis, 68
Corticosteroids, 126
Costochondral junction
  beading of, 23
  rickets in, 26f, 27f, 28f
Cranial nerve palsies, osteopetrosis and, 74
Crush artifact, in malignant lymphoma, 359f
Cushing's disease, osteoporosis in, 16f
Cystic degeneration, in fibrous dysplasia, 152,
  154f, 157f
Cysts
  aneurysmal. *See* Aneurysmal bone cysts.
  simple. *See* Unicameral bone cysts.
  subchondral
    in osteoarthritis, 100, 101f, 102f,
      103f, 104f
    in rheumatoid arthritis, 112, 114f
Cytopenias, in Gaucher's disease, 93

D

Degenerative joint disease, and avascular
  necrosis, 498f, 499f
Dentinogenesis imperfecta, 82
Diabetes, Charcot's joint and, 108f, 109f
Dialysis, renal osteodystrophy and, 17
Diaphyseal dysplasia, progressive.
  See Camurati-Engelmann disease.
Dual-energy x-ray absorptiometry (DEXA)
  scanning, 11

E

Earlobes, ochronosis and, 121
Eburnation, 101f
Eddowes' syndrome, 81
Ekman-Lobstein disease, 81
Elbow, pigmented villonodular synovitis in, 186f
Enchondroma, 267f

Enchondroma *(Continued)*
  chondromas vs., 270f, 271f
  dedifferentiated chondrosarcoma vs., 318f
  vs. unicameral bone cyst, 464f
Endochondral ossification
  in ankylosing spondylitis, 168, 170f
  osteogenesis imperfecta in, 86f
  osteopetrosis and, 78f
Endosteal erosion, in renal osteodystrophy, 17
Endosteal hyperostosis, in melorheostosis, 68
Eosinophilic granuloma, angiosarcoma vs., 392f
Eosinophils
  in angiosarcoma, 394f
  in histiocytosis X, 374, 375f
Epidermoid cyst, unicameral bone cyst vs., 464f
Epiphyses
  in Camurati-Engelmann disease, 55f
  in osteogenesis imperfecta, 83, 86f
  rickets and, 27f, 28f
  slipped, in renal osteodystrophy, 17
Epithelioid hemangioendothelioma, 387–395
  differential diagnosis of, 387, 388
  pathology of, 388
    gross, 388, 389f
    histologic, 388, 389f, 390f, 391f, 392f,
      393f, 394f, 395f
  radiography of, 387, 389f, 390f, 391f
  signs and symptoms of, 387
  treatment of, 388
Epithelioid hemangiomas, 386f
Epithelioid islands, in adamantinoma, 416, 417f
Erdheim-Chester disease, 533–538
  differential diagnosis of, 533, 534
  incidence of, 533
  pathology of, 534, 537f, 538f
  radiography of, 533, 535f, 536f
  signs and symptoms of, 533
  treatment of, 534
Ergocalciferol
  for osteomalacia, 32
  for rickets, 24
Erlenmeyer flask-like appearance, 74
  in Gaucher's disease, 94, 96f
Estrogen receptor modulators, 12
Ewing's sarcoma, 427–436
  atypical, 435f
  differential diagnosis of, 428
  hemangiopericytoma vs., 401f
  histiocytosis X vs., 375f
  malignant lymphoma vs., 354f
  osteomyelitis vs., 491f
  pathology of, 428
    gross, 428, 429f
    histologic, 428, 429f, 430f, 432f, 433f,
      434f, 435f, 436f
  radiography of, 427–428, 429f, 431f, 432f
  small cell osteosarcoma vs., 252, 253f, 256f
  signs and symptoms of, 427
  treatment of, 428

F

Factor VIII deficiency. *See* Hemophilia.
Fasciitis, avulsive cortical irregularity vs., 480f
Femur, 451f
  amyloidosis in, 142
  angiosarcoma in, 391f, 393f
  avascular necrosis of, 94, 96f, 97f, 98f, 498f,
    499f, 500f
  avulsive cortical irregularity of, 479f
  Charcot's joint and, 107f
  chondroblastoma in, 275f
  chondroma in, 267f, 269f, 271f
  chondromyxoid fibroma in, 282f
  chondrosarcoma in, 290f, 300f

Femur (Continued)
   clear cell, 327f, 329f
   dedifferentiated, 317f
   mesenchymal, 323f
   Erdheim-Chester disease in, 535f, 536f
   Ewing's sarcoma in, 431f
   fibrocartilaginous dysplasia in, 270f
   fibroma in, 474f, 475f
   fibrosarcoma in, 339f, 340f
   fibrous dysplasia in, 155f, 157f
   fluorosis and, 92f
   fractures, and avascular necrosis, 495
   Gaucher's disease and, 94, 96f, 97f, 98f
   giant cell tumor of, 406f, 408f
   hemangioma in, 385f
   hemangiopericytoma of, 400f
   infarcts in, 502f
   lytic lesion in, 9f
   malignant fibrous histiocytoma of,
      345f, 346f, 347f, 348f
   malignant giant cell tumor in, 413f, 414f
   malignant lymphoma of, 356f, 357f
   massive osteolysis in, 506f, 507f, 508f
   mastocytosis in, 369f, 370f
   melorheostosis in, 69f, 70f
   metastatic carcinoma in, 515f, 518f
   multiple chondromas in, 289f
   myeloma in, 363f
   osteoarthritis in, 101f, 102f
   osteoblastoma in, 206f, 208f
   osteochondroma in, 262f, 263f
   osteoid osteoma in, 197f, 198f, 199f
   osteomyelitis in, 487f, 488f, 491f
   osteopetrosis in, 76f, 77f
   osteoporosis in, 13f, 16f
   osteosarcoma in, 213f, 215f, 217f
      high-grade surface, 238f, 239f
      parosteal, 221f, 223f, 224f, 225f
      periosteal, 230f
      small cell, 253f, 256f
      telangiectatic, 243f, 244f
   Paget's disease in, 48f, 50f, 52f
   periosteal chondroma in, 295f
   postradiation sarcoma of, 445f
   prosthesis, 508f
   in renal osteodystrophy, 19f, 20f
   rickets in, 26f, 27f, 30f
   rheumatoid arthritis in, 117f
   synovial chondromatosis in, 175f
Fibrilization, 102f
Fibrocartilaginous dysplasia, 155f
   vs. chondroma, 270f
Fibrochondroid matrix, in chondroblastoma,
   274, 275f, 276f
Fibroma, 471-475
   benign fibrous histiocytomas vs., 335f, 336f
   chondromyxoid, 279-284
      differential diagnosis of, 279-280
      gross pathology of, 280, 281f
      histology of, 280, 281f, 282f, 283f, 284f
      oncogenic osteomalacia in, 41f
      radiography of, 279-280, 281f, 282f, 283f
      signs and symptoms of, 279
      treatment of, 280
   desmoplastic, fibrosarcoma vs., 342f
   differential diagnosis of, 472, 473
   pathology of, 472
      gross, 472, 473f
      histologic, 472, 473f, 474f, 475f
   radiography of, 471, 473f, 474f, 475f
   signs and symptoms of, 471
   treatment of, 472
Fibromatosis, congenital, and hemangiopericytoma, 402f

Fibrosarcoma, 337-342
   dedifferentiated chondrosarcoma
      vs., 314, 316f, 317f, 318f
   differential diagnosis of, 338
   and malignant giant cell tumor, 413f, 414f
   vs. Paget's sarcoma, 442f
   pathology of, 338
      gross, 338, 339f
      histologic, 338, 339f, 341f, 342f
   as postradiation sarcoma, 444, 445f, 446f
   radiography of, 337-338, 339f, 340f
   signs and symptoms of, 337
   treatment of, 338
Fibrous cortical defect, 477-480
   differential diagnosis of, 477
   pathology of, 477
      gross, 477, 478f
      histologic, 477, 478f, 479f, 480f
   radiography of, 477, 478f, 479f, 480f
   signs and symptoms of, 477
   treatment of, 477
Fibrous dysplasia, 151-157
   differential diagnosis of, 152
   low-grade osteosarcoma vs., 247, 248, 250f
   neurilemmoma vs., 451f
   osteomalacia in, 38, 40f
   Paget's disease vs., 51f
   parosteal osteosarcoma vs., 222f, 223f
   pathology of, 152
      gross, 152, 154f, 157f
      histologic, 152, 154f, 155f, 156f, 157f
   radiography of, 151-152, 154f, 155f, 156f
   signs and symptoms of, 151, 154f
   treatment of, 152
   xanthomatosis and, 148f
Fibrous histiocytoma
   benign, 333-336
      differential diagnosis of, 333, 334
      fibroma vs., 475f
      gross pathology of, 334, 335f
      histology of, 334, 335f, 336f
      radiography of, 333, 335f, 336f
      signs and symptoms of, 333
      treatment of, 334
   dedifferentiated chondrosarcoma vs.,
      314, 316f, 317f
   vs. giant cell tumor, 409f
   malignant, 343-349
      differential diagnosis of, 344
      gross pathology of, 344, 345f
      histology of, 344, 345f, 346f, 347f,
         348f 349f
      malignant giant cell tumor vs., 414f
      malignant lymphoma vs., 352, 358f
      vs. Paget's sarcoma, 442f
      as postradiation sarcoma, 444
      radiography of, 343, 345f, 346f, 347f
      signs and symptoms of, 343
      treatment of, 344
Fibrovascular connective tissues, in Paget's
   disease, 50f
Fibula
   adamantinoma in, 417f, 418f
   aneurysmal bone cyst of, 456f
   chondroma in, 267f, 268f, 270f
   Erdheim-Chester disease in, 535f
   Ewing's sarcoma in, 429f
   fibroma in, 474f
   giant cell tumor of, 409f
   hemangioma in, 383f, 386f
   hypertrophic osteoarthropathy in, 61f
   melorheostosis in, 69f
   multiple chondromas in, 288f, 289f
   myeloma in, 364f

Fibula (Continued)
   osteochondroma in, 261f
   in osteogenesis imperfecta, 85f
   Paget's disease in, 49f
   pulmonary hypertrophic osteoarthropathy
      in, 64f
Finger
   multiple chondromas in, 287f
   osseous epidermoid cyst of, 464f
Fish scale appearance of bone, 82
Flame sign, 46
Fluorosis, 89-92
   differential diagnosis of, 89
   pathology of, 89, 92f
   radiography of, 89, 91f, 92f
   signs and symptoms of, 89
   treatment of, 89
Follicular carcinoma of thyroid, metastatic, 517f
Foot
   Charcot's joint and, 109f
   in melorheostosis, 71f
   multiple chondromas in, 288f
   pigmented villonodular synovitis in, 182f
   postradiation osteosarcoma of, 447f
Forearm, osteogenesis imperfecta in, 84f
Fracture(s)
   and avascular necrosis, 495
   with bone cyst, 459, 461f, 462f
   fibroma and, 471, 472, 475f
   with fibrosarcoma, 340f
   in Gaucher's disease, 94
   malignant lymphoma and, 353f
   and massive osteolysis, 506f, 507f
   in myeloma, 361, 363f
   in osteogenesis imperfecta, 82, 85f, 86f, 87f
   in osteomalacia, 34f
   osteoporosis and, 11, 12, 13f, 14f
   with Paget's sarcoma, 441f
   in Paget's disease, 46, 48f, 49f
   in renal osteodystrophy, 17
Frontal bossing, 24

G
Ganglion cyst, 463f, 464f
Gaucher's disease, 93-98
   differential diagnosis of, 94
   inheritance pattern and types, 93
   pathology of, 94, 97f, 98f
   radiography of, 94, 96f, 98f
   signs and symptoms of, 93-94
   treatment of, 94
Ghost tumor cells, 409f
Giant cell reaction, 465-469
   differential diagnosis of, 465
   in myeloma, 362, 365f
   pathology of, 465, 468f, 469f
   radiography of, 465, 467f
   signs and symptoms of, 465
   treatment of, 465-466
Giant cells
   in benign fibrous histiocytoma, 336f
   in chondroblastoma, 274, 275f, 278f
   in chondromyxoid fibroma, 280, 281f
   in clear cell chondrosarcoma, 326, 328f
   in dedifferentiated chondrosarcoma, 318f
   in fibroma, 472, 474f, 475f
   in fibrous dysplasia, 156f
   in giant cell tumor, 404, 405f, 406f, 408f
   in Langerhans' cell histiocytosis, 376f
   in lymphoma, 358f
   in malignant fibrous histiocytomas,
      344, 348f
   in osteosarcoma, 212, 213f
   in phosphaturic mesenchymal tumors, 42f

Giant cells *(Continued)*
 in pigmented villonodular synovitis, 180, 184f, 185f
 in telangiectatic osteosarcoma, 242, 244f, 245f
 in xanthomas, 147f, 149f
Giant cell tumor(s), 403–409
 aneurysmal bone cyst vs., 455f
 brown tumor vs., 8f, 9f
 chondroblastoma vs., 274, 275f, 276f
 differential diagnosis of, 404
 fibroma vs., 474f
 fibrous dysplasia vs., 156f
 fibrous histiocytoma vs., 344, 346f
 vs. giant cell reaction, 468f
 of hyperparathyroidism, 4, 5f, 6f
 malignant, 411–414
  dedifferentiated chondrosarcoma vs., 318f
  differential diagnosis of, 412
  pathology of, 412, 413f, 414f
  radiography of, 411–412, 413f, 414f
  signs and symptoms of, 411
  treatment of, 412
 vs. metastatic carcinoma, 518f
 osteomalacia and, 38, 43f
 osteosarcoma vs., 212, 217f
 pathology of, 404
  gross, 404, 405f, 408f
  histologic, 404, 405f, 406f, 407f, 408f, 409f
 pigmented villonodular synovitis vs., 186f
 radiography of, 403, 405f, 406f, 407f
 and renal osteodystrophy, 17
 signs and symptoms of, 403
 telangiectatic osteosarcoma vs., 245f, 246f
 treatment of, 404
 xanthomatosis and, 146, 148f, 149f
Glomus tumors, 401f
Glycogen, 252
Gorham's disease, 385f, 503–508
 differential diagnosis of, 504
 pathology of, 504, 506f, 507f
 radiography of, 503–504, 505f, 506f, 507f, 508f
 signs and symptoms of, 503
 treatment of, 504
Gout, 125–133
 differential diagnosis of, 126
 pathology of, 126
  gross, 128f, 129f, 133f
  histologic, 130f, 131f, 132f, 133f
 radiography of, 126, 127f, 132f, 133f
 signs and symptoms of, 125–126, 127f
 tophi in, 125, 126, 127f, 129f, 131f
 treatment of, 126
Granulocytic sarcoma, vs. malignant lymphoma, 355f
Granuloma(s)
 giant cell. *See* Giant cell reaction.
 infectious, 120f
 rheumatoid, 118f, 120f
Granulomatous infectious disease, gout vs., 133f
Granulomatous reaction, to arthroplasty, 189
Greater trochanter, chondroblastoma in, 277f
Growth lines, in fluorosis, 90
Growth plates, in osteogenesis imperfecta, 83, 86f

H

Hamartoma, chest wall, 481–484
 differential diagnosis of, 481
 pathology of, 481, 483f, 484f
 radiography of, 481, 483f
 signs and symptoms of, 481
 treatment of, 481

Hand
 amyloidosis and, 143f
 BPOP in, 528f, 529f, 530f
 chondroma in, 269f
 enchondroma in, 267f
 Ewing's sarcoma in, 435f, 436f
 giant cell reaction in, 467f, 468f, 469f
 multiple chondromas in, 287f, 288f
 osteoarthritis in, 101f
 osteogenesis imperfecta in, 84f
Hand-Schüller-Christian disease, 373, 374
Harrison's groove, 23, 24, 26f
Hearing loss, in osteogenesis imperfecta, 82
Heberden's nodes, 99, 100, 101f
 in chondrocalcinosis, 135
Hemangioendothelioma, 387–395
 differential diagnosis of, 387, 388
 pathology of, 388
  gross, 388, 389f
  histologic, 388, 389f, 390f, 391f, 392f, 393f, 394f, 395f
 radiography of, 387, 389f, 390f, 391f
 signs and symptoms of, 387
 treatment of, 388
Hemangioma, 381–386
 differential diagnosis of, 382
 in Maffucci's syndrome, 285, 289f
 vs. massive osteolysis, 506f
 pathology of, 382
  gross, 382, 383f, 384f, 385f
  histologic, 382, 383f, 386f
 radiography of, 381–382, 383f, 384f, 385f
 signs and symptoms of, 381
 treatment of, 382
Hemangiopericytoma, 397–402
 differential diagnosis of, 397, 398
 mesenchymal chondrosarcoma vs., 322f, 323f
 myeloma vs., 366f
 pathology of, 397–398
  gross, 397, 399
  histologic, 398, 399f, 400f, 401f, 402f
 radiography of, 397, 399f, 400f
 signs and symptoms of, 397
 treatment of, 398
Hemangiopericytomatous pattern, 42f, 43f
 in mesenchymal chondrosarcoma, 320, 322f, 324f
 in small cell osteosarcoma, 252, 255f
Hemarthroses, 509
Hemophilia, 509–512
 differential diagnosis of, 509
 pathology of, 509, 511f, 512f
 radiography of, 509, 511f, 512f
 signs and symptoms of, 509
 treatment of, 510
Hepatocellular carcinoma, metastatic, 517f
Herringbone pattern, in fibrosarcoma, 338, 339f
Hip
 Charcot's joint and, 109f
 juvenile rheumatoid arthritis in, 114f
 melorheostosis in, 70f
 osteoporosis in, 16f
 pigmented villonodular synovitis in, 182f
 synovial chondromatosis in, 175f, 178f
 tuberculous osteomyelitis in, 490f
Hip arthroplasty, osteolysis and, 190f
Histiocytes
 in benign fibrous histiocytoma, 334, 335f
 in Erdheim-Chester disease, 533, 537f, 538f
 in Gaucher's disease, 94, 96f, 97f, 98f
 in periprosthetic osteolysis, 191f
 in xanthomatosis, 145, 146, 147f, 148f

Histiocytoma. *See* Fibrous histiocytoma.
Histiocytosis X. *See* Langerhans' cell histiocytosis.
HLA-B27, 167
Hodgkin's disease, and granulomatous reaction, 493f
Hodgkin's lymphoma, 359f
Homogentisic acid, 121, 122
Humerus
 angiosarcoma in, 389f
 avascular necrosis in, 497f
 BPOP in, 531f
 Charcot's joint and, 109f
 chondroblastoma in, 276f
 chondromyxoid fibroma of, 283f
 chondrosarcoma in, 299f
  clear cell, 327f, 329f
  dedifferentiated, 315f, 316f
 fibrosarcoma in, 340f
 fibrous dysplasia in, 156f
 in Gaucher's disease, 94, 96f
 giant cell tumor in, 406f, 409f
 malignant lymphoma in, 353f
 multiple chondromas in, 287f
 osteoarthritis of, 104f
 osteomalacia in, 43f
 osteomyelitis in, 488f
 osteosarcoma in, 215f
  parosteal, 222f, 224f
  small cell, 253f
  telangiectatic, 245f
 periosteal chondroma in, 293f, 294f
 postradiation sarcoma of, 445f, 446f, 447f
 unicameral bone cyst in, 461f, 462f
Hyaline cartilage. *See* Cartilage.
Hyaline cartilage tumor
 epithelioid hemangioendothelioma vs., 393f
 features of, 299f
 pattern of, 294f
Hypercalcemia, in hyperparathyroidism, 3
Hypergammaglobulinemia, 361
Hyperostosis, in melorheostosis, 68, 69f
Hyperostosis generalisata with pachyderma, 54
Hyperparathyroidism, 3–9
 differential diagnosis of, 4
 osteomalacia and, 32
 pathology of, 4
  gross, 6f
  histologic, 6f, 7f, 8f, 9f
 radiography of, 4, 5f, 7f, 8f, 9f
 renal osteodystrophy vs, 17, 18f
 signs and symptoms of, 3–4
 treatment of, 4
Hyperuricemia
 in chondrocalcinosis, 135
 in gout, 125

I

Ilium
 angiosarcoma in, 395f
 benign fibrous histiocytoma in, 336f
 brown tumor of, 8
 chondromyxoid fibromas in, 281f
 epithelioid hemangioendothelioma in, 393f
 Ewing's sarcoma in, 434f
 fibrosarcoma in, 340f
 fibrous dysplasia in, 154f, 155f
 Hodgkin's lymphoma of, 359f
 malignant lymphoma of, 356f
 mastocytosis in, 369f
 oncogenic osteomalacia in, 43f
 osteochondroma in, 262f
  with chondrosarcoma, 308f, 309f
 osteomalacia in, 35f

Ilium (Continued)
    osteomyelitis in, 494f
    Paget's sarcoma in, 441f
    xanthomatosis in, 147f
Ilizarov gradual distraction, 68
Immunohistochemical stains, for lymphoid
    markers, 352, 354f, 355f
Infants, osteopetrosis in, 73
Interphalangeal joints, osteoarthritis in, 101f
Ischium
    aneurysmal bone cyst of, 455f
    hemangiopericytoma of, 399f, 401f
    Paget's sarcoma in, 441f

J

Joint(s)
    Charcot's. *See* Charcot's joint.
    effusions, in hypertrophic
        osteoarthropathy, 59
    in chondrocalcinosis, 135, 136, 137f
    melorheostosis and, 67
    in ochronosis, 122
    in osteoarthritis, 100, 101f
    pigmented villonodular synovitis in,
        179, 180
    subluxation, in rheumatoid arthritis,
        115f, 116f
Juvenile rheumatoid arthritis (JRA), 114f

K

Kidney, hyperparathyroidism and, 7f
Knee
    avulsive cortical irregularity in, 478f
    Charcot's joint and, 106, 107f
    chondroblastoma in, 275f
    chondrocalcinosis in, 137f
    giant cell tumor in, 405f
    gout in, 128f
    with hemophilia, 511f, 512f
    infarcts in, 502f
    in melorheostosis, 71f
    in ochronosis, 124f
    pigmented villonodular synovitis
        in, 182f
    rheumatoid arthritis in, 114f
    synovial chondromatosis in, 175f
Knee prosthesis, 508f
Kyphoscoliosis, in osteogenesis imperfecta, 82

L

Langerhans' cell histiocytosis, 373–378
    chondroblastoma vs., 274, 276f
    chondromyxoid fibroma vs., 282f
    differential diagnosis of, 374
    pathology of, 374
        gross, 374, 375f
        histologic, 374, 375f, 376f, 377f, 378f
    radiography of, 374, 375f, 376f, 377f
    signs and symptoms of, 373
    treatment of, 374
    xanthomatosis vs., 146
Langerhans' cells, 374, 377f
Lead poisoning, sclerosis of, 79f
Leiomyosarcomas, fibrosarcoma vs., 342f
Lethal osteogenesis imperfecta congenita, 81
Lethal perinatal osteogenesis imperfecta, 81
Letterer-Siwe disease, 373, 374
Ligaments
    calcification of
        in ankylosing spondylitis, 168
        in chondrocalcinosis, 136, 137f
    laxity of, in rheumatoid arthritis, 116f
Loose bodies, with osteoarthritis, 104f

Looser's zones
    in osteomalacia, 32
    in renal osteodystrophy, 17, 18f
    in rickets, 24
Lumbar spine
    aneurysmal bone cyst in, 457f
    metastasis in, 518f
    pigmented villonodular synovitis in, 187f
Lung carcinoma
    osteoarthropathy in, 63f, 64f
    metastases with, 515f
Lymph nodes, sarcoidosis in, 521f
Lymphoid nodules, 116f
Lymphoma
    Ewing's sarcoma vs., 436f
    Hodgkin's, 359f
    immunoblastic, myeloma vs., 364f
    malignant, 351–359
        differential diagnosis of, 352
        gross pathology of, 352, 353f
        histology of, 352, 353f, 354f, 355f,
            357f, 358f, 359f
        myeloma vs., 363f, 365f
        radiography of, 351–352, 353f, 356f,
            357f
        signs and symptoms of, 351
        treatment of, 352
    non-Hodgkin's, 353f

M

Macroglossia, amyloidosis and, 143f
Macrophages, in pigmented villonodular
    synovitis, 184f, 185f
Maffucci's syndrome, 285,289f
Magnetic resonance imaging (MRI)
    in Paget's disease, 46
    of pigmented villonodular synovitis,
        180, 182f, 183f
    of synovial chondromatosis, 174
Mandible, 451f, 452f
    mesenchymal chondrosarcoma in, 324f
    osteoblastoma in, 207f
    postradiation osteosarcoma in, 446f
Marble bone disease, 73. *See also*
    Osteopetrosis.
Mastocytosis, 367–371
    differential diagnosis of, 367
    pathology of, 367
        gross, 367, 369f
        histologic, 367, 369f, 370f, 371f
    radiography of, 367, 369f, 370f, 371f
    signs and symptoms of, 367
    treatment of, 367
Maxilla
    fibrosarcoma in, 339f
    osteoblastoma in, 207f
Mazabraud's syndrome, 151, 152
Melorheostosis, 67–71
    differential diagnosis of, 68
    pathology of, 68, 69f, 70f
    radiography of, 68, 69f, 70f, 71f
    signs and symptoms of, 67–68
    treatment of, 68
Meninges, hemangiopericytoma of, 401f
Meningioma, fibrous dysplasia vs., 155f, 156f
Mesenchymal hamartoma of the chest wall.
    See Hamartoma, chest wall.
Metacarpals
    BPOP in, 529f
    giant cell reactions in, 467f, 469f
    massive osteolysis in, 506f
    rheumatoid arthritis in, 115f, 116f
Metadiaphyseal region, in Gaucher's
    disease, 94

Metaphyses
    fibrous defect, osteomalacia in, 38
    in osteopetrosis, 74, 76f
    in rickets, 23, 26f, 27f
Metastases
    Erdheim-Chester disease vs., 536f
    pulmonary. *See* Pulmonary metastases
Metastatic carcinoma. *See* Carcinoma,
    metastatic.
Metatarsals
    giant cell reaction in, 467f
    gout and, 125, 126, 127f, 133f
Milkman's syndrome, 32
MRI. *See* Magnetic resonance imaging.
Multinucleated giant cells. *See* Giant cells.
Multiple myeloma. *See* Myeloma.
Muscle
    amyloidosis and, 143f
    chondrosarcoma and, 310f
Myeloma, 361–366
    amyloidosis and, 141f, 142f
    differential diagnosis of, 362
    Erdheim-Chester disease vs., 536f
    osteomyelitis vs., 492f
    pathology of, 362
        gross, 362, 363f, 365f
        histologic, 362, 363f, 364f, 365f, 366f
    radiography of, 362, 363f, 364f, 365f
    signs and symptoms of, 361
    treatment of, 362
Myxoid matrix, in phosphaturic mesenchymal
    tumors, 44f

N

Nasal bones, hemangioma in, 384f
Necrosis
    avascular. *See* Avascular necrosis.
    in histiocytosis X, 374
Neurilemmoma, 449–452
    differential diagnosis of, 449, 450
    pathology of, 450, 451f, 452f
    radiography of, 449, 451f, 452f
    signs and symptoms of, 449
    treatment of, 450
Neuroblastoma, metastatic, 516f
Nidus, in osteoid osteoma, 196, 197f,
    198f, 200f
Noncaseating granulomatous inflammation, in
    sarcoidosis, 519, 521f
Non-Hodgkin's lymphoma, 353f
Nonsteroidal anti-inflammatory drugs (NSAIDs)
    for chondrocalcinosis, 136
    for gout, 126

O

Ochronosis, 121–124
    differential diagnosis of, 122
    inheritance and, 121
    pathology of, 122, 123f, 124f
    radiography of, 122, 123f, 124f
    signs and symptoms of, 121–122
    treatment of, 122
Ollier's disease, 270f
    chondroma in, 285, 287f, 288f, 289f, 290f
Onion skin periostitis, 60
    in Ewing's sarcoma, 429f, 431f
Ossification
    anterior spinal ligament, 168
    as osteosarcoma, 216f
Osteitis, dissecting, with hyperparathyroidism,
    6f, 7f
Osteoarthritis, 99–104
    Charcot's joint vs., 108f
    classification of, 99

Osteoarthritis *(Continued)*
 differential diagnosis of, 100
 pathology of, 100
  gross, 101f, 102f, 104f
  histologic, 102f, 103f, 104f
 radiography of, 100, 101f, 104f
 signs and symptoms of, 99–100
 treatment of, 100
Osteoarthropathy, hypertrophic, 59–65
 classification of, 59
 differential diagnosis of, 60
 pathology of, 60, 61f, 62f
 radiography of, 60, 61f, 63f, 64f, 65f
 signs and symptoms of, 59, 63f
 treatment of, 60
Osteoblastic activity, in Paget's disease,
  46, 50f, 51f
Osteoblastoma, 203–210
 aneurysmal bone cyst vs., 458f
 differential diagnosis of, 204
 osteomalacia in, 38
 osteosarcoma vs., 218f
 pathology of, 204
  gross, 205f
  histologic, 205f, 206f, 207f,
   208f, 209f, 210f
 radiography of, 203–204, 205f, 206f, 207f
 signs and symptoms of, 203
 treatment of, 204
Osteochondroma, 259–263
 BPOP vs., 525, 527f, 529f, 530f
 chondrosarcoma in, 305–311
  differential diagnosis of, 305, 306
  gross pathology of, 306, 307f, 309f
  histology of, 306, 307f, 308f, 310f, 311f
  radiography of, 305, 307f, 308f, 309f
  signs and symptoms of, 305
  treatment of, 305
 differential diagnosis of, 259–260
 vs. parosteal osteosarcoma, 220, 224f
 pathology of, 260
  gross, 260, 261f, 263f
  histologic, 260, 261f, 262f, 263f
 radiography of, 259–260, 261f, 262f
 signs and symptoms of, 259
 treatment of, 260
Osteoclastic activity
 in Paget's disease, 50f, 51f, 52f
 in renal osteodystrophy, 18, 20f, 21f
Osteodystrophy, renal, 17–21
Osteofibrous dysplasia, 159–165
 differential diagnosis of, 159, 160
 pathology of, 160
  gross, 160, 161f, 163f
  histologic, 160, 163f, 164f, 165f
 radiography of, 159, 161f, 162f
 signs and symptoms of, 159
 treatment of, 160
Osteogenesis imperfecta, 81–87
 classification of, 81, 82
 differential diagnosis of, 83
 pathology of, 83
  gross, 83, 85f
  histologic, 83, 86–87f
 radiography of, 82–83, 84f, 85f, 87f
 signs and symptoms of, 82
 treatment of, 83
Osteogenesis imperfecta congenita, 85f
Osteogenesis imperfecta letalis type Vrolik, 81
Osteogenesis imperfecta tarda, 85f
Osteoid
 in Camurati-Engelmann disease, 56f
 in dedifferentiated chondrosarcoma, 314
 in fibrosarcoma, 341f

Osteoid *(Continued)*
 in fibrous dysplasia, 152, 154f, 155f
 and malignant fibrous histiocytoma, 348f
 in osteoblastoma, 204
 osteoid osteoma, 196, 198f
 osteomalacia and, 32, 35f, 36f
 in osteosarcoma, 212, 216f
  high-grade surface, 236, 237f, 239f
  low-grade central, 248, 250f
  periosteal, 228, 230f, 233f
  small cell, 252, 254f, 255f, 256f
 in postradiation sarcomas, 444
Osteoid osteoma, 195–201
 and Brodie's abscess, 493f
 differential diagnosis of, 196
 osteoblastoma vs., 203, 204
 osteomyelitis vs., 487f
 pathology of, 196
  gross, 196, 197f
  histologic, 196, 197f, 198f, 200f, 201f
 radiography of, 195–196, 197f, 198f, 199f
 signs and symptoms of, 195
 treatment of, 196
Osteolysis
 massive, 385f, 503–508
  differential diagnosis of, 504
  gross pathology of, 504
  histology of, 504, 506f, 507f
  radiography of, 503–504, 505f, 506f,
   507f, 508f
  signs and symptoms of, 503
  treatment of, 504
 in osteofibrous dysplasia, 161f
 in Paget's disease, 46, 47f
 periprosthetic, 189, 190f, 191f
Osteoma, osteoid. *See* Osteoid osteoma.
Osteomalacia, 31–36
 differential diagnosis of, 32
 oncogenic, 37–44
  differential diagnosis of, 38
  pathology of, 38, 41f, 42f, 43f, 44f
  radiography of, 38, 40f, 41f
  signs and symptoms of, 37
  treatment of, 39
 pathogenesis of, 32
 pathology of, 33
  gross, 34f
  histologic, 35f, 36f
 radiography of, 32, 34f
 renal osteodystrophy vs, 17
 signs and symptoms of, 31–32
 treatment of, 32–33
Osteomyelitis, 485–494
 differential diagnosis of, 485
 Ewing's sarcoma vs., 428, 429f
 histiocytosis X vs., 375f, 376f
 osteopetrosis and, 74
 pathology of, 485
  gross, 485, 488f, 489f, 490f
  histologic, 485, 489f, 491f, 492f,
   493f, 494f
 radiography of, 485, 487f,
  488f, 490f, 491f
 signs and symptoms of, 485
 squamous cell carcinoma in, 419f
 treatment of, 485–486
 tuberculous, 489f, 490f, 491f
 xanthogranulomatous, 494f
Osteopenia
 in fluorosis, 90, 92f
 in hyperparathyroidism, 4, 5f
 with osteomalacia, 32, 34f
 and osteoporosis, 13f
 in rheumatoid arthritis, 115f

Osteopetrosis, 73–79
 differential diagnosis of, 74
 pathology of, 74
  gross, 74
  histologic, 77f, 78f, 79f
 radiography of, 74, 76f, 77f, 79f
 signs and symptoms of, 73–74
 treatment of, 74–75
Osteophytes, in osteoarthritis,
  100, 101f, 102f
Osteoporosis, 11–16
 fluoride and, 91f
 inactive, 15f
 pathology of, 11
  gross, 13f, 14f, 15f
  histologic, 15f
 radiography of, 11, 13f, 16f
 signs and symptoms of, 11
 transient, 16f
 treatment of, 11–12
Osteoporosis circumscripta, 46
Osteopsathyrosis idiopathica of Lobstein, 81
Osteosarcoma, 211–218
 aneurysmal bone cyst vs., 456f, 458f
 chondroblastic, 214f, 216f
  chondrosarcoma vs., 303f
  clear cell chondrosarcoma vs., 329f
 conventional, small cell osteosarcoma
  vs., 255f
 differential diagnosis of, 212
 fibroblastic
  fibrosarcoma vs., 341f
  malignant fibrous histiocytoma vs., 348f
 high-grade surface, 235–239
  differential diagnosis of, 235, 236
  gross pathology of, 235–236, 237f
  histology of, 236, 237f, 238f, 239f
  periosteal osteosarcoma vs., 232f
  radiography of, 235, 237f, 238f, 239f
  signs and symptoms of, 235
  treatment of, 236
 intramedullary, 237f, 239f
 low-grade central, 247–250
  differential diagnosis of, 247, 248
  pathology of, 247, 248, 249f, 250f
  radiography of, 247, 249
  signs and symptoms of, 247
  treatment of, 248
 oncogenic osteomalacia in, 40f
 osteoblastic, 214f, 216f
 osteoblastoma vs., 204, 206f, 208f, 209f
 within osteochondroma, 311f
 osteofibrous dysplasia vs., 164f
 osteoid osteoma vs., 198f
 osteosclerotic, 239f
 vs. Paget's sarcoma, 441f, 442f
 parosteal, 219–225
  differential diagnosis of, 219–220
  gross pathology of, 220, 221f
  histology of, 220, 221f, 222f, 223f,
   224f, 225f
  radiography of, 219–220, 221f, 222f, 223f
  signs and symptoms of, 219
  treatment of, 220
 pathology of, 212
  gross, 212, 213f
  histologic, 212, 213f, 214f, 216f, 217f,
   218f
 periosteal, 227–233
  differential diagnosis of, 227, 228
  gross pathology of, 228, 229f
  histology of, 228, 229f, 230f, 231f,
   232f, 233f
  radiography of, 227, 229f, 230f, 231f

Osteosarcoma *(Continued)*
    signs and symptoms of, 227
    treatment of, 228
    postchemotherapy, 217f
    radiography of, 211–212, 213f, 215f
    signs and symptoms of, 211
    vs. simple bone cyst, 459
    small cell, 251–256
        differential diagnosis of, 252
        Ewing's sarcoma vs., 430f
        gross pathology of, 252, 253f
        hemangiopericytoma vs., 401f
        histology of, 252, 254f, 255f, 256f
        mesenchymal chondrosarcoma vs.,
          322f, 323f
        radiography of, 251–252, 253f
        signs and symptoms of, 251
        treatment of, 252
    telangiectatic, 241–246
        differential diagnosis of, 241, 242
        giant cell tumor vs., 404, 406f
        gross pathology of, 242, 243f
        histology of, 242, 243f, 244f, 245f, 246f
        radiography of, 241, 243f, 244f, 245f
        signs and symptoms of, 241
        treatment of, 242
    treatment of, 212
Osteosclerosis
    in fibrous dysplasia, 156f
    in fluorosis, 90, 91f, 92f
    in renal osteodystrophy, 17, 18f, 21f
    in Gaucher's disease, 96f
    in malignant lymphoma, 357f
    in mastocytosis, 369f, 370f, 371f
    in osteofibrous dysplasia, 161f
    in Paget's disease, 52f
    in pigmented villonodular synovitis, 182f
    in rickets, 30f

P

Pachyderma, in hypertrophic
    osteoarthropathy, 59
Pagetoid bone, osteoid osteoma vs., 201f
Paget's disease, 45–52
    Camurati-Engelmann disease vs., 56f
    differential diagnosis of, 46, 47
    incidence of, 45
    malignant fibrous histiocytoma with, 343
    osteomalacia vs., 34f
    pathology of, 46
        gross, 49f, 50f
        histologic, 50f, 51f, 52f
    phases of, 46
    radiography of, 46, 48f, 49f, 52f
    renal osteodystrophy vs, 21f
    sarcoma in. *See* Paget's sarcoma.
    with small cell osteosarcoma, 253f
    signs and symptoms of, 45–46
    treatment of, 47
Paget's sarcoma, 439–442
    differential diagnosis of, 440
    pathology of, 440, 441f, 442f
    radiography of, 439, 441f, 442f
    signs and symptoms of, 439
    treatment of, 440
Pain
    in hyperparathyroidism, 3, 4
    in osteomalacia, 31, 32
    in Paget's disease, 46
Pannus
    in osteoarthritis, 100
    in rheumatoid arthritis, 112, 117f
Papillary carcinoma, metastatic, 516f
Papillary tufting, in angiosarcoma, 393f

Parathyroid adenoma, 7f
Parosteal osteosarcoma, 219–225
    dedifferentiated, 224f
    differential diagnosis of, 219–220
    low-grade central osteosarcoma vs.,
        248, 249f
    vs. osteochondroma, 263f
    osteomyelitis vs., 492f
    pathology of, 220
        gross, 220, 221f
        histologic, 220, 221f, 222f, 223f,
          224f, 225f
    radiography of, 219–220, 221f, 222f, 223f
    signs and symptoms of, 219
    treatment of, 220
Pelvis
    aneurysmal bone cyst of, 455f, 456f
    chondrosarcoma arising in osteochon-
        droma of, 309f
    fibrosarcoma in, 340f
    fibrous dysplasia in, 40f
    fluorosis and, 91f
    Gaucher's disease and, 98f
    massive osteolysis in, 505f
    mastocytosis in, 369f, 370f, 371f
    melorheostosis in, 69f, 70f
    metastatic carcinoma in, 518f
    osteochondroma in, 262f
    osteomalacia in, 34f
    osteopetrosis in, 76f
    osteoporosis in, 16f
    Paget's sarcoma in, 441f
Perinuclear hof, 362
Periodic acid-Schiff (PAS) stain, for Ewing's
    sarcoma, 430f
Periosteal desmoid, 477–480
    differential diagnosis of, 477
    pathology of, 477
        gross, 477, 478f
        histologic, 477, 478f, 479f, 480f
    radiography of, 477, 478f, 479f, 480f
    signs and symptoms of, 477
    treatment of, 477
Periosteal new bone formation
    in Camurati-Engelmann disease, 54
    in hypertrophic osteoarthropathy, 60, 61f,
        62f, 63f, 65f
Periostitis, onion skin, 60
    in Ewing's sarcoma, 429f, 431f
Peripheral nerves, neurilemmomas of, 451f
Peripheral neuropathy
    and Charcot's joint, 105, 107f, 108f, 109f
    in myeloma, 361
Phalangeal erosion
    in hyperparathyroidism, 4, 5f, 9f
    in renal osteodystrophy, 17, 21f
Phalangeal sarcoidosis, 521f, 522f
Phalangeal tufts, in renal osteodystrophy, 21f
Phalanx
    BPOP in, 527f, 528f
    distal
        giant cell reaction of, 467f
        hemangiopericytoma in, 401f
        in Paget's disease, 52f
Phantom bone disease, 385f, 386f
Phenylalanine catabolism disorder, 121
Phosphate deficiency
    and osteomalacia, 32
    and rickets, 24
Phosphaturic mesenchymal tumor, 37–44, 38,
    41f, 42f. *See also* Osteomalacia, oncogenic.
Phosphorus, in hyperparathyroidism, 3
Physaliferous cells, 422, 424f, 425f
Pigmentation, cutaneous, 151, 154f

Pigmented villonodular synovitis, 179–187
    chondroblastoma vs., 278f
    differential diagnosis of, 180
    hemophilia vs., 511f
    pathology of, 180
        gross, 180, 183f, 184f
        histologic, 180, 184f, 185f, 186f
    radiography of, 180, 182f, 183f, 186f, 187f
    signs and symptoms of, 179
    treatment of, 180
Plasma cell dyscrasias, and amyloidosis,
    139, 141f, 142f
Plasma cells
    in myeloma, 364f
    in osteomyelitis, 492f
Plasmacytoma, 142f
Polyostotic disease, 151, 154f, 155f
Postradiation sarcoma, 443–447
    differential diagnosis of, 444
    pathology of, 444, 445f, 446f
    signs and symptoms of, 443
    treatment of, 444
Primitive neuroectodermal tumor (PNET),
    Ewing's sarcoma vs., 436f
Pseudofractures
    in osteomalacia, 32, 34f
    in renal osteodystrophy, 17
    in rickets, 24
Pseudogout. *See* Chondrocalcinosis.
Pseudotumor, hemophilia and, 512f
Pubis
    aneurysmal bone cyst of, 455f
    benign fibrous histiocytoma of, 335f, 336f
    Ewing's sarcoma in, 431f
    fracture, from mastocytosis, 370f
    Paget's sarcoma in, 441f
Pulmonary fibrosis, osteoarthropathy in, 62f
Pulmonary hypertrophic osteoarthropathy.
    See Osteoarthropathy, hypertrophic.
Pulmonary metastases
    with chondroblastoma, 278f
    with clear cell chondrosarcoma, 330f
    with fibrosarcoma, 339f
    and giant cell tumor, 408f

R

Rachitic rosary, 23, 24, 27f, 28f
Radius
    fibrous dysplasia in, 40f
    giant cell tumor of, 407f
Reed-Sternberg cells, 359f
Renal cell carcinoma
    malignant fibrous histiocytoma vs., 349f
    metastatic, 516f, 518f
Renal failure, amyloidosis and, 139, 143f
Renal osteodystrophy, 17–21
    differential diagnosis of, 17, 18
    pathology of, 17–18
        gross, 19f, 20f
        histologic, 20f, 21f
    radiography of, 17, 19f, 21f
    signs and symptoms of, 17
    skull appearance in, 7f
    treatment of, 18
Renal stones
    in gout, 125, 126, 127f
    in hyperparathyroidism, 3
Reticulin fibers, in malignant lymphoma,
    352, 354f
Reticulin stain, 388, 393f, 400f
    for Ewing's sarcoma, 430f
Rheumatoid arthritis, 111–120
    Charcot's joint vs., 106
    differential diagnosis of, 112, 113

Rheumatoid arthritis *(Continued)*
    osteoarthritis vs, 100
    pathology of, 112, 113
        gross, 115f, 119f
        histologic, 116f, 117f, 118f, 120f
    prevalence of, 111
    pulmonary hypertrophic osteoarthropathy
        vs., 61f
    radiography of, 112, 114f, 115f
    signs and symptoms of, 111–112, 114f
    treatment of, 112
Rheumatoid factor, 111
Rheumatoid nodules, 111, 112, 114f, 118f,
    119f, 120f
Rib(s)
    chest wall hamartoma and, 483f
    fibrous dysplasia in, 156f, 157f
    hemangiopericytoma in, 399f
    mesenchymal chondrosarcomas in, 322f
    myeloma in, 365f, 366f
    neurilemmoma of, 451f
    osteoblastoma in, 205f
    small cell osteosarcoma in, 254f
Rice bodies of osteoarthritis, 175f
Rickets, 23–30
    differential diagnosis of, 24
    pathogenesis of, 24
    pathology of, 24
        gross, 27f, 28f, 29f
        histologic, 28f, 29f, 30f
    radiography of, 24, 26f, 27f, 30f
    in renal osteodystrophy, 17
    signs and symptoms of, 23–24
    treatment of, 24, 32, 33
Rosai-Dorfman disease, 146. *See also* Sinus
    histiocytosis with massive lymphadenopathy
    (SHML).
Rugger jersey spine, 46
    in osteopetrosis, 74
    in renal osteodystrophy, 17, 18f

S
Sacroiliac joint
    ankylosing spondylitis and, 168
    chondrosarcoma in, 300f
Sacrum
    benign fibrous histiocytoma in, 336f
    chordomas in, 421, 422, 423f, 424f, 425f,
        426f
    fibrosarcoma in, 340f
    giant cell tumor of, 407f, 408f
    neurilemmoma in, 450, 452f
    SHML in, 494f
Sarcoidosis, 519–523
    differential diagnosis of, 519, 520
    incidence of, 519
    pathology of, 519, 521f, 523f
    radiography of, 519, 521f, 522f
    signs and symptoms of, 519
    treatment of, 520
Sarcoma
    aneurysmal bone cyst vs., 456f
    Charcot's joint vs., 107f
    from benign giant cell tumor, 413f
    hemangioma vs., 382
    malignant lymphoma vs., 358f
    neurilemmomas vs., 452f
    Paget's, 46, 47. *See also* Paget's sarcoma.
    Paget's disease and, 48f, 50f
    postradiation, 443–447
        differential diagnosis of, 444
        gross pathology of, 444, 445f
        histology of, 444, 445f, 446f
        radiography of, 443, 445f, 447f

Sarcoma *(Continued)*
        signs and symptoms of, 443
        treatment of, 444
Scapula, angiosarcoma in, 389f
Sclerae
    blue, 81, 82
    ochronosis and, 121
Sclerosis. *See* Osteosclerosis.
Scoliosis
    in Charcot's joint, 106
    in osteogenesis imperfecta, 83
    in rickets, 24
Sequestrae
    and avascular necrosis, 495
    in osteomyelitis, 485, 488f, 489f
SHML. *See* Sinus histiocytosis with massive
    lymphadenopathy.
Shoulder
    Charcot's, 108f
    mastocytosis in, 371f
    osteoarthritis in, 101f, 104f
    synovial chondromatosis in, 175f, 178f
Sinus histiocytosis with massive lymphadenopathy
    (SHML)
    and osteomyelitis, 494f
    xanthomatosis vs., 146
Skeletal deformities, in rickets, 23
Skin rash, in mastocytosis, 367
Skull
    chondroblastoma in, 277f
    fibrous dysplasia in, 156f
    hemangioma in, 381, 384f
    hemangiopericytomatous pattern in, 402f
    Langerhans' cell histiocytosis in, 376f
    myeloma in, 364f
    in Paget's disease, 46, 49f
Slipped epiphyses, in renal osteodystrophy, 17
Small blue cell tumor, metastatic neuroblastoma
    vs., 516f
Small round cell tumor, small cell osteosarcoma
    vs., 253f
Soft tissue
    in gout, 126, 127f
    in hypertrophic osteoarthropathy, 61f, 62f
    mesenchymal chondrosarcoma of, 324f
Spheno-occipital chordomas, 421, 422, 426f
Spinal cord degenerative diseases, and Charcot's
    joint, 105, 108f
Spindle cell(s)
    in avulsive cortical irregularity,
        478f, 479f, 480f
    in benign fibrous histiocytoma, 335f
    in dedifferentiated chondrosarcoma,
        314, 316f, 317f
    in fibroma, 472, 474f
    in fibrosarcoma, 338, 339f
    in malignant giant cell tumor, 412, 414f
    in neurilemmoma, 450, 451f
    in osteosarcoma, 212, 213f, 216f
        high-grade surface, 236
        low-grade central, 248
        parosteal, 221f, 222f, 224f, 225f
        periosteal, 228, 229f, 232f
    in Paget's sarcoma, 440
    sarcoma
        adamantinoma vs., 420f
        and dedifferentiated chondrosarcoma,
            315f, 317f
    tumor
        and chondrosarcomas, 311f
        as postradiation sarcoma, 444, 445f
Spine. *See also* Lumbar spine; Thoracic spine;
    Vertebrae.
    in ankylosing spondylitis, 167, 168, 169f, 171f

Spine *(Continued)*
    hemangioma in, 382, 385f
    rickets and, 23
Splenomegaly, in Gaucher's disease, 93
Sprue, 35f
Squamous cell carcinoma, adamantinoma vs.,
    418f, 419f
Stellate reticulum, in adamantinoma,
    416, 417f
Steroids
    and avascular necrosis, 495
    for gout, 126
    for histiocytosis X, 374
Storiform pattern
    in fibroma, 472, 474f, 475f
    in malignant fibrous histiocytoma,
        344, 345f, 347f
Subchondral bone, in osteoarthritis, 100, 101f
Subchondral sclerosis, in ochronosis, 122
Subungual exostoses, osteochondroma vs., 263f
Synovectomy
    for pigmented villonodular synovitis, 180
    for synovial chondromatosis, 174
Synovial chondromatosis, 173–178
    differential diagnosis of, 174
    pathology of, 174
        gross, 174, 175f
        histologic, 174, 176f, 177f, 178f
    and periosteal chondroma, 295f
    radiography of, 173–174, 175f, 178f
    signs and symptoms of, 173
    treatment of, 174
Synovial fluid
    in gout, 125, 127f
    in rheumatoid arthritis, 111
Synovitis, metallic, 183f, 190f
Synovium
    in ankylosing spondylitis, 168
    in Charcot's joint, 106, 109f
    in gout, 126
    in hemophilia, 509, 511f, 512f
    in ochronosis, 124f
    in pigmented villonodular synovitis, 180
    rheumatoid arthritis and, 112, 115f, 116f,
        117f, 119f
    villous hyperplasia of, 116f, 119f
        hemophilia and, 511f, 512f
    villous hypertrophy in, 103f, 109f
Syphilis, Charcot's joint and, 108f
Syringomyelia, Charcot's joint and, 108f
Systemic lupus erythematosus, avascular
    necrosis and, 495, 500f

T
Temporal bone, chondroblastoma in, 277f, 278f
Temporomandibular joint, pigmented
    villonodular synovitis of, 278f
Teriparatide, 12
Thoracic spine
    chordoma in, 426f
    Langerhans' cell histiocytosis in, 376f
    osteogenesis imperfecta in, 84f
    osteopetrosis in, 76f
Thumb, chondromas in, 270f, 288f
Thyroid carcinoma, 517f
Tibia, 223f
    adamantinoma in, 417f, 418f, 419f
    aneurysmal bone cyst of, 456f
    benign fibrous histiocytoma of, 335f
    bone infarction in, 347f
    brown tumor of, 6f
    chondroblastoma in, 276f
    chondromyxoid fibroma in, 41f, 284f
    chondrosarcomas in, 290f, 307f

Tibia *(Continued)*
　　Erdheim-Chester disease in, 535f
　　Ewing's sarcoma in, 431f
　　fibroma in, 473f, 474f, 475f
　　Gaucher's disease and, 98f
　　giant cell tumor in, 405f
　　hemangioma in, 383f
　　hypertrophic osteoarthropathy in, 61f, 63f
　　intraosseous ganglion of, 463f
　　Langerhans' cell histiocytosis in, 377f
　　malignant fibrous histiocytoma of, 347f
　　melorheostosis in, 69f, 71f
　　multiple chondromas in, 288f
　　myeloma in, 364f
　　osteoarthritis in, 101, 103f
　　osteochondroma in, 261f, 307f
　　in osteofibrous dysplasia, 159, 161f,
　　　　162f, 163f
　　osteogenesis imperfecta in, 84f, 85f
　　osteomyelitis in, 487f, 488f
　　osteopetrosis and, 79f
　　osteosarcoma in, 40f, 218f
　　　　high-grade surface, 237f, 238f
　　　　low-grade central, 249f
　　　　periosteal, 229f, 231f
　　　　postradiation, 447f
　　Paget's disease in, 48f, 49f
　　Paget's sarcoma in, 441f
　　pulmonary hypertrophic osteoarthropathy
　　　　in, 64f
　　rheumatoid arthritis in, 114f
　　rickets in, 27f, 30f
Tissue discoloration, ochronosis and, 121
Toe
　　chondroma in, 268f
　　sarcoid in, 522f
Tongue, amyloidosis and, 143f
Tophi
　　in gout, 125, 126, 127f, 129f, 131f
　　urate, calcium pyrophosphate deposition
　　　　vs., 137f
Tophaceous pseudogout, 136
Total hip arthroplasty, osteolysis and, 190f
Total knee arthroplasty, 508f
　　osteolysis and, 190f
Trabeculae. *See* Bone trabeculae.
Transient osteoporosis, 16f

Tuberculous osteomyelitis, 489f, 490f, 491f
Tyrosine catabolism disorder, 121

U

Ulna
　　angiosarcoma in, 390f
　　BPOP in, 527f
　　fibrous dysplasia in, 40f
　　multiple chondromas in, 289f
　　neurilemmoma in, 452f
Unicameral bone cyst (simple cyst), 459–464
　　differential diagnosis of, 459
　　pathology of, 460
　　　　gross, 460, 463f, 464f
　　　　histologic, 460, 462f, 463f, 464f
　　radiography of, 459, 461f, 462f, 463f, 464f
　　signs and symptoms of, 459
　　treatment of, 460
Urate crystals, 128f, 129f, 130f, 131f, 132f, 133f
Urate tophi, calcium pyrophosphate deposition
　　vs., 137f
Urine, ochronosis and, 121
Urticaria pigmentosa, 367

V

van der Hoeve's syndrome, 81
Vascular calcification, in renal
　　osteodystrophy, 17
Vascular pattern, in oncogenic
　　osteomalacia, 42f
Vascular tumor(s)
　　adamantinoma vs., 417f
　　metastatic carcinoma vs., 516f
　　osteomalacia in, 38
　　Paget's disease vs., 51f
Verocay bodies, 450
Vertebrae
　　amyloidosis and, 139, 141f, 142f
　　in ankylosing spondylitis, 167, 168,
　　　　169f, 170f, 171f
　　corduroy, 385f
　　hemangiopericytoma of, 399f
　　in fluorosis, 91f
　　in Gaucher's disease, 94, 96f, 97f
　　Langerhans' cell histiocytosis in, 377f
　　lumbar. *See* Lumbar spine.

Vertebrae *(Continued)*
　　myeloma in, 366f
　　in ochronosis, 122, 123f
　　osteoblastoma in, 207f
　　in osteogenesis imperfecta, 83
　　in osteomalacia, 32
　　osteopetrosis in, 74, 77f
　　osteoporosis of, 13f, 14f, 16f
　　Paget's disease and, 46, 48f, 50f, 442f
　　picture frame, 48f
　　renal osteodystrophy and, 19f, 20f, 21f
　　striped pattern of, 74, 77f
　　thoracic. *See* Thoracic spine.
Vertebral chordomas, 421
Vertebral compression fractures, in Gaucher's
　　disease, 94
Vertebral disks
　　in ochronosis, 122, 123f, 124f
　　in osteomalacia, 32
Vertebral hemangioma, 385f
Vertebra plana, 376f
Vertebroplasty, 12
Villonodular synovitis, pigmented.
　　See Pigmented villonodular synovitis
Vitamin D abnormalities
　　and osteomalacia, 32
　　and rickets, 24
Vitamin D supplementation, 24, 33

W

Wormian bone, in osteogenesis imperfecta, 83
Wrist
　　chondrocalcinosis in, 137f
　　multiple chondromas in, 287f

X

Xanthomatosis, 145–149
　　differential diagnosis of, 146
　　pathology of, 146
　　　　gross, 148f
　　　　histologic, 147f, 148f, 149f
　　radiography of, 145–146
　　signs and symptoms of, 145
　　treatment of, 146

CONTENTS

Body parts 8

Fueling the body 20

Brainpower 30

Pumping blood 40

Life story 50

Index 60

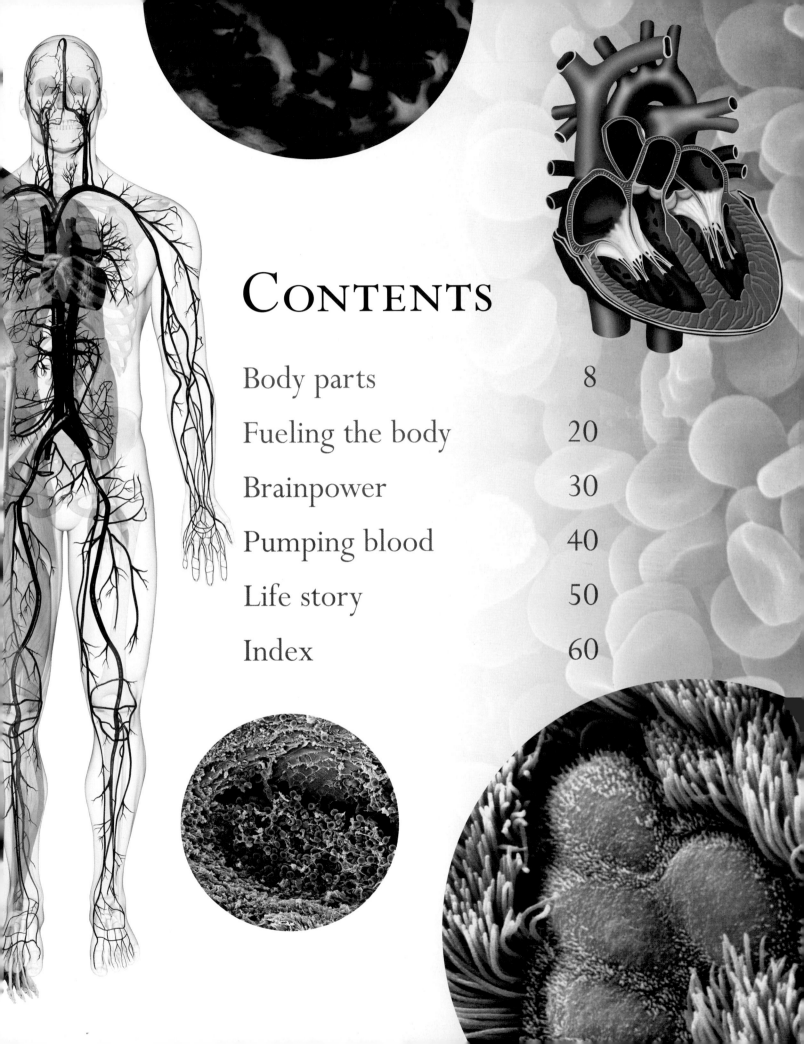

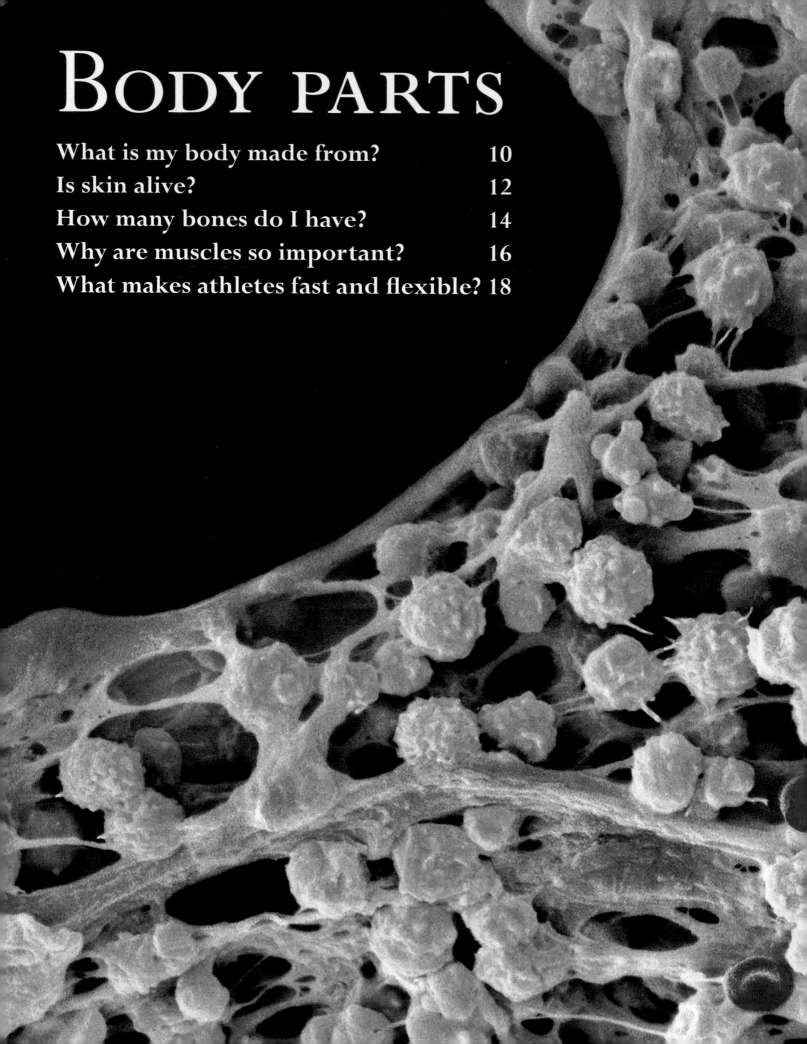

BODY PARTS

What is my body made from?   10

Is skin alive?   12

How many bones do I have?   14

Why are muscles so important?   16

What makes athletes fast and flexible? 18

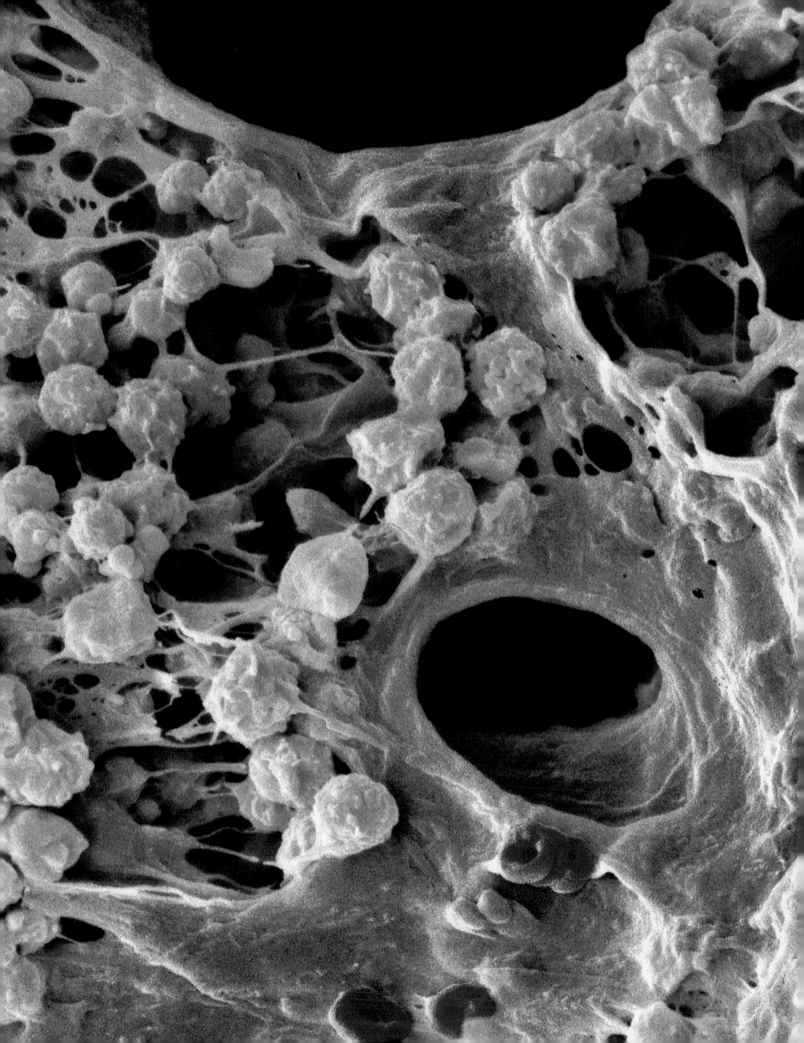

What is my body made from?

It takes about 100 trillion (100,000,000,000,000) microscopic living units called cells to make a human body. There are many different types of cells, and these are organized into the tissues and organs that make up your major body systems. These include the skeletal and muscular systems, which support and move the body, and the digestive and respiratory systems, which supply food and oxygen.

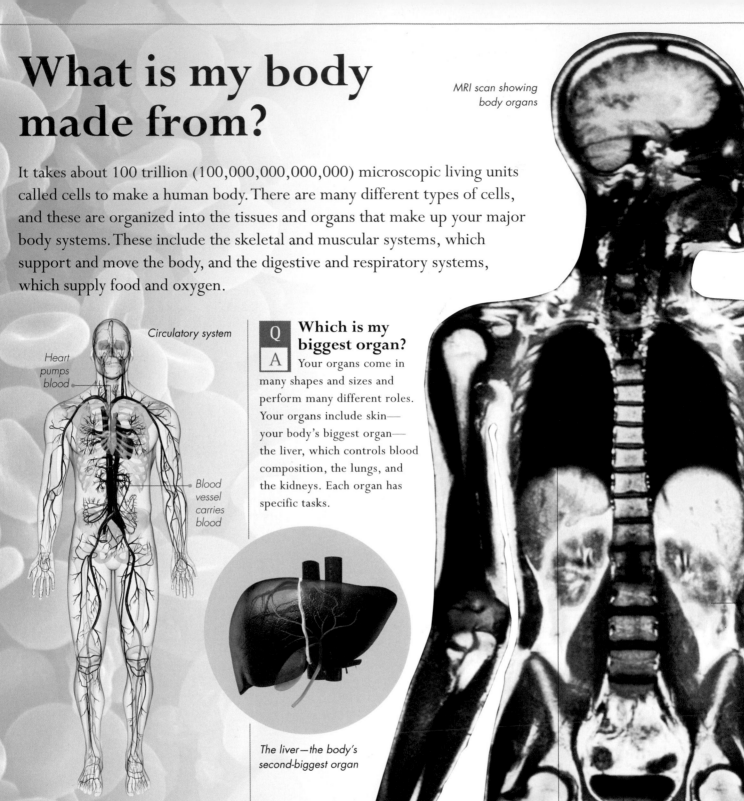

MRI scan showing body organs

Circulatory system

Heart pumps blood

Blood vessel carries blood

Q A Which is my biggest organ? Your organs come in many shapes and sizes and perform many different roles. Your organs include skin— your body's biggest organ— the liver, which controls blood composition, the lungs, and the kidneys. Each organ has specific tasks.

The liver—the body's second-biggest organ

Q A How does my body work? At the simplest level, cells of the same type work together in groups to form tissues. Different tissues cooperate to make organs, such as the heart, and linked organs work together to form one of the body's 12 systems. In the circulatory system, for example, the heart and blood vessels work together to carry blood all around the body.

Lung takes in oxygen

Bladder stores urine produced by the kidneys

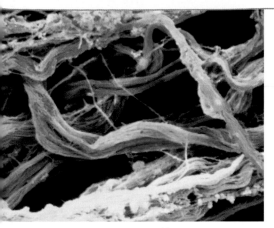

Connective tissue fibers

Q A What holds my body together?

There are four basic types of tissues in your body—epithelial, nervous, muscular, and connective. Epithelial tissues are protective; they cover the skin and line the mouth, stomach, and other organs. Nervous tissues form your body's control system—the brain and nervous system. Muscular tissues form the muscles that move you. And connective tissues, as their name suggests, hold together other tissues and your entire body.

- Bone supports the upper arm
- Kidney
- Muscle moves the fingers

Q A Are cells alive?

Although they are microscopic, cells have a complex structure. A membrane surrounds the cell and controls what enters and leaves it. Tiny structures, called organelles, float and move in the jellylike cytoplasm. Organelles each have their own jobs, but they work together to make the cell a living unit. For example, mitochondria release energy in order to power the cell's activities, while the nucleus contains the cell's operating instructions.

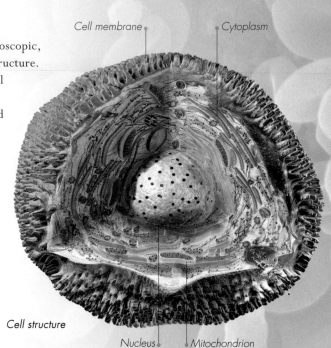

Cell membrane · Cytoplasm

Cell structure

Nucleus · Mitochondrion

Cell division

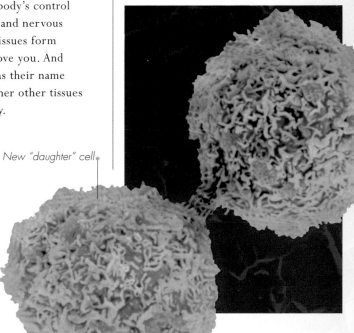

New "daughter" cell·

Q A How do cells multiply?

Right now, some of your cells are dividing by a process called mitosis. Highly organized and precisely timed, mitosis enables your cells to multiply so that you can grow, maintain yourself, and replace worn-out cells. During mitosis, the instructions inside the nucleus, which are needed in order to build and run a cell, are copied and separated into two equal packages. Then the "parent" cell divides into two identical "daughter" cells, each with its own complete set of instructions.

Stem cell

More Facts

- There are more than 200 different types of cells in the body, including red blood cells, nerve cells, fat cells, and muscle cells.

- A cell lining the small intestine has a life span of just 36 hours, while a red blood cell lives for four months, and a brain cell can last a lifetime.

- An egg, or ovum, released from a woman's ovary, is at least 0.0039 in (0.1 mm) across and is the biggest cell in the body.

- Stem cells are found in various body tissues. They multiply rapidly to produce cells that become specialized to do a specific job. In red bone marrow, for example, stem cells produce blood cells

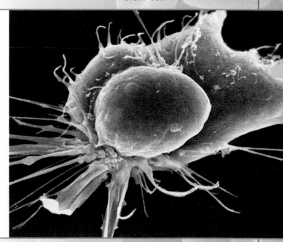

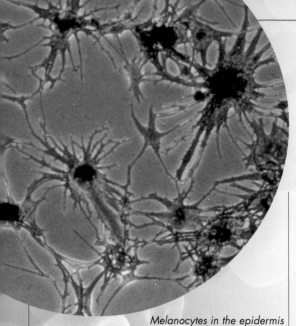

Melanocytes in the epidermis

Is skin alive?

Enclosing your body like a winter coat, skin is a tough, waterproof, germ-proof barrier that separates your insides from the harsh outside world. It also houses receptors that detect touch, pressure, heat, cold, and pain. The skin has two parts: the epidermis and the dermis. The protective epidermis constantly produces cells that migrate upward to the skin's surface where they flatten, die, and are worn away as skin flakes. Very much alive, the lower dermis contains blood vessels, hair follicles, sweat glands, and sensory receptors.

Q A **What makes skin the color it is?**
Deep in the epidermis, cells called melanocytes release melanin—a brown pigment that colours your skin. Melanin also filters out harmful ultraviolet radiation in sunlight that can damage skin cells. We all have the same number of melanocytes, but they produce more melanin in people with darker skin.

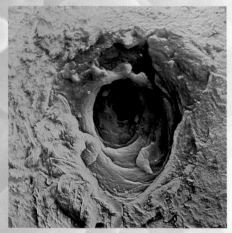

Sweat pore

Q A **Why do I sweat when it's hot?**
Your skin helps keep your body temperature at a steady 98.6°F (37°C). If it's hot, sweat released onto your skin's surface evaporates and cools you down. At the same time, blood vessels near the skin's surface widen and release heat. If it's cold, you stop sweating and the blood vessels narrow to cut heat loss.

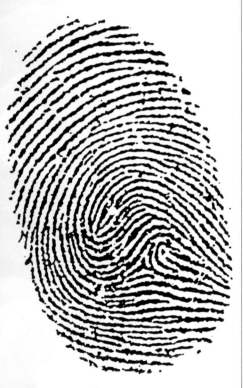

Fingerprint

Q A **What makes my fingerprints unique?**
Tiny, swirling ridges on your fingers help you grip things. They also leave behind sweaty patterns called fingerprints. These ridges form before you are born, shaped by the conditions around you in your mother's uterus. Those conditions are different for each person, even for identical twins, making your fingerprints unique.

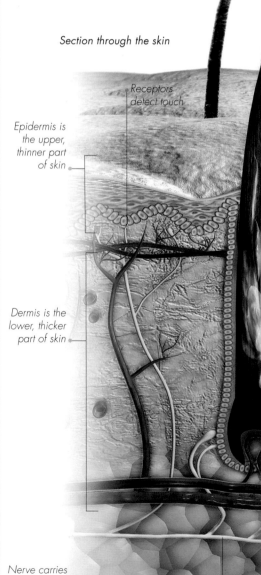

Section through the skin

Receptors detect touch

Epidermis is the upper, thinner part of skin

Dermis is the lower, thicker part of skin

Nerve carries signals from the receptors

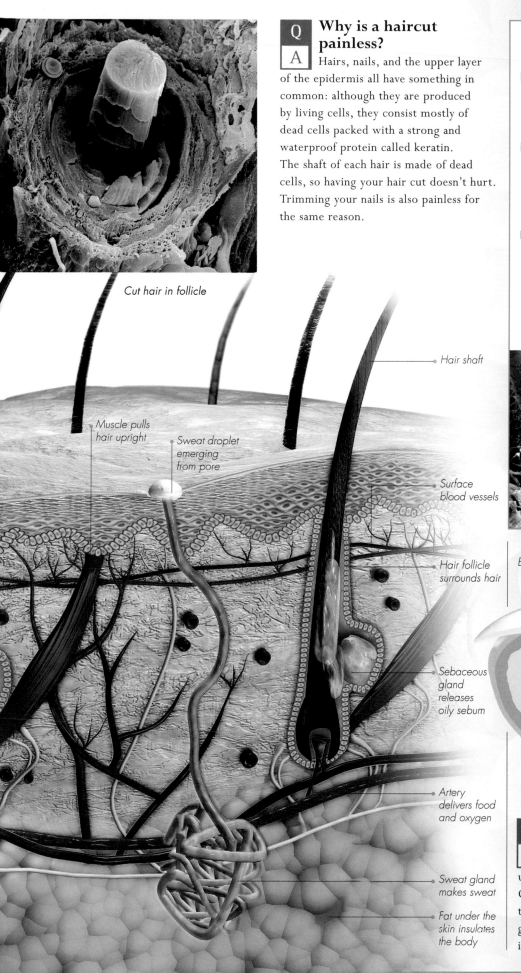

Q | A | Why is a haircut painless?

Hairs, nails, and the upper layer of the epidermis all have something in common: although they are produced by living cells, they consist mostly of dead cells packed with a strong and waterproof protein called keratin. The shaft of each hair is made of dead cells, so having your hair cut doesn't hurt. Trimming your nails is also painless for the same reason.

Cut hair in follicle

Hair shaft

Muscle pulls hair upright

Sweat droplet emerging from pore

Surface blood vessels

Hair follicle surrounds hair

Sebaceous gland releases oily sebum

Artery delivers food and oxygen

Sweat gland makes sweat

Fat under the skin insulates the body

More Facts

- Although very thin, at 11 lbs (5 kg) skin is the heaviest body organ, despite losing 50,000 skin flakes every minute.

- You have approximately 100,000 head hairs that grow about 0.4 in (10 mm) every month. Between 75 and 100 head hairs are lost and replaced daily.

- Head lice are small, wingless insects, common among young children, that grip hairs with their pincers and pierce the scalp to feed on blood.

Head louse gripping hairs

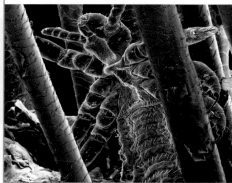

Body of nail   Nail bed   Nail root   Finger bone

Section through a fingertip

Q | A | How quickly do fingernails grow?

Nails protect fingertips, help pick up small objects, and scratch itches. Growing from the nail root, the body of the nail slides forward over the nail bed, growing by about 0.2 in (5 mm) a month in the summer, but slower in the winter.

13

How many bones do I have?

Without its skeleton, your body would collapse in a floppy heap. This supportive framework is constructed from 206 bones and makes up about 20 percent of your body weight. Each bone is a living organ with a structure that makes it as strong as steel, but at a fraction of the weight. Your skeleton also surrounds and protects delicate organs, such as the brain and heart, and, when pulled by muscles, makes you move.

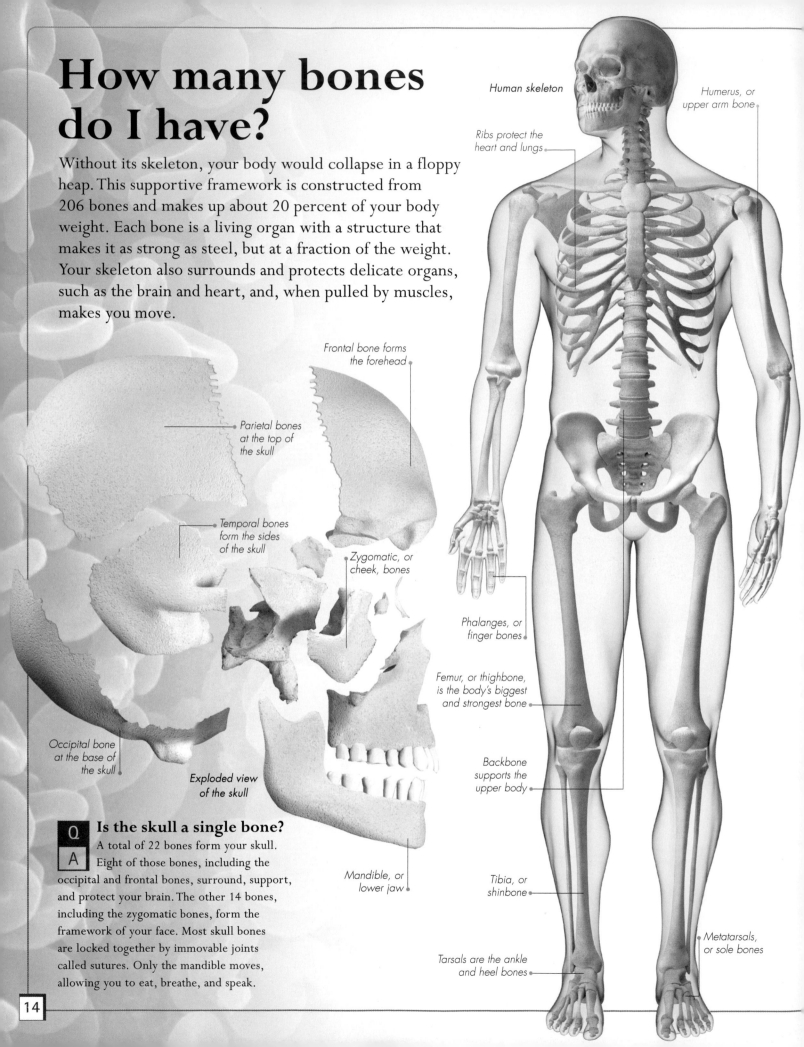

Human skeleton

Ribs protect the heart and lungs

Humerus, or upper arm bone

Frontal bone forms the forehead

Parietal bones at the top of the skull

Temporal bones form the sides of the skull

Zygomatic, or cheek, bones

Occipital bone at the base of the skull

Exploded view of the skull

Phalanges, or finger bones

Femur, or thighbone, is the body's biggest and strongest bone

Backbone supports the upper body

Mandible, or lower jaw

Tibia, or shinbone

Metatarsals, or sole bones

Tarsals are the ankle and heel bones

Q A **Is the skull a single bone?**
A total of 22 bones form your skull. Eight of those bones, including the occipital and frontal bones, surround, support, and protect your brain. The other 14 bones, including the zygomatic bones, form the framework of your face. Most skull bones are locked together by immovable joints called sutures. Only the mandible moves, allowing you to eat, breathe, and speak.

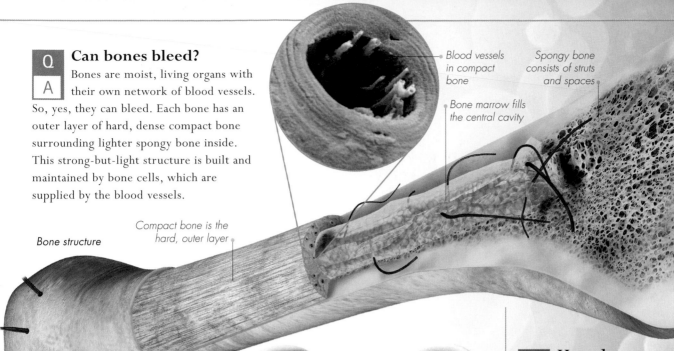

Q. A. Can bones bleed?

Bones are moist, living organs with their own network of blood vessels. So, yes, they can bleed. Each bone has an outer layer of hard, dense compact bone surrounding lighter spongy bone inside. This strong-but-light structure is built and maintained by bone cells, which are supplied by the blood vessels.

Blood vessels in compact bone

Spongy bone consists of struts and spaces

Bone marrow fills the central cavity

Bone structure

Compact bone is the hard, outer layer

Q. A. Are male and female skeletons the same?

You can distinguish between male and female skeletons by looking at the pelvis. This basin-shaped structure attaches the thighbones to the body and supports organs in the abdomen. In women the opening in the center of the pelvis is wider than in men. This provides room for a baby's head to squeeze through during childbirth.

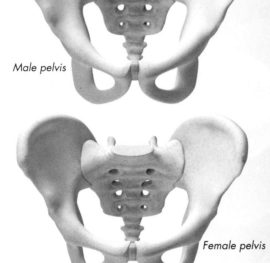

Male pelvis

Female pelvis

Q. A. How do x-rays work?

By projecting this invisible type of radiation through the body and onto a photographic plate, doctors can see hard structures such as bones. Even though bones are very tough, fractures can happen if, for example, they suffer a sudden impact.

Artificially colored x-ray of fractured arm bones

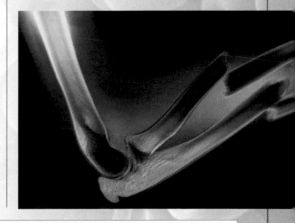

How do bones heal themselves?

If a bone is fractured, a self-repair system immediately springs into action. Blood leaking from damaged blood vessels clots in order to stop further bleeding. Then the rebuilding process, which takes weeks or months, begins. Doctors often line up the broken ends of the bones to make sure that the repair works correctly and is not the wrong shape.

1 Within hours of the fracture, a blood clot forms between bone ends, sealing off cut blood vessels.

2 After three weeks, fibrous tissue replaces the clot. New blood vessels supply bone-building cells.

3 After three months, new bone has replaced the fibrous tissue and the repair is almost complete.

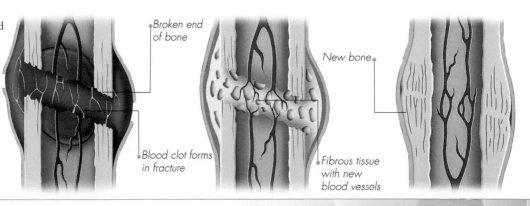

Broken end of bone

New bone

Blood clot forms in fracture

Fibrous tissue with new blood vessels

Why are muscles so important?

Eating your lunch or riding a bike would be impossible without muscles. They produce every movement that you make. Muscles are unique in their ability to contract, or get shorter, in order to create pulling power. There are three types of muscles. Skeletal muscles pull bones to move your body. Smooth muscles squeeze the walls of organs to, for example, push food along the small intestine. Cardiac muscle, found only in the heart, pumps blood.

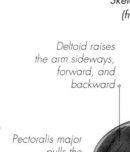

Skeletal muscles (front view)

Deltoid raises the arm sideways, forward, and backward

Pectoralis major pulls the arm forward

Rectus abdominis bends the body forward

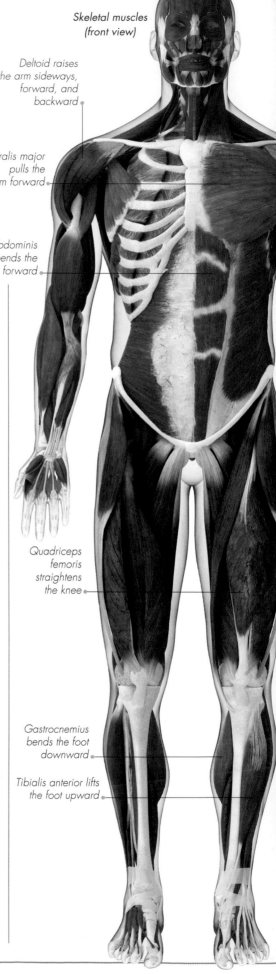

Quadriceps femoris straightens the knee

Gastrocnemius bends the foot downward

Tibialis anterior lifts the foot upward

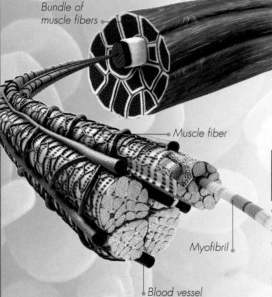

Bundle of muscle fibers

Skeletal muscle

Muscle fiber

Myofibril

Blood vessel

Skeletal muscle structure

Q&A What is inside a muscle?
Your skeletal muscles are made from long, cylindrical cells called muscle fibers. These are organized into bundles that run lengthwise down the muscle, and each fiber is packed with parallel, rodlike strands called myofibrils. These, in turn, contain overlapping filaments that interact to make muscles contract.

Q&A How do muscles work?
Skeletal muscle contracts when your brain tells it to. Signals are carried from the brain by neurons or nerve cells (green), the ends of which form junctions with muscle fibers (red). The arrival of a nerve signal makes filaments inside the myofibrils slide over each other so that their muscle fibers, and therefore the muscle, get shorter and "pull" on a part of your body so that you move.

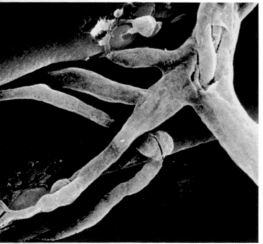

Nerve-muscle junction

How are muscles attached to bones?

A At each end of a muscle, a cord or sheet called a tendon attaches it firmly to a bone. Each tendon is reinforced with parallel bundles of tough collagen fibers. This makes it incredibly strong so that, when a muscle contracts to pull a bone, its tendon does not tear. A tendon extends from a muscle, through the periosteum, and into the bone's outer layer, where it is firmly anchored.

Biceps femoris bends the arm at the elbow

Flexor carpi radialis bends the wrist

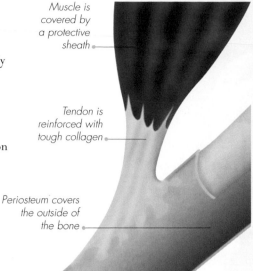

Muscle is covered by a protective sheath

Tendon is reinforced with tough collagen

Periosteum covers the outside of the bone

Connecting muscle to bone

What happens when I sleep?

A As well as moving your body, muscles also maintain your posture. Muscles in your neck, back, and hips partially contract to keep your body upright and your head steady, whether you are standing or sitting. Called muscle tone, this partial contraction is constantly adjusted by your brain. When you fall asleep, muscle tone almost disappears. That's why, if you happen to fall asleep in a chair, your head flops to the side.

Falling asleep

Which muscles make me smile?

A You have about 30 small muscles that produce a vast range of facial expressions and reveal to others how you are feeling. One end of your facial muscles are attached to the skin of your face, which they tug to create a particular look, be it grinning or frowning. Smiling muscles include the risorius, the two zygomaticus muscles, which pull the corner of your mouth upward and outward, and the levator labii superioris, which raises your upper lip.

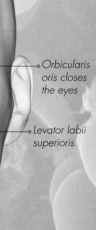
Facial muscles

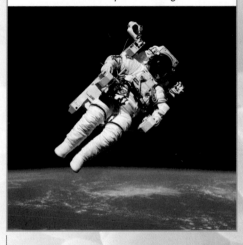

Frontalis raises the eyebrows

Zygomaticus minor

Zygomaticus major

Risorius pulls the mouth to the side

Orbicularis oris closes the eyes

Levator labii superioris

What makes athletes fast and flexible?

Anyone who exercises regularly and correctly can improve their fitness, which is a measure of how efficiently their body works. Athletes are very good examples of how this can be done. The joints between their bones, which allow the body to move, are very flexible. The muscles that pull on those bones in order to create movement are very strong. Athletes also have great stamina because their heart works efficiently to supply the muscles with energy.

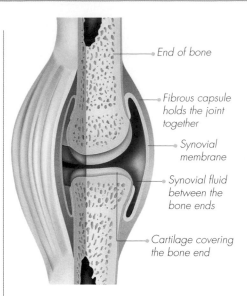

End of bone

Fibrous capsule holds the joint together

Synovial membrane

Synovial fluid between the bone ends

Cartilage covering the bone end

Q A How do joints move smoothly?

Most of your body's 400 joints are free-moving synovial joints. They all share the basic structure that you can see above. The ends of the bone are coated with slippery cartilage and are separated by oily synovial fluid, released by the synovial membrane. The combination of cartilage and fluid allows the joint to move smoothly, without the bone ends rubbing together.

Athlete in action

Thigh muscle contracts to straighten the knee joint

Are there different types of joints?

There are six different types of synovial joints in your body. The shapes of their bones' ends and the way in which they fit together determine the range and freedom of movement allowed by each joint type. The ball and socket joint, for example, allows all-around movement.

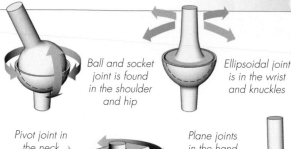

Ball and socket joint is found in the shoulder and hip

Ellipsoidal joint is in the wrist and knuckles

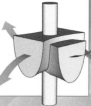
Hinge joint in the knee and elbow is like a hinge

Pivot joint in the neck allows the head to shake

Plane joints in the hand allow limited movement

Saddle joint allows the thumb to move freely

Q/A How do muscles work with joints to move my body?

Muscles are attached to bones on either side of a joint. However, they can only pull, not push, so opposing sets of muscles are needed in order to produce movements in different directions. In the arm, for example, the biceps brachii contracts to bend the elbow joint, while the triceps brachii contracts to straighten it.

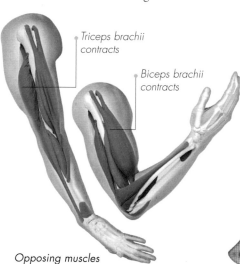
Triceps brachii contracts
Biceps brachii contracts

Opposing muscles

Q/A Why do I get hot when I exercise?

To move your body, muscles convert chemical energy, in the form of fuels such as glucose, into movement energy. A byproduct of this conversion is heat. The more you exercise, the more heat your muscles release and the hotter you get. Thermography is a type of imaging that produces color-coded "heat pictures" called thermograms, which show how much heat is being released by the body.

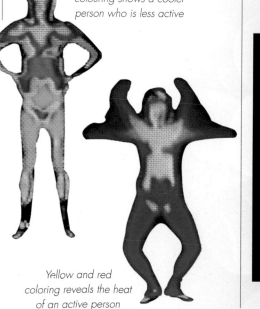
Green and blue colouring shows a cooler person who is less active

Yellow and red coloring reveals the heat of an active person

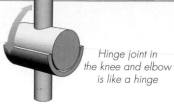

X-ray of a dislocated finger joint

Q/A What is a dislocated joint?

This x-ray shows two finger bones that have been forced out of line so that they no longer meet at a joint. In this situation the joint is said to be "dislocated". Dislocated joints are often caused by sporting injuries or falls. They are treated by a doctor who carefully moves the bones back into place.

Q/A Do joints wear out?

The cartilage that covers the ends of the bones in a joint can wear away with age. This makes the joint painful and much less flexible. One solution is to replace the worn-out joint with an artificial joint. Joints that can be replaced in this way include those in the knee, hip, shoulder, and finger.

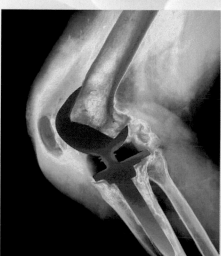

X-ray of an artificial knee joint

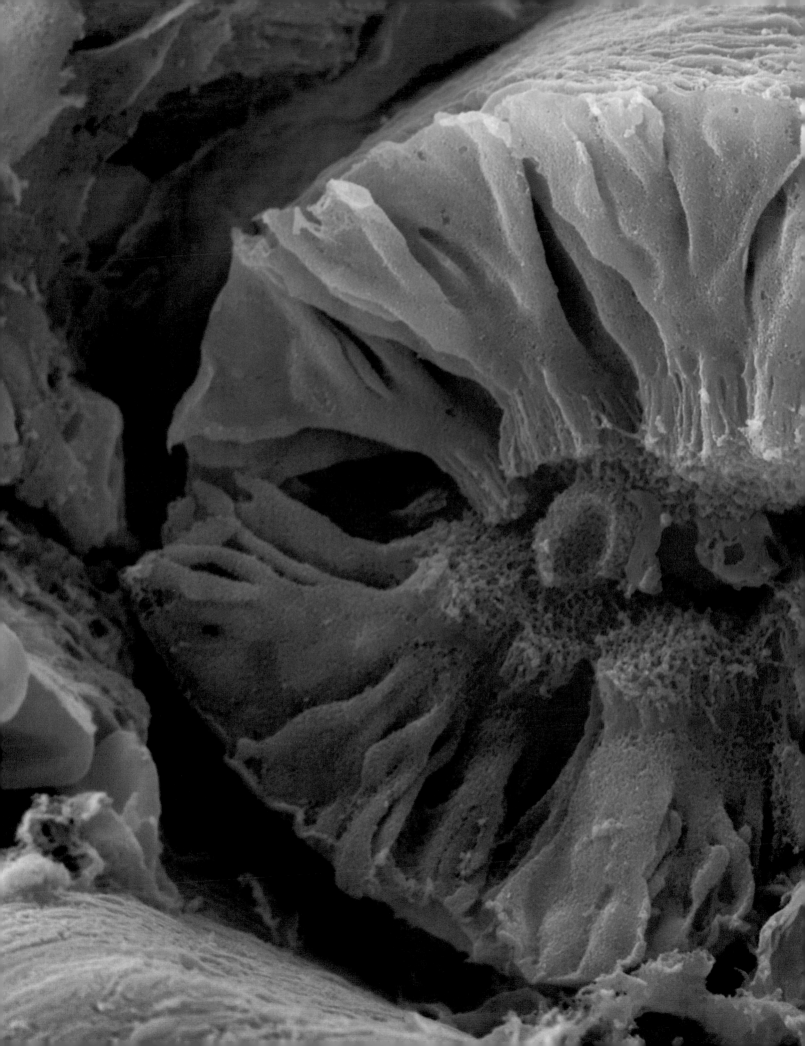

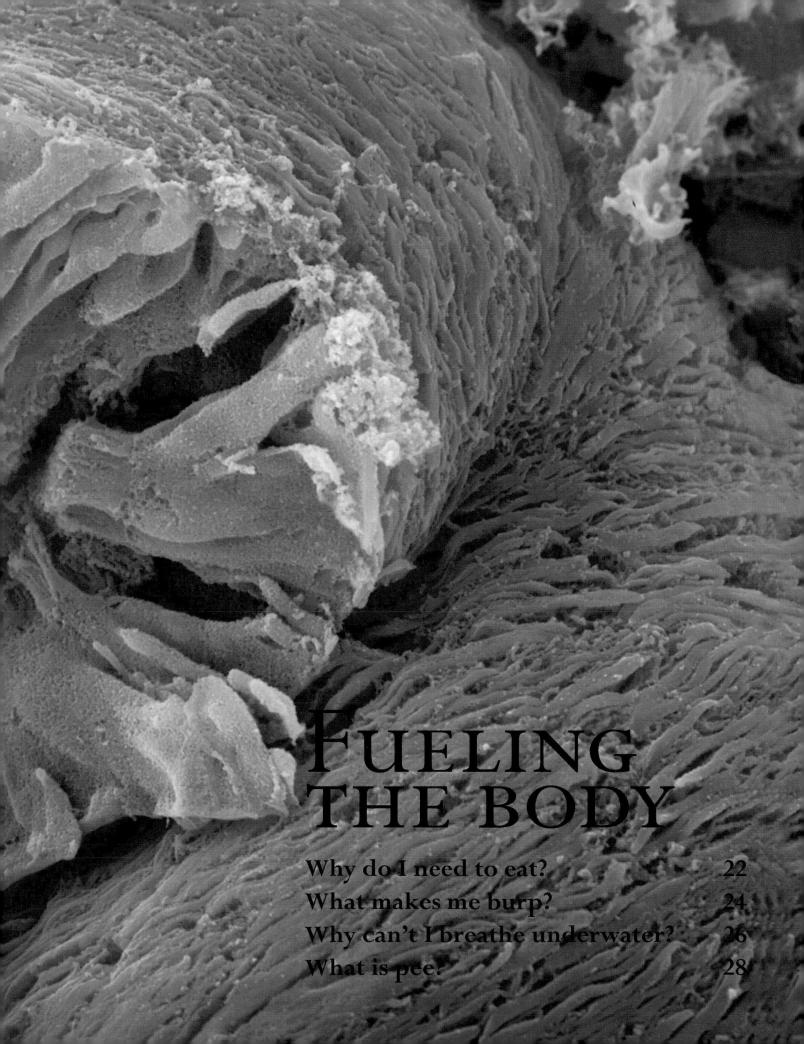

FUELING THE BODY

Why do I need to eat?   22
What makes me burp?   24
Why can't I breathe underwater?   26
What is pee?   28

Why do I need to eat?

Every few hours we are driven by a feeling of hunger to eat food. Eating is essential because food contains the nutrients that the body needs in order to stay alive. Nutrients include carbohydrates and fats, which supply energy, proteins, which provide the raw materials for growth and repair, and vitamins and minerals, which cells need to work correctly. The body's digestive system digests, or breaks down, the complex molecules in food to release simple nutrients that the body can use. This process starts in the mouth.

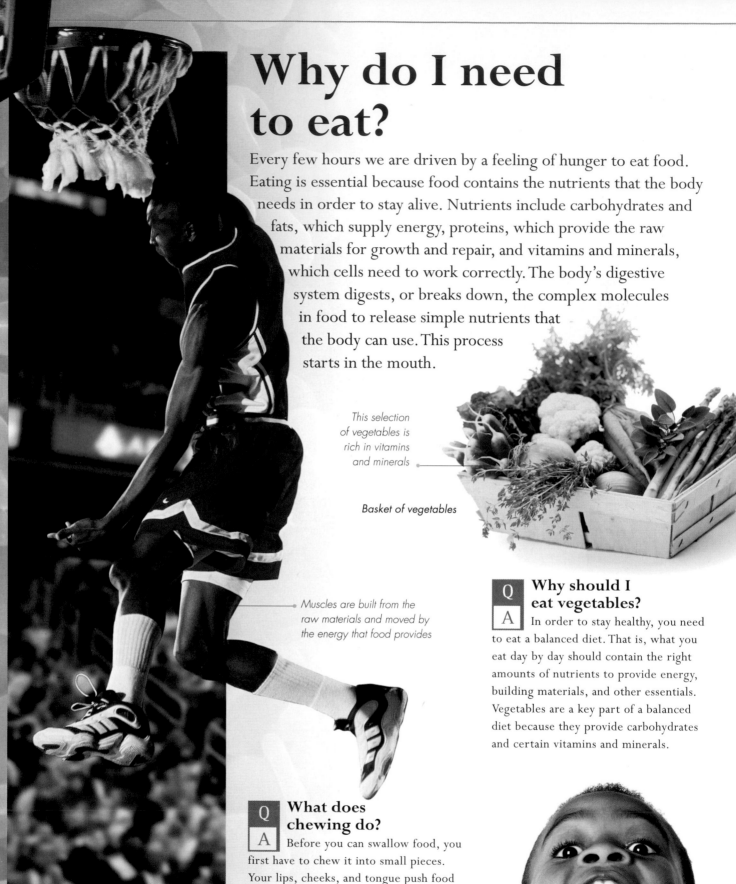

This selection of vegetables is rich in vitamins and minerals

Basket of vegetables

Muscles are built from the raw materials and moved by the energy that food provides

Q A Why should I eat vegetables?

In order to stay healthy, you need to eat a balanced diet. That is, what you eat day by day should contain the right amounts of nutrients to provide energy, building materials, and other essentials. Vegetables are a key part of a balanced diet because they provide carbohydrates and certain vitamins and minerals.

Q A What does chewing do?

Before you can swallow food, you first have to chew it into small pieces. Your lips, cheeks, and tongue push food between your teeth. Powered by strong jaw muscles, front teeth slice food, while bulkier back teeth crush it into a paste. At the same time, your tongue mixes food with saliva.

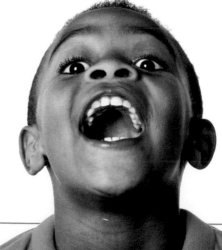

How is food broken down?

Your teeth and stomach use muscle action to break down food into small particles. These particles are then targeted by chemical digesters called enzymes, especially in the small intestine. Enzymes speed up the breakdown of large food molecules into simple nutrients, such as glucose, that can be absorbed into the bloodstream.

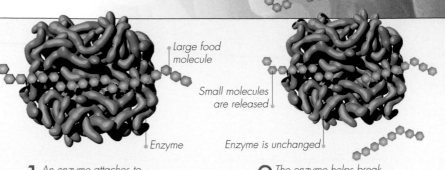

Large food molecule

Small molecules are released

Enzyme is unchanged

Enzyme

1 An enzyme attaches to a complex food molecule and locks it in place.

2 The enzyme helps break down the complex molecule into simpler nutrients.

More Facts

- In an average lifetime a person will eat about 25 tons of food, equivalent to the combined weight of five African bull elephants.

- We have two sets of teeth during our lifetime. The first set contains 20 milk, or baby, teeth. These are gradually replaced during childhood and teenage years by 32 adult teeth.

- We release two pints (one litre) of saliva daily. Saliva also cleans the mouth and contains a bacteria-killing chemical called lysozyme.

- Plaque is a mixture of food and bacteria that builds up and sticks to teeth that are not brushed regularly. Plaque bacteria feed on food remains, releasing acids that eat away at teeth and cause decay.

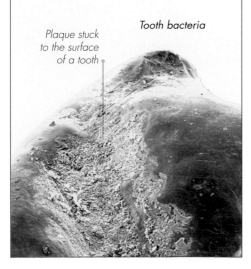

Plaque stuck to the surface of a tooth

Tooth bacteria

Salivary gland

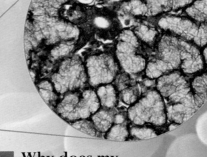

Q A Why does my mouth water?

If you are hungry, the sight, smell, or thought of food triggers the release of saliva. This watery liquid is squirted into your mouth by three pairs of salivary glands (left, yellow). Saliva moistens food during chewing. It also contains an enzyme that digests starchy food and slimy mucus that binds chewed food particles together and makes them easier to swallow.

Q A What happens when I swallow?

Once food has been thoroughly chewed, your tongue pushes it backward. As soon as the slimy ball of food touches the back of your throat, it sets off an automatic reflex action. You briefly stop breathing, to stop food from going "down the wrong way," while food is pushed down your throat and into the esophagus. Muscles in the wall of your esophagus alternately contract (squeeze) and relax to move food downward to your stomach—a journey that takes just 10 seconds.

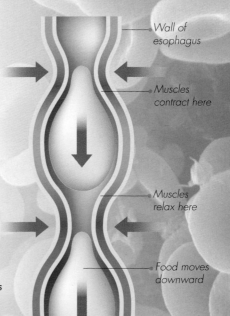

Wall of esophagus

Muscles contract here

Muscles relax here

Food moves downward

Food in the esophagus

23

What makes me burp?

Digestion really gets started in your stomach. There, chewed-up lumps of food are turned into a soupy mixture—a process that may produce gases that cause you to burp. Digestion is completed in the small intestine, where complex food substances are broken down into simple nutrients such as glucose. In the large intestine any leftover waste is turned into feces, ready to be pushed out of the body.

Q A What is stomach acid?

Ten seconds after being swallowed, food arrives in the stomach, where it is mixed with gastric (stomach) juice. This highly acidic liquid is produced by millions of gastric glands deep in the stomach's lining. As well as a strong acid, gastric juice contains a protein-digesting enzyme called pepsin that only works in acidic conditions. Stomach acid also kills most harmful bacteria in food and drink.

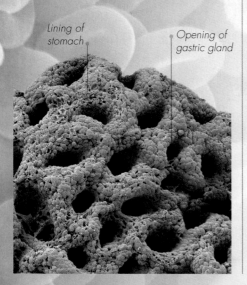

Lining of stomach

Opening of gastric gland

Q A What's the point of a pancreas?

Tucked under the stomach, your pancreas plays a key role in digestion. It releases pancreatic juice through a duct (tube) into the duodenum, the first section of the small intestine. This juice contains several enzymes that digest different types of food. The nearby gallbladder stores and releases bile, made by the liver, through the same duct, and this aids fat digestion.

Q A How big is the small intestine?

The most important part of the digestive system, the small intestine is narrower but much longer than the large intestine. Its inner surface is folded and covered with tiny fingerlike villi. Enzymes on their surface complete the process of digestion, and villi provide a massive surface across which simple nutrients are absorbed into the bloodstream.

Gallbladder

Pancreas releases several enzymes

Villi lining the small intestine

Small intestine

How does the stomach work?

When food arrives in the stomach, its lower end—the exit into the small intestine—is closed off by a ring of muscle called the pyloric sphincter. The stomach's muscular walls mix food with gastric juice and churn it into a creamy paste. After three or four hours of mixing, partially digested food is released in small amounts into the small intestine.

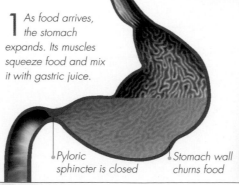

1 As food arrives, the stomach expands. Its muscles squeeze food and mix it with gastric juice.

2 After hours of processing, creamy food is released in squirts into the small intestine.

Pyloric sphincter is open

Pyloric sphincter is closed

Stomach wall churns food

Muscles push out food

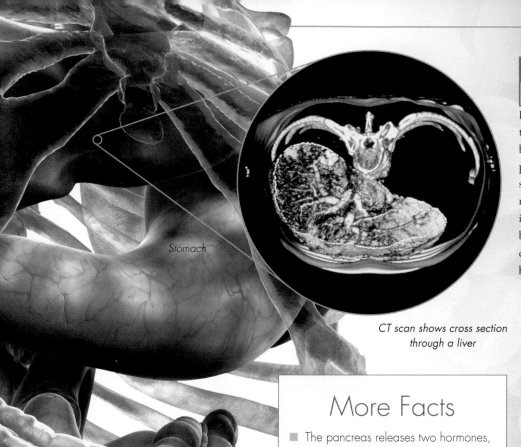

Stomach

CT scan shows cross section
through a liver

Could I live without a liver?

Q

A Your liver is essential for life. Its busy cells perform more than 500 jobs that balance the chemical makeup of your blood. Those jobs include storing and processing recently digested nutrients—such as glucose, fats, vitamins, and minerals—arriving from the small intestine, removing poisons from the blood, and recycling worn-out red blood cells. These activities also release heat that helps keep your body's insides warm.

Large intestine

More Facts

- The pancreas releases two hormones, insulin and glucagon, into the bloodstream. These chemical messengers control levels of glucose—the body's main energy supply—in the blood.

- The liver is your body's largest internal organ. Only your skin is bigger and heavier.

- The small intestine is about 20 ft (6 m) long and 1 in (2.5 cm) wide. The large intestine is about 5 ft (1.5 m) long and 2 in (5 cm) wide.

- Billions of bacteria live harmlessly inside the colon, the longest part of the large intestine. They feed on undigested waste, give feces (poop) their color and smell, and make farts.

Video pill contains a tiny camera

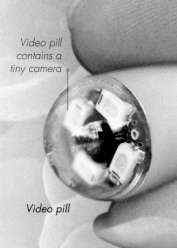

Video pill

How long does digestion take?

Q

A The entire digestive process, from food being chewed to waste emerging from the other end, takes between one to two days. A device called a video pill takes a similar time, once swallowed, to travel from the mouth to the anus. It contains a tiny camera, a light source, and a transmitter that sends images of the inside of the intestines to a receiver outside a patient's body. Doctors then look at the images to see if the patient has any problems.

Bacteria inside the colon

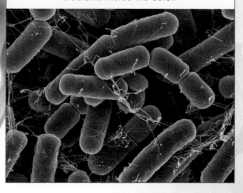

Why can't I breathe underwater?

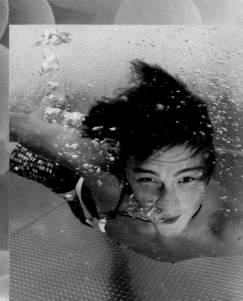

Every time you breathe in, air is carried by your airways to your lungs. There, oxygen from the air enters your bloodstream to be carried to all your body cells. Cells need constant supplies of oxygen to release the energy that keeps them and you alive. That process also releases waste carbon dioxide, which you then breathe out. Your lungs only work in air —in order to breathe underwater, you would need gills like a fish.

Q | A Is it windy inside the windpipe?

As you breathe in and out, air rushes up and down your trachea, or windpipe, so it is very breezy in there. At its lower end, the trachea splits into two bronchi, one for each lung. Each bronchus then divides into smaller and smaller branches inside the lungs, getting air to every part.

Q | A What goes on inside the lungs?

The smallest branches of the bronchi, called bronchioles, end in bunches of tiny air sacs. There are 150 million of these microscopic air sacs, called alveoli, in each lung. Oxygen passes from the alveoli into the bloodstream to be carried to all the body's cells, while carbon dioxide moves in the opposite direction.

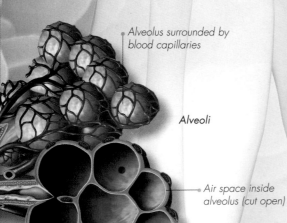

Alveolus surrounded by blood capillaries

Alveoli

Air space inside alveolus (cut open)

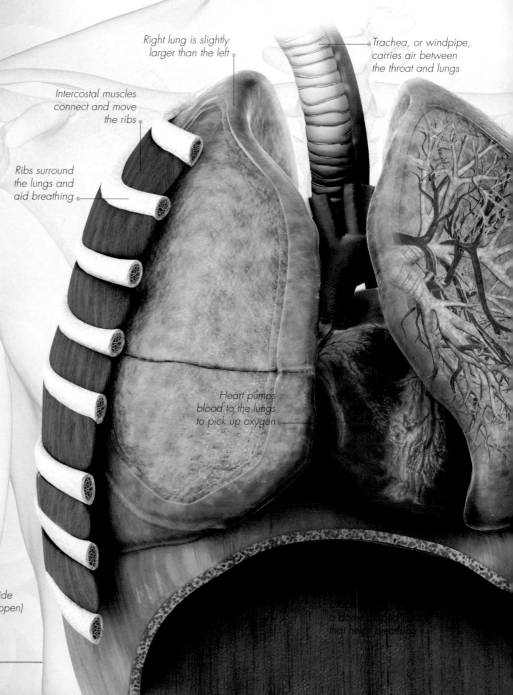

Right lung is slightly larger than the left

Trachea, or windpipe, carries air between the throat and lungs

Intercostal muscles connect and move the ribs

Ribs surround the lungs and aid breathing

Heart pumps blood to the lungs to pick up oxygen

a dome-shaped muscle that helps breathing

Should I breathe through my nose?

It is preferable to inhale through your nose rather than through your mouth. Air passing through the nasal cavity—the space behind your nose—is automatically cleaned, moistened, and warmed. Sticky mucus and hairlike cilia lining the nasal cavity trap and dispose of dust and other particles that might otherwise damage your lungs.

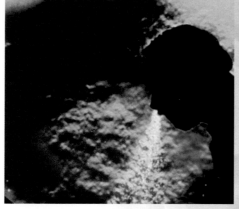

Air turbulence caused by a sneeze

What causes hay fever?

We all inhale particles, such as pollen grains, when we breathe in. But some people react to these particles and develop an allergy called hay fever. This results in watery eyes, a runny, itchy nose, and sneezing. When somebody sneezes, a surge of air, released suddenly from the lungs, blasts through the nasal cavity to remove any irritations.

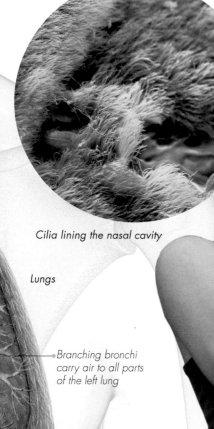

Cilia lining the nasal cavity

Lungs

Branching bronchi carry air to all parts of the left lung

Musician blows into a trumpet

How do musicians play and breathe at the same time?

Some musicians who play wind instruments, such as the trumpet or oboe, are able to use a technique called circular breathing. This allows them to play music without interruption for longer periods of time than they could with normal breathing. They learn to use their cheeks like bellows in order to maintain a flow of air through the instrument while at the same time inhaling air through their nose.

Why does my chest move when I breathe?

Your lungs cannot expand and shrink on their own. When you inhale, your diaphragm flattens and pushes downward while your ribs and chest move upward and outward. This makes your lungs expand so that air is sucked in. During exhalation, the diaphragm is pushed upward, the ribs move downward, your chest and lungs get smaller, and air is pushed out.

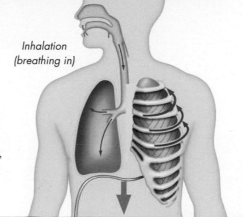

Inhalation (breathing in)

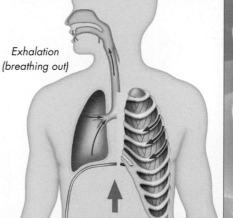

Exhalation (breathing out)

What is pee?

Your body's built-in waste disposal service, the urinary system, consists of two kidneys, two ureters, a bladder, and a urethra. The kidneys constantly process blood to keep its composition the same. They remove poisonous wastes produced by cells and surplus water from food and drink. Mixed together, the wastes and water form urine, which is released from your body when you pee.

Right kidney

Urinary system

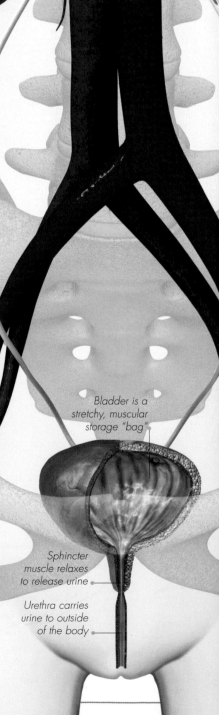

Q / A How is urine made?
Inside each kidney there are a million tiny, coiled tubes called nephrons. At one end of the nephron, fluid is filtered from the blood. As this fluid passes along the nephron, useful substances, such as glucose, pass back into the bloodstream. The remaining waste liquid, now called urine, flows out of the kidney and down the ureter to the bladder, where it is stored.

Q / A What makes us feel the need to go to the bathroom?
Your bladder has a stretchy wall that expands as it fills up with urine. You can see how much the bladder (green) expands in these x-rays (below). As the bladder fills up, stretch sensors in its wall send messages to your brain telling you that it's time to go to the bathroom.

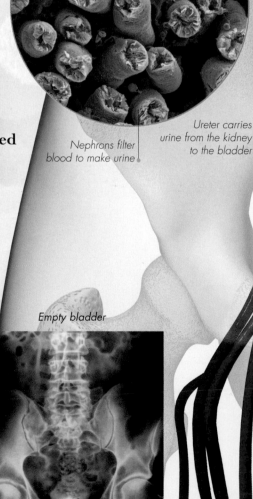

Nephrons filter blood to make urine

Ureter carries urine from the kidney to the bladder

Bladder is a stretchy, muscular storage "bag"

Sphincter muscle relaxes to release urine

Urethra carries urine to outside of the body

Full bladder

Empty bladder

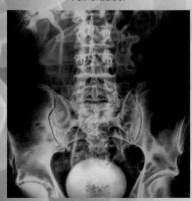

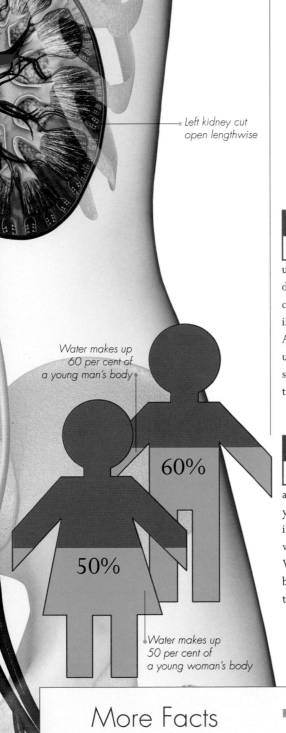

Left kidney cut open lengthwise

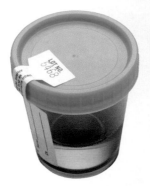

A urine sample, ready for testing

Q A Why is urine yellow?

Urine contains various dissolved substances, one of which gives urine its yellow color. To help them discover why patients are sick, doctors check the levels of certain substances in urine to see if they are abnormal. A test stick is dipped into a patient's urine sample. Its colored bands detect specific substances and change colour to show how much of each is present.

Water makes up 60 per cent of a young man's body

60%

50%

Water makes up 50 per cent of a young woman's body

Q A How much water is in my body?

Water is very important. It is a major part of blood, and without water, your cells would not work. A child's body is around 65 percent water. After puberty, water content depends on a person's sex. Women contain less water than men because they have more body fat—a tissue that contains little water.

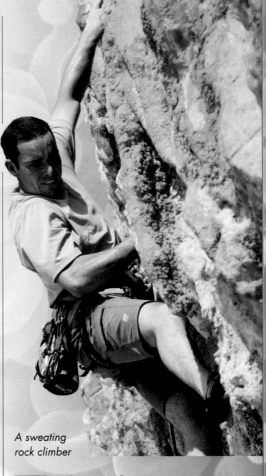

A sweating rock climber

Q A What makes me feel thirsty?

Whenever you sweat, pee, or breathe out, your body loses some of its water. This makes your mouth feel dry and your blood more concentrated, which is detected by the "thirst center" in your brain. This thirst center is makes you feel thirsty, so that you feel the need to drink. The drink wets your mouth, quenches your thirst, and replaces the lost water.

More Facts

- Babies can't control when they pee. Once a baby's bladder is full, it empties automatically.

- Your kidneys process 3,080 pints (1,750 litres) of blood and filter about 317 pints (180 litres) of fluid into the nephrons, but release just 2.6 pints (1.5 litres) of urine per day.

- Water makes up about 95 percent of urine. The major waste dissolved in urine is urea—a substance produced by liver cells.

- To keep your water content the same, the kidneys release more, diluted urine if you have drunk lots of fluid and less urine that is more concentrated if you are dehydrated and sweating.

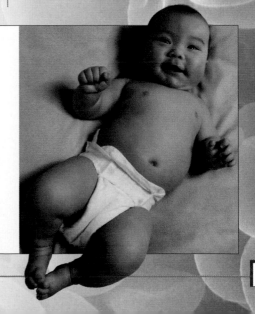

BRAINPOWER

Do smart people have bigger brains?   32
Why can't I see in the dark?   34
How did I hear what you said?   36
Why does candy taste sweet?   38

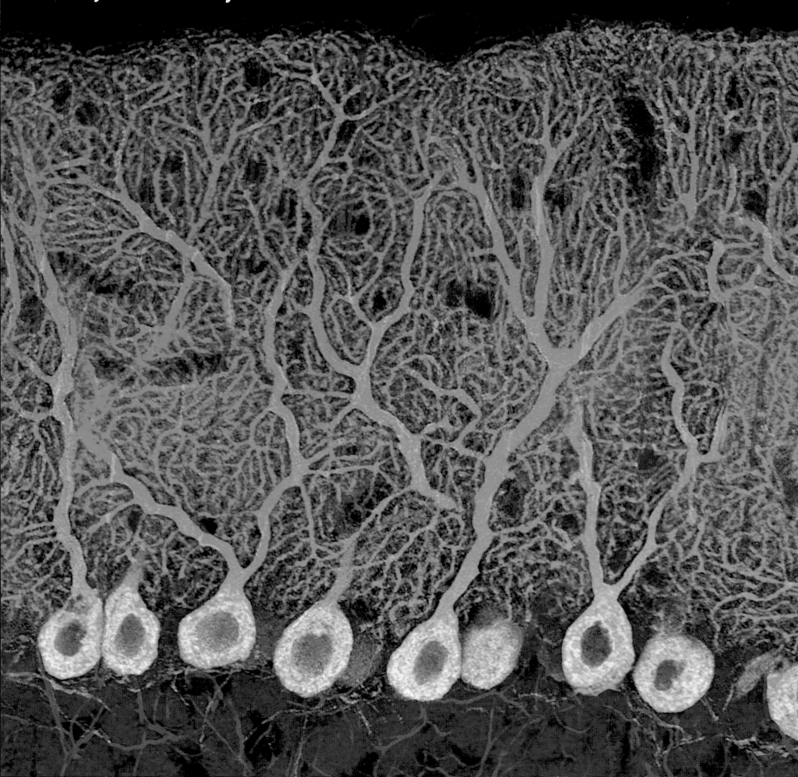

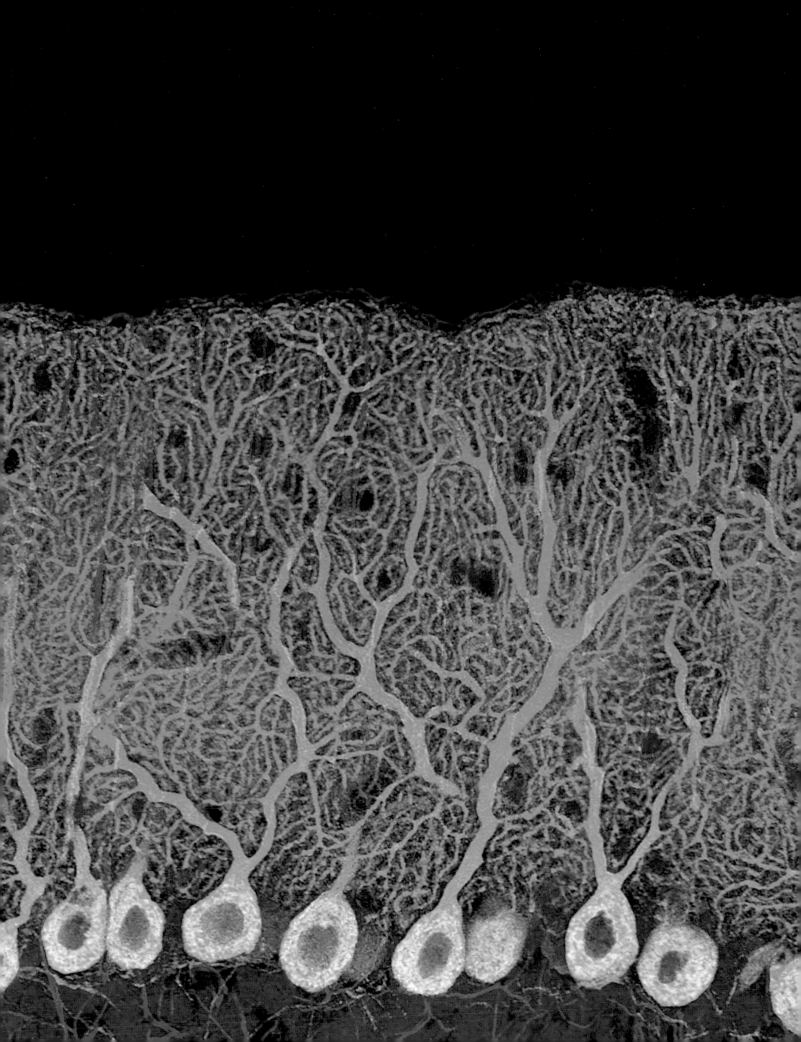

Do smart people have bigger brains?

The nervous system controls and coordinates your body's activities with split-second timing. It collects information about what is happening inside and outside your body and sends it along nerves and the spinal cord to your brain. There, the information is processed, enabling you to think, feel, remember, and move. Your brain's size doesn't affect any of this—having a bigger brain does not make you any smarter.

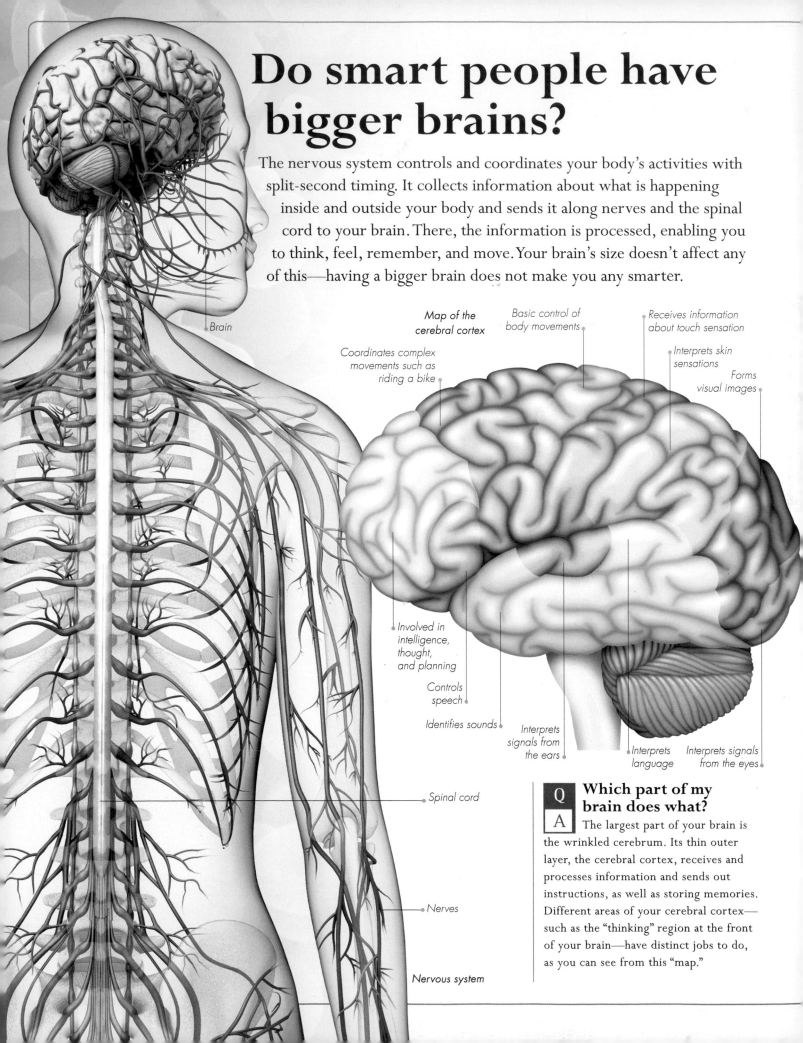

Brain

Map of the cerebral cortex

Coordinates complex movements such as riding a bike

Basic control of body movements

Receives information about touch sensation

Interprets skin sensations

Forms visual images

Involved in intelligence, thought, and planning

Controls speech

Identifies sounds

Interprets signals from the ears

Interprets language

Interprets signals from the eyes

Spinal cord

Nerves

Nervous system

Q **Which part of my brain does what?**

A The largest part of your brain is the wrinkled cerebrum. Its thin outer layer, the cerebral cortex, receives and processes information and sends out instructions, as well as storing memories. Different areas of your cerebral cortex— such as the "thinking" region at the front of your brain—have distinct jobs to do, as you can see from this "map."

How do I react so quickly?

Your nervous system is constructed from a massive network of interconnected cells called neurons. The brain alone contains 100 billion neurons. Each neuron has a long, narrow extension called a nerve fiber that generates and transmits electrical signals, called impulses, at very high speeds. This allows you to instantly react to events, even when the signal has to travel all the way from your big toe to your brain.

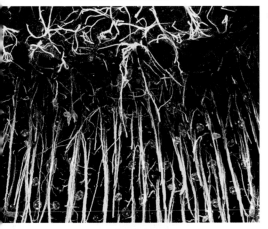

Neurons in the brain

Painting with the left hand

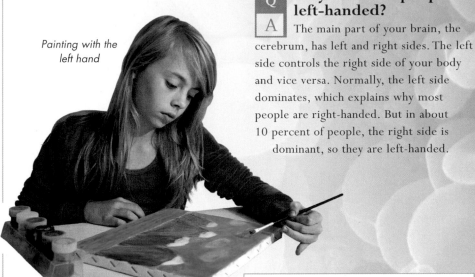

Why are some people left-handed?

The main part of your brain, the cerebrum, has left and right sides. The left side controls the right side of your body and vice versa. Normally, the left side dominates, which explains why most people are right-handed. But in about 10 percent of people, the right side is dominant, so they are left-handed.

How can reflexes protect me from danger?

If you touch something sharp or very hot, you automatically pull your hand away without thinking about it. This is an example of a reflex—an action that is rapid, unchanging, and protects us from harm. Pain signals from your fingers travel to your spinal cord. This sends instructions to your arm muscles to move your hand at the same time that signals reach your brain so that you feel pain.

Withdrawal reflex

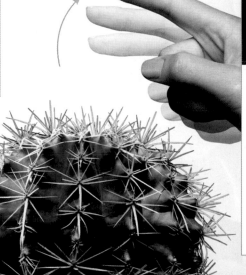

More Facts

- Your brain makes up just 2 percent of your body weight but uses 20 percent of your oxygen intake to release energy to keep it working.

- Busy brain neurons create patterns of electrical activity called brain waves, which can be detected by attaching electrodes to the scalp.

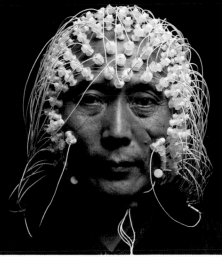

Detecting brain waves

- Your brain doesn't turn off when you sleep, although its brain waves change. At night your brain sorts and stores information, making you dream.

- The left side of your cerebrum deals with math, language, and problem solving. The right side focuses on art, music, and creativity.

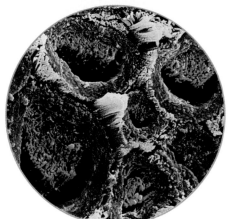

Cross section through nerve

What is a nerve?

Nerves are the cables of the nervous system. Their "wires" are the long nerve fibers (green) that carry high-speed signals. Bundles of nerve fibers are protected by tough but bendable sheaths (purple). Nerves relay information from sensors to the spinal cord and brain about what is happening to the body. They also carry instructions the opposite way to muscles and other organs.

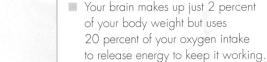

Why can't I see in the dark?

Vision is our most important sense. It allows us to see our surroundings. The sense organs responsible for vision are the eyes. Moving constantly, the eyes collect light and focus it onto receptor cells. These cells send signals to the brain, which creates images that we can see. In the dark there is little or no light, so we are unable to see.

Retina contains light receptors

Optic nerve carries nerve signals to the brain

Fovea is the most sensitive part of the retina

Structure of the eye

Q A Why do my pupils change size?

Your colored irises automatically control the size of your pupils and, therefore, the amount of light that enters your eyes. Without this control, you would be dazzled in bright light and unable to see in dim light. Circular muscle fibers in your irises close your pupils in bright light, and spokelike radial muscle fibers contract to open your pupils in dim light.

Radial muscle fibers relax

Circular muscle fibers contract

Radial muscle fibers contract

Circular muscle fibers relax

Sclera is the tough outer layer

Muscle moves the eyeball

Light receptor cells

Cone

Rod

Q A How do we see in color?

The retina contains two types of light receptor cells. About 120 million rods work best in dim light and enable you to see in shades of gray. Seven million cones, mostly found in the fovea directly behind the lens, allow you to see the color and detail of what you are looking at.

Q A Is an eye similar to a camera?

Cameras use lenses to focus light rays from an object to form an image on a light-sensitive surface. The eyes are no different. Light rays from an object are focused automatically, whatever its distance from the eyes, by the cornea and lens to form an upside-down image on the retina. This sends signals to the brain, which enables you to "see" the object the right way around.

Lens

Cornea

Object

Retina

Light rays

Upside-down image

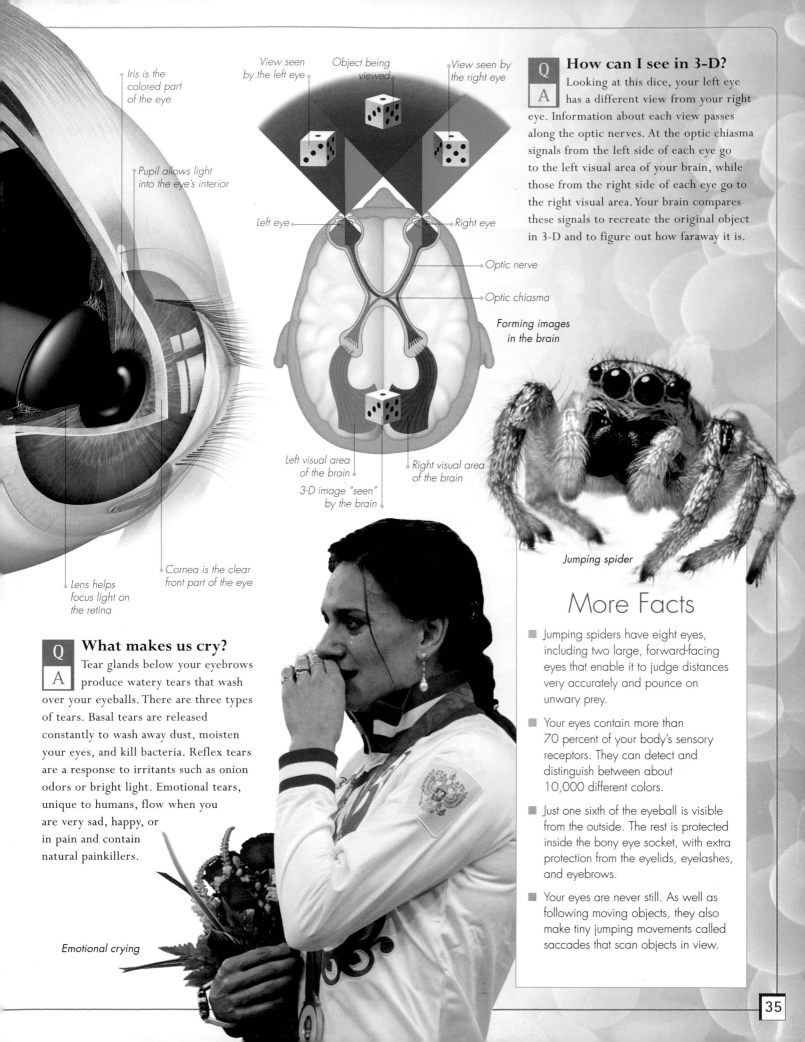

Iris is the colored part of the eye

Pupil allows light into the eye's interior

View seen by the left eye

Object being viewed

View seen by the right eye

Left eye

Right eye

Optic nerve

Optic chiasma

Forming images in the brain

Left visual area of the brain

Right visual area of the brain

3-D image "seen" by the brain

Lens helps focus light on the retina

Cornea is the clear front part of the eye

How can I see in 3-D?

Looking at this dice, your left eye has a different view from your right eye. Information about each view passes along the optic nerves. At the optic chiasma signals from the left side of each eye go to the left visual area of your brain, while those from the right side of each eye go to the right visual area. Your brain compares these signals to recreate the original object in 3-D and to figure out how faraway it is.

Jumping spider

What makes us cry?

Tear glands below your eyebrows produce watery tears that wash over your eyeballs. There are three types of tears. Basal tears are released constantly to wash away dust, moisten your eyes, and kill bacteria. Reflex tears are a response to irritants such as onion odors or bright light. Emotional tears, unique to humans, flow when you are very sad, happy, or in pain and contain natural painkillers.

Emotional crying

More Facts

■ Jumping spiders have eight eyes, including two large, forward-facing eyes that enable it to judge distances very accurately and pounce on unwary prey.

■ Your eyes contain more than 70 percent of your body's sensory receptors. They can detect and distinguish between about 10,000 different colors.

■ Just one sixth of the eyeball is visible from the outside. The rest is protected inside the bony eye socket, with extra protection from the eyelids, eyelashes, and eyebrows.

■ Your eyes are never still. As well as following moving objects, they also make tiny jumping movements called saccades that scan objects in view.

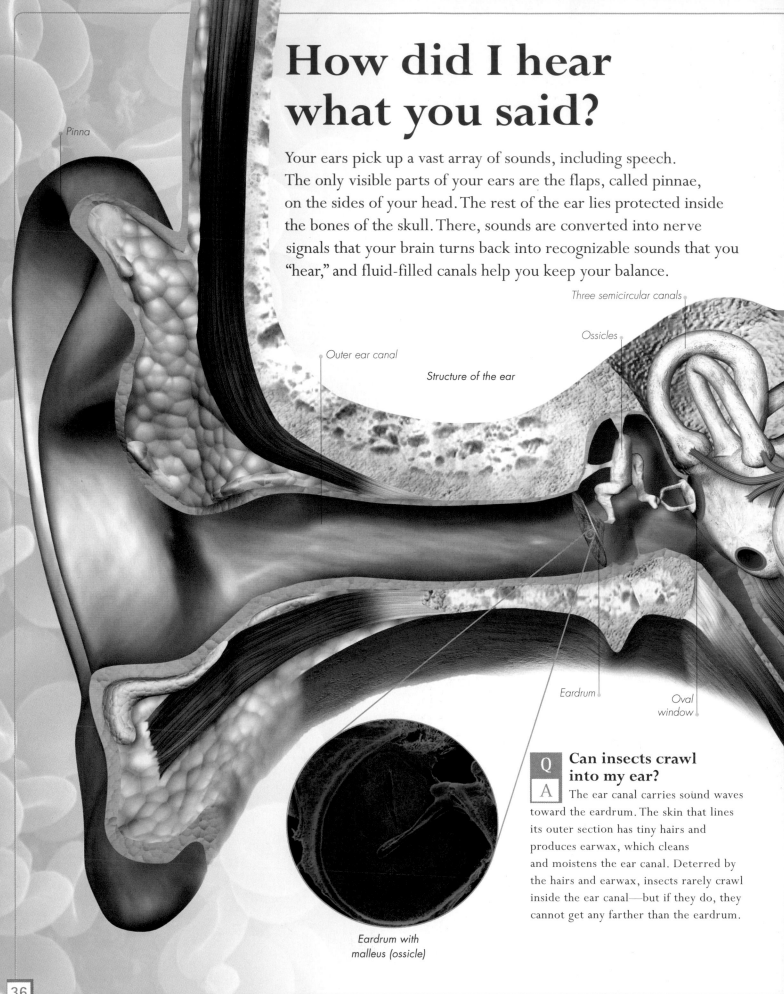

How did I hear what you said?

Your ears pick up a vast array of sounds, including speech. The only visible parts of your ears are the flaps, called pinnae, on the sides of your head. The rest of the ear lies protected inside the bones of the skull. There, sounds are converted into nerve signals that your brain turns back into recognizable sounds that you "hear," and fluid-filled canals help you keep your balance.

Pinna

Three semicircular canals

Ossicles

Outer ear canal

Structure of the ear

Eardrum

Oval window

Eardrum with malleus (ossicle)

Q **Can insects crawl into my ear?**

A The ear canal carries sound waves toward the eardrum. The skin that lines its outer section has tiny hairs and produces earwax, which cleans and moistens the ear canal. Deterred by the hairs and earwax, insects rarely crawl inside the ear canal—but if they do, they cannot get any farther than the eardrum.

Q/A What are sound waves?

Anything that moves or vibrates creates waves of pressure, called sound waves, that travel through the air. On entering your ear, they make the eardrum vibrate. This, in turn, sets up pressure waves in the fluid-filled cochlea of the inner ear. These bend the tiny "hairs" on the cochlea's hair cells, causing them to send signals to the hearing part of your brain.

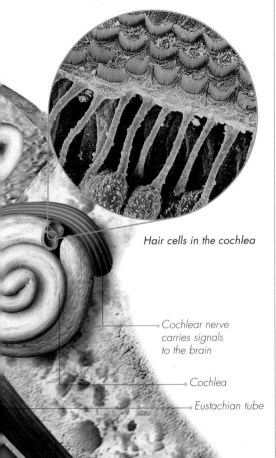

Hair cells in the cochlea

Cochlear nerve carries signals to the brain

Cochlea

Eustachian tube

Q/A Are there any bones in my ear?

Linking the eardrum to the inner ear are three small bones, or ossicles, individually named the malleus (hammer), incus (anvil), and stapes (stirrup) after their shapes. The smallest, the stapes is even tinier than the incus shown here. The ossicles form a bony chain that transmits sound vibrations from the eardrum to the oval window—the entrance to the inner ear.

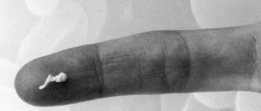

Incus bone on a fingertip

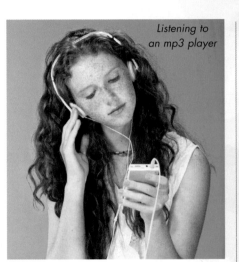

Listening to an mp3 player

Q/A Can loud noise damage my ears?

Your ears can distinguish between a massive range of sound volumes and have a built-in mechanism to protect the inner ear from sudden loud noises. But long-term exposure to loud sounds, such as constantly listening to loud music through earphones, can damage the cochlea's delicate hair cells and lead to deafness.

Q/A How do ears help us balance?

The inner ear contains three semicircular canals, arranged at right angles to each other. These, and other inner ear sensors, keep your brain updated about the movement and position of your head. Your brain uses this information, together with input from your eyes, to tell your muscles what to do, in order to keep you balanced.

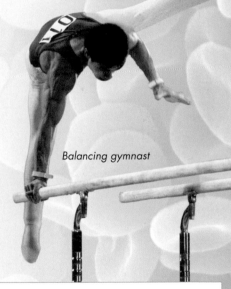

Balancing gymnast

More Facts

■ The Eustachian tube connects your ear to your throat and keeps air pressure inside and outside the ear equal. A sudden pressure change, such as when a plane takes off, makes hearing difficult. But if you yawn or swallow, the tube widens to equalize pressure, causing your ears to pop.

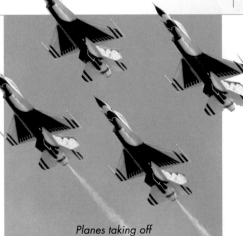

Planes taking off

■ Sounds reach one ear a split second before the other. This allows your brain to figure out which direction the sounds came from.

■ Younger people can hear a much wider range of sounds than older people can.

■ Animals such as cats and bats can hear very high-pitched sounds that we cannot.

Why does candy taste sweet?

Being able to smell and taste allows us to enjoy food and drink and many other aspects of life. The senses of smell and taste are closely linked; both are located in the head—one in the nose and the other in the mouth. Both detect chemicals that are carried in the air (smell) or in food (taste). They also help us distinguish between the sweetness of candy, and the bitterness of foods that might be poisonous.

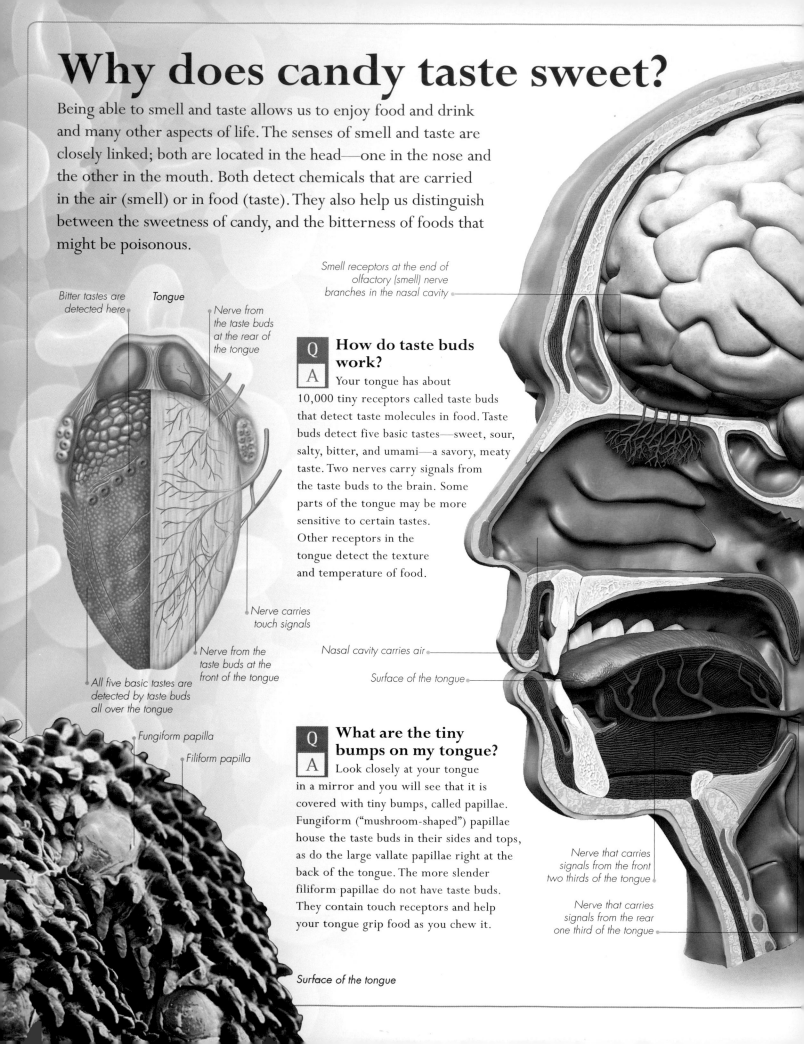

Bitter tastes are detected here

Tongue

Nerve from the taste buds at the rear of the tongue

Smell receptors at the end of olfactory (smell) nerve branches in the nasal cavity

Nerve carries touch signals

Nerve from the taste buds at the front of the tongue

All five basic tastes are detected by taste buds all over the tongue

Fungiform papilla

Filiform papilla

Nasal cavity carries air

Surface of the tongue

Nerve that carries signals from the front two thirds of the tongue

Nerve that carries signals from the rear one third of the tongue

Surface of the tongue

Q A How do taste buds work?

Your tongue has about 10,000 tiny receptors called taste buds that detect taste molecules in food. Taste buds detect five basic tastes—sweet, sour, salty, bitter, and umami—a savory, meaty taste. Two nerves carry signals from the taste buds to the brain. Some parts of the tongue may be more sensitive to certain tastes. Other receptors in the tongue detect the texture and temperature of food.

Q A What are the tiny bumps on my tongue?

Look closely at your tongue in a mirror and you will see that it is covered with tiny bumps, called papillae. Fungiform ("mushroom-shaped") papillae house the taste buds in their sides and tops, as do the large vallate papillae right at the back of the tongue. The more slender filiform papillae do not have taste buds. They contain touch receptors and help your tongue grip food as you chew it.

How do I smell things?

Smelling happens in the lining of the roof of your nasal cavity—the space behind your nose. Sticking out from the lining are the tips of smell receptors, which look like this (see below). Each tip has several hairlike cilia. Breathed-in molecules dissolve in watery mucus and stick to these cilia. This causes the smell receptors to send signals to the brain, which identifies what you are smelling.

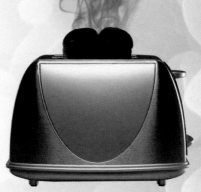

Can we smell danger?

As well as helping you enjoy delicious food or pick up the scent of flowers, your sense of smell has another important role to play. The smell of smoke, for example, warns you that something may be on fire and that you need to take action. Food that looks fine but smells terrible should put you off eating it in case it is poisonous.

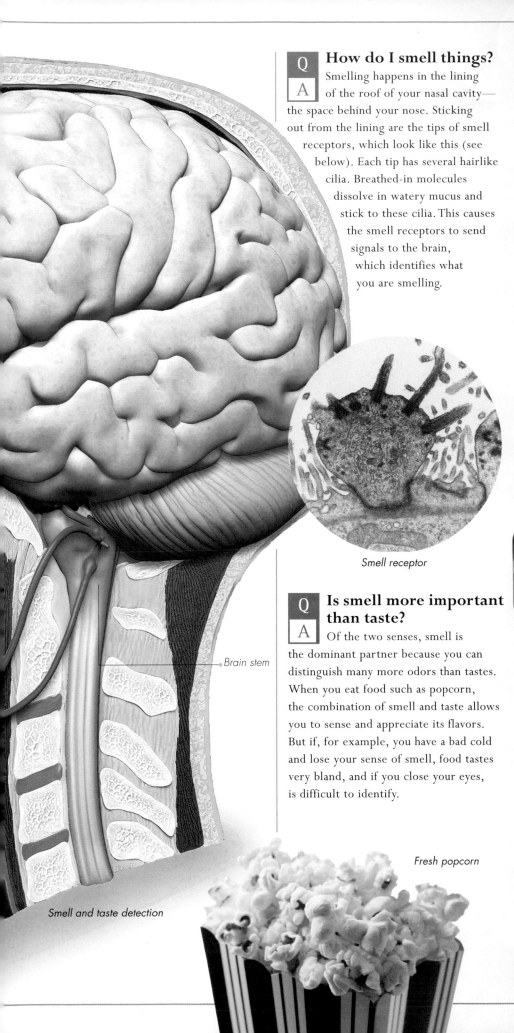

Smell receptor

Is smell more important than taste?

Of the two senses, smell is the dominant partner because you can distinguish many more odors than tastes. When you eat food such as popcorn, the combination of smell and taste allows you to sense and appreciate its flavors. But if, for example, you have a bad cold and lose your sense of smell, food tastes very bland, and if you close your eyes, is difficult to identify.

Brain stem

Smell and taste detection

Fresh popcorn

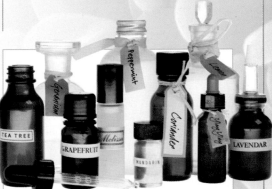

More Facts

- People who work as perfumers have a "super sense" of smell that enable them to identify and distinguish between subtle fragrances.

- Other people with smell and taste "super senses" are employed as tea, wine, or food tasters. They are born with this exceptional ability.

- Your millions of smell receptors can detect more than 10,000 different smells, but your taste buds can only detect five different tastes.

- Some scents can be detected at very low concentrations, including methyl mercaptan—the chemical added to odorless natural gas to make it smell.

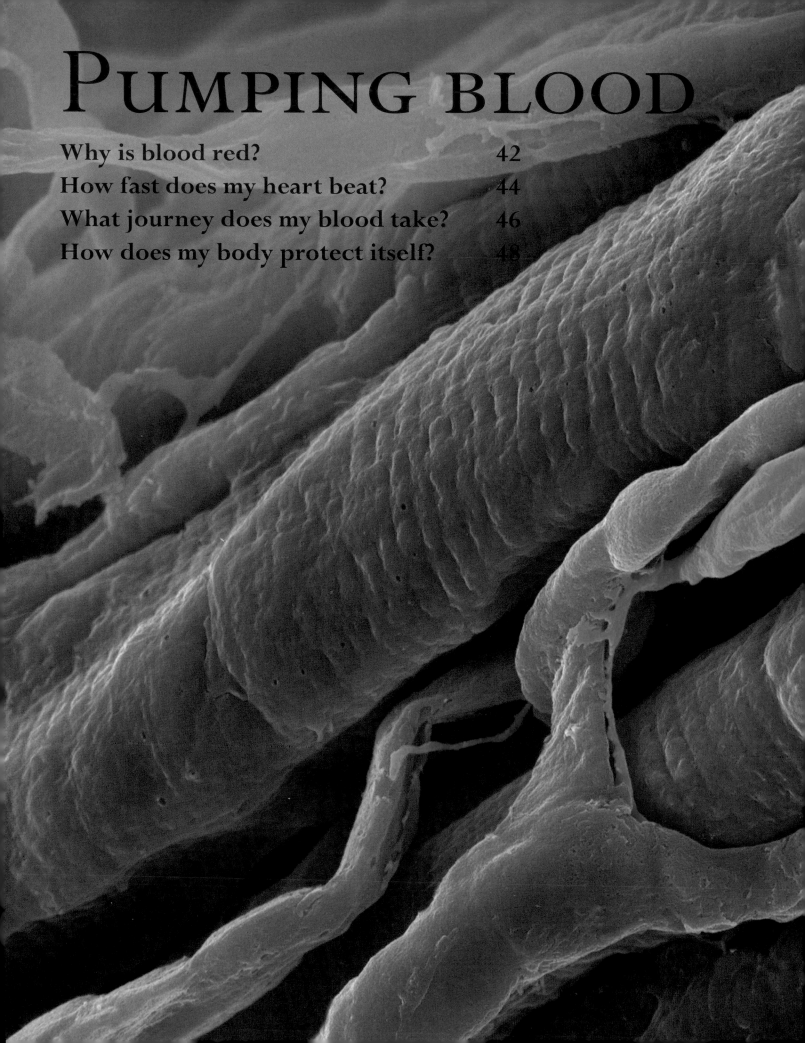

PUMPING BLOOD

Why is blood red?   42

How fast does my heart beat?   44

What journey does my blood take?   46

How does my body protect itself?   48

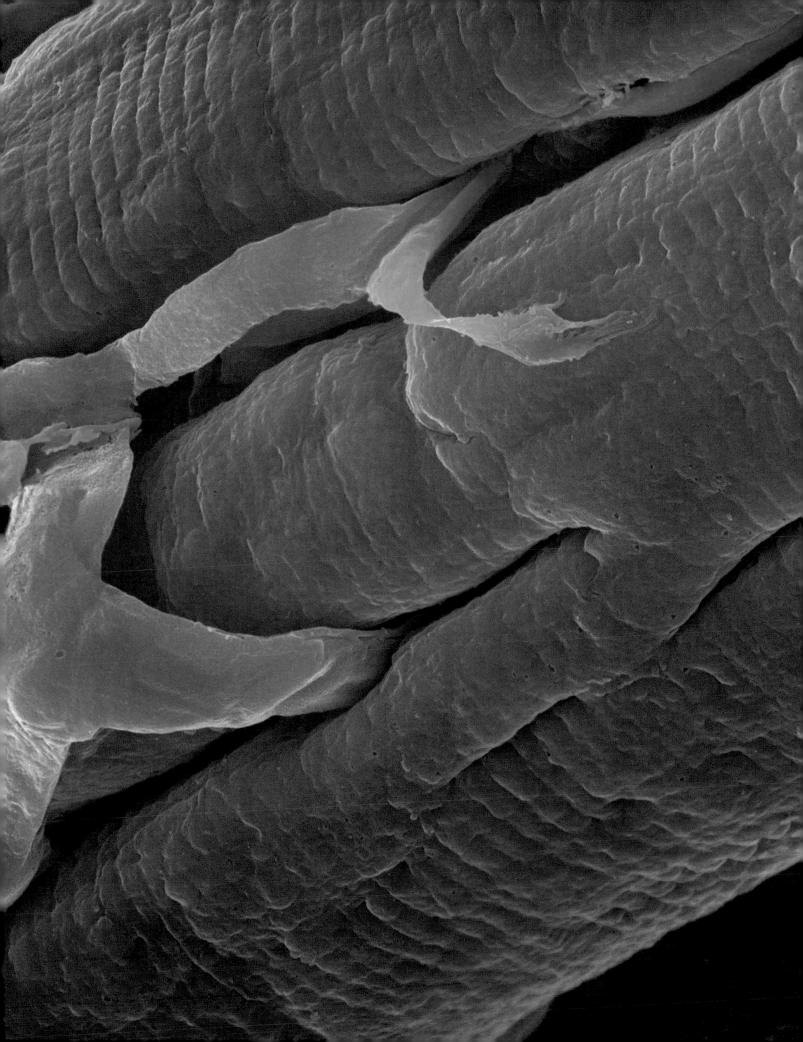

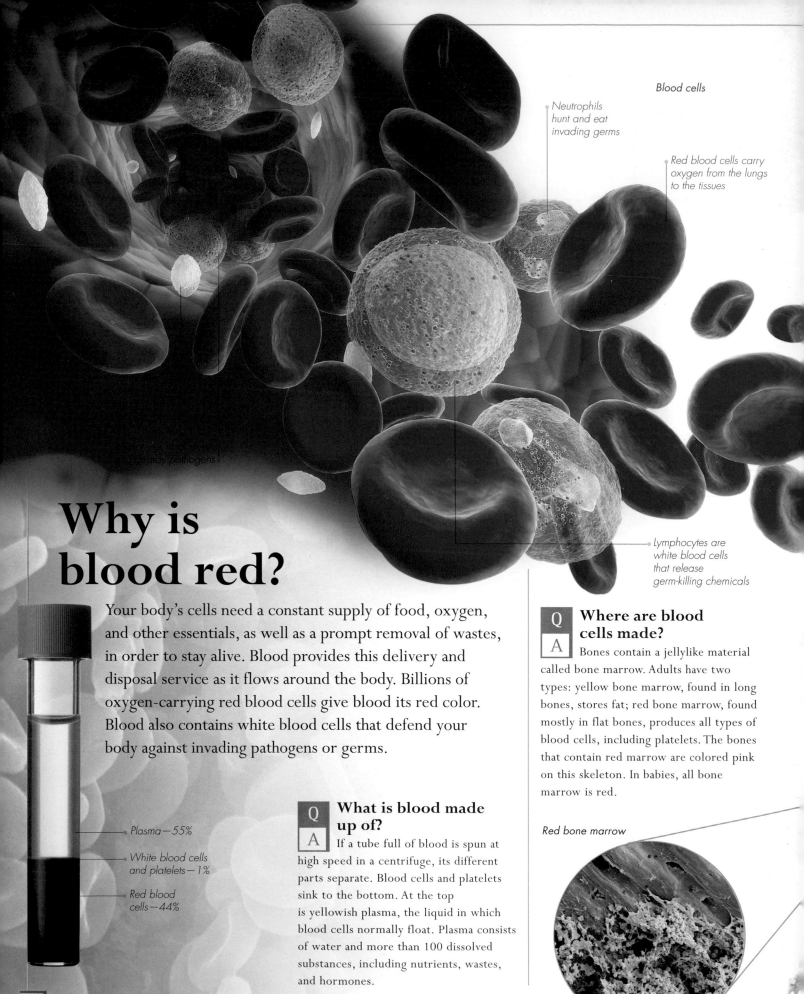

Blood cells

Neutrophils hunt and eat invading germs

Red blood cells carry oxygen from the lungs to the tissues

Lymphocytes are white blood cells that release germ-killing chemicals

Why is blood red?

Your body's cells need a constant supply of food, oxygen, and other essentials, as well as a prompt removal of wastes, in order to stay alive. Blood provides this delivery and disposal service as it flows around the body. Billions of oxygen-carrying red blood cells give blood its red color. Blood also contains white blood cells that defend your body against invading pathogens or germs.

Plasma—55%

White blood cells and platelets—1%

Red blood cells—44%

Q/A What is blood made up of?

If a tube full of blood is spun at high speed in a centrifuge, its different parts separate. Blood cells and platelets sink to the bottom. At the top is yellowish plasma, the liquid in which blood cells normally float. Plasma consists of water and more than 100 dissolved substances, including nutrients, wastes, and hormones.

Q/A Where are blood cells made?

Bones contain a jellylike material called bone marrow. Adults have two types: yellow bone marrow, found in long bones, stores fat; red bone marrow, found mostly in flat bones, produces all types of blood cells, including platelets. The bones that contain red marrow are colored pink on this skeleton. In babies, all bone marrow is red.

Red bone marrow

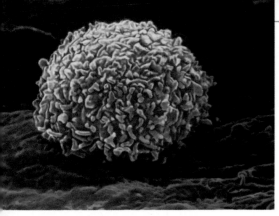

White blood cell

Q A Are white blood cells really white?

This neutrophil has been colored to make it stand out, but in real life it is transparent, like other types of white blood cells. They are called "white" because they are not red, and also because they form a thin, white layer when blood is spun in a centrifuge tube. Like other white blood cells, neutrophils protect the body against infections.

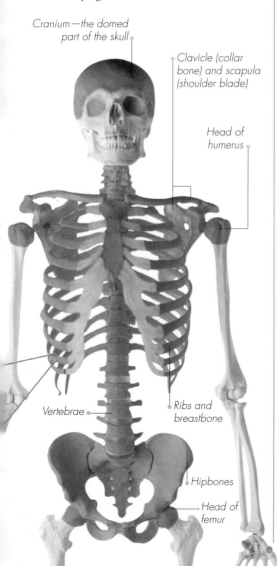

Cranium—the domed part of the skull

Clavicle (collar bone) and scapula (shoulder blade)

Head of humerus

Vertebrae

Ribs and breastbone

Hipbones

Head of femur

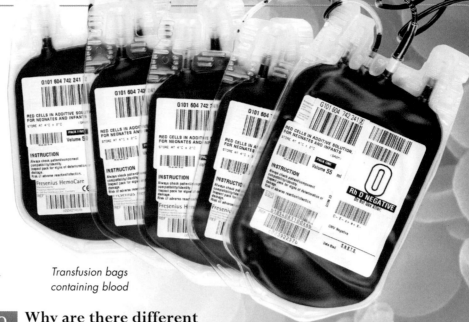

Transfusion bags containing blood

Q A Why are there different blood groups?

Your red blood cells carry one, both, or neither of two tiny markers called A and B. Whether you do or don't have these markers determines whether you belong to blood group A, B, AB, or O. To avoid problems during blood transfusions (transfers), a person should receive blood from someone of the same blood group.

Q A How much blood do I have?

If all the blood was drained out of your body, you would be about 8 percent lighter in weight. In adults this percentage amounts to between 7 and 8.8 pints (4 and 5 litres) of blood in women and, because they are bigger on average, 8.8 to 10.5 pints (5 to 6 litres) in men. The volume of blood in your body is controlled by your kidneys.

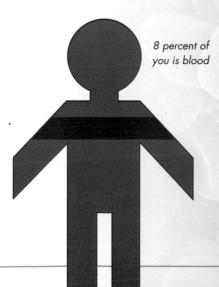

8 percent of you is blood

More Facts

■ A single tiny drop of blood contains 250 million red blood cells, 375,000 white blood cells, and 16 million platelets.

■ Red blood cells have no nucleus and a life span of 120 days. Two million new red blood cells are made by bone marrow every second.

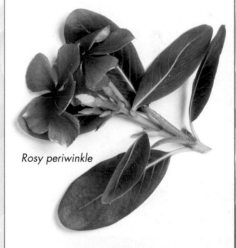

Rosy periwinkle

■ Leukemia is a disease, sometimes fatal, in which too many abnormal white blood cells are produced. Drugs extracted from the rosy periwinkle, a rainforest plant, have been used to successfully treat leukemia.

■ Red blood cells contain hemoglobin, a red-colored protein that carries oxygen. A single red blood cell contains 250 million hemoglobin molecules.

How fast does my heart beat?

At the core of your body's blood transportation system is a muscular pump—the heart. The heart has two sides, left and right, each with an upper and lower chamber , the atrium and ventricle. The heart beats about 70 times per minute to pump blood to your cells, speeding up when necessary to meet increased demand. During an average lifetime, the heart beats more than 2.5 billion times without taking a rest.

Superior vena cava brings oxygen-poor blood from the upper body

Valve guards the exit from the right ventricle

Right atrium receives oxygen-poor blood

Cardiac (heart) muscle

Valve between the atrium and ventricle

Right ventricle pumps blood to the lungs

Inferior vena cava carries oxygen-poor blood from the abdomen and legs

Q A Does the heart have its own blood supply?

The muscular wall of your heart needs an uninterrupted supply of fuel and oxygen to keep it beating. But it can't get these supplies from the blood that gushes through its chambers. Instead, it has its own special supply: two coronary arteries, shown here in this cast, branch repeatedly to carry oxygen-rich blood throughout the heart's wall.

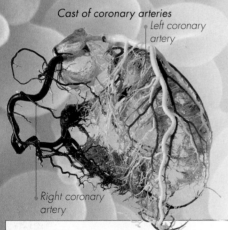
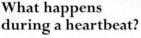

Cast of coronary arteries

Left coronary artery

Right coronary artery

Q A What's special about heart muscle?

In a lifetime of beating your heart never takes a break. Cardiac muscle never tires, contracting regularly and automatically to pump blood. A tiny section of the wall of the right atrium acts as a "pacemaker." It sends out signals that make the network of cardiac muscle cells contract at the same rate.

What happens during a heartbeat?

If you listen to, or feel, your heart beating, every heartbeat probably feels like a single event. In fact, each one is made up of three separate, precisely timed stages. Electrical signals spread through the heart's muscular wall, ensuring that first the atria and then the ventricles contract to pump blood through and out of the heart. Valves ensure that blood flow is always in the same direction.

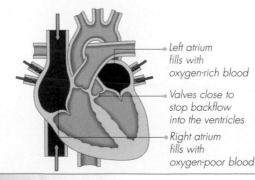

1 Your heart's muscular wall is relaxed, and blood from the lungs and the body flows, respectively, into the left and right atria.

Left atrium fills with oxygen-rich blood

Valves close to stop backflow into the ventricles

Right atrium fills with oxygen-poor blood

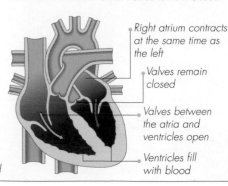

2 Left and right atria contract together, forcing blood through the valves that separate them from their ventricles. Other valves remain closed.

Right atrium contracts at the same time as the left

Valves remain closed

Valves between the atria and ventricles open

Ventricles fill with blood

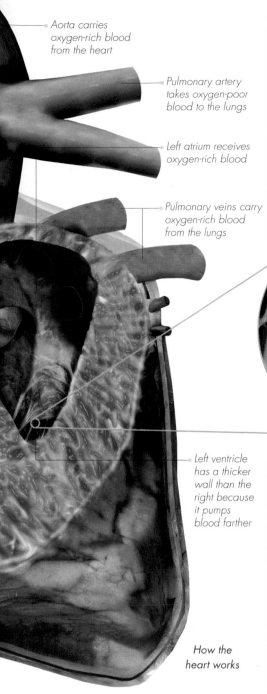

Aorta carries oxygen-rich blood from the heart

Pulmonary artery takes oxygen-poor blood to the lungs

Left atrium receives oxygen-rich blood

Pulmonary veins carry oxygen-rich blood from the lungs

Left ventricle has a thicker wall than the right because it pumps blood farther

How the heart works

3 The two ventricles contract together, pushing blood to the lungs and body. Valves between atria and ventricles close to prevent backflow.

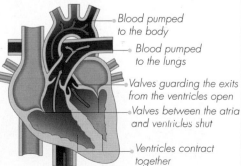

Blood pumped to the body

Blood pumped to the lungs

Valves guarding the exits from the ventricles open

Valves between the atria and ventricles shut

Ventricles contract together

Do heartstrings really exist?

Q A If someone "tugs at your heartstrings," it means that you feel sympathy for them. It's just an expression, but there are also real heartstrings. When your ventricles contract, these cords tug at the valves between the atria and ventricles. This stops the valves from turning inside out like umbrellas in a gale.

Heartstrings

Why does my heart beat faster when I run?

Q A Your muscles need energy to move you. This energy is generated using glucose and oxygen, which are delivered by the blood. The more active you are and the more strenuous the exercise, the harder your muscles work and the more energy they need. To supply this demand, your heart beats faster in order to pump more blood to your muscles to meet their need for extra glucose and oxygen.

Strenuous exercise

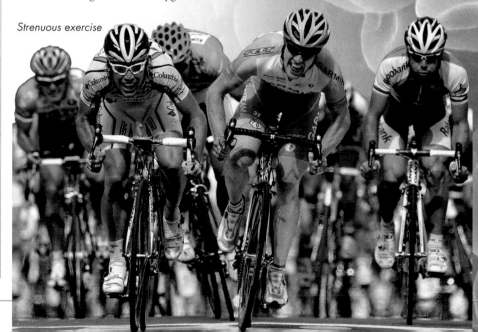

What do doctors hear through a stethoscope?

Q A Every time your heart beats, it produces sounds. A short "dup" sound is created when the valves guarding the heart's exits close as the ventricles relax. A longer "lub" sound is made when the ventricles contract and valves between atria and ventricles slam shut. By listening to heart sounds, doctors can check whether valves are doing their job correctly.

Scan of relaxed heart

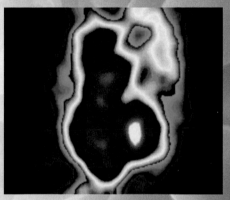

Scan of contracted heart

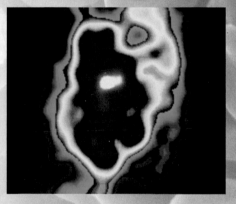

What journey does my blood take?

Pumped by the heart, blood circulates in one direction around the body to deliver supplies to all body cells. This circulatory system has two "loops." One carries oxygen-poor blood (blue) from the heart to the lungs to pick up oxygen. The other sends out oxygen-rich blood (red) to the tissues through the aorta and returns oxygen-poor blood to the heart through the large vena cava veins.

Circulatory system

Common carotid artery carries blood to the head and brain

Subclavian artery carries blood to the arm

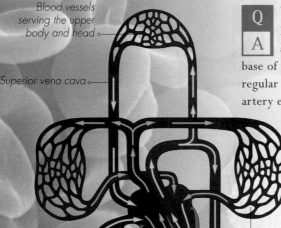

Blood vessels serving the upper body and head

Superior vena cava

Right side of the heart pumps oxygen-poor blood to the lungs

Blood vessels in the liver

Inferior vena cava

Blood vessels in the lower body and legs

Blood vessels in the lung

Left side of the heart pumps oxygen-rich blood to the body

Aorta is the biggest artery

Blood vessels in the stomach and intestines

Blood flow around the body

Q A What is a pulse?

If you hold the tips of two fingers against your wrist, just below the base of your thumb, you should feel a regular "pulse." This is produced by an artery expanding every time your heart beats and forcing blood along it. You have a vast network of blood vessels, made up of arteries (red), veins (blue), and tiny capillaries. Altogether these blood vessels stretch for more than 60,000 miles (100,000 km).

Inferior vena cava returns blood from the lower body to the heart

Aorta carries blood to the abdomen and lower body

What is the difference between arteries and veins?

There are three types of blood vessels in your body—arteries, veins, and capillaries—each one with their own distinct structure. Arteries and veins are linked by a network of capillaries that pass through all body tissues.

1 Arteries carry oxygen-rich blood from the heart to the tissues. They have a thick wall that is both muscular and stretchy to withstand the high blood pressure created when the heart beats.

2 Veins have thin walls and carry oxygen-poor blood under low pressure from the tissues toward the heart. Valves inside veins prevent blood from flowing backward.

Inner lining

Muscle layer

Outer protective layer

Muscle layer

Stretchy layer

Inner lining

Valve flap stops blood flowing the wrong way

Outer layer

3 Capillaries have a wall that is just one cell thick and relatively leaky. Food and oxygen pass from blood flowing along the capillaries to the surrounding tissue cells.

Capillary wall allows some substances to pass through easily

Nucleus of a cell in a capillary wall

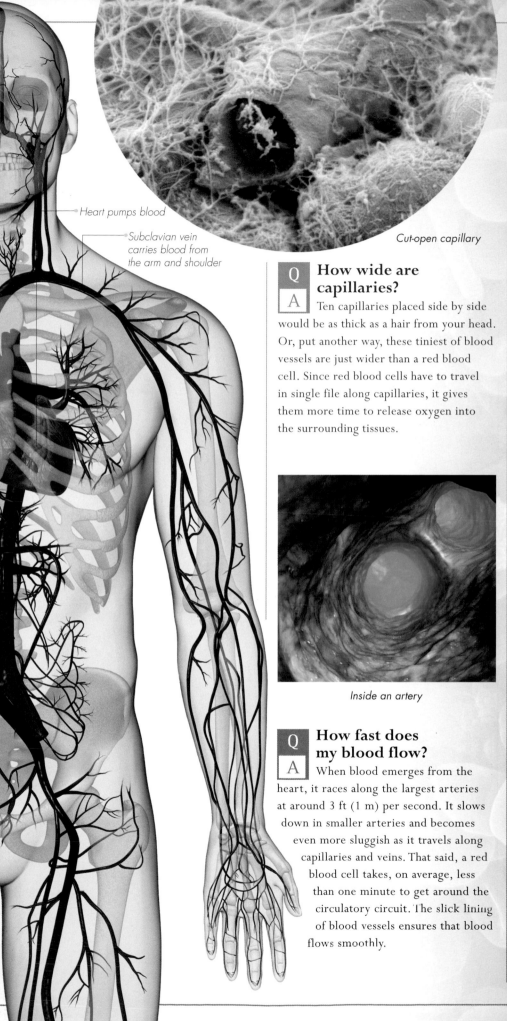

Heart pumps blood

Subclavian vein carries blood from the arm and shoulder

Cut-open capillary

Why do people get frostbite?

When it's cold, the blood vessels supplying your skin temporarily get narrower so that less blood flows through them. This reduces heat loss through the skin, especially from exposed parts such as the fingers. But if the body is exposed to freezing conditions for long periods, narrowed blood vessels starve skin cells of vital supplies, resulting in painful frostbite.

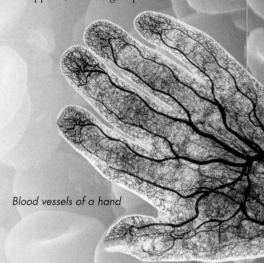

Blood vessels of a hand

How wide are capillaries?

Ten capillaries placed side by side would be as thick as a hair from your head. Or, put another way, these tiniest of blood vessels are just wider than a red blood cell. Since red blood cells have to travel in single file along capillaries, it gives them more time to release oxygen into the surrounding tissues.

Inside an artery

What is blood pressure?

It may have a long name but this machine (below) has a straightforward role, measuring your blood pressure. This is the pressure, or "push", on an artery's wall, produced when your heart beats. Blood pressure provides the driving force that keeps blood moving around your body. But if it is too high for long periods, it can cause health problems.

Sphygmomanometer

How fast does my blood flow?

When blood emerges from the heart, it races along the largest arteries at around 3 ft (1 m) per second. It slows down in smaller arteries and becomes even more sluggish as it travels along capillaries and veins. That said, a red blood cell takes, on average, less than one minute to get around the circulatory circuit. The slick lining of blood vessels ensures that blood flows smoothly.

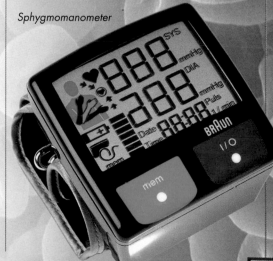

How does my body protect itself?

You are constantly exposed to germs that will make you sick if they get inside your body. Various defense mechanisms stop this from happening. Your skin, for example, is a germ-proof barrier. If germs do get in, they are destroyed by macrophages and lymphocytes—white blood cells found in your blood—and in your body's drainage network, the lymphatic system (below).

Q **What are germs?**

A Also called pathogens, germs are microorganisms—living things that can only be seen using a microscope—that cause disease. That is, they stop your body from working normally. Germs include the viruses that give you the flu or a cold and the bacteria that cause stomachaches. Left to their own devices, they would multiply inside your body and cause great harm.

Flu virus particle

Tonsils trap breathed-in germs

Lymph drains into this vein

Thymus gland "trains" defense cells

Thoracic duct collects lymph from the legs and abdomen

Lymph vessel carries lymph toward the main ducts

Lymph node "filters" lymph and contains macrophages and lymphocytes

Lymph capillary collects lymph from the tissues

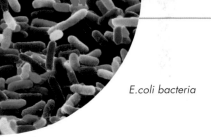
E.coli bacteria

How do white blood cells kill bacteria?

Macrophages like this one are white blood cells that specialize in destroying bacteria by eating them. This ruthless hunter tracks down invaders by following the chemical trails that they leave behind. The macrophage then sends out projections that stick to and surround a bacterium and pulls the germ inside it. Once inside the macrophage, the bacterium us doused in powerful enzymes that digest and kill it.

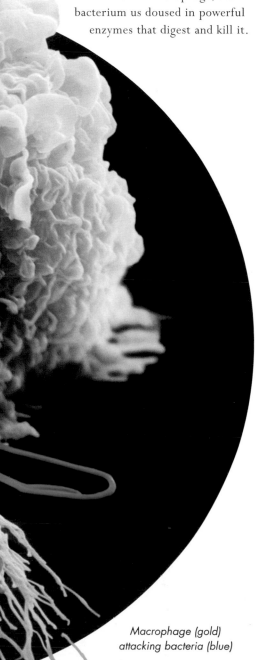
*Macrophage (gold)
attacking bacteria (blue)*

More Facts

- Protists are single-celled organisms, and some of them are germs. Plasmodium, for example, is a protist that causes malaria. Biting mosquitoes spread it from person to person, and it multiplies inside their red blood cells.

- Once you have had a particular disease, your immune system responds much faster to another attack of the same pathogens, so you rarely get the same disease twice.

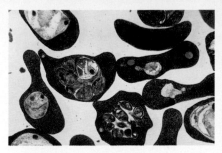
Plasmodium protists inside red blood cells

- Your tears, saliva, and sweat contain germ-killing chemicals, while stomach acid destroys bacteria or viruses that you swallow in food or drink.

Why does a doctor take your temperature?

Under normal conditions, your body's internal temperature is about 98.6°F (37°C). But if you are infected by bacteria or viruses, your body gets hotter, producing a fever. This helps fight infection because germs cannot multiply and spread at higher temperatures.

Taking a temperature

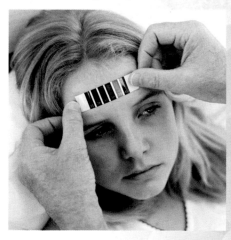

Does my body remember different germs?

Your body has an army of powerful defenders. Lymphocytes are a type of white blood cell that "remember" a germ's identity and release disease-fighting chemicals called antibodies to target specific germs. Antibodies do not destroy germs; they bind to their prey and mark them for destruction by macrophages.

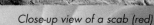
Close-up view of a scab (red)

How does a scab form?

A built-in repair mechanism acts swiftly to plug leaks from damaged blood vessels. If, for example, you cut yourself and start bleeding, a jellylike clot forms at the wound site to seal the holes in blood vessels. The clot dries out to form a protective scab that stays in place on the skin until the tissues underneath it have been repaired.

*Antibodies (blue and pink)
surround a bacterium*

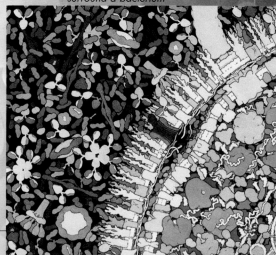

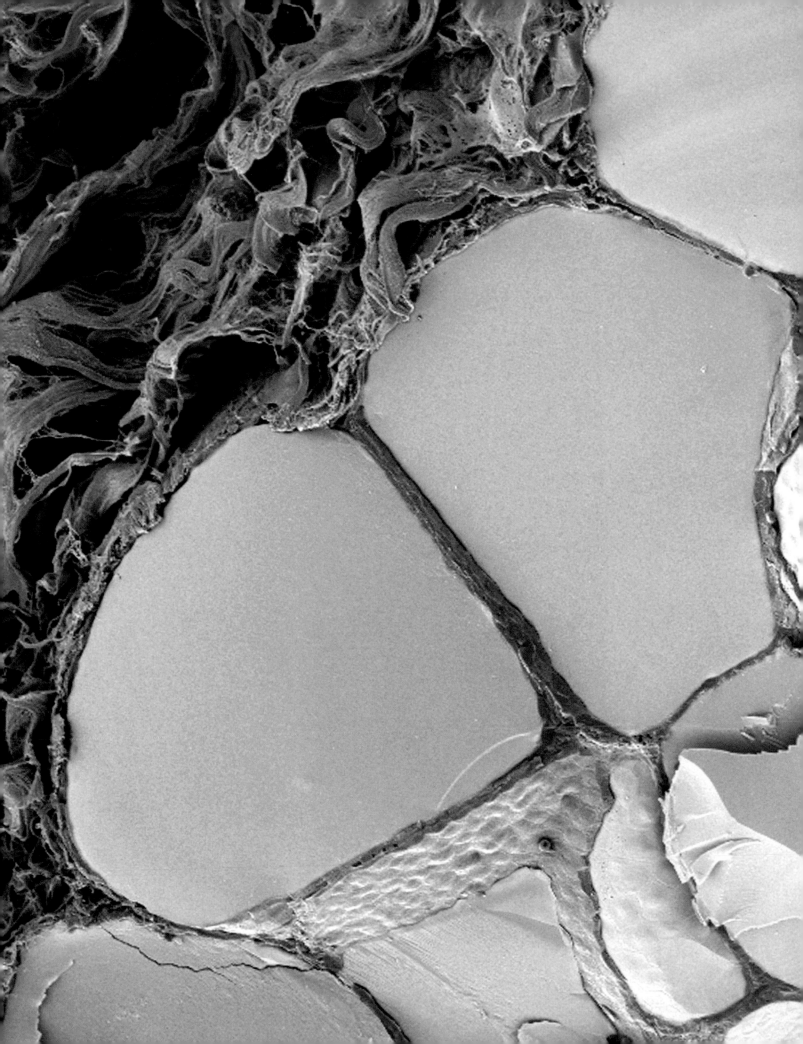

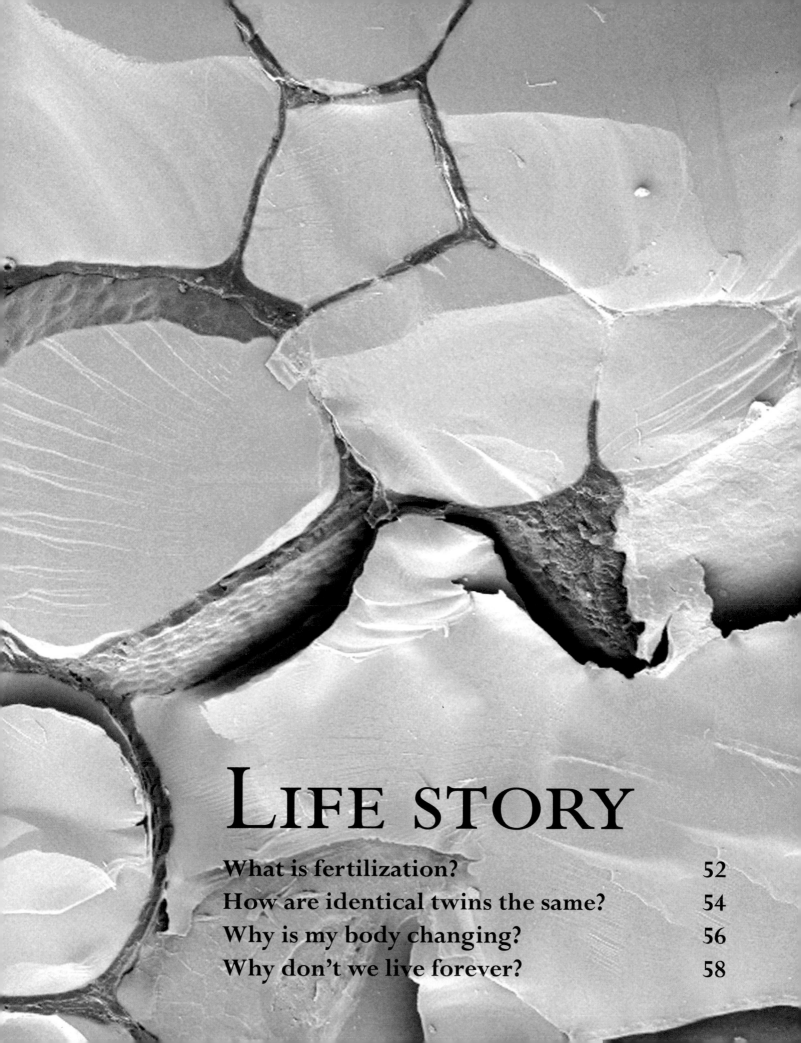

LIFE STORY

What is fertilization?   52

How are identical twins the same?   54

Why is my body changing?   56

Why don't we live forever?   58

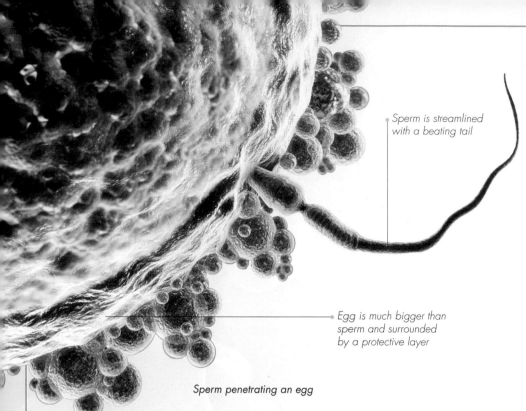

*Sperm is streamlined
with a beating tail*

*Egg is much bigger than
sperm and surrounded
by a protective layer*

Sperm penetrating an egg

Q | **Where does
A | fertilization occur?**

The female reproductive system
consists of two ovaries, two fallopian
tubes, the uterus, and the vagina—a tube
that connects the uterus to outside of the
body. Each month one of the ovaries
releases a mature egg into the fallopian
tube. If the egg meets sperm within one
day of its release, fertilization will happen.
Once a sperm has penetrated the outer
covering of the egg, its nucleus fuses
with the egg's nucleus to form
a fertilized egg.

*Female reproductive
system*

*Fallopian tube carries
egg from the ovary
to the uterus*

What is fertilization?

The job of the reproductive system is to produce babies. Unlike
other body systems, male and female reproductive systems are
very different. But, in adults, both produce special sex cells—eggs
in women and sperm in men—that contain the genetic material
to make a person. If sperm and egg meet and fuse, fertilization
occurs. Genetic instructions from both parents combine to
produce a new individual. The female reproductive system also
provides a safe place for the baby to develop during the nine
months of pregnancy.

*Ovaries produce and store
eggs, then release them*

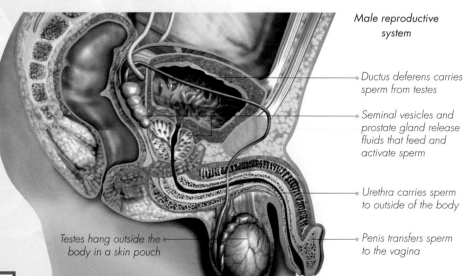

*Male reproductive
system*

*Ductus deferens carries
sperm from testes*

*Seminal vesicles and
prostate gland release
fluids that feed and
activate sperm*

*Urethra carries sperm
to outside of the body*

*Penis transfers sperm
to the vagina*

*Testes hang outside the
body in a skin pouch*

Q | **Where are sperm made?**
A | Males have two plum-sized testes
that contain masses of tiny, coiled
tubules. These are the sperm "factories"
inside which cells divide to produce
immature sperm. It takes 20 days for
sperm to mature before they are pushed
into the ductus deferens—the tube that
delivers them to the penis. Together, the
testes, penis, and the tubes that link them
make up the male reproductive system.

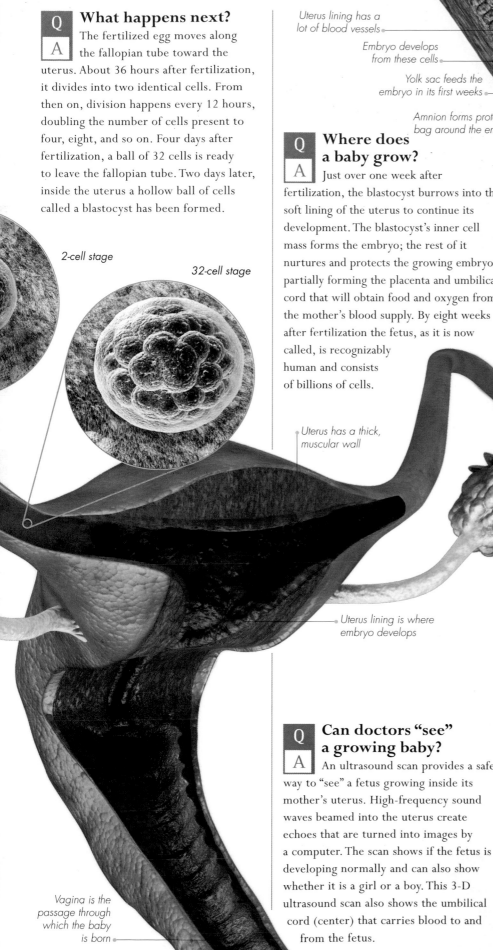

Q A What happens next?

The fertilized egg moves along the fallopian tube toward the uterus. About 36 hours after fertilization, it divides into two identical cells. From then on, division happens every 12 hours, doubling the number of cells present to four, eight, and so on. Four days after fertilization, a ball of 32 cells is ready to leave the fallopian tube. Two days later, inside the uterus a hollow ball of cells called a blastocyst has been formed.

2-cell stage

32-cell stage

Uterus has a thick, muscular wall

Uterus lining is where embryo develops

Vagina is the passage through which the baby is born

Q A Where does a baby grow?

Just over one week after fertilization, the blastocyst burrows into the soft lining of the uterus to continue its development. The blastocyst's inner cell mass forms the embryo; the rest of it nurtures and protects the growing embryo, partially forming the placenta and umbilical cord that will obtain food and oxygen from the mother's blood supply. By eight weeks after fertilization the fetus, as it is now called, is recognizably human and consists of billions of cells.

Uterus lining has a lot of blood vessels

Embryo develops from these cells

Yolk sac feeds the embryo in its first weeks

Amnion forms protective bag around the embryo

Ten days after fertilization

More Facts

- When a baby girl is born, her two ovaries already contain more than one million immature eggs, some of which will be released after she reaches puberty.

- In adult men the testes produce around 250 million sperm each day. If they are not released, sperm are broken down and recycled.

- Only a few hundred sperm survive the journey to the fallopian tube.

- The uterus normally resembles an upside-down pear. But during pregnancy, as a fetus grows, the uterus expands massively to the size of a basketball, returning to its original size after birth.

Inside a uterus

Q A Can doctors "see" a growing baby?

An ultrasound scan provides a safe way to "see" a fetus growing inside its mother's uterus. High-frequency sound waves beamed into the uterus create echoes that are turned into images by a computer. The scan shows if the fetus is developing normally and can also show whether it is a girl or a boy. This 3-D ultrasound scan also shows the umbilical cord (center) that carries blood to and from the fetus.

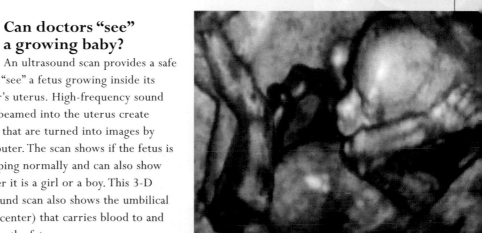

3-D ultrasound scan

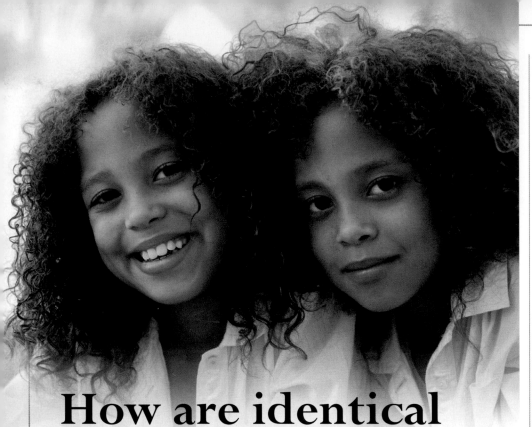

How are identical twins the same?

The nucleus of every body cell contains structures called chromosomes that are made from DNA. This master molecule holds the instructions that make you look human but also give you individual features that make you stand out from the crowd. You inherit DNA from both your parents. When humans reproduce, slightly different DNA instructions from each parent come together in the fertilized egg to create a unique individual. Occasionally, a fertilized egg splits into two separate cells. These develop into twin babies that look identical because they share exactly the same DNA.

Q A What are genes?

A set of 23 chromosomes contains the instructions, called genes, required to build and run cells and, therefore, the human body. Every chromosome carries many genes. Each gene consists of a short section of the long, coiled DNA molecule that makes up the chromosome. A gene's DNA holds the coded information needed to make one of the many proteins that make your body work.

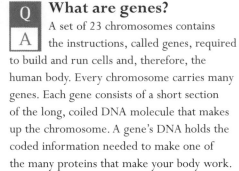

Computer model of a chromosome

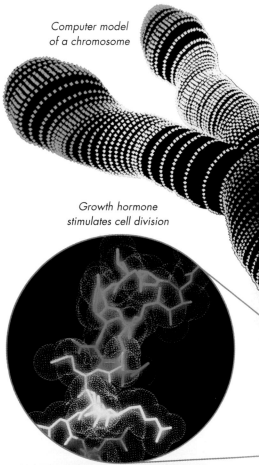

Growth hormone stimulates cell division

Q A How many chromosomes do I have?

There are 23 pairs of chromosomes inside a body cell, which are here arranged and numbered in order of size from 1 (longest) to 22 (shortest). The 23rd pair is the sex chromosomes —XY in males and XX in females —which determine a person's sex. One member of each chromosome pair comes from your mother and one from your father. When a man's sperm and a woman's egg fuse at fertilization, each contributes 23 chromosomes, making 46 chromosomes in the fertilized egg that develops into a baby.

Human chromosomes

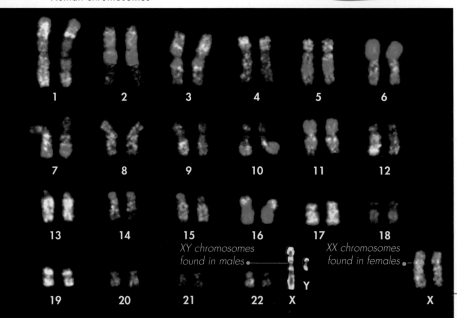

1 2 3 4 5 6

7 8 9 10 11 12

13 14 15 16 17 18

XY chromosomes found in males *XX chromosomes found in females*

19 20 21 22 X X

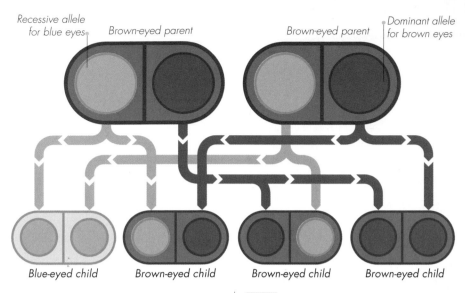

Recessive allele for blue eyes · Brown-eyed parent

Brown-eyed parent · Dominant allele for brown eyes

Blue-eyed child   Brown-eyed child   Brown-eyed child   Brown-eyed child

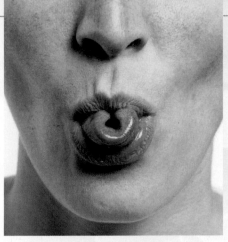

A tongue roller

Different genes shown as colored bands

Q A Why don't I look the same as my parents?

Both chromosomes—one from each parent—in a pair contain the same genes, although one of the chromosomes in the pair may carry different versions, or alleles, of those genes. While one allele (dominant) will always have an effect on the person's makeup, the other one (recessive) won't unless it is present on both chromosomes. That's why you could have blue eyes when both of your parents have brown eyes.

Reading the genome

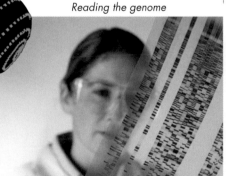

Q A Why can some people roll their tongue?

Most of your features are each controlled by several genes. But a few depend on a single gene, including being able—or not—to roll your tongue like this. If you inherit the dominant tongue-rolling allele (version) of the gene from one or both parents, you can roll your tongue. But if you inherit the non-tongue-rolling allele from both parents, you can't.

Q A What was the Human Genome Project?

The human genome is all the DNA contained in one set of 23 chromosomes. During the Human Genome Project (1990–2003), scientists around the world discovered the sequence of the "letters" in DNA molecules that make up the "words" of the instructions (genes) that control our cells. They did this by breaking up DNA molecules in order to "read" the "letters" in order. This also allowed them to locate the position of genes on chromosomes.

More Facts

■ It was once believed that there were 100,000 genes in the human genome. The Human Genome Project suggests that there are only 20,000–25,000.

■ Stretched out, the DNA in the chromosomes of one tiny cell would extend more than 6.5 ft (2 m). All the DNA in your body would extend across 124 billion miles (200,000,000,000 km).

■ If you can't see an eye shape here, you are probably colorblind, meaning that you can't distinguish certain colors. This is caused by a gene carried on the X sex chromosome. Boys have just one X chromosome, so if they inherit the gene, they are colorblind. But to become colorblind, girls have to inherit the gene on both of their X chromosomes, which is why it's much rarer in girls.

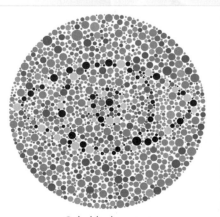

Colorblindness test

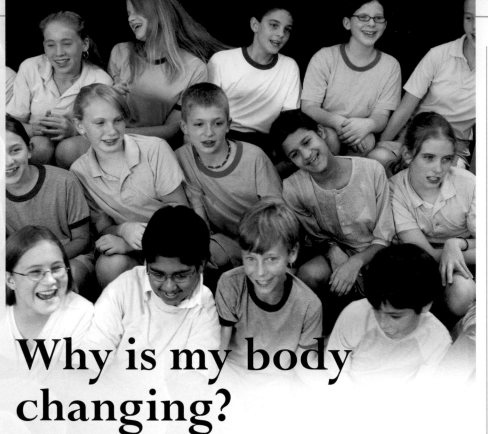

How fast does a child's brain grow?

When a baby is born, its brain contains the adult complement of 100 billion neurons (nerve cells), but it is just one quarter of the size of an adult's. That is because those neurons have few interconnections and have yet to link up to form the massive network that makes us so smart. Gaps between the skull bones that surround a child's brain allow the brain to expand as the network grows.

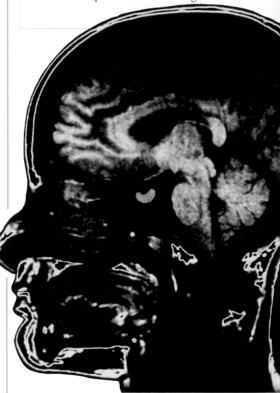

Pituitary gland at the base of the brain

MRI scan of brain

Why is my body changing?

As we get older, each of us follows the same sequence of changes. Our bones grow as we do, and our brains become increasingly more complex as we experience the world around us. But possibly the most dramatic change is during puberty, when children become young adults. Puberty starts in late childhood, earlier in girls than in boys. During puberty, both girls and boys get taller, their body shapes change, and their reproductive systems "turn on" and start working; girls start having their period and release eggs, while boys start making sperm.

Q **A** **What happens to a teenager's body?**
Both girls and boys show a growth spurt at the same time as their body shapes change to resemble an adult woman or an adult man. A girl's body becomes more rounded, and she develops breasts, while a boy's body becomes more muscular. Both sexes grow hair in their armpits and around their genitals.

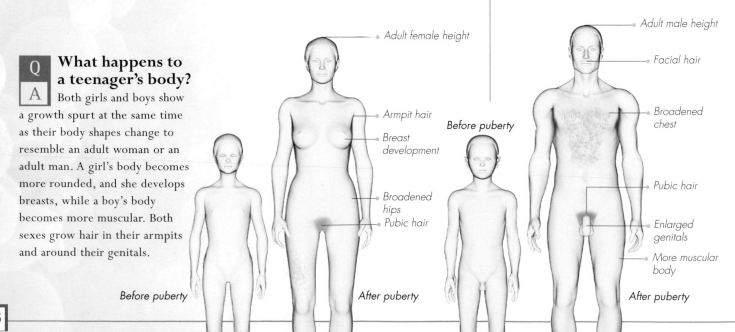

Adult female height

Armpit hair

Breast development

Before puberty

Broadened hips
Pubic hair

Adult male height

Facial hair

Broadened chest

Pubic hair

Enlarged genitals

More muscular body

Before puberty

After puberty

Before puberty

After puberty

1 *Brain neurons (green) have few links between them. Membranes span the gaps between skull bones that allow the brain to expand.*

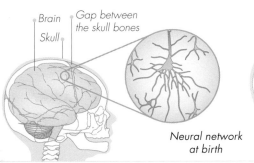

Brain
Skull
Gap between the skull bones

Neural network at birth

2 *As a result of learning and experience, connections between neurons greatly increase, making the brain almost adult sized.*

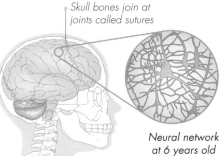

Skull bones join at joints called sutures

Neural network at 6 years old

3 *The full-sized brain has a complete neural network, and immovable sutures lock the skull bones together.*

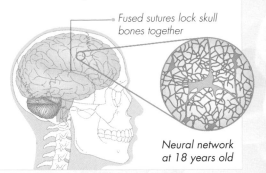

Fused sutures lock skull bones together

Neural network at 18 years old

Q A Why does puberty start?

The events of puberty are initially started by two hormones released from the pituitary gland. In girls these hormones target the ovaries, causing the release of eggs and female sex hormones. In males they target the genitals, causing the release of male sex hormones and stimulating sperm production. It is the sex hormones that trigger the changes in girls' and boys' bodies.

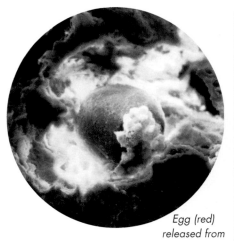

Egg (red) released from an ovary

More Facts

- In girls puberty generally begins between the ages of 10 and 12, while in boys it is between 12 and 14.

- Adolescence is the word that describes all the changes to a person, including puberty and changes in behavior, that are completed by the late teens.

- Special sweat glands in the armpits only start working at puberty. They release a thicker sweat that, when broken down by bacteria, produces body odor.

Sweat on skin

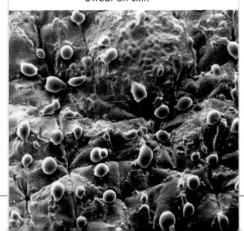

Q A What is the menstrual cycle?

This sequence of events, which repeats itself every 28 days, on average, prepares the uterus to receive a fertilized egg. During a menstrual cycle, the lining of the uterus thickens, and around day 14, an egg is released from an ovary. If the egg is fertilized, it implants in the thick uterus lining. If not, the lining is shed during a period.

Hand of a 1-year-old

Q A How do bones get bigger?

The skeleton forms as a baby grows in the uterus. At first the skeleton is made of flexible cartilage, but gradually this is replaced by harder bone. This process, called ossification, continues into the teenage years, as shown by these two x-rays. In the one-year-old's hand, many "bones" are still largely cartilage—which continues to grow in length. In the 20-year-old's hand, growth and ossification are complete.

Hand of a 20-year-old

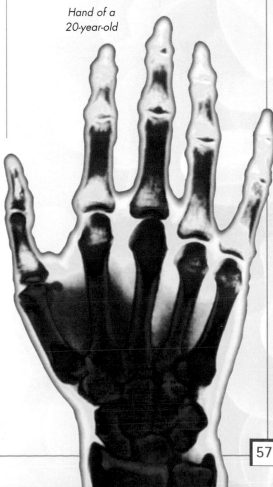

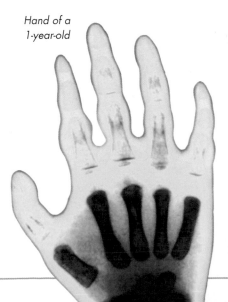

Why don't we live forever?

Aging and death are natural parts of the human life cycle that is "programmed" into our cells. By the time we reach our 60s, the first signs of wear and tear appear. The skin wrinkles, hair thins and whitens, eyesight and hearing can get worse, thinking slows down, and we get more aches and pains. But many changes can be kept at bay by a good diet and by regular exercise such as the gentle movements of tai chi.

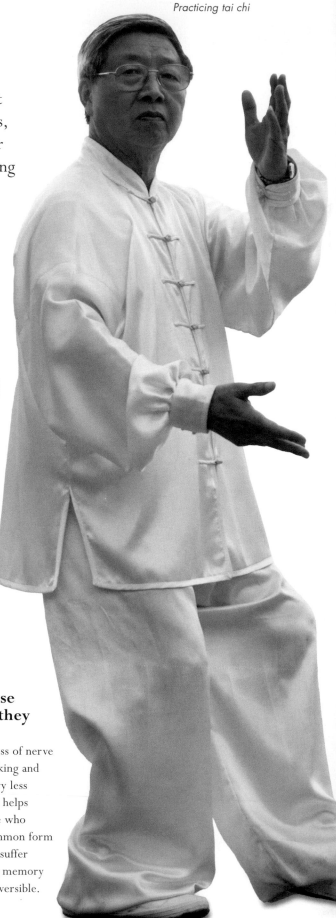

Practicing tai chi

Q A What makes our body age?

Our cells, and their instruction-carrying chromosomes, regularly divide in order to repair and maintain our bodies. But the number of times they can divide in a lifetime is limited. Chromosomes have protective tips called telomeres, which get shorter with every division. When they eventually disappear, cell division is no longer possible, which leads to signs of aging.

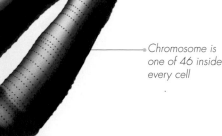

Telomeres cap the ends of a chromosome

Chromosome is one of 46 inside every cell

Chromosome

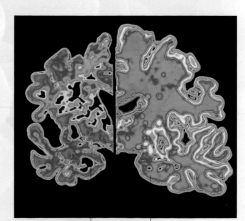

Brain cross section with Alzheimer's

Healthy brain cross section

Q A Does everyone lose their memory as they get older?

It isn't inevitable. Although the loss of nerve cells in old age usually make thinking and reaction times slower and memory less efficient, keeping the mind active helps reverse these changes. But people who develop dementia—the most common form of which is Alzheimer's disease—suffer dramatic brain shrinkage, causing memory loss and confusion that are not reversible.

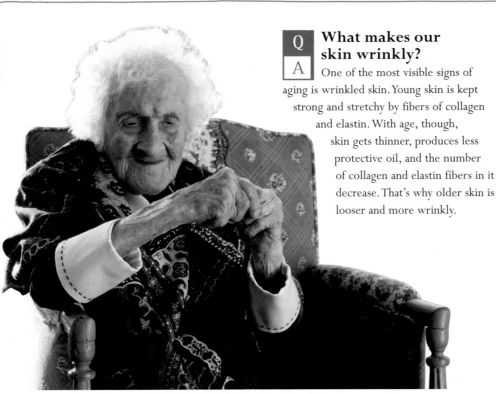

What makes our skin wrinkly?

One of the most visible signs of aging is wrinkled skin. Young skin is kept strong and stretchy by fibers of collagen and elastin. With age, though, skin gets thinner, produces less protective oil, and the number of collagen and elastin fibers in it decrease. That's why older skin is looser and more wrinkly.

Jeanne Calment (1875–1997)—the oldest person ever

Why do older people's bones break more easily?

Throughout life our bones constantly reshape by breaking down and rebuilding themselves. As we age, bone breaks itself down faster than it can be replaced. This makes bones less dense and weaker so that they fracture more easily. Loss of bone density is the most dramatic in osteoporosis, a condition found mainly in older women. In addition, joints between bones tend to get stiffer with age.

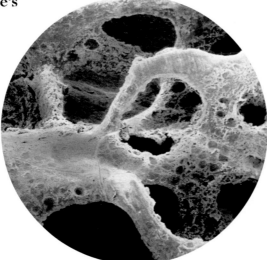

Osteoporosis in bone

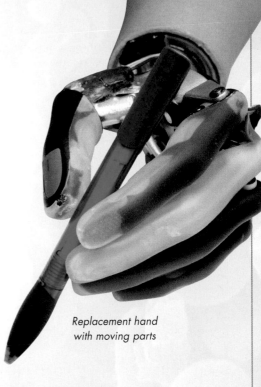

Replacement hand with moving parts

Can we replace body parts?

If we lose a hand, leg, or other body part, either through a disease or an accident, it will not grow back. But it can probably be replaced. This bionic hand, for example, is "wired up" so that the fingers move as instructed by its owner's brain. This enables it to grip a pen just like a normal hand. Internal organs, such as kidneys or the heart, that have been damaged or are diseased can be replaced by healthy organs provided by donors.

Artificial skin

More Facts

■ Most of us will live for much longer than our ancestors because we have better diets, live in cleaner, healthier surroundings, and receive superior medical care.

■ On average, women live longer than men. Life expectancy in the Western world is about 83 for women and 78 for men.

■ Men can produce sperm for a lifetime, but women stop releasing eggs at the time of menopause, which occurs, on average, at the age of 51.

■ Skin that is damaged may soon be able to be replaced by artificial skin grown in a laboratory. It would be made with a patient's own cells so that it is not rejected by the patient's body.

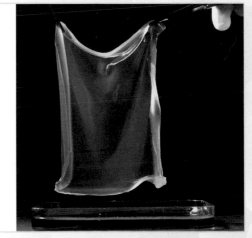

INDEX

A, B

adolescence 57
aging 19, 58—59
alleles 55
alveoli 26
Alzheimer's disease 58
antibodies 49
aorta 45, 46
armpits 56, 57
arteries 13, 44—45, 46, 47
athletes 18
atria 44—45
babies 52—53
    bladder control 29
    bone development 57
    bone marrow 42
    brain 56
bacteria 24, 48—49
    and body odor 57
    harmless 25
balance 37
biceps 17, 19
bile 24
bladder 10, 28—29
blastocyst 53
blood 29, 42—43
    in bones 15
    circulation 10, 46—47
blood cells
    bone marrow and 42
    red 25, 42, 43, 47
    white 42, 43, 48, 49
blood clotting 15, 49
blood groups 43
blood pressure 47
blood transfusions 43
blood vessels 46—47
body odor 57
bone marrow 15, 42—43
bones 14—15
    in the ear 37
    fractures 15, 59
    growth, ossification 57
    muscles fixed to 17, 19
    osteoporosis 59
brain 32—33
    Alzheimer's disease 58
    and balance 37
    growth 56—57
brain waves 33
breathing 26—27
bronchi and bronchioles 26
burping 24

C

cameras 34
capillaries 46, 47
carbon dioxide 26
cartilage 18, 19, 57
cells 10, 11
    and aging 58
    division (mitosis) 11

nucleus 11, 54
skin 12
    see also blood cells; neurons
cerebral cortex 32
cerebrum 32, 33
chest 27, 56
chewing 22, 23
children
    bone development 57
    hearing 37
    water content 29
    see also babies; puberty
chromosomes 54—55, 58
cilia 27, 39
circulatory system 10, 46—47
clavicle 43
cochlea 37
collagen 59
colon 25
color
    of eyes 55
    seeing in 34, 35
    of skin 12
    of urine 29
colorblindness 55
cones 34
connective tissues 11
cornea 34, 35
crying 35
cytoplasm 11

D, E

dementia 58
dermis 12
diaphragm 26—27
digestive system 22—25
DNA (deoxyribonucleic acid) 54—55
dreaming 33
ductus deferens 52
duodenum 24
ears 17, 36—37
egg (ovum) 11, 52—53, 54
    menopause and 59
    puberty and 56, 57
elastin 59
embryo 53
energy 45
enzymes 23, 24, 49
epidermis 12—13
epithelial tissues 11
esophagus 23
Eustachian tube 37
exercise 18, 45
eyes 34—35
    color of 55
    colorblindness 55
    muscles 17, 34

F, G

facial muscles 17

fallopian tubes 52—53
farting 25
fat 13
feces 25
femur 14, 43
fertilization 52—53, 54, 57
fetus 53
fever 49
fingernails 13
fingerprints 12
fingers
    bones (phalanges) 14
    dislocated joint 19
    see also hand
flu virus 48
food 22—23
fovea 34
fractures 15, 59
freckles 55
frostbite 47
gallbladder 24
genes 54—55
genitals 52, 56, 57
germs 48—49
glucagon 25
glucose 19, 23, 24, 25, 28, 45
gravity 17
growth 56, 57

H

hair 12—13, 56
hammer bone 36, 37
hand
    bionic 59
    blood vessels 47
    bone development 57
    see also fingers
hay fever 27
head lice 13
hearing 36—37
heart 16, 26, 44—45, 46—47
heartbeat 44—45
heartstrings 45
heat
    released by liver 25
    released by muscles 19
    and sweat 12, 13
hemoglobin 43
hormones 57
Human Genome Project 55

I, J, K, L

immune system 49
injuries
    dislocation 19
    fractures 15
    scabs 49
insulin 25
intestines

large 24, 25
small 23, 24—25
iris 34, 35
jaw muscles 17, 22
joints 18—19
    artificial 19
    dislocated 19
keratin 13
kidneys 10—11, 28—29, 43
left-handedness 33
lens 34, 35
leukemia 43
limbs, false 59
liver 10, 25, 46
lungs 10, 26—27, 46
lymph and lymph nodes 48
lymphatic system 48
lymphocytes 48, 49

M

macrophages 48—49
malaria 49
melanin 12
melanocytes 12
memory 58
men
    chromosomes 54, 55
    life expectancy 59
    reproductive system 52, 53, 56, 57, 59
    skeleton 15
    volume of blood 43
    water content 29
menopause 59
menstrual cycle 57
mitochondria 11
mitosis 11
mucus 27, 39
muscle fibres 16
muscle tone 17
muscles 11, 16—17, 22, 56
    diaphragm 26—27
    exercise and 18, 45
    eye 17, 34
    fixed to bones 17, 19
    heart 16, 44—45
    intercostal 26
    produce heat 19
    stomach 24
muscular tissues 11
music, loud 37
musicians (wind players) 27
myofibrils 16

N, O

nails 13
nephrons 28—29
nerves 33
nervous system 32, 33
nervous tissues 11
neurons (nerve cells) 16, 33,

56—57
neutrophils 43
nose 27, 38—39
optic nerve 34, 35
organelles 11
organs 10
    transplants 59
osteoporosis 59
ovaries 52—53, 57
    see also egg
oxygen 26
    blood and 42, 43, 46, 47
    brain and 33
    heart and 44—45

P

pain 33
pancreas 24, 25
papillae 38
pathogens see germs
pelvis 15
penis 52
periods 57
periosteum 17
pituitary gland 56, 57
placenta 53
plaque 23
plasma 42
plasmodium 49
platelets 42, 43
pregnancy 52—53
prostate gland 52
protists 49

puberty 56—57
pulse 46
pupil 34, 35
pyloric sphincter 24

R, S

receptors 12
reflexes 33
reproductive system
    52—53, 56, 57, 59
retina 34
ribs 14, 26, 43
rods 34
saliva 22, 23, 49
scab 49
scapula 43
sebaceous gland 13
semicircular canals 37
skeletal muscles 16—17
skeleton 14—15
    see also bones
skin 12—13
    and aging 59
    artificial 59
    color 12
skull 14, 43
sleep 17, 33
smell 38—39
smiling 17
smooth muscles 16
sneezing 27
sound 37
sperm 52, 53, 54, 56, 57, 59
sphygmomanometer 47

spinal cord 32, 33
stem cells 11
stethoscope 45
stirrup bone 37
stomach 23, 24—25, 46
    acid 24, 49
sutures 14, 57
swallowing 23
sweat 12, 13, 29, 49, 57
sweat glands 13, 57
synovial fluid 18

T

tai chi 58
tarsals 14
taste 38—39
taste buds 38
tears 35, 49
teeth 22, 23
telomeres 58
temperature, body 49
tendons 17
thermography 19
thighs 14, 18
thirst 29
thymus gland 48
tissues 11
tongue 22, 23, 38, 55
tonsils 48
trachea see windpipe
triceps 19
twins 54

U, V, W, X

ultrasound scan 53
umbilical cord 53
ureter 28—29
urethra 28—29, 52
urinary system 28—29
urine 28—29
uterus 52—53, 57
vagina 52—53
valves
    heart 44—45
    in veins 46
veins 46
    pulmonary 45
    subclavian 47
    vena cava 44, 46
ventricles 44—45
vertebrae 43
video pill 25
viruses 48, 49
water 29
windpipe 26
women
    chromosomes 54, 55
    life expectancy 59
    reproductive system
        52—53, 56, 57, 59
    skeleton 15
    volume of blood 43
    water content 29
wrinkles 59
x-rays 15
vision see eyes
    3-D vision 35

CREDITS

Dorling Kindersley would like to thank Caitlin Doyle for proof-reading and Americanization, and Jackie Brind for the index.

The publisher would like to thank the following for their kind permission to reproduce their photographs: (Key: a-above; b-below/bottom; c-center; l-left; r-right; t-top)

2-3 Corbis: Photo Quest Ltd / Science Photo Library. 4 Corbis: Steve Gschmeissner / Science Photo Library (bl); Visuals Unlimited (cl) (tl). 4-7 Corbis: Visuals Unlimited (background). 5 Corbis: Steve Allen / Brand X (cr); Visuals Unlimited (br). Getty Images: Spike Walker (tr). 6 Corbis: Kurt Kormann (cl); Photo Quest Ltd / Science Photo Library (tl). Getty Images: Sandra Baker (bl). 7 Corbis: Visuals Unlimited (tc). Getty Images: Steve Gschmeissner / Science Photo Library (bl); Dr. Kessel & Dr. Kardon / Tissues & Organs (br). 8-9 Science Photo Library: Steve Gschmeissner. 10 Science Photo Library: Simon Fraser (cr). 10-19 Corbis: Visuals Unlimited (background). 11 Science Photo Library: (br); A. Dowsett, Health Protection Agency (c); Prof. P. Motta / Dept. Of Anatomy / University "La Sapienza", Rome (tr). 12 Science Photo Library: Dr Jeremy Burgess (cl); L'oreal / Eurelios (tl). 13 Science Photo Library: Steve Gschmeissner (tl) (cr). 15 Science Photo Library: Dept. Of Clinical Radiology, Salisbury District Hospital (cr); Andrew Syred (tc). 16 Science Photo Library: Don Fawcett (bc). 17 Corbis: (cr). Getty Images: Mike Kemp (cl). 18 Corbis: Wally McNamee (c). 19 Corbis: Dan McCoy - Rainbow/

Science Faction (bc). Science Photo Library: DU Cane Medical Imaging Ltd (cr); Zephyr (br). 20-21 Corbis: Dennis Kunkel Microscopy, Inc./ Visuals Unlimited. 22 Corbis: Dimitri Lundt/ TempSport (cl). 22-29 Corbis: Visuals Unlimited (background). 23 Corbis: Image Source (cr). Science Photo Library: Dr Tony Brain (bl). 24 Corbis: MedicalRF.com (cra); Science Photo Library/ Photo Quest Ltd (cl) (cr). 24-25 Getty Images: 3D4Medical.com. 25 Corbis: Dennis Kunkel Microscopy, Inc./ Visuals Unlimited (bc); Reuters (br). Science Photo Library: BSIP GEMS / Europe (tc). 26 Corbis: Oliver Rossi (tl). Getty Images: Nucleus Medical Art, Inc. (bl). 27 Getty Images: Jupiterimages (c). Science Photo Library: Dr Gary Settles (tc); Eye Of Science (cl). 28 Corbis: Visuals Unlimited (c). Science Photo Library: (bl) (bc). 29 Corbis: Mod Art / CSA Images (tc); Roy Hsu/ Blend Images (br). 30-31 Getty Images: Thomas Deerinck. 32-39 Corbis: Visuals Unlimited (background). 33 Alamy Images: Chuck Franklin (tc). Getty Images: Iconica / Brick House Pictures (bc). National Geographic Stock: Cary Wolinsky (cr). Science Photo Library: Steve Gschmeissner (clb); C. J. Guerin, PHD, MRC Toxicology Unit (cl). 34 Science Photo Library: Omikron (bl). 35 Getty Images: Fabrice Coffrini / AFP (bc). 36 Science Photo Library: Steve Gschmeissner (c). 37 Corbis: Wally McNamee (cr). Getty Images: Digital Vision / James Woodson (c); Workbook Stock / Thierry Grun (bc). Science Photo Library: Susumu Nishinaga (cl); Amanaimages (bc). Getty Images: Iconica / Jeffrey Coolidge (tr); StockFood Creative / Ian Garlick (cr). Science Photo Library: Steve Gschmeissner (c). 40-41 Corbis: Visuals Unlimited. 42 Science Photo Library: Steve Gschmeissner (br). 43 Science Photo Library: NIBSC (tl); Antonia Reeve (tr). 44 Getty Images: Visuals Unlimited / Dr. Fred Hossler (c).

45 Getty Images: Jasper Juinen (br). Science Photo Library: CNRI (cr) (crb); Susumu Nishinaga (c). 47 Alamy Images: Hugh Threlfall (br). Corbis: Frans Lanting (cr). Science Photo Library: Eye Of Science (tc); Roger Harris (c). 48 Science Photo Library: Pasieka (cra). 48-49 Science Photo Library: Eye Of Science (bc); NIBSC (tc). 49 Getty Images: Stockbyte (cb). Science Photo Library: David Goodsell (br); Steve Gschmeissner (cr); Dr Gopal Murti (tr). 50-51 Science Photo Library: Steve Gschmeissner. 52-59 Corbis: Visuals Unlimited (background). 53 Corbis: Visuals Unlimited (crb). Science Photo Library: GE Medical Systems (br). 54 Corbis: Tim Pannell (tl). Science Photo Library: CNRI (br/XY); Dept. Of Clinical Cytogenetics, Addenbrookes Hospital (br); Pasieka (cr). 54-55 Science Photo Library: Pasieka. 55 Corbis: Andrew Brookes (cr). Science Photo Library: David Nicholls (br). 56 Corbis: Randy Faris (tl). Science Photo Library: Scott Camazine (cr). 57 Science Photo Library: (br); Professors P.M. Motta & J. Van Blerkom (c); Richard Wehr / Custom Medical Stock Photo (tr). 58 Getty Images: Mike Kemp (cr). Science Photo Library: Pasieka (bl) (c). 59 Corbis: EPA / Waltraud Grubitzsch (tr); Pascal Parrot (tl). Science Photo Library: Mauro Fermariello (br); Prof. P. Motta / Dept. Of Anatomy / University "La Sapienza", Rome (c). 60-61 Corbis: Visuals Unlimited. 62-63 Corbis: Photo Quest Ltd/ Science Photo Library

Jacket images: Front: Science Photo Library: Susumu Nishinaga (background); Pasieka c (skull). Back: Corbis: Jens Nieth bl; Visuals Unlimited cla; Science Photo Library: Mehau Kulyk cl; Bill Longcore tl; Susumu Nishinaga clb

All other images © Dorling Kindersley
For further information see: www.dkimages.com

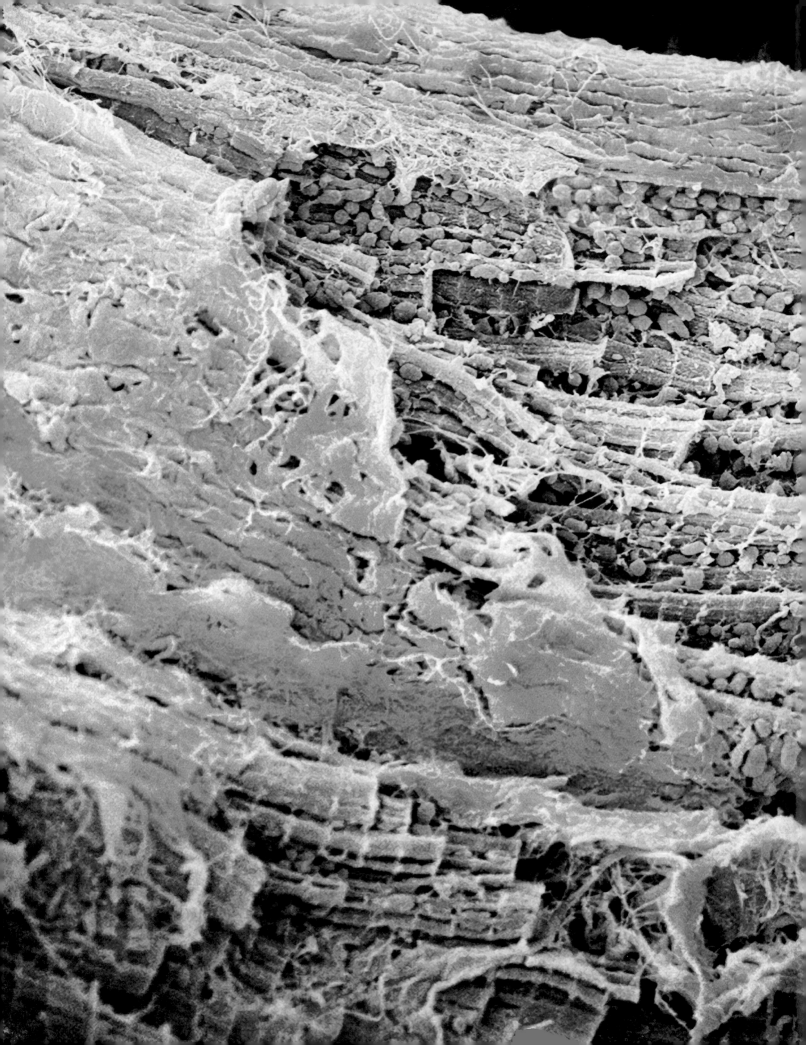